Ethics in Critical Care Medicine

Ethics in Critical Care Medicine

James P. Orlowski, MD

University Publishing Group
Hagerstown, Maryland

University Publishing Group, Inc.
Hagerstown, Maryland 21701
1-800-654-8188

Materials in Exhibit 3-4 are reprinted from J. Fletcher et al., ed., *Introduction
to Clinical Ethics,* 2nd ed. (Frederick, Md.: University Publishing Group,
1997), 13. © University Publishing Group. All rights reserved. Used with
permission. Exhibit 19-1 is reprinted from P. Appelbaum and T. Gutheil,
Clinical Handbook of Psychiatry and the Law, 2nd ed. (Baltimore, Md.:
Lippincott Williams & Wilkins, 1991), 239-40. © by Lippincott Williams &
Wilkins, 1991. Used with permission. An earlier version of Exhibit 24-1
appeared in S.H. Imbus and B.E. Zawacki, "Encouraging Dialogue and
Autonomy in the Burn Intensive Care Unit," *Critical Care Clinics* 2, no. 1
(1986): 53-60. © 1996 by W.B. Saunders Company. Used with permission.
Exhibit 25-3 and Exhibit 25-5 © 1989 by Ginger Schafer Wlody. Used with
permission. Exhibit 25-6 1986 by Ginger Wlody. Used with permission.
Exhibit 28-1 and Exhibit 28-2 are reprinted from K.V. Iserson, A.B. Sanders,
and D. Mathieu, *Ethics in Emergency Medicine,* 2nd ed. (Tucson, Ariz.: Galen
Press, 1995). © 1995 by Galen Press. Used with permission.
Photo on the front cover used with the kind permission of the University
Community Hospital Pediatric Care Unit, Tampa, Florida.

ISBN (cloth): 1-55572-080-3
ISBN (paper): 1-55572-055-2

Contents

Preface

James P. Orlowski

Having spent a number of years as both a critical care physician and a medical ethicist, I am acutely aware of the important and frequent interaction of these two specialties and their complementary natures. *Ethics in Critical Care Medicine* seeks to synthesize these two areas into a single textbook.

The critical care environment encompasses the multiple intensive care units (ICUs) in a hospital—including the medical, surgical, neurological, neurosurgical, coronary, cardiothoracic, pediatric, neonatal, burn, shock/trauma, respiratory, and transplant units—as well as the emergency department and other areas where critically ill patients are cared for and managed. As such, the critical care areas are often hotbeds of ethical dilemmas. Most hospital ethicists and hospital ethics committees find that the majority of ethics consults, ethical dilemmas, and ethical moments occur in the ICUs. For these reasons, a reference textbook that addresses these ethical dilemmas is needed. *Ethics in Critical Care Medicine* is designed to fill this need and to address the myriad of ethical issues encountered in critical care.

Ethics in Critical Care Medicine is intended to be both a reference and an orientation to the multitude of ethical issues that care providers encounter in the ICU and emergency department. Its audience is anticipated to include students from all healthcare disciplines, residents, nurses, social workers, respiratory therapists, clergy, ethicists, physicians, and anyone else who must face and help resolve these ethical dilemmas.

A number of outstanding individuals in the fields of critical care and ethics have contributed chapters for *Ethics in Critical Care Medicine*. Chapter 1 provides a historical perspective on both disciplines—critical care medicine and medical ethics. Both of these disciplines are relatively young and were conceived at about the same time. These disciplines have become interdependent because of their frequent interfaces when ethical issues arise in critical care. The presence of an ethicist on rounds in the ICU is now standard practice at many institutions. Many hospital ethics committees around the country are chaired by intensive care clinicians.

This book is a logical out-growth of the collaboration between these two disciplines.

Chapter 2 addresses ethical theory and practice as it applies to critical care. This chapter forms the theoretical basis for much of what follows in the textbook. Chapter 3 addresses the ethics of care and the importance of caring in critical care. Humaneness and humanity require an ethics of care in the critical care environment, which leads us to the importance of the environment and the milieu of the critical care unit in providing humane care to patients. The milieu includes not only the physical environment, but also the nonphysical atmosphere of the ICU. Are families made to feel welcome or are they treated as intruders? Is there a collaborative approach to caring for the patient that appreciates the input of multiple disciplines to the holistic care of the patient, or are ancillary personnel such as social workers, chaplains, and dieticians tolerated but not appreciated? Do consulting services feel they are contributing to the overall care of the patient, or do they feel they have entered into a foreign, unfamiliar, and unfriendly area of the hospital? ICUs are technology-intense and frequently seem like a science-fiction environment—not only to patients and families, but also to healthcare providers unfamiliar or uncomfortable with all of the tubes, monitors, alarms, noises, and machines.

Chapter 4 deals with who makes decisions in the ICU and what decisions are frequently made. These include decisions about cardiopulmonary resuscitation (CPR), do-not-resuscitate (DNR) orders, withdrawal of life support, diagnosis of brain death, and organ donation. This chapter also addresses the ethics of urgency versus the ethics of common sense in decision making in the ICU and emergency room. Chapter 5 addresses the ethics of withholding and withdrawing life-sustaining therapies in the ICU, which could be referred to as "orchestrating death in the ICU." This chapter addresses the decisions to be made and whose decisions they are, along with strategies for dealing with conflicts involving patients, families, or other healthcare providers. It also addresses the "how-to" of humanely and compassionately withdrawing life supports and allowing patients to die with dignity in the ICU.

An important part of the management of any patient in the ICU, and especially during the withdrawal of life-sustaining therapies, is the humane and appropriate use of pain-control and pain-relief agents. Suffering is also an important aspect of the human experience of critical care, and the physical and psychological aspects of suffering and its recognition and treatment are addressed in chapter 6.

Chapter 7 discusses the topic of triage and the responsible use of ICU resources. It addresses the use of scoring systems and outcome predictors as guides to the appropriate and responsible use of critical care resources and technology. Scoring systems are an increasingly popular and important tool in critical care as a means of characterizing patients and comparing ICUs. But scoring systems carry the risk of inappropriate utilization when applied to individual patients.

Critical care units are often the site of new and experimental technologies and therapies. Chapter 8 discusses the ethical issues in performing research in critical care and employing new or experimental approaches on highly vulnerable patients. Important new changes in federal regulations governing emergency and critical care research have been promulgated recently. Patients in the ICU are often the subjects of new and experimental therapies and technologies, and they are also often the objects for the education and training of students and residents who may be unfamiliar with the technologies and the critical illnesses they encounter in the ICU.

Brain death is almost always a prerequisite for organ donation, and brain death by definition can only be diagnosed in the ICU in the absence of cardiorespiratory death. Chapter 9 discusses the important aspects of defining death in the ICU and critical care units, the criteria for brain death, and the importance of organ donation. Also discussed is the acceptance of brain-death criteria by the medical community and the public as well as by patients and families.

The role of religion in the critical care setting is an often-neglected issue. Religious beliefs of patients, families, and healthcare providers can affect the care provided in critical care areas. Patients and families can have unusual beliefs that stress the already stressful environment of the ICU. Watching a Jehovah's Witness patient refuse transfusions and bleed to death can place a tremendous strain on the ICU team. At the other end of the spectrum are families who insist on all heroic measures because they believe in miracles, despite the obvious futility of the situation. In addition, it is important for care providers to recognize sociocultural death rituals to assist in the humane aspects of facilitating dying in the ICU or dealing with death in the emergency department. Russ Connors presents a fascinating thesis in chapter 10, in which he discusses "The ICU as Holy Ground."

Chapter 11 deals with the confusion surrounding the terms *coma, persistent vegetative state, permanent vegetative state,* and *unconsciousness* in the ICU. The definitions and diagnostic criteria for each of these conditions are elucidated, and the prognostic and ethical implications of the diagnoses are explained.

The appropriate use of dialysis technologies in the ICU are covered in chapter 12, including the ethical issues of withholding or withdrawing this life-sustaining technology in ICU patients. Guidelines for making these difficult decisions are elaborated.

Chapter 13 addresses the importance of humanizing technology in the ICU and the importance that a humane approach to patients will have on the future of critical care. Much can be done to make the ICU a more humane and caring environment, and much can be done to make the technology of critical care more humane and less intrusive.

ICUs are often accused of being cold, uncaring, and emotionless places. Chapter 14 emphasizes the important role that emotions can and should play—not only for patients and families, but also for healthcare providers.

Legal issues provide another source of conflict in the ICU that can place its players on the offensive or defensive. Medicolegal issues occasionally conflict with ethical issues in the ICU, and are often a source of confusion. Chapter 15 clarifies these ethical-legal issues and suggests appropriate resolutions.

As in many other specialty areas inside and outside of medicine, there is a unique language to critical care with connotations and nuances that often escape the uninitiated. Chapter 16 examines humanizing and dehumanizing language in the ICU and suggests ways to improve communication.

Chapter 17 addresses a major ethical issue in this age of limited resources—luxury care, or the demanding of care above and beyond the standard of care. This care has been termed unaffectionately as "Bubbacare." This chapter discusses how to meet the needs and demands of individual patients, families, healthcare providers, and society.

Advance directives are playing an increasing role in decisions about whether to admit patients to an ICU and decisions about the degree and aggressiveness of care to provide in the ICU. Surrogates often become the primary decision makers in the ICU, because most ICU patients are no longer capable of making decisions. Surrogates' appropriate role and their right to contradict previously expressed decisions of patients are discussed in chapter 18.

The need to determine whether a patient is capable of decision making and whether he or she is competent comes up frequently in the ICU and in ethics consultation in general. Painkillers, sedatives, and other medications can interfere with a patient's decision-making capacity but do not necessarily make a patient permanently incapable of participating in decisions about treatment. ICU psychosis, which is a frequent cause of incapacity, should be better addressed. These issues are discussed in chapter 19.

Disputes among patients, families, surrogates, and healthcare providers are not uncommon in the stressful environment of the ICU, and dispute resolution and mediation are new areas of attention to resolve these problems. The authors of chapter 20 have a great deal of experience in this area, especially in a neurological/neurosurgical ICU.

Chapters 21 through 28 focus on issues unique to individual critical care areas including obstetrics-gynecology, pediatrics, neonatology, shock-trauma, prehospital care, and the emergency department. Chapters 25 and 26 address ethical issues unique to nursing and social work. Chapter 29 summarizes a worldview of the ethical issues facing critical care now and in the future.

One of the humorous aspects of editing this book was discovering all of the similes and metaphors used by authors to characterize the ICU.

The most intricate was Russ Connor's discussion of the ICU as a sacred place or "holy ground"—a place of mystery, wonder, and awe as well as ultimate terror and dread.

Many other authors had equally poetic ways of describing the ICU. Smith and Frank related entering an ICU to entering a foreign land or country which provokes "culture shock." Candilis characterized the ICU as a "crucible," which conjures an image of alchemy. Taylor calls the ICU a "body parts repair shop," which is more a mechanical than a mystical image.

Utilizing a battle or war imagery, Powderly refers to the ICU as a place of "constant bombardment" with stress, which quickly leads to burn-out. Zawacki names it a "battleground for the war on death." Silverman calls the ICU an "emotional hazard" and a "crisis-loaded terrain." Utilizing a rescue fantasy, Marshall and Perlmutter state that patients in an ICU are "frequently rescued from biological death with advanced resuscitative techniques" and refer to it as a "high-tech hospice."

One of the most poignant metaphors is made by David Beyda, who refers to the intensivist as a "conductor of a technologic orchestra, much of which is out of tune with the patient."

This book is dedicated to all the hard-working individuals who must face these ethical issues in their daily care of critically ill patients, and to the patients and their families who have taught us so much about critical illness and the ethical issues that are a necessary part of caring humanely for the critically ill.

1

A History of Critical Care Medicine and Medical Ethics

James A. Christensen and James P. Orlowski

INTRODUCTION

Critical care medicine and medical ethics have shared an amazingly similar history. Both are relatively new specialties that have been formally recognized only within the past 25 years. And yet both have been practiced since antiquity.

Critical care medicine came into its own with the founding of the Society of Critical Care Medicine in 1970.[1] It was formally approved as a new medical subspecialty by the American Board of Medical Specialties in 1980. Critical care medicine became a subspecialty of the board-certified specialties of pediatrics, internal medicine, anesthesiology, and surgery at that time. Its roots extend back to early research on cardiopulmonary resuscitation, military studies on resuscitation of shock victims, and the mechanical ventilation or "iron lung" therapy for individuals with polio. Biblical references to what might be called critical care and resuscitation include the resurrection of Lazarus (John 11:1-44) and the resurrection of the 12 year-old daughter of Jairus, the president of the synagogue (Matthew 9:18-26, Mark 5:21-43, Luke 8:40-56).

Similarly, medical ethics gained formal recognition with the founding of the Hastings Center in 1969 and the Kennedy Institute of Ethics in

1971. Although medical ethics has not yet been formally approved as a medical specialty, a number of legal and legislative initiatives requiring the establishment of institutional review boards, infant care review committees, and ethics committees point to the importance and recognition of medical ethics. Its recent underpinnings include the "god committees" that decided which persons would receive dialysis when this technology first became available in the 1950s. Its roots extend back to the writings of Aristotle, the oath of Hippocrates, and the ethical writings of Hippocrates.

Just as medical ethics and critical care medicine had their modern origins around 1970, the merging and interrelationship of critical care medicine and medical ethics began in 1970 with the publication of Paul Ramsey's landmark book, *The Patient as Person*, which articulated the need for ethics in medical practice.[2] Then in 1976 came the Karen Ann Quinlan case, which emphasized the need for cogent and consistent societal, legal, and moral guidelines to meet the ethical moments that arise in critical care medicine.

Critical care medicine is often the source of many ethical issues and dilemmas, and ethical questions are confronted in critical care areas more often than in any other area of medical practice. The interplay of medical ethics and critical care medicine has enriched both areas.

HISTORICAL ASPECTS OF CRITICAL CARE MEDICINE

Critical care medicine's origins were in the development of mechanical ventilation for poliomyelitis in the 1950s, the research by the military into resuscitation of shock victims in the Korean and Vietnam wars, and the synthesizing of many studies into what became modern cardiopulmonary resuscitation in 1960.

The first respiratory Intensive Care Units (ICUs) were established in Scandinavia to treat victims of the polio epidemic in the early 1950s. The first ICU in the United States was the multidisciplinary, medical-surgical ICU at Baltimore City Hospital in the early 1960s.

The idea of a specialty of critical care medicine arose at a time when medical knowledge had so expanded that individual specialties had developed in vertical fashion around individual organ systems such as cardiology, nephrology, gastroenterology, and pulmonology. It was nothing short of revolutionary to propose a specialty that would cut across these traditional vertical lines of specialization and result in a specialist who managed the total patient, prioritized organ systems, watched for interactions in the treatment of one organ system that might adversely affect other organ systems, and coordinated the multiple specialists managing a critically ill patient. The specialist in critical care medicine was envisioned to be a supervising and coordinating physician, trained in resuscitation and life support, who would not usurp the role of the admitting physician or consulting specialists; instead the critical care specialist would coordinate the medical information and treatment plan and provide the continuous surveillance and vigilance necessary to manage critically ill patients effectively.

The Society of Critical Care Medicine was founded on February 10, 1970, when a "Conference Group on Critical Care Medicine" met at the Los Angeles Hilton Hotel in Los Angeles, California.[3] The idea of organizing such a group was the brainchild of Burton Waisbren in discussion with Will Shoemaker and a number of other physicians.[4] The purpose of the inaugural meeting was to combine thoughts, plans, and experiences that would help bring order to the new field of critical care medicine. Twenty-nine members originally attended, with seven members in absentia.[5]

The leaders in this new field recognized the formidable organizational problems that evolved from segmentation of critical care services in hospitals. They also recognized the important role of nurses, paramedical staff, and medical technologists in the operation of critical care facilities and the need for close liaison with engineering, computer, and related technical resources in lifesaving efforts.

The leaders in this field also discussed the qualifications of professionals who direct critical care units, as well as the need for training and certification of specialists in critical care. They also explored priorities in the care of the most critically ill patients, who at that time were left to the supervision of the least experienced physicians (namely interns and junior resident staff). There was uniform agreement on the potential advantages of a formal, interdisciplinary approach to the treatment of the critically ill. Meeting participants also focused on nursing, burnout, and the rotation of nurses through other units to preserve their interest and broaden their skills.

Participants at this initial meeting generally recognized the economic and utilization advantages gained from pooling facilities for laboratory measurements, respiratory therapy, resuscitation equipment, and monitoring equipment. They expressed considerable concern about the efficacy and safety of major items of equipment that were on the market and suggested that the government should play a greater role in regulating medical equipment and its manufacturers.

Representatives of government and other societies called attention to the need for additional information that would document the advantages and disadvantages of various staffing and facility configurations in the critical care environment. They also called for studies to document what an "optimal" facility is and to document that critical care actually saves lives.

Participants at the meeting uniformly agreed on the important role of biomedical engineers at the bedside and on the potential value of computer technologies to help monitor and manage patient care. However, they regarded computer applications as still largely experimental rather than operational for routine care.

They also discussed the role of emergency medicine in relation to critical care medicine and expressed the sentiment that the elements of emergency medicine were fundamentally different from those of critical care. One participant reported that fewer than 5 percent of patients who enter emergency rooms are critically ill or injured; thus, the operational commitment of emergency rooms is largely to the care of an outpatient population rather than to emergency management of the most critically ill. Participants at the meeting assumed that the immediate transfer of such critically ill or injured patients to critical care units imposes a primary triage function of the emergency room rather than a definitive role of critical care medicine.[6]

At this initial meeting, Max Harry Weil was elected ("drafted," according to him) chairperson.[7] A secretary transcribed the deliberations of the conference group and the subsequent business meeting during which the Society of Critical Care Medicine (SCCM) was established, but unfortunately the transcriber died of a "coronary episode" only three days after the meeting had taken place. Therefore, the report of the original meetings had to be based on relatively sketchy notes taken by the chairperson without the benefit of specific quotations from the various speakers.[8]

Alan Nahum was elected chairperson of the publications committee and charged with investigating and bringing before the society a proposal for an official journal, including specific plans for publication. The journal *Critical Care Medicine* was inaugurated in January 1973, with William C. Shoemaker as editor.[9]

The first annual meeting of the SCCM was held in Los Angeles on February 27, 1972, and Max Harry Weil was elected as the society's first president.[10] The primary commitments of the society were defined as developing educational programs and establishing standards of practice. Educational goals included basic training for physician-trainees, fellowship programs, and continuing medical education. Peter Winter presented proposed guidelines on education of critical care physicians, including qualifications of candidates prior to entering critical care training programs, basic curriculum, and duration of training.

The guidelines committee, chaired by John J. Downes, drafted organizational guidelines concerning standards of practice for critical care units, which were adopted by the society and published in the *Journal of the American Medical Association*.[11] These guidelines defined the purpose and set standards for staffing and organizing clinical facilities for the care of the critically ill.

A number of issues were discussed at the initial meetings in February and July 1970, including whether the practice of critical care medicine should be regarded exclusively as a specialty or as an area open to all physicians and surgeons responsible for acutely ill patients. Other issues discussed included whether critical care medicine should be a separate specialty, whether there should be a new specialty board, whether critical care should have departmental status in a university medical school, and to what extent critical care practitioners should be politically active on the local and national scene. Meeting participants also decided that membership should be open to specialists in foreign lands and to individuals from related disciplines including critical care nurses, respiratory therapists and technicians, biomedical engineers, and other medical and paramedical scientists.

Dedication to patient care was defined as the central purpose of the SCCM. The purpose, as stated by the second president of the society, Peter Safar, was "to improve the care of patients with acutely life-threatening illnesses and injuries and promote the development of optimal facilities for such care."[12] By 1974, the definition of critical care medicine encompassed the triad of (1) resuscitation, (2) emergency care for life-threatening conditions, and (3) intensive care.[13]

In 1973, the SCCM supported the request of the American College of Emergency Physicians to the American Medical Association Council on Medical Education for residency and specialty status in emergency medicine and requested approval for critical care medicine fellowship programs and the certification of special competence in critical care medicine. On behalf of the American Board of Anesthesiologists, William Hamilton proposed the joint creation of certification of special competence in critical care medicine to the boards of internal medicine, surgery, and pediatrics. The original intent was to have a single board examination in critical care medicine, encompassing all of the specialty areas. The intent was for critical care medicine to be a multidisciplinary specialty.[14]

At the same time, the SCCM began collaborating informally with the rapidly growing American Association of Critical Care Nurses (AACN). In late 1972 and early 1973 SCCM published guidelines in the *Journal of the American Medical Association* and *Critical Care Medicine* for organizing critical care units and for training physicians in critical care medicine.[15]

In 1980 the efforts of the individual boards of anesthesiology, internal medicine, pediatrics, and surgery to create a multidisciplinary subspecialty of critical care medicine, with a single board examination covering all four specialties, fell apart over the issue of whether pulmonary medicine specialists should automatically be considered intensivists, or whether they should take additional training in critical care. The American Board of Internal Medicine, under the leadership of C.C.J. Carpenter, withdrew from the joint application and filed a separate application for a subspecialty certification in critical care medicine for internal medicine (including pulmonary medicine). Shortly thereafter, the boards of pediatrics, surgery, and anesthesiology each filed separate applications to the American Board of Medical Specialties. The status quo of the vertical structuring of American medicine had been preserved to a degree. Anesthesiology went on to offer the first independent examination in critical care medicine in 1986; internal medicine, surgery, and pediatrics followed suit.[16]

The Section on Bioethics of the SCCM was formed in 1988, and the Ethics Award of the SCCM, named in memory of Christer Grenvik, was initiated in 1990. James P. Orlowski and his critical care fellow, Sharon Stern, were the first recipients of this award.

HISTORICAL ASPECTS OF MEDICAL ETHICS

Bioethics had its beginnings as a discipline in the late 1960s. Before the inception of bioethics, moral philosophy and science were considered separate domains. Medicine had no need for philosophical discourse because medical science was viewed as impersonal and exact. However, advances in biomedical technology during the twentieth century created ethical dilemmas for society. The phenomenal advances in medical technology and societal changes in the 1960s precipitated the birth of bioethics.

The 1960s was a decade marked by cultural and societal change. It was an era defined by the rebirth of moral values and practical ethics, which inspired several important cultural movements. The feminist movement achieved improved rights for women. The civil rights movement set new precedents for the rights of minorities and spawned the patient's rights movement. The patient's rights movement became a voice of public concern for the well-being of the patient and asserted the patient's right to full knowledge of prognosis to make decisions concerning treatment.

Since the early 1900s, medical science had been gaining new respect and ability through discoveries in bacteriology, pathology, physiology, and biomedical engineering. At the same time, people were gradually becoming aware of societal and environmental hazards that could result from advancing scientific knowledge and technology. Medical science made several extraordinary advances around the 1960s. Suddenly, the full power and potential of medicine were realized. The new medical technology altered the traditional views about the bounds of nature and the meaning of human life. Medicine could suddenly offer longer life expectancy, new options for lifestyles, the control of procreation, powerful new medications to control diseases, and cures for diseases that had caused morbidity and mortality for centuries.

Although medical science offered society many positive advances in the 1960s, some medical advances created ethical dilemmas. For example, the development of birth control and medically safe abortions created intense ethical controversy between science and religion. The advent of prenatal diagnosis not only allowed the option of therapeutic abortion if genetic defects were detected, but also made possible the abortion of a healthy fetus if it was of undesired sex.

The development of ICUs and mechanical ventilation gave medicine the ability to prolong life almost indefinitely. This new lifesaving technology raised questions about whether it is acceptable to terminate extraordinary efforts to prolong life and about when such terminations are considered euthanasia.

Scientific change was creating new moral puzzles and perplexities. Our society was challenged to develop new methods and rules with which to deal with the new moral dilemmas created by biotechnology. It was necessary for the scientific and philosophical aspects of medicine to merge and form a field of bioethics.

One of the key issues in the early medical ethics debates concerned the availability of scarce medical treatments. When important new technologies and treatments are introduced, the number of people in need of treatment often exceeds the amount of resources and the number of trained professionals available to provide the treatment. Therefore, decisions concerning how to allocate scarce medical resources must be made. When dealing with scarce, lifesaving technology, such decisions become very controversial. In these cases, choosing who will receive treatment means selecting who will live and die.

With the development of the hemodialysis machine by Willem Kolff at the Cleveland Clinic in the late 1950s, and the development of the vascular shunt by Belding Scribner in 1960, long-term hemodialysis became a reality. The limited availability of dialysis machines created the first ethical dilemma to receive national attention—who would be selected to receive this lifesaving therapy and, conversely, who would be denied this rationed therapy and therefore sentenced to death. In 1960, roughly 15,000 people were in need of this lifesaving procedure. A number of major medical centers performing dialysis formed multidisciplinary committees to select the candidates for dialysis. One such committee in Seattle, Washington, received national attention when *Life* magazine ran a cover story on this nine-member "God Committee" and its selection process.[17] This committee, which included a majority of public representatives, decided who would receive dialysis, based on social contributions, citizenship, and personal and family factors. The public concern and national controversy over who and how someone was selected for this lifesaving therapy eventually resulted in congressional amendment of the Social Security Act in 1972 to include medical coverage for all individuals with end-stage renal disease, thereby ending the necessity for rationing dialysis.[18]

Much of the foundation of bioethics was formed through the influence of religious and theological ethics. In 1954, the Episcopal theologian Joseph Fletcher wrote the revolutionary tome, *Morals and Medicine*.[19] Fletcher proposed that bioethics should revolve around the rights of the patient. *Morals and Medicine* supported the patient's rights to use contraceptives, artificial insemination, and euthanasia. Fletcher emphasized the patient's right to full knowledge of his or her diagnosis and options for treatment. In 1970 the Methodist theologian Paul Ramsey wrote *The Patient as Person*, which addressed the issues of organ transplantation, life support, mechanical ventilation, and human experimentation.[20] Fletcher and Ramsey agreed on several key issues that became foundational for modern bioethics. Both of these authors invoked the traditional moral disciplines of religion in making ethical decisions, recognized the positive and negative effects of modern medicine and technology, and emphasized the dominance of the patient's rights in medical ethics.

As medical research efforts expanded in the mid-twentieth century, the public became aware of several incidents of unethical human experimentation. Media coverage of these incidents raised public concerns which resulted in legislation to protect human subjects of biomedical research. The most infamous of these unethical experiments were the Tuskegee syphilis experiments, the Jewish Chronic Disease Hospital Studies, and the Willowbrook School studies.

From 1932 to 1972, the U.S. Public Health Service and the Centers for Disease Control sponsored an experiment to study the effects and time course of untreated syphilis on human test subjects. This study, known as the Tuskegee Experiment, involved 399 patients who had contracted syphilis, all of whom were poor, black Americans. Although all of the test subjects were volunteers and had signed consent forms, most of the subjects were illiterate and were obviously not aware of the health risks involved in the study. Although the antibiotic penicillin had been developed in the 1940s and was highly effective in treating syphilis, the subjects in the Tuskegee Experiment were not offered or notified of the availability of this treatment. By 1969, 28 of the men had died from untreated syphilis.

In 1963, at the Jewish Chronic Disease Hospital in Brooklyn, New York, researchers injected chronically ill, elderly patients with viable liver-cancer cells, without consent from the subjects or their immediate families. The purpose of the experiment was to study the effects of the cancer cells on the patients and to determine if the cells could survive in chronically ill patients who did not already have cancer.

From 1965 to 1971 Dr. Saul Krugman conducted studies on hepatitis at the Willowbrook State School in New York, a school for retarded children. He infected incoming students with hepatitis by feeding them samples of the hepatitis virus extracted from the stool of infected students. Although the school had obtained parental consent for the experiment, the consent was coerced; parents knew that it was unlikely that their children would be admitted to the state school unless they agreed to the experiments.

Another stimulus for the development of the field of medical ethics was Henry Beecher's report in the *New England Journal of Medicine* of 22 research studies published in prestigious medical journals that involved unethical or questionably ethical practices. Beecher had accumulated 50 examples over a short period of time, but he reported on only 22 of them because of space limitations in the journal. Beecher estimated that 12 percent of 100 studies that he examined in an "excellent journal" were probably unethical.[21]

In response to the disclosure of these unethical experiments, the National Commission for the Protection of Human Research Subjects was formed, and in 1979 the commission published the *Belmont Report*, which called for ethical guidelines for human experimentation and established institutional review boards (IRBs) to evaluate all research projects in institutions that receive federal funding to guarantee the protection of the research subjects.[22]

Most recently, disclosure of abuses of human research subjects in radiation research studies conducted by the U.S. government under the auspices of the Atomic Energy Commission and the Department of Defense have come to light. These studies, conducted during the Cold War period of 1947 to 1974, included injecting plutonium or uranium into patients, some but not all of whom were terminally ill, without their knowledge or consent.[23]

Bioethics gained formal recognition in medicine with the establishment of the Hastings Center in Hastings on Hudson, New York, in 1969, by Willard Gaylin and Daniel Callahan.[24] In 1971 the Kennedy Institute of Ethics was established at Georgetown University in Washington, DC. Both the Hastings Center and the Kennedy Institute regularly published ethics-related materials, developed model legislation, and provided advice on landmark cases.[25]

Many of the historical developments in medical ethics centered around landmark legal cases that had far-reaching ethical and legal implications. The first such case was the *Tarasoff* case, which involved a psychiatrist who determined that a patient was intent on killing his girlfriend. The psychiatrist notified the police, but he did not notify the woman of the potential threat. The police claimed they were powerless to act, since no crime had been committed. The patient carried out his threat, and the family subsequently sued the psychiatrist for failing to warn the woman. In 1974 the California Supreme Court stated, "When a doctor or psychotherapist, in the exercise of his professional skill and knowledge, determines, or should determine, that a warning is essential to avert danger arising from the medical or psychological condition of his patient, he incurs a legal obligation to give that warning."[26] This decision continues to be widely debated as a threat to patient-physician relationships and confidentiality.

One of the foremost landmark cases was the *Quinlan* case in 1976.[27] The parents of Karen Ann Quinlan sought permission to discontinue life support of their daughter, who had been injured in an automobile accident and left in a persistent vegetative state, dependent on mechanical ventilation. The Supreme Court of New Jersey ruled that the Quinlan family should consult an ethics committee in deciding whether to remove their daughter from life support. Hospitals began establishing ethics committees, especially in New Jersey, where the case had the force of law. Karen Ann Quinlan was subsequently removed from mechanical ventilation; she did not immediately die and, in fact, survived for seven more years.

In 1978 the U.S. Congress created the President's Commission for the Study of Ethical Problems in Medicine and Biomedical and Behavioral Research (The President's Commission).[28] President Jimmy Carter appointed the initial 11 commissioners, with attorney Morris B. Abram as chairperson. Congress specifically limited the commission's tenure with a termination date of December 1982; this date was later extended by Congress to March 1983.[29] Congress charged the commission to undertake the study of the ethical and legal implications of five subjects—informed consent and the protection of human subjects, the definition of death, access to healthcare, compensation for research injuries, and making healthcare decisions. The commission also studied other issues that arose during their tenure, including forgoing life-sustaining treatment, genetic engineering and screening, and whistle-blowing in biomedical research.[30]

In 1978 the first edition of the *Encyclopedia of Bioethics* was published,[31] and in 1979 Beauchamp and Childress published their *Principles of Biomedical Ethics*.[32]

In 1982 the first "Baby Doe" case occurred when a Down's Syndrome baby with esophageal atresia died in Monroe County, Indiana, after his parents refused to permit the surgery necessary to correct his congenital malformation. A second case occurred in 1983 in New York, when parents decided to treat their baby's abscess infection with antibiotics rather than the more aggressive surgical treatment and the baby died. This case further fueled the controversy about decisions that involve the treatment of deformed, or less than perfect, babies.

In 1983, the President's Commission issued a report calling for hospitals to establish ethics committees to "promote effective decision-making" for mentally incompetent patients and handicapped newborns.[33]

Spurred by the Baby Doe cases, Surgeon General C. Everett Koop and the U.S. Department of Health and Human Services (DHHS) in 1984 announced that newborns were protected under the 1973 Rehabilitation Act and issued specific "Baby Doe Regulations."

These regulations took on Orwellian proportions of "Big Brother is watching you"; they required hospitals to post signs in nurseries warning that withholding treatment from deformed newborns was illegal and listing an 800 number that any individual could call anonymously to report neglect or abuse of newborns where treatment was being withheld. If an anonymous report or tip was received, a team of child-protection workers would descend on the hospital to investigate. Government agencies subsequently investigated 49 hospitals, but no facility was charged with infringement. The Baby Doe rules also required hospitals that provide care to newborns to create infant-care-review committees to review decisions regarding the treatment of handicapped newborns.

Also in 1984, the first book on institutional ethics committees, *Institutional Ethics Committees and Health Care Decision Making*, was published by Ronald E. Cranford and A. Edward Doudera.[34]

In 1986 the U.S. Supreme Court overturned the DHHS "Baby Doe" regulations in the case of the *American Hospital Association v. Otis Bowen*, Secretary of DHHS.[35] The highest court stated that the subject of mandating care for defective newborns was to be regulated under state laws. Also in 1986, Maryland passed a bill requiring all hospitals to setup ethics committees by June 1987, although the bill included no sanctions for noncompliance.

In 1988 the Joint Commission on Accreditation of Hospitals (subsequently the Joint Commission on Accreditation of Healthcare Organizations—JCAHO) required hospitals to establish formal policies on do-not-resuscitate (DNR) orders.

In 1990 the U.S. Supreme Court decided the case of *Cruzan v. Director, Missouri Department of Health*. The highest Court decided on the case of a young woman who had been in a persistent vegetative state for at least four years as the result of an automobile accident. The Court determined that a competent person has a constitutionally protected liberty under the 14th Amendment to refuse unwanted medical treatment including "lifesaving nutrition and hydration," but left the decision to the individual states as to the burden of proof necessary when the individual was incompetent and had not executed a living will or other written proof of his or her wishes.[36]

The year 1990 also saw the passage of the Patient Self-Determination Act by the U.S. Congress, as part of the Budget Reconciliation Act of 1990. This federal law required institutions receiving Medicare/Medicaid payments for services to solicit advance directives from adult patients upon admission to the institution, to provide patients with information about advance directives upon admission, and to provide community education on advance directives.[37]

In 1991 the first case of medical futility versus patient or family autonomy and surrogate decision making was heard with the case of Helga Wanglie. This case involved an 86-year-old woman at the University of Minnesota, Hennepin County Hospital, who was in a persistent vegetative state. Her physicians and the ethics committee considered continued mechanical ventilation, resuscitation, intensive care, and nutrition and hydration to be futile therapies and sought to discontinue these life-sustaining therapies. The patient's family, including her husband, demanded continued therapies; they were motivated by religious beliefs and by the earlier expressed wishes of the patient. The hospital went to court to seek the appointment of a guardian *ad litem* to make healthcare decisions in place of the husband and family. The court ruled that the patient's husband was the proper surrogate decision maker for his wife.[38]

In 1991 the Hemlock Society's Derek Humphrey published the book, *Final Exit: The Practicalities of Self-Deliverance and Assisted Suicide for the Dying.*[39]

JCAHO began requiring in 1991 that hospitals have a mechanism in place for the discussion of ethical issues arising in the care of patients.

Futile care came to the forefront again in 1993 in a case involving the care of an anencephalic infant referred to as "Baby K." The baby's mother demanded repeated resuscitation and continued care of an anencephalic infant, which most considered futile. Even a guardian *ad litem* appointed by the court had recommended that further prolongation of Baby K's dying process was futile and inhumane. But on July 1, 1993, Federal Judge Claude Hilton ruled that the hospital and physicians had a duty to provide full medical care, including resuscitation and ventilatory support, to Baby K under the Federal Rehabilitation Act of 1973, the Americans with Disabilities Act of 1990, and the Emergency Medical Treatment and Active Labor Act. The judge stated that he did not believe that Congress had intended these laws to require treatment of anencephalics or futile cases but that it was up to Congress to change the laws and correct the wording. The judge made no findings regarding a standard of care for anencephaly or pertaining to the issue of the best interest of the infant.[40]

In 1994 the state of Oregon passed "Measure 16," which legalized physician-assisted suicide under certain circumstances. Similar measures had failed by narrow margins in California and Washington in prior years. The Oregon law did not result in any assisted suicides in the state until 24 March 1998, largely because of legal challenges to the law. In June of 1997, the United States Supreme Court ruled that there was no constitutional right to physician-assisted suicide. In doing so, the Court upheld laws in New York and Washington state which made it illegal for doctors to give drugs to terminally ill patients who want to speed the end of their lives. The justices distinguished between the state bans on physician assisted suicide—which they upheld—and laws that permit dying patients to refuse life-saving medical treatment, which the Supreme Court had supported in the Cruzan decision in 1990. The decision still allows states to enact laws prohibiting or permitting assisted suicide.[41]

In 1995 *Gilgunn v. Massachusetts General Hospital* was decided. An ethics committee authorized the placement of a DNR order on an elderly, hospitalized patient whose daughter had demanded all therapies, including resuscitation. In this case, the court sided with the hospital and physicians, citing the futility of resuscitation in the patient's case and the appropriate steps of obtaining ethics consultation using the hospital's Optimum Care Committee on two occasions. The case is currently under appeal.[42]

In 1995 the JCAHO began requiring hospitals to have codes of ethics for organizational behavior. The JCAHO also required that such codes address access to care and criteria for admission, transfer, and discharge.

CONCLUSION

Critical care medicine and medical ethics are intricately linked. Each contributes to the body of knowledge of the other. Each has experienced an amazingly similar beginning and growth, and both are presently struggling with their adolescence. It is hoped that critical care medicine and medical ethics will continue to exert an important influence on each other.

NOTES

1. M.H. Weil, "Minutes from the Founding Meeting of the Society of Critical Care Medicine," 10 February 1970; Society of Critical Care Medicine, *Coming of Age: A Collection of Historical Documents Commemorating Two Decades of the Society of Critical Care Medicine* (Anaheim, Calf.: Society of Critical Care Medicine, 1990).

2. P. Ramsey, *The Patient as Person: Explorations in Medical Ethics* (New Haven, Conn.: Yale University Press, 1970).

3. See note 1 above.

4. M.H. Weil, "The Society of Critical Care Medicine: Its History and Its Destiny," *Critical Care Medicine* 1 (1973): 6-8.

5. See note 1 above.

6. Ibid.

7. Ibid.

8. See notes 1 and 4 above.

9. See note 4 above; W.C. Shoemaker, "Interdisciplinary Medicine: Accommodation or Integration?" *Critical Care Medicine* 3 (1975): 14-17.

10. See note 4 above.

11. Society of Critical Care Medicine, "Guidelines for Organization of Critical Care Units," *Journal of the American Medical Association* 222 (1972): 1532-35.

12. P. Safar, "Critical Care Medicine—Quo Vadis?" *Critical Care Medicine* 2 (1974): 9-13.

13. Ibid.

14. Ibid.

15.See note 11 above; Society of Critical Care Medicine, "Guidelines for Training of Physicians in Critical Care Medicine," *Critical Care Medicine* 1 (1973): 23-26.

16. J.W. Hoyt et al., "History of the Society of Critical Care Medicine," *Critical Care Medicine* 24 (1996): S3-S9.

17. S. Alexander, "They Decide Who Lives, Who Dies," *Life*, 9 November 1962, 102-12.

18. M.B. Abram and S.M. Wolf, "Public Involvement in Medical Ethics: A Model for Government Action," *New England Journal of Medicine* 310 (1984): 627-32.

19. J. Fletcher, *Morals and Medicine* (Princeton, N.J.: Princeton University Press, 1954).

20. See note 2 above.

21. H.K. Beecher, "Ethics and Clinical Research," *New England Journal of Medicine* 274 (1966): 1354-60.

22. National Commission for the Protection of Human Subjects of Biomedical and Behavioral Research, *The Belmont Report: The Ethical Principles and*

Guidelines for the Protection of Human Subjects of Research (Washington, DC: U.S. Government Printing Office, 1979).

23. Advisory Committee on Human Radiation Experiments, "Research Ethics and the Medical Profession: Report of the Advisory Committee on Human Radiation Experiments," *Journal of the American Medical Association* 276 (1996): 403-09.

24. The Hastings Center, "The Hastings Center: A Short and Long 15 Years," *Hastings Center Report* (1984); The Hastings Center, "The Hastings Center: Ethics in the 80s," *Hastings Center Report* 11, no. 6 (1981): S1-S16.

25. E.D. Pellegrino, "The Metamorphosis of Medical Ethics: A 30-Year Retrospective," *Journal of the American Medical Association* 269 (1993): 1158-62.

26. *Tarasoff v. Regents of the University of California*, 529 P2d, 189 (Cal. 1974); ¶ 551 P2d, 334

27. *In re Quinlan*, 70 N.J. 10, 355 A.2ed 647 (1976).

28. A. Helm, "Summary of the President's Commission for the Study of Ethical Problems in Medicine and Biomedical and Behavioral Research," *Military Medicine* 152 (1987): 425-30.

29. Ibid.

30. Ibid.

31. W. T. Reich, ed., *Encyclopedia of Bioethics* (New York: Free Press, 1978).

32. T.L. Beauchamp and J.F. Childress, *Principles of Biomedical Ethics* (New York: Oxford University Press, 1979).

33. President's Commission for the Study of Ethical Problems in Medicine and Biomedical and Behavioral Research, *Deciding to Forego Life-Sustaining Treatment* (Washington, D.C.: U.S. Government Printing Office, 1983), 160-70.

34. R.E. Cranford and A.E. Doudera, *Institutional Ethics Committees and Health Care Decision Making* (Ann Arbor, Mich.: Health Administration, 1984).

35. *Bowen v. American Hospital Association*, 476 U.X. 610, 106 S.Ct. 2101 (9 June 1986).

36. *Cruzan v. Director, Missouri Department of Health*, 110 S. Ct. 2841 (1990).

37. Omnibus Budget Reconciliation Act of 1990, Public Law No. 100-508 (1990).

38. M. Angell, "The Case of Helga Wanglie; A New Kind of Right to Die Case," *New England Journal of Medicine* 325 (1991): 511-12.

39. D. Humphrey, *Final Exit: The Practicalities of Self-Deliverance and Assisted Suicide for the Dying* (Secaucus, N.J.: Hemlock Society, 1991).

40. G. T. Annas, "Asking the Courts to Set the Standard of Emergency Care—The Case of Baby K," *New England Journal of Medicine* 330 (1994): 1542-45.

41. See note 36 above.

42. *Gilgunn v. Massachusetts General Hospital*, no. 92-4820 (Massachusetts Supreme Court, Suffolk County, 1995).

2

The Construction of Ethics and Its Reconstruction in Critical Care: Ethical Theory and Practice

Mary Faith Marshall and Martin Perlmutter

INTRODUCTION

It is no accident that neither the first nor the second edition of the Society of Critical Care Medicine's classic *Textbook of Critical Care* contained a chapter dealing with ethical issues. Legal issues were addressed, and significant attention was directed at defining death. But ethical consideration of whether and how new medical technologies should be applied, and the problems that attend their application, were absent. This troubling omission mirrored what was happening in the clinical setting, where consideration of ethical questions regarding the nature and goals of critical care medicine lagged far behind the ever-insistent application of life-sustaining technology. Newly discovered means to preserve life overwhelmed any consideration of when and at what cost a life should be saved. In 1995, 25 years after the dawning of the new field of critical care medicine, a chapter on ethical issues appeared in the third edition of the *Textbook of Critical Care*, reflecting a widely shared perception that life-and-death issues depend in large part on concerns about quality of life, costs, and the desires of the patient.[1]

The disciplines of bioethics and critical care medicine have evolved simultaneously. Both fields result from new clinical options available to healthcare providers and consumers. Until recently, limited options for successful medical intervention provided a limited context for ethical decision making; when there are no real options to consider, there are no real choices to make. As options burgeoned, so did the field of biomedical ethics, which addressed concerns about the various choices that became available. Advanced technology offered new choices that needed to be made from an ethical perspective. So too with critical care medicine. New resources became available that fostered the discipline of critical care medicine. Closed-chest cardiac massage, mechanical ventilation, invasive monitoring, organ transplantation, and treatment of the syndromes of shock gave healthcare practitioners the wherewithal to intervene in ways that had previously been unavailable.

The availability of these interventions spawned a new medical paradigm—the technological imperative—which called for aggressive application of new technologies whenever there was a chance that they might be successful. The application of these technologies sometimes resulted in situations in which patients could not be weaned from the ventilator or patients' lives continued without any considerations of quality. New issues, such as assessing quality of life and deciding whether to initiate treatment when the outcome might be a severely compromised patient, have been created by these new technological options. Technologic developments in critical care medicine guide the development of bioethics more generally. As more and more options become available to healthcare providers and consumers, explicit ethical decisions must be made about which options to choose.

Historically, paternalism worked well as the primary model of clinical decision making. Because there were not many fundamental decisions to be made, physicians were well suited to make life-or-death choices on behalf of their patients. Advanced technological options were not available, so the clinical goals of preserving or expanding life posed few dangers. There were relatively few long-term abuses of aggressive therapy because the technology to sustain life did not exist. As a result, there was little to consult the patient about. The expertise of the caregivers in such a limited arena of technology provided a good structure for paternalism. Because of technological advances, the model of paternalism is no longer successful, and today the preferences of the patient must inform the real choices that are available.

Quite separately from advances in critical care technology, social movements in the 1960s generated a new interest in individual rights, specifically civil rights and women's rights. Discussion of rights was extended to the patient in the medical context. The patient had a crucial voice that needed to be heard separately from the healthcare worker's judgment about appropriate treatment. As a result, patients and clinicians became more concerned about respecting decisional autonomy—because there were more decisions to be made that profoundly affected the quality of patients' lives and because individuals were thought to be entitled to determine their own destinies.

One result of these changes is that the main distinctions that dominated bioethics for many years no longer receive the same attention. For example, the distinction between *withholding* treatment and *withdrawing* it, which was supposed to reflect the fundamental ethical distinction between letting die and killing, no longer holds the importance it once had when medical treatments were more rudimentary. Removing sophisticated technology often seems the same as allowing the patient to die, most often mercifully, so that it no longer seems that care providers who withdraw such treatment have "dirty hands." So too, the distinction between *ordinary* and *extraordinary* care. It is difficult to have a clear sense of what is extraordinary when organs can be replaced, ventilation can be provided mechanically, and brain-dead corpses can be maintained for long periods of time. Even the distinction between *life* and *death* has lost much of its significance in biomedical ethics contexts; it remains important in determining when organs can be harvested to give to other patients, but it is no longer so central a concern when treating the patient from whom the organs can be harvested.

All of these older distinctions have counterparts in the contemporary debate. Withholding and withdrawing life-sustaining treatment has a counterpart in the discussion regarding artificial hydration and nutrition; some have argued that keeping food and water from the patient is killing the patient, not merely allowing the patient to die. Concerns about ordinary and extraordinary care are discussed as "standards of care." The appropriateness of treatment is no longer governed by the notion of the ordinary; rather, professional standards of treatment should determine what is provided to the patient. The futility of a treatment relates to standards of care, not to the distinction between the ordinary and the extraordinary. Issues about life and death have been preempted by questions about quality of life. Absolute criteria such as "brain death" or "heart-lung function" play less of a role than the judgment about what sort of life is worth living.

THE GOALS OF CRITICAL CARE MEDICINE AND THE TECHNOLOGICAL IMPERATIVE

A necessary preliminary in relating ethical theory to critical care practice is determining the appropriate goals of critical care medicine. Historically, physicians have defined their primary duties as healing the sick, promoting health, and relieving suffering. Prolongation of life as a medical goal is a modern phenomenon (first articulated in the eighteenth century by Sir Francis Bacon) and has no foundation in the Hippocratic tradition.[2] Before the discovery of antibiotics, most Americans died of infectious diseases. Prior to World War II, most Americans died at home. Today, the majority of Americans die in acute care hospitals, and many of these deaths occur in intensive care units (ICUs). Until recently, patients did not survive the failure of single or multiple organ systems. Today, even patients who are brain dead, permanently unconscious, or anencephalic can be maintained biologically with high-technology supportive devices. Patients in multiple-organ-system failure are repeatedly rescued from biological death with advanced resuscitative techniques. The results of these efforts, measured in terms of quality of life, productivity, or length of life remaining, are often questionable.

Today, almost all acute care hospitals have one or more ICUs. According to recent estimates, there are more than 65,000 ICU beds in more than 6,000 acute care hospitals.[3] In 1990, 1 percent of the gross domestic product was spent caring for 6 million patients in ICUs across the country. Even though ICU beds comprise only 8 percent of all acute care beds, 17 percent of all hospital patients are admitted to ICUs, and such units account for 28 percent of acute care hospital costs.[4]

The structure of ICUs and the expertise of critical care clinicians vary widely. Less than half of all ICUs have full-time medical directors, a medical director who is certified in critical care, an assigned respiratory therapist, nurses who are certified by the American Association of Critical Care Nurses, or mechanisms for resolving triage conflicts at the level of medical director or attending physician.[5] These data raise troubling questions about the nature and purpose of critical care medicine. Inherent are issues of benefits and risks to patients, medical effectiveness, distributive justice, medical paternalism, and the appropriate use of technology in treating patients who are terminally ill.

Decisions regarding care at the end of life are often the catalyst for value conflicts. The classic dilemma in critical care decision making encompasses one of two scenarios: (1) when patients or families demand medically ineffective care and clinicians are reluctant to provide it, or (2) when clinicians force unwanted or medically inappropriate care on unwilling or decisionally incapable patients. In a seminal study, Solomon and colleagues reported that half of all physician and nurse respondents in five hospitals (and 70 percent of house officers) had "acted against their conscience in providing care to the terminally ill."[6] In an early study of ICU effectiveness, Knaus and colleagues reported that 25 percent of ICU treatment was provided to patients who had no need for ICU care or were too sick to benefit from it.[7] More recent data from Knaus are even less reassuring. Of a cohort of 571 mechanically ventilated patients in 12 ICUs, 48 percent of the patients had a 75 percent risk of hospital death at the time of admission. After four days in the ICU, their mortality risk had increased to 97 percent.[8]

These data reflect only certain subpopulations of critical care patients. Raffin and colleagues have reported that the death rate of all patients admitted to critical care units is between 15 to 20 percent.[9] Included in these statistics, however, are patients with low mortality rates of 4 to 6 percent (such as patients undergoing coronary artery bypass graft surgery or vascular surgery and patients who attempt suicide by overdose). Eliminating these patient populations results in an overall ICU mortality rate of between 30 to 40 percent.[10] Other patient populations fare less well. Those with adult respiratory distress syndrome have mortality rates of 65 to 100 percent.[11] Patients with hematologic malignancies who are admitted to ICUs have mortality rates of 80 to 100 percent.[12]

Exhibit 2-1
Factors Affecting a Decision to Admit or Discharge from the ICU

1. Likelihood of a successful outcome
2. Patient's life expectancy due to disease
3. Patient's anticipated quality of life
4. Preferences of the patient/surrogate
5. Burdens for those affected
6. Health and other needs of the community
7. Individual and institutional moral and religious values

Knaus and his colleagues have identified two primary functions of the ICU: "(1) life support of organ system failure in critically ill patients; or (2) close monitoring of stable non-critically ill patients in case the need for life support suddenly occurs."[13] Raffin has also proposed two major goals of the critical care team. The first goal, to save the salvageable, qualifies and appropriately narrows Knaus's objective of life support of the critically ill. Raffin's second goal, to help the dying have a peaceful and dignified death, raises serious questions about the purpose of critical care medicine.[14] As Angell and others have observed, too often the ICU, rather than serving only patients with reversible acute illness, is used as a "high-tech hospice."[15] Angell urges that we jettison the notion that "more is better" where healthcare is concerned, especially in the context of intensive therapy for terminally ill patients.[16]

Any seasoned intensive care physician or nurse will attest that critical care comprises two things: (1) the application of high technology and advanced medical science, and (2) the provision of specialized, intensive nursing care. Critical care medicine is delivered in team fashion. The clinicians who practice it—physicians, nurses, respiratory therapists, pharmacists, and others—are more interdependent in this arena than in any other setting in the acute care hospital. The milieu is high energy, high stress, and high technology. The ICU can be simultaneously exhilarating and dehumanizing for the critical care clinician. Decision making turns rapidly on a stream of technologically generated data toward the clinical goal of achieving and maintaining the patient in a steady state of physiological equilibrium. The patient as person is often lost in this flow of information and its attendant tasks. According to Bulger and coauthors, "Advanced technology and the increasingly complex organizational styles it has engendered tend to isolate patients as human beings just at the time when and in the settings where their confrontation with suffering and death may be most intense."[17]

Since its inception, modern critical care medicine has been closely influenced by the technological imperative and its partner—the use or abuse of medical power. The medical economist Victor Fuchs first coined the term *technological imperative* in 1974. It is "the desire of the physician to do everything that he has been trained to do, regardless of the benefit/cost ratio."[18] Some 20 years later, Howard Brody, a physician and philosopher, posited that "medical ethics is about power and its responsible use." He observed: "When the medical equivalent of the Vietnam War tragedy occurs and the physician reports that he had to destroy the village in order to save it, we assume that the intention was benign.

But this comforting story denies that physicians are too human and that they have buried within them this same impulse to relish the unresisted use of power."[19]

Application of life-sustaining technology as an instrument of physicians' power was never prospectively or deliberately chosen as a driving force behind critical care medicine. Only a retrospective review brings it, and its implications, to light. In a classic essay in the *Hastings Center Report*, physician Eric Cassell warns: "If there is one thing that can be singled out as the engine of the medical economic inflation now occurring everywhere in the world, it is the seeming irresistible spread of technology into every level of medicine—irresistible to doctors, patients, and nations alike. . . . As a class, technologies are reductive, oversimplifying, impatient, intolerant of ambiguity and democratic. They spread much more quickly than the ideas that inform them."[20] The immediacy of technology lures us because it is unrelated to our own reasoning, and therefore neater, or simpler. Cassell suggests a dichotomy between human sophistication, characterized by a tolerance for ambiguity, and technological sophistication, which eliminates ambiguity. Technology removes ambiguity "by narrowing down the field of difference between what is good and what is bad, so that ultimately one test result is taken to be good and another result bad. And that is how the state of the coronary arteries became accepted as the equivalent of a disease of the heart itself."[21]

Cassell points out the inverse relationship in the clinical environment between the importance of a medical decision (and its attendant need for knowledge) and uncertainty. One method of eliminating uncertainty is by oversimplifying the patient and his or her clinical problem to a problem with a particular organ. This reductionism perpetuates a collapsing spiral of data generation and problem redefinition. In this manner, patients and their complaints and symptoms become less important than technologically generated "hard" data. The care of the person, the ultimate meaning of prognosis and outcome, is lost as the clinical aperture narrows to focus on salvaging and maintaining an organ. Cassell warns that technology is self-perpetuating: "Doctors who have mastered a technology tend to use it as often as possible not necessarily for reasons of profit, but because they love their skills and technologies. . . . Problems tend to be redefined so that a technology becomes appropriate when it might otherwise not be. A saying that makes the point has become popular among physicians, 'To the man with a hammer, everything is a nail.' "[22]

Oversimplification of the goals of critical care medicine can result in the misapplication of sophisticated technology and the abuse of the clinician's power. In this context, patients are vulnerable and at risk of receiving unwanted or futile care. The ends of critical care medicine are best served by assessing the patient's survivability and quality of life and by paying special attention to the patient's preferences. The goals of relieving suffering at the end of life and of providing patients with a good death might best be achieved in a hospice setting rather than an ICU. Hospice care is best provided in a more humane environment, one more welcoming to family members, with professionals trained to help patients and their families through the dying process.

PROFESSIONAL ETHICS AND ETHICAL THEORY

In an introduction to the field of healthcare ethics, it is important to distinguish between professional ethics and ethical theory and to provide a brief history of each.

PROFESSIONAL ETHICS

Professional ethics is a code of conduct suitable for persons within a field. Indeed, professions are defined by a code of conduct. There are standards for clergy, accountants, nurses, and academicians that describe what constitutes professional conduct within the field. Confidentiality is crucial for ministers, accuracy for accountants, caring for nurses, and honesty for academicians. These particular "virtues" are especially appropriate for different professionals.

The best-known example of a professional code of conduct is the Hippocratic oath. The tradition it embodies has guided Western medicine for generations. Its simplicity bespeaks the limited abilities of physicians, but its focus on benefitting the patient is still the guiding principle of healthcare; in fact, the focus on benefitting the client is central to professional ethics in general.

The Hippocratic corpus, which dates from the fourth century B.C., is a collection of writings by mostly unknown authors who were members of family guilds of physicians. The Hippocratic oath comprises two essential parts. The first governs the student's responsibilities to his teachers and forbears and precludes sharing medical knowledge with nonmembers of the guild. This part of the code attempts to protect the profession and is not particularly directed at the patient. Professions are concerned with their continuation and their integrity. The second part articulates rules of the physician's behavior with regard to the patient. The most important precept of the code, which has come to be known as the Hippocratic principle, states: "Whatever houses I may visit, I will come for the benefit of the sick." A principle of beneficence is the central tenet with respect to the physician's treatment of the patient.

The obligation not to inflict a harm is often erroneously invoked as the first principle of the Hippocratic oath. The maxim *primum non nocere* (above all, do no harm) does not appear in the Hippocratic corpus. However, the principle of nonmaleficence is implied in the oath: "I will use treatment to help the sick according to my ability and judgement, but I will never use it to injure or wrong them."[23] Other rules ordained by the oath concern physicians' relations with their patients, such as the protection of confidentiality and prohibitions against sexual relations with patients and against the use of poisons or abortifacients to end life. As a professional code, the Hippocratic oath proposes standards suitable for a particular profession by which individual practitioners can be judged.

Codes of conduct have become far more elaborate since the fourth century B.C. The two functions of protecting the profession and protecting the client remain central concerns. Setting standards for admission into the profession, guaranteeing that certain activities are performed only by members of the profession, and providing a code of conduct for the profession have become important activities for all professional groups. The code of conduct always speaks of the obligations of the professional to the client. Each profession has particular concerns that are addressed in the code of conduct. The code has a descriptive function and prescriptive one, describing the activities of the professional and prescribing appropriate behavior by the professional. Trial lawyers, tax accountants, surveyors, and architects are no different in this regard than physicians, nurses, social workers, respiratory therapists, or hospital administrators.

ETHICAL THEORY

In addition to professional codes of ethics, there is the more general and abstract field of ethics that has been a central field within Western philosophy since the writings of Plato and Aristotle, with their concern with the good life, justice, and human excellence. The focus of philosophical ethics is broader than professional ethics; it looks at the rightness of human behavior in general, without restricting it to a particular activity or profession.

Clearly, a survey of the history of ethical theory is beyond the purview of this chapter. However, the two competing post-Enlightenment traditions of philosophical ethics that inform the discussion of critical care ethics should be introduced briefly. The Enlightenment's aim of dislodging human institutions from their religious foundations and of grounding activities and practices in reason revived interest in ethical theory and generated two comprehensive theories of ethics. The first is associated with the European continent, is identified with Rousseau and Kant, and emphasizes the universality of morality. For an action to be right for me to do, it has to be the sort of action that I can will for others to do as well. So in acting (morally), I am "legislating" behavior for other agents, since I have to be willing to accept others acting on the same principle that I acted on. The moral enterprise is to consider whether the action qualifies as being part of a desirable world. So, for example, lying is morally wrong because I cannot will others to lie and, specifically, I cannot will to be lied to. This ethical tradition focuses on the nature of the act done, rather than its consequences. It emphasizes the centrality of autonomy and respect for persons, since our actions toward others must be compatible with their personhood or self-direction. One is precluded from treating persons as merely a means to an end, because that is demeaning to their personhood. This is the *deontological* tradition; it emphasizes obligations, duties, and rights that stem from the value of persons.

The second ethical tradition is associated with Great Britain, is identified with Bentham and Mill, and emphasizes the desirability of the consequences of the action. Human beings seek pleasure and avoid pain, so actions that produce the most pleasure and the least pain are good. An action that produces pain for no good reason is the paradigmatic bad action. Because all human beings count equally, a calculus can be constructed that examines the short- and long-term consequences of actions in terms of pleasures and pains to give guidance about those actions that are good and bad. Benefits are to be sought, and harms are to be avoided. The only justification of a harm is that a future benefit will come from it that outweighs the harm. As a central human institution, morality is designed to maximize the good and minimize the bad. This tradition is *consequentialist*, emphasizing the consequences of actions. It is also utilitarian, attempting to maximize total utility, while focusing less on its distribution.

Both of these traditions are philosophical in a broad sense. They are systematic attempts to develop theories of right and wrong or good and bad that are based on features of personhood. The deontological theory focuses on persons as self-governing agents, thereby emphasizing notions such as autonomy and self-determination, whereas the utilitarian theory emphasizes the important fact that persons desire pleasure and do not desire pain. Both theories recommend behavior appropriate to their view of persons.

Both traditions have been influential in Anglo-American legal history. Natural, inalienable rights that inhere in individuals fit in well with the deontological tradition. Persons have special status and deserve to be respected by allowing them freedom from interference in their pursuits. Utilitarianism has been an important legal reform tradition. Child labor was a harm to children, so laws were passed restricting it; compulsory education was a benefit and so was enacted into law. Utilitarians emphasize that institutions, such as morality and the law, serve human needs, so they must be reformed when they produce more harm than good. Cost-benefit analyses are models of utilitarian thought.

Justice or fairness is an interesting and historically important ethical notion that has received a lot of attention within both traditions. The deontological tradition emphasizes the wrong done to someone in treating them in a way that you would not want to be treated, and grounds justice on this feature of universalizability. So taking another's umbrella, discriminating against the poor, or favoring your oldest child are all unjust because the umbrella owner, the poor, and your other children are being treated in ways that you yourself would not want to be treated. Treating them unfairly is treating them in ways incompatible with universal laws of morality.

The utilitarian discussion of justice is less direct. The most prominent version of that discussion distinguishes between rules and their application. Rules are justified by considerations of utility for all those affected by the rules. Moral behaviors such as telling the truth, keeping promises, and respecting parents are all types of actions that have good consequences, so moral laws require them. Similarly, immoral actions such as killing, stealing, or coveting typically have bad consequences and so are enjoined by moral laws. Thus, utilitarians think that the consequences justify the rules, with each person counting as one. Applying the rules is more straightforward. Taking another's umbrella, discriminating against the poor, and favoring your oldest child violate the rules, which are themselves justified by the good consequences produced by conforming to them. So, the wrongness of individual acts of theft is in virtue of rules prohibiting the theft; the wrongness of theft is in virtue of the benefits of allowing persons to own property. Unfairness or injustice is a particular form of partiality within the personal and impartial moral system of rules.[24]

Not surprisingly, the crucial terms that inform the contemporary discussion of bioethics came from these traditions, though they had a long life even before these traditions. *Autonomy* is perhaps the central notion within bioethics. It is almost always connected with the patient or surrogate, and attending to the patient's will should govern his or her options for treatment. It is a formal notion, emphasizing who makes the choice, while not addressing what the appropriate choice is. *Beneficence* and *nonmaleficence* are substantive notions addressed at the caregiver, and date back to the Hippocratic tradition. These notions focus on the good and bad results of medical treatment and urge the caregiver to do good and not harm. *Justice* is a distributional notion that arises in situations in which the demand for resources outstrips their availability. Triage in critical care is an excellent example of a procedure to distribute limited resources in an equitable way.

ETHICAL PRINCIPLES

RESPECT FOR AUTONOMY

Persons should be entitled to govern their own lives; they should be able to make decisions based on their own values, beliefs, and prejudices. Self-determination is essential for being a person. This dimension of autonomy is not an endorsement of the decision, but an endorsement of the right to make a decision. One may disagree with a Jehovah's Witness's refusal of a blood transfusion but agree that she has the right to refuse unwanted treatment. In fact, respect for autonomy gives little substantive direction about which choice should be made. In the clinical context, this means that individuals have the right to consent to or refuse any form of medical treatment. Consent and refusal are corollaries of one another; they are flip sides of the same coin, each meaningless without the other.

The elements of informed consent can be broken down into two categories: elements of information and elements of consent.[25] Information elements comprise adequate disclosure by the healthcare provider of all information that the patient or surrogate decision maker needs to make an informed decision regarding medical treatment, and subsequent understanding of that information by the patient or surrogate. It is difficult to specify how much information is necessary for a particular individual and how much needs to be understood, but there should be enough information and understanding that the benefits, risks, and alternatives to treatment are available for review. A physician's recitation of a litany of risks and benefits, coupled with the patient's signature on a consent document, does not constitute adequate informed consent. Often it is difficult to know whether the patient or his/her surrogate understands the information adequately. Consent elements also involve voluntariness (freedom from coercion) and decisional capacity. Critically ill patients are often obtunded, unconscious, narcotized, sedated, rendered speechless by endotracheal tubes, pharmacologically paralyzed, in pain, or afraid. Family members may be in emotional distress, fearful, or feeling guilty. Adequate disclosure by the clinician of the nature of the therapy; its purpose; its benefits, risks, and consequences; the probability that it will be successful; the feasible alternatives; and the prognosis if the therapy is not given is often impossible in an emergency situation when the patient is in a life-threatening condition and no surrogate decision maker is available. Even if circumstances allow for adequate disclosure of the nature of therapy, the patient or surrogate may not meet the criteria for capable decision making: he or she may not understand the information relevant to the decision, might not be able to reason about alternatives and consequences against a background of personal values and goals, and may be iatrogenically (or otherwise) unable to communicate with caregivers about the decision. In addition, the decision maker may not be free of coercion from controlling influences such as pain; fear; or manipulative family members, clinicians, clergy, or others.[26]

The notion of informed consent seems uncontroversial. In fact, Ahronheim, Moreno, and Zuckerman recently suggested that informed consent is the overarching value in modern clinical ethics. "The principle of self-determination is commonly regarded as the first principle of contemporary biomedical ethics. . . . No doctrine, principle, or proposition has been more influential than the idea that the competent, adult patient has the right to determine the course of his or her own medical treatment. In the standard account of clinical ethics theory, this is the touchstone."[27] But there are both theoretical and practical problems with informed consent, especially in critical care. On the theoretical level, it conflicts with the model of paternalism, which emphasizes the expertise of the healthcare providers and the relative ignorance of the patient and his or her family. This imbalance of power in a high-stakes, critical care setting often results in the patient's relying on the expertise of the healthcare team to determine his or her choice. Typically, the patient or family will respond to a detailed account of the alternatives available by asking what the healthcare worker would recommend and agreeing with the recommendation.

On the practical level, the standard elements of informed consent are difficult to achieve in the critical care setting. It is difficult for a clinician to disclose completely and for the patient to comprehend adequately. The patient may lack decision-making capacity, and the context may be coercive. Furthermore, in the critical care setting, clinicians generally take the patient's physical presence in an ICU bed as evidence of consent to life-sustaining therapy. Given these facts, it is important that the healthcare team be aware of substantive considerations that ought to inform the plan for treatment. The doctrine that the patient's wishes should be honored is important, but the patient will often defer to the judgment of the healthcare professional. As a result, the professional must know how to respond to questions about the desirability of further treatment. Respect for autonomy carries a lot more weight in the ideal decision-making context than it does in the critical care setting.

BENEFICENCE AND NONMALEFICENCE

The Hippocratic tradition often distinguishes between nonmaleficence and beneficence. The reason for the distinction is to elevate the duty to do no harm above the duty to do good. That is, professionals ought to make special efforts to do no harm—to guarantee that their client's are not made worse off by professionals' actions. Of course, professionals have a duty to benefit their clients as well, but that obligation is more nebulous and less urgent. Part of the motivation for the distinction is dirty hands. If persons suffer because I fail to help them, there is clearly a harm that I can prevent. So, my not feeding the hungry and my not donating blood or organs results in a harm that I can prevent. The world would clearly be a better place if there were more Good Samaritans reaching out to help others in need. But if I actually cause them harm, the responsibility is more clearly mine, because the harm is directly attributable to my actions. It is this sort of reasoning that leads practitioners to conclude that withholding treatment is less objectionable than withdrawing it, since withdrawing treatment is causing a harm in a way that withholding it is not.

Nonetheless, it is best to view the obligation not to cause a harm as part of a continuum that includes the obligation to prevent a harm, the obligation to remove a harm, and the obligation to promote a good. Viewing it as a continuum is especially appropriate in professional contexts when there is a relationship between the parties, the goods and harms are relatively clearly defined by the professional relationship, and the results are intentional. That is, it might be important to distinguish between not feeding the hungry and taking food from the hungry; the second is clearly more objectionable morally than the first because it is intentionally harming another person in a way that neglecting to feed might be merely indirection. But, in the context of critical care, the distinction is far less important, because the patient is there to be helped, the help has to do with illness, and intentionally not helping in a critical care context is actually harming. Refusing to stabilize a patient in shock, when such stabilization is possible and desirable, is actually causing a harm. Under these circumstances, dirty hands apply equally to withholding treatment and withdrawing it. So, there is no important moral distinction between withdrawing and withholding life support in the context of critical care.

As a general rule, beneficence is a more demanding principle than nonmaleficence, because there are countless good things that we can do to benefit others. In fact, some have objected to beneficence because it has endless scope, requiring us always to feed the hungry and help the needy. And there is always more we can do, forgoing more and more of our own desires in order to help the needy even more. It gives us the responsibility to benefit the world as if we were responsible for the plight of the destitute. Nonmaleficence is a much more modest requirement.

Contextualizing beneficence to a professional relationship—whether that of critical care provider, tax accountant, or divorce lawyer—eliminates much of the problem of scope. Even beneficence is not an endless requirement, since it is relative to the profession and its goals. So the intensive care practitioner must stabilize a patient to allow for successful treatment outside the ICU, the tax accountant must help put the client in the best possible tax situation, and the divorce lawyer must provide the best outcome with respect to the divorce.

The professional must live up to a standard of due care that determines which harms are worth the risk and which are not. Benefits and harms are less abstract in a professional context, since the context clarifies what is to count as a benefit or harm. Many medical procedures might result in harm to the patient, but the possible harm is not adequate reason to refrain from the procedure. Risk-averse policies are often not best for the patient, especially in a critical care setting where a more aggressive policy is often called for. Professionals should be made aware of standards for the profession, since malpractice suits often turn on judgments about whether the practitioner acted within the guidelines of the profession. So, if the standards of care no longer distinguish between withdrawing therapies and withholding them, or between ordinary and extraordinary care, then the practitioner within that field must abandon those distinctions. Of course, practitioners must live with their conscience and so must refer the patient to other professionals when they feel that the professional standards of care violate their own moral standards.

Clearly, consequentialist notions such as benefits and harms require judgments about whether the benefits are worth the risks, if the likelihood of success justifies the treatment, or if the harms that might result from the treatment require a more conservative strategy. These are often difficult determinations that depend on details of the case, such as the patient's preferences, the quality of life that the patient will enjoy, the length of life predicted after recovery, and so on. Futility is one not-so-subtle way to deal with these determinations; it includes not only hopeless treatment for a dying patient—which is clearly inappropriate—but also a procedure that is highly unlikely to be effective, treatment with a qualitatively poor outcome that is virtually certain, and treatment that is speculative or untried.[28] All these dimensions raise questions of proportionality—questions about whether the treatment is worth undertaking. Of course, there are other issues involved in proportionality that are seldom mentioned, such as the financial cost of the treatment, the age of the patient, and the availability of a support network for the patient after the treatment. These are all important considerations that need to be addressed before aggressive therapies are provided. These are difficult judgments, and it is not easy to weigh all of these dimensions to arrive at the best decision, even when one knows what the ethical concerns are.

Ethics committees and ethics consultation services are available at many hospitals with ICUs. These provide an excellent opportunity for discussing hard cases with professionals who are familiar with the ethics literature governing healthcare. Discussions with ethics committees or ethics consultants are confidential and advisory only, and should be initiated early when there are real decisions to be made, when the issues are not yet moot. These discussions are often reassuring to the practitioner, since hard cases often create self-doubt, uncertainty, and regret on the part of the healthcare provider. There is no reason for the intensive care practitioner to bear the burden of his or her decisions alone. Such discussions can also serve to reassure patients' families.[29]

JUSTICE

The U.S. healthcare system is faced with growing pressures regarding the allocation of scarce resources. There are at least two reasons for these pressures. First, the percentage of Gross National Product in the United States devoted to healthcare is rapidly increasing; this phenomenon raises the specter that the United States will become less competitive in the global marketplace as it commits more and more of its resources to healthcare. If U.S. employers must pay higher labor costs because of healthcare coverage than employers elsewhere, they will either relocate their industries abroad or lose out to foreign competitors. Managed care is one attempt to deal with this inefficiency by using gatekeepers who restrict access, by limiting which therapies are covered by insurance policies, and by developing other cost-control strategies for healthcare delivery. Second, healthcare dollars are allocated inefficiently. Expensive one-on-one care is the model for healthcare delivery. Critical care, for example, is an inefficient way to save lives. Public health, preventive care, and fitness and nutrition programs provide much more "bang for the buck" than critical care or organ transplants. Managed care companies are beginning to address such issues.

These issues of efficiency and cost are related to issues of justice. Such issues were the central theme of a 1995 report commissioned by the Institute of Medicine of the National Academy of Sciences. The report, *Society's Choices: Social and Ethical Decision Making in Biomedicine,* quoted Representative George Brown, Jr., Chairman of the Committee on Science, Space, and Technology of the U.S. House of Representatives, who bemoans the misalliance between medical technology that is driven by the free market and the goal of improved quality of life for all. According to the report:

[Brown maintains that] freewheeling market forces and the drive for high-technology solutions to our society's problems may in fact displace nontechnological, readily distributed preventive solutions in favor of inequitable, expensive, and sometimes even less effective solutions. Implied in his argument is the notion that high-technology solutions to biotechnological problems are more likely to produce ethically contorted and difficult situations than are the simpler, low-technology solutions that are driven by concern for the fair and equitable access for all to elemental human needs.[30]

Vaccination programs raise fewer problems of equity than do organ transplants.

In the United States, for example, the elderly consume a bigger and bigger chunk of the disproportionately large piece of the economy that is devoted to healthcare. The amount spent on healthcare for the elderly in their last year of life is staggering. Intergenerational equity is a concern of justice. Disproportionate allocation of healthcare dollars to the elderly restricts the resources that are available to younger generations for education, environmental protection, or payment of the federal debt.

These macro-level issues are matters of public policy, removed from the day-to-day decisions of the intensive care clinician. It is not the intensivist's purview to worry whether money spent on an individual patient can be better spent on a vaccination program. Nonetheless, pressures of this sort do affect healthcare delivery and those who provide it, because the context of healthcare delivery is informed by large-scale issues about efficiency and justice. As pressures to control costs mount, there will be increasing pressures on critical care clinicians to restrict what types of patients are admitted to ICUs, what procedures are available to patients, and how long patients are able to stay in ICU beds. Thus, macro-level concerns of justice and efficiency affect clinicians' micro-level choices. Not all of the scarcities confronted by patients and clinicians are financial. The lack of sufficient available organs for transplantation necessitates choosing between potential recipients. Inherent in the development of any new technology is its initial limited availability; experimental procedures and new pharmacologic agents will be parsed out just as penicillin and hemodialysis were when they first became available.

As with any sort of rationing, the fair distribution of scarce resources depends upon fair and explicit procedures for their allocation. Within the context of critical care, triage has been the paradigmatic mechanism of patient selection. The historical origin of modern medical triage is the military system; the concept of triage was first introduced by Baron Dominique Jean Larrey, Napoleon's chief surgeon. Larrey devised a system of removing wounded soldiers from the battlefield using the primary selection criterion of severity of injury—not the soldier's rank or office as had previously been the case. Since then, military triage systems have reflected a more utilitarian calculus; a higher priority for treatment is assigned to wounded soldiers who need limited treatment and can easily be returned to battle than to soldiers with life-threatening wounds. During the North African campaign in the Second World War, for example, limited supplies of the newly discovered antibiotic penicillin were given to American soldiers infected with venereal disease rather than to those wounded in battle. Combat readiness and winning the war were the objectives that informed this decision.

Civilian triage mechanisms also reflect a utilitarian calculus, but the objectives of treatment are different than those of the military. Individual benefits weigh more heavily in the civilian context. The severity of an individual's illness, or need, is generally tempered by survivability or chance of a successful outcome. In a 1994 consensus statement on the triage of critically ill patients, the Ethics Committee of the Society of Critical Care Medicine (SCCM) recognized specific principles that should govern triage decisions in critical care.[31] ICU admission should be based on the premise that the patient will benefit from ICU care "substantially" more than from non-ICU care. Certain types of patients, such as those who have good prospects with or without ICU care or those with poor prospects of benefit even with ICU care, should not be admitted to the ICU. The SCCM Ethics Committee identified seven factors that should weigh in the benefit—utility calculus, that governs admission to or discharge from the ICU: (1) likelihood of a successful outcome; (2) the patient's life expectancy due to disease(s); (3) the patient's anticipated quality of life; (4) preferences of the patient/surrogate; (5) burdens for those affected, including financial and psychological costs and missed opportunities to treat other patients; (6) health and other needs of the community; and (7) individual and institutional moral and religious values.

Too often, critical care is distributed by default, rather than by prospectively devised, concrete criteria that are equitably applied. Numerous studies have reported that critical care resources may be distributed inequitably.[32] Inappropriate cost considerations, conflicts over medical turf, or inattention to outcomes data may unjustifiably influence triage decisions. A recent survey of critical care practitioners reported that quality of life as viewed by the patient, probability of surviving hospitalization, reversibility of the acute disorder, and the nature of the chronic disorder were the most important factors governing admission to the ICU. However, few of the respondents believed that age should be a criterion for limiting critical care, and more than 40 percent of the respondents said they would admit patients in a chronic vegetative state or with a metastatic carcinoma and a superimposed life-threatening event.[33] It is crucial for institutions to have a policy governing admission to and discharge from the ICU. Healthcare dollars should not be spent supporting those in chronic vegetative states in an ICU, and prospective policies prohibiting such use of healthcare resources is the best way to guarantee that the pressures of the moment do not overwhelm those entrusted to make the right decision. Once the policy is in place, it would be unjust to make exceptions without very strong reasons.

REFLECTIONS

The discussion of moral principles might lead to the conclusion that there is a science of moral decision making in the context of critical care. That is hardly the case. There is no algorithm or calculus according to which one can apply considerations of autonomy, beneficence, nonmaleficence, and justice to all medical situations to reach a determinate conclusion. Nonetheless, these values indicate the considerations that healthcare practitioners should use in determining appropriate care.

Critical care poses special problems in the application of these principles. The first problem is that there is often great uncertainty in the environment of critical care. Second, there is often a sense of urgency that precludes appropriate reflection and consultation about the propriety of care. Immediate physiological stabilization often precedes long-term outcomes assessment. Third, the professional staff in critical care typically do not know the patient or family. The patient presents without a life story and without the ability to relate his or her life story, preferences for care, or concerns about feared outcomes. There is no familiarity with which to establish the trust necessary for a meaningful dialogue with family members. As a result, the dynamics of the presenting situation in critical care often require clinicians to start treatment, if only to achieve a situation in which they can reflect upon how to proceed. Withholding therapy has a finality to it that might well be premature when the patient first presents in an emergency situation. For this reason, it is vital to remember that, from a moral perspective, withholding and withdrawing life support are not fundamentally different. If they were different, there would be significant pressure not to begin critical care treatment at all for fear that there would be no way to stop treatment once it is begun. For this reason, critical care units should have explicit procedures for routine, periodic review of the plan of care and goals of treatment for all patients. Some benefit is gained by having explicit guidelines about admission to the ICU, whether the ICU is to be used as a hospice unit to care for the vegetative patient, or to treat patients with reversible organ-system failure.

Policies that require automatic review of patients on life support and rules that govern resuscitation are necessary to ensure that critical care is delivered ethically. They give important guidelines for appropriate critical care and they also protect the critical care team from litigation. But such policies cannot eliminate the hard cases that often arise in critical care settings. Formal moral frameworks that involve deductive reasoning and the application and balancing of general principles can point clinicians in the right direction; however, they often do not provide sufficient guidance to resolve moral dilemmas, especially when competing principles are involved. In such cases, other less formal theoretical approaches may help supplement formal moral reasoning. Such approaches often rely on the context, or circumstances, of situations to provide helpful information that may guide decision making. Feminist ethics is an example of such an approach; it is concerned with interpersonal relationships, with concrete acts of caring, and with freedom from oppression or coercion. Casuistical ethics also compares the relevant similarities and differences among cases and carefully examines the historical elements of a given case. Virtue ethics challenges the moral agent or decision maker to place a particular moral decision or act within the context of the sort of life that he or she might choose to live, or the sort of person that he or she might choose to be. The development of moral character involves consecutive moral choices that reflect "this sort of life" or "that particular person." All these views are attempts to supplement the principle-based views on which this chapter has focused.[34] It is important to realize that a particular person is being cared for, that this particular case has similarities to and differences from analogous cases that may be more clear, and that different decisions reflect different virtues.

Narrative ethics uses elements of each of these less formal, theoretical approaches. Within this framework, the lives of patients and clinicians are viewed as narratives. Critical care is a crucial juncture in these life stories. The complex interplay of past, present, and future provides a rich medium for choice and decision making. Questions such as what sort of life the patient has lived until the present moment inform queries about what sort of life the patient might want to live in the future, and this in turn informs assessments about quality of life. Focusing only on the present moment in the ICU robs decision makers of important information and, consequently, of important options. The critical care environment tends to foster a tunnel vision that precludes placing the patient, family, and clinicians within a broader context. As Eric Cassell observes, "The numbers of the readout, images on film, dexterity required for its deployment, technical complexities, tubes, wires, plugs, valves, needles, gauges, mirrors, focusing devices, and on and on exist in the here and now the immediate moment. . . . How different from the patient. A bundle of large questions, a life that exists only in the most fragmentary sense in the here and now. Look at a patient, see only the here and now, and you have missed the truth of a sick person."[35] The same must be said of the family members, significant others, and clinicians involved in the case. Look at an intensive care practitioner or a family member, see only the here and now, and you have also missed the truth of that person.

Howard Brody, in an essay entitled "The Four Principles and Narrative Ethics," has outlined the way in which the formal "principalist" approach to moral reasoning can be complemented by a narrative ethics approach.[36] He recommends that the application of moral principles be informed by the following three factors:

1. The choice that the patient is now making, or the way the clinician now behaves toward the patient, is going to become one episode in the unfolding narrative of the patient's life, and will acquire meaning within the context of that narrative.
2. The action the clinician is now about to take will also become an episode in the clinician's life narrative, and will reflect upon the clinician's core commitments and values.
3. The action that the clinician and patient are about to take is embedded in a context that consists of their life histories, the lives of other involved parties, and the customs and practices of the community and the institution (such as the hospital). A full understanding of the action requires that it be interpreted within that context. The "right course of action" to resolve a problem is not necessarily the action that conforms to an abstract principle; rather, it may be the action which, without violating any moral principles, most successfully navigates all the contextual factors to move the situation in a direction that best serves the major interests of all involved parties.[37]

AIKEN'S LEVELS OF MORAL DISTINCTION

Critical care clinicians may be familiar with major theoretical approaches to ethics such as *deontological* or duty-based theories, which are informed by fundamental respect for persons (or the intrinsic worth of others), or *teleological* or ends-based theories (such as utilitarianism), which are concerned with the outcomes of moral action or the application of general principles to particular cases. However, most clinicians lack working knowledge of ethical theory and do not systematically apply it to medical decision making. A useful tool for understanding moral decision making is the framework provided by the philosopher Henry David Aiken, who sees determinations of right and wrong as occurring on several levels. Aiken's "levels of moral discourse" acknowledge the complexity of moral decision making and the many factors that influence it.[38] Aiken's levels are not hierarchical, but might best be conceived of as a circular account of moral argumentation and justification. The circle can be entered at any point, and most moral arguments occur on more than one level given the changes in context as a situation evolves. Each level of moral discourse informs the level that precedes or follows it.

EXPRESSIVE-EVOCATIVE LEVEL

Aiken begins with the "expressive-evocative" level or the level of the emotions. This involves expressions of personal feelings and nonreflective reactions to situations, with a simple gut-level determination of like versus dislike, good versus bad. No moral justification is required for the observation, "What a beautiful Saturday morning! Too bad I have to spend it making rounds in the ICU rather than playing soccer." Nonetheless, the emotions play an important role in the process of moral analysis.[39] Without nonreflective reactions to people, things, or situations, we would be incapable of experiencing the initial emotional and subsequent cognitive dissonance required for the recognition of ethical problems or dilemmas. That vague discomfort or sixth sense that something "feels wrong" about a particular situation is a prerequisite for determining that a moral problem exists, that something *is* wrong.

THE LEVEL OF MORAL RULES

It is at the second level, the level of "moral rules," that the normative question, "What should I do in this situation?" arises. The answer generally hinges on the "communal code" or "standards of propriety" that hold in one's society. Such standards are not universal, but relative to the social context in which the issue is raised. The answer to the query, "Should I tell this patient that he has terminal cancer?" might be very different when posed to a Japanese oncologist versus an American oncologist. In Japan, tradition may dictate that an unfortunate diagnosis should be disclosed only to family members, not to the patient himself. In America, attitudes toward telling patients bad news are different. Over the last 40 years, sequential surveys of physicians have demonstrated a change in attitudes toward disclosing directly to a patient the diagnosis of cancer. In 1953, 69 percent of physicians favored not disclosing the diagnosis of cancer directly to a patient;[40] in 1961, a full 90 percent of physicians favored nondisclosure;[41] by 1979 a turnabout had occurred, and 97 percent of physicians surveyed *favored* direct disclosure of the diagnosis of cancer.[42]

THE LEVEL OF ETHICAL PRINCIPLES

By way of the above example, it is obvious that morality changes and evolves. One reason it does so is that people question or challenge the conventional wisdom. The question, "What should I do?" suggests the next question, "Why is that what I should do?" Aiken identifies this third level of moral discourse as the level of "ethical principles." Here, persons may question the rightness or wrongness of an action that is dictated by a moral rule, and may ultimately challenge their continued allegiance to that rule. Such queries often arise when moral rules conflict or when societal conditions change. The duty to save lives takes on different meaning, and has richer moral content, within the context of modern critical care medicine than at any previous time. When deciding whether to admit a patient with metastasized cancer and multisystem organ failure to the ICU, the triage officer may feel a conflict between the duty to save or prolong life and the duty not to impose a harm. He or she may question the conventional wisdom that dictates that the physician's duty is to save lives. The conditions that exist in the modern ICU are not those that existed when the duty to prolong life was first articulated.

THE POST-ETHICAL OR HUMAN LEVEL

At the fourth level, the "post-ethical" or "human" level, Aiken raises a paradoxical question: "Why should I be moral?" The answer to this question can only be made by a gratuitous decision—that I honor my commitments only as long as I am motivated to do so. I act as a moral agent because I am a "rational moral being" but am free at any time to break free of the constraints of rationality. In this sense, Aiken observes, the existentialist philosophers were correct in their assessment that in any given situation humans choose to act morally, to be bound by moral constraints. Within that same situation, humans also possess the freedom to choose not to act morally. The answer to the question, "Why be moral?" involves the same sort of consecutive moral choice that inheres in the development of moral character. "Why be moral?" is essentially the same question as "What sort of person do I choose to be?" or "What sort of life do I choose to live?"

CONCLUSION

In a classic article, "Pediatric Intensive Care Training: Confronting the Dark Side," Jellinek and colleagues contrast the rewards and gratifications of practicing critical care medicine with the personal burdens and costs that it imposes on clinicians.[43] Providing critical care is a privilege, an opportunity to enter the lives of patients and families during portentous moments and to employ hard-won skills and knowledge for the benefit of others. Frequently, clinicians experience joy, relief, exultation, and a sense of great accomplishment. Alternatively, the "dark side" of critical care includes feelings of fallibility, anger, frustration, loss, and pain that is shared with anxious or grieving families. Such feelings may result in unhealthy psychological detachment or signs of depression that characterize the well-known "burnout" that is frequently experienced by critical care clinicians. There is no avoiding the intensity associated with critical care. It is a high-stakes situation with individual lives on the line, with families who are dependent on clinicians eagerly listening to their every word. There will be successes and failures.

Unresolved ethical dilemmas are part of the dark side of critical care. Critical care clinicians must acknowledge that ethical problems are inherent in their practice and should prepare themselves to work toward effective resolution of such problems. Unrealistic expectations about easy ethical solutions should be avoided. As bioethicist John Fletcher observes, "The ethics business is not the happiness business."[44] Critical care practitioners should enter into the resolution of ethical dilemmas with the goal of achieving the best possible outcome in the case. There is generally not a single "right" or "good" answer to a difficult ethical question. Ultimately, effective resolution depends on an effective problem-solving process that takes account of clinical facts, the patient's preferences, open communication, medical uncertainties and a range of human values. The problem-solving process should be multifaceted. Answers to the questions "What should I do?" and "Why?" depend upon situational context, the balancing of moral rules and principles, anticipating the consequences of actions, and a prospective decision about what sort of intensive care clinician one wants to be.

Intensive care is best conceived of as a team effort, with each team member participating in the resolution of hard choices. Including members of the ethics committee or the ethics consultation service in this process enlarges the community of professionals who are familiar with the ethical issues confronting critical care. Such a team effort is likely to make for better choices, better community, and a more humane intensive care environment.

NOTES

1. S.M. Ayres et al., eds., *Textbook of Critical Care*, 3rd ed. (Philadelphia: W.B. Saunders, 1995).

2. D. Mayo and M. Bennett, "The Role of Burden/Benefit Analysis in the Orchestration of Death in the ICU," in *Human Values in Critical Care Medicine*, ed. S.J. Youngner (New York: Praeger, 1986), 35.

3. T.A. Raffin, "Ethical Concerns in Managing Critically Ill Patients," in *Critical Care Medicine: Principles of Diagnosis and Management*, ed. J.E. Parrillo and R.C. Bone (St. Louis, Mo.: Mosby, 1995), 1447.

4. A.H. Combs, "Critical Care Practice in the Era of Consumerism," in *Textbook of Critical Care*, 3rd ed., ed. S.M. Ayres et al. (Philadelphia: W.B. Saunders, 1995), 1817.

5. J.S. Growger et al., "Descriptive Analysis of Critical Care Units in the United States: Patient Characteristics and Intensive Care Unit Utilization," *Critical Care Medicine* 20 (1992): 727.

6. M.E. Solomon et al., "Decisions Near the End of Life: Professional Views on Life-Sustaining Treatments," *American Journal of Public Health* 83, no. 1 (1993): 14-22.

7. W. Knaus, E. Draper, and D.P. Wagner, "The Use of Intensive Care: New Research Initiatives and Their Implications for National Health Policy," *Milbank Memorial Fund Quarterly* 61 (1983): 561, as cited in J. Paris and F. Reardon, "An Ethical and Legal Analysis of Problems in Critical Care Medicine," in *Intensive Care Medicine*, 3rd ed., ed. J.M. Rippe (Boston: Little, Brown and Company, 1996), 2549.

8. W.A. Knaus, "Prognosis with Mechanical Ventilation: The Influence of Disease, Age and Chronic Health Status on Survival from an Acute Illness," *American Review of Respiratory Disease* 140 (1989): S8, as cited in Paris and Reardon, "An Ethical and Legal Analysis," see note 7 above.

9. T.A. Raffin, J. Shurkin, and W.S. Sinkler, *Intensive Care: Facing Critical Choices* (New York: W.H. Freeman, 1988); Freeman cited in Raffin, "Ethical Concerns," see note 3 above.

10. Ibid.

11. T.A. Raffin, "Survival of Patients with Systemic Illness," *American Review of Respiratory Disease* 140 (1989): S28; A.B. Montgomery et al., "Causes of

Mortality in Patients with ARDS," *American Review of Respiratory Disease* 132 (1985): 485, as cited in Raffin, "Ethical Concerns," see note 3 above.

12. D.P. Schuster and J.M. Marion, "Precedents for Meaningful Recovery During Treatment in a Medical Intensive Care Unit: Outcome in Patients with Hematologic Malignancy," *American Journal of Medicine* 75 (1983): 402, as cited in Raffin, "Ethical Concerns," see note 3 above.

13. Knaus et al., see note 7 above, p. 562.

14. Raffin, see note 3 above.

15. Paris and Reardon, "Ethical and Legal Analysis," see note 7 above, p. 2549.

16. M. Angell, "Cost Containment and the Physician," *Journal of the American Medical Association* 254 (1985): 1203.

17. R.E. Bulger, E.M. Bobby, and H.V. Fineberg, eds., "Introduction," in *Society's Choices: Social and Ethical Decision Making in Biomedicine* (Washington, D.C.: National Academy Press, 1995), 36.

18. V.R. Fuchs, *Who Shall Live? Health, Economics, and Social Choice* (New York: Basic Books, 1974), 60.

19. H. Brody, *The Healer's Power* (New Haven, Conn.: Yale University Press, 1992), 21-22.

20. E.J. Cassell, "The Sorcerer's Broom: Medicine's Rampant Technology," *Hastings Center Report* 23, no. 2 (1993): 32-39.

21. Ibid, 35.

22. Ibid.

23. T.L. Beauchamp and J.F. Childress, "Nonmaleficence," in *Principles of Biomedical Ethics*, 4th ed. (New York: Oxford University Press, 1995), 189.

24. See, for example, J. Rawls, "Two Concepts of Rules," *Philosophical Review* 64 (1995): 3-32.

25. R.J. Boyle, "The Process of Informed Consent," in *Introduction to Clinical Ethics*, ed. J.C. Fletcher et al. (Frederick, Md.: University Publishing Group, 1995), 84-87.

26. R.J. Boyle, "Determining Patients' Capacity to Share in Decision Making," in *Introduction to Clinical Ethics*, ed. J.C. Fletcher et al. (Frederick, Md.: University Publishing Group, 1995), 74.

27. J.C. Ahronheim, J. Moreno, and C. Zuckerman, *Ethics in Clinical Practice* (Boston: Little, Brown and Company, 1994), 13-14.

28. Ibid, 22 and 213.

29. M.S. Jellinek et al., "Pediatric Intensive Care Training: Confronting the Dark Side," *Critical Care Medicine* 21, no. 5 (1993): 775-79.

30. Bulger et al., see note 17 above, p. 39.

31. Society of Critical Care Medicine Ethics Committee, "Consensus Statement on the Triage of Critically Ill Patients," *Journal of the American Medical Association* 271, no. 15 (1994): 1200-03.

32. D. Crane, *The Sanctity of Social Life: Physicians' Treatment of Critically Ill Patients* (New York: Russell Sage Foundation, 1975); R.A. Perlman, T.S.

Invi, and W.B. Canter, "Variability in Physician Bioethical Decision-Making," *Annals of Internal Medicine* 97 (1982): 420-25; H.S. Perkins, A.R. Jonsen, and W.V. Epstein, "Providers as Predictors: Using Outcome Predictions in Intensive Care," *Critical Care Medicine* 14 (1986): 105-10; M.F. Marshall et al., "The Influence of Political Power: Medical Provincialism and Economic Incentives on the Rationing of Surgical Intensive Care Unit Beds," *Critical Care Medicine* 20, no. 3 (1992): 387-94; Society of Critical Care Medicine Ethics Committee, "Attitudes of Critical Care Medicine Professionals Concerning Distribution of Intensive Care Resources," *Critical Care Medicine* 22, no. 2 (1994): 358-62.

33. Society of Critical Care Medicine Ethics Committee, "Attitudes of Critical Care," see note 32 above.

34. S. Sherwin, *No Longer Patient: Feminist Ethics and Health Care* (Philadelphia: Temple University Press, 1992); A.R. Jonsen and S. Toulmin, *The Abuse of Casuistry: A History of Moral Reasoning* (Berkeley, Calif.: University of California Press, 1988); A. Macintyre, *After Virtue* (Notre Dame, Ind.: Notre Dame Press, 1981).

35. Cassell, see note 20 above, p. 340.

36. H. Brody, "The Four Principles and Narrative Ethics," in *Principles of Health Care Ethics*, ed. R. Gillon (New York: John Wiley & Sons, 1994), 207-15.

37. Ibid, 214-15.

38. H.D. Aiken, *Levels of Moral Discourse in Reason and Conduct: New Bearings in Moral Philosophy* (Westport, Conn.: Greenwood Press, 1961), 65-87.

39. S. Callahan, "The Role of Emotion in Ethical Decisionmaking," *Hastings Center Report* 18 (June-July 1988): 9-14.

40. W.T. Fritts and I.S. Ravdin, "What Philadelphia Physicians Tell Patients about Cancer," *Journal of the American Medical Association* 15 (1953): 901.

41. D. Oken, "What to Tell Cancer Patients: A Study of Medical Attitudes," *Journal of the American Medical Association* 175 (1961): 1120.

42. D.H. Novack et al., "Changes in Physicians' Attitudes Toward Telling the Cancer Patient," *Journal of the American Medical Association* 241 (1979): 897.

43. Jellinek et al., see note 29 above.

44. John Fletcher, personal communication with M.F. Marshall.

3

The Ethics of Care
in Critical Care

Carol Taylor

INTRODUCTION

Many healthcare ethicists are eagerly exploring the literature on caring and advancing arguments defending care as a distinct moral orientation. Among the factors contributing to the ethics of care's new popularity are (1) attentiveness to Carol Gilligan's groundbreaking work in moral development;[1] (2) recognition of the limitations of the justice orientation to ethics, which is grounded in universality, impartiality, and fairness; (3) growing dissatisfaction with rote applications of the principle-based approach to clinical ethics; and (4) respect for the results of nursing theories that ground clinical practice in professional, caring relationships. Central to care as a distinct moral orientation for caregivers is the nature of the healthcare professional-patient relationship and attention to the "particulars" of individual patients, viewed within the context of their life's narrative. Rejecting a reductionistic, mechanistic approach to healing, the ethics of care calls for a phenomenological methodology that invites caregivers to empathically enter the patient's world.

What becomes immediately apparent when one begins to read the literature on caring is the confusion that surrounds the term itself. *Care* is a term with multiple meanings. I can "take care," "care for," "care about," or simply "care." Morse, Bottorff, Neander, and Solberg offer a careful delineation and comparison of various definitions of caring according to five major conceptualizations of caring: caring as a human trait, caring as a moral imperative, caring as affect, caring as an interpersonal interaction, and caring as an intervention.[2] They conclude that the concept of caring is relatively undeveloped and that it has not been fully explicated. Although most clinicians and certainly the public would place a high value on professional caring, they are liable to find it difficult to describe the nature of professional caring (how it differs from more generic types of caring) and its related moral obligations. If they are unable to do this, it is impossible for clinicians to hold themselves and their colleagues accountable for caring. Before reading further, it may be helpful to try to respond to the following questions:

1. Is professional care essential to healing?
2. Is the obligation to care central to the professional ethics of those in all helping professions? What grounds this obligation?
3. What does a model of professional caring, as opposed to more generic forms of caring, look like? Describe the type of caring that is a core competence for members of your discipline/profession.
4. Have healthcare professionals defined caring in a sufficiently precise manner to allow us to hold ourselves and one another accountable to care? Can it be quantified in a manner that allows the use of professional caring as a criterion for admission to practice, hiring, promoting, and firing?
5. What factors have contributed to what Benner calls "the privatization of caring?"[3] If we are unsatisfied with the privatization of caring, what are our options?
6. What practical strategies can be used to teach caring (if we believe that caring can be taught!) and to transform cultures of caregiving institutions to caring cultures?
7. Is it needlessly frustrating and hopelessly romantic to suggest in today's healthcare culture that all healthcare professionals are obligated to care?
8. What is caring's "dark side"? Ought there be constraints placed on professional caring?

This chapter expands earlier writings[4] and offers a conceptualization of the ethics of care as a moral imperative for healthcare professionals in general, and for those engaged in critical care specifically. The central thesis is that professionals who accept responsibility for the well-being of individuals entrusted to their charge incur obligations to care in certain ways. After a brief review of the literature, the chapter introduces a model of professional caring and describes related moral obligations and virtues, describes characteristics of an ethics of care, drawing examples from critical care, outlines the fundamental moral skills dictated by an ethics of care, and contrasts the principle- and care-based approaches to clinical ethics.

REVIEW OF THE LITERATURE

The newly revised *Encyclopedia of Bioethics* offers an excellent introduction to care with sections devoted to the history of the notion of care, historical dimensions of an ethics of care in healthcare, and contemporary ethics of care.[5] Because the Kohlberg-Gilligan debate resulted in widespread acceptance of care as a distinct moral orientation and provided the groundwork for the development of a systematic, philosophic ethic of care beyond the world of healthcare professionals, Gilligan's groundbreaking work in moral development is essential.[6] Sharpe explores the implications of the Kohlberg-Gilligan debate for medical ethics.[7] Important voices in feminine ethics are Noddings,[8] who focuses on caring as a practical activity, and Ruddick,[9] who emphasizes "maternal thinking." Kierkegaard and Heidegger provided the philosophic grounding for caring's existentialist and phenomenological methodologies, and May and Erikson are credited with important psychological components. Mayeroff's 1971 book *On Caring* offers a detailed description and explanation of the experiences of caring and being cared for.[10] Before Gilligan, nurse theorists, educators, and philosophers explored and applied a more extensive theory and ethics of care than any other group.[11] Important physician voices include Cabot and Peabody and more recently Tisdale and Pellegrino.[12] A collection of essays entitled *The Crisis of Care* eloquently makes the case for affirming and restoring caring practices in the helping professions.[13]

ELEMENTS OF PROFESSIONAL CARING

Professional caring presumes an ability to care in a manner that is substantially affective, cognitive, volitional, imaginative, motivated, and expressive. A description of the role these six elements play in professional caring follows. For each element, the continuum of outcomes sought is specified, as well as the problems associated with the deficiency or excess of that element. When evaluation results in a judgment of deficiency or excess in any of the elements of professional caring, continued practice should be contingent on the remediation of the problematic behaviors.

1. Affection
   - *Definition*: feeling of positive regard that is experienced as a response to the presence or thought of the one cared for; feelings may range from a simple regard of kinship that acknowledges another human in need, to feelings of loving and tender regard.
   - *Continuum*: from simple regard to tender solicitude.
   - *Deficiency and excess*: too little feeling for another can result in the recipient of care feeling objectified and depersonalized; too much feeling may overwhelm the recipient of care, incapacitate the caregiver, and make needed therapeutic intervention impossible.

2. Cognition
   - *Definition*: intellectual grasp of what is essential to the well-being of the one cared for.
   - *Continuum*: from general knowledge of essential components of health and well-being to very precise knowledge of the same.
   - *Deficiency and excess*: absent, incomplete, or inaccurate knowledge of what is essential to the object of care's well-being results in ineffective caring;   knowledge of the elements of well-being and the strategies to produce them—the need always to explore "one more option"—may unnecessarily delay needed intervention.

3. Volition
   - *Definition*: commitment to use one's expertise and energy to secure the well-being of the one(s) cared for.
   - *Continuum*: from a general commitment to fill role responsibility to full-hearted commitment to patient's well-being.
   - *Deficiency and excess*: caregivers who are volitionally deficient arbitrarily commit their expertise and energy to securing the well-being of those entrusted to their care; there is no guarantee that the patient's well-being will be served in a reliable fashion, and the trust that should exist between caregivers and the patient breaks down; an excess of volition may result in caregivers' assuming responsibility for aspects of pa-

tients' well-being beyond their control or authority; the caregiver may exceed the appropriate limits of self-sacrifice and assume responsibility that rightfully belongs to the patient or other parties.

4. Imagination
   - *Definition*: empathic ability to enter into and share the world of the other sufficiently to understand the other's unique existential situation and needs.
   - *Continuum*: from basic ability to experience patient's life situation and needs to proficient ability to experience patient's life situation and needs.
   - *Deficiency and excess*: deficient imagination may result in uniform or substandard care that treats all persons with similar health problems alike; imagination may result in overidentification with patients and an inability to maintain the critical reflective stance and distance that is essential to practice.

5. Motivation
   - *Definition*: that which influences the will in a manner that predisposes one to act altruistically to promote the patient's well-being; that which explains action.
   - *Continuum*: from well-being of patient is not compromised by other professional motivations to well-being of patient is the primary professional motivation.
   - *Deficiency and excess*: caregivers with deficient motivation cannot be trusted when unsupervised to act responsibly to ensure the patient's well-being; ly motivated caregivers are prone to burnout because of their willingness to assume unrealistic responsibilities and to neglect personal, family, and other demands not related to work.

6. Expressiveness of action
   - *Definition*: verbal and nonverbal behaviors used to communicate caring.
   - *Continuum*: from behaviors in which interventions generally communicate caring to interventions consistently are perceived as communicating caring
   - *Deficiency and excess*: deficient expressiveness resulting from the caregiver's inattention to caring behaviors and to how these are being perceived may result in the patient's objecti-

fication and the patient's feeling unworthy of care; excesses in expressiveness generally communicate a smothering effect, which overwhelms the patient.

Each element of professional caring has related virtues and moral obligations (see Exhibit 3-1). Because the ethics of care is rooted in relationality and responsiveness, it should not be surprising that virtues are given primacy. Caregivers operating from the ethics of care are consistently predisposed to interact in certain ways with patients. The ethics of care is thus both a character-guiding and action-guiding theory of ethics.

A model of professional caring based upon these six elements of care offers a way to distinguish the caring of clinicians from that of patients' family members and friends. Although all caring others have an obligation to be moved by the experiences of the patient, clinicians must also have knowledge of what is essential to the patient's recovery or ability to cope with illness and be committed to using their skills to achieve desired patient outcomes. In addition to knowing what a hypothetical patient with condition X requires, clinicians must individualize their knowledge to this particular patient with his or her unique needs, be motivated to secure the patient's well-being, and communicate caring in a manner that is understood by the patient. Unless all six elements are present in each act of professional caring, the caring is deficient. This understanding of professional caring makes the old question, "Would you rather have a doctor/nurse who cares or one who is competent?" meaningless. A caring clinician *is* competent.

Using this model, a clinician cares professionally only if he or she:

1. experiences positive regard for the person being cared for (affection)
2. intellectually grasps what is essential to the well-being of the person cared for (cognition)
3. commits expertise and energy to secure the well-being of the person cared for (volition)
4. is empathically able to enter and share in the world of the one cared for (imagination)
5. is moved to care primarily because of a commitment to secure the well-being of the person cared for (motivation)
6. demonstrates caring behaviors that are perceived as such by the one cared for (expression).

If these elements are accepted as the necessary and sufficient conditions for professional caring, the next step will be the development of

Exhibit 3-1
The Essential Elements of a Model of Professional Caring: Related Virtues and Moral Obligations

Element	Related Virtues	Related Moral Obligations
Affective	Respect (regard), solicitude, compassion	To practice in a manner that leaves one open to be moved by the experience of patients and their significant other
Cognitive	Intellectual honesty	To practice with the knowledge demanded by professional responsibilities
		To seek assistance when one's competence is unequal to new and changing professional responsibilities
		To hold other members of the caregiving team accountable for responsible practice
		To critique scientific advances in light of their ability to contribute to human well-being
		To evaluate treatment regimens, systems of care, and health policy in light of their ability to affect the well-being of patients and population aggregates
Volitional	Accountability, trustworthiness	To hold oneself accountable for the human well-being of patients assigned to one's care
		To respond to human need to a degree commensurate with professional responsibilities
Imaginative	Empathy	To share empathically in the experiences of patients and their significant others
Motivational	Altruism	To make the well-being of patients one's primary professional concern
		To balance appropriate self-care with professional care responsibilities in a manner that does not jeopardize the well-being of patients or colleagues
Expressive	Caring	To interact with patients, their significant others, and colleagues in a manner that is perceived as being respectful and affirming of human dignity

measurement tools to enable educators and supervisors to use these elements as criteria for grading, hiring, promoting and firing.

CHARACTERISTICS OF AN ETHICS OF CARE

In their concise survey of ethical orientations and theories, Wicks, Spielman, and Fletcher offer the following description of care and justice as distinct bases for ethics:

> The care perspective begins from the network of relationships one has with others and the sense of connection which grows out of them. The source of the moral life is in the human capacity to extend care to others, to nurture attachments and to develop the communication and psychological skills needed to sustain these networks of care. Moral problems arise out of disruptions in or conflicts between responsibilities to others and require a type of thinking which is contextual and narrative. . . . In contrast, the justice perspective begins from the standpoint of separation and individuality and emphasizes autonomy. Morality is conceived as involving conflicting rules or abstract principles which require a formal, deductive logic to achieve some balance between them. Rules, rights and concepts of fairness are emphasized while relationships and specific persons tend to be of much less importance.[14]

According to Rollo May, care must be at the root of ethics, for the good life comes from what we care about.[15] Clinicians who operate from an ethics of care share the following characteristics:
1. Care about people and human flourishing
2. Believe in the centrality of the caring relationship
3. Promote the dignity and respect of patients as people
4. Cultivate responsiveness and responsibility
5. Accept particular patient and healthcare professional variables (beliefs, values, relationships) as morally relevant factors in ethical decision making
6. Pay attention to the ecology (contextual factors) of the moral choice/act.

PEOPLE AND HUMAN FLOURISHING MATTER
The moral orientation based on caring counters any forces operating in healthcare that objectify and dehumanize patients. These forces in-

clude a mechanistic approach to healthcare that reduces patients to body systems (or increasingly to a genetic profile) to be probed and studied by strangers and the rote application of ethical systems grounded in the principles of universalizability, impartiality, and autonomy. The many high-tech interventions required to manage acutely ill patients make it easier to lose sight of the patient in his or her totality in a critical care unit than in any other healthcare setting. In this case, the critical care unit is based on the model of a body parts-car repair shop; it focuses on wholeness of body (cure) rather than wholeness of being (care). The ethics of care offers a helpful corrective that keeps caregiving centered on the person. It challenges a task orientation to practice that isolates "the doing of things" (albeit with excellent technical proficiency) from their purpose—promoting the well-being of particular individuals. The care perspective reminds clinicians to ask constantly if the professional lens they are using is focused correctly. It reminds clinicians that behind a patient's "numbers"—the blood chemistries, viral titres, the tidal volume —is a person with beliefs, values, and interests. Health is an important good, instrumental to our enjoyment of most other goods, but it is not an absolute.

Citing a study in which nurses who were asked for an account of their current day offered descriptions of what they had done rather than stories of care for particular patients and their families, Benner writes: "They had become technicians doing tasks rather than practitioners engaged in care and restoration. It is not hard to understand why practice would deteriorate to this 'job description' level given the overwork and institutional press for efficiency and the societal taboos against getting 'too involved.' This loss of engagement and loss of narrative memory is encouraged by the loss of public space for narrative accounts of patient care and diminished shared dialogue between practitioners."[16]

Critical care clinicians are as obligated as any other caregivers to be concerned about issues related to quality of life. Recognizing the subjective dimension of quality of life—no two persons define it exactly the same—and its multidimensionality—the fact that it encompasses physical, functional, emotional, social, and spiritual well-being—the ethics of care directs critical care clinicians to blend the clinical and social sciences paradigms.

In the *clinical paradigm* (the "biomedical" model), the focus is on etiologic agents; pathological processes; and biological, physiological, and clinical outcomes. The principal goal is to understand causation in order to guide diagnosis and treatment. Controlled experiments are its principal methodology, and current biomedical research is directed at fundamental molecular, genetic, and cellular mechanisms of disease. Its intellectual roots are in biology, biochemistry, and physiology.

In contrast, the *social sciences paradigm* (the "quality-of-life" model) focuses on dimensions of functioning and overall well-being, and current research examines ways to measure complex behaviors and feelings accurately. Experimental research designs are rarely possible, since the focus of social science is on the way numerous social structures and institutions influence individuals. Models of health based on the social sciences paradigm have their foundations in sociology, psychology, and economics and use concepts and methods foreign to physicians and clinical researchers.[17]

The evaluation of professional competency in critical care is often based on outcomes criteria such as amelioration of clinical manifestations of disease, reduced inpatient stays, or decreased incidence of complications. Language such as "resource utilization measures" to describe these criteria suggests that it is the economic costs of illness rather than the human costs of illness that shape the way we understand the patient and his or her experience. Whether to interact personally with patients and their families in meaningful ways and to bring to clinical decision making a sense of the patient that transcends the "clinical picture" is increasingly viewed as an option to be decided by individual caregivers. The ethics of care changes this approach dramatically, arguing that it is the responsibility of each caregiver involved in a patient's care to work collaboratively to deliver holistic care that is responsive to the patient and his or her priorities.

Guided reflection. Reflection questions follow for clinicians who are committed to keeping a clear clinical focus on people and human well-being:

1. What does the way I allocate my professional time and the content of my orders, reports, and documentation about patients communicate about my clinical priorities?
2. If asked to describe a patient, would I be able to report on anything other than the patient's physical condition? Am I person oriented or problem oriented?
3. Do I know my patients well enough to promote anything more than the well-being of their body? Can I articulate what they

consider to be essential to their quality of life? Do patient outcomes include criteria related to quality of life?

4. Which of my professional interventions specifically counter the depersonalizing and dehumanizing effects of critical care?

5. Do the structures of care in my setting support care that is holistic, individualized, prioritized according to medical need *and* the patient's interests, and continuous? Or is this meaningless rhetoric? In what ways do the culture of my institution and health policy in general need to change to remedy deficiencies?

RELATIONSHIPS MATTER

The fundamental unit of the ethics of care is not the individual, but the individual in relationship. Human well-being is intrinsically linked to our ability to relate to others. The ethics of care directs professional caregivers to pay attention to the web of relationships linking the patient to family, friends, concerned others, and the healthcare team. The collaborative relationships between professional caregivers are also a subject of concern.

Experience repeatedly demonstrates that the quality of one's relationship with another person is the most significant element in determining the effectiveness of helping. Studies have also linked improved patient outcomes with respectful, collaborative relationships among members of the caregiving team. Of all the problems that can arise in professional caregiving, perhaps the most common is failure to establish rapport and trustful relationships. As the marketplace continues to transform healthcare into a new and often cutthroat corporate entity, trust is quickly squandered, and each participant in the process—including patients, families, professional caregivers, healthcare administrators and payers—is counseled to take care of self.

The ethics of care rejects the business model of professional relationships among equals and assigns moral weight to the particulars of the different parties in relationships. If it is true that illness results in certain patient vulnerabilities that render healthcare professional-patient relationships asymmetrical, then ethical models that assume equality between participants in relationships will provide an inadequate basis for healthcare ethics. In critical care settings where all the patients are acutely ill and most families are experiencing tremendous stress and disruption of their usual lifestyles, the inequality in knowledge, power, resources, comfort, and ease, are readily apparent. Acknowledging the unequal relationships that exist between healthcare professionals and patients, the ethics of care directs healthcare professionals to be trustworthy, to develop caring relationships directed to the patient's healing, and to advocate for patients competently and willingly. This is very different from an obligation simply to "be fair." The justice orientation to ethics proposes contractual agreements viewing the participants in a caregiving relationship as equals. The emphasis is on formal equality, reciprocity, and individual rights. The care orientation replaces the contractual model with a fiduciary model that emphasizes interdependence and mutual obligations. The crucial difference between these two models may be illustrated by contrasting what it means to respect a patient's autonomy in both models. Operating within the contractual model, an obligation to refrain from interfering in the decisions made by competent patients suffices. There is no obligation to "protect" patients from poor or ill-advised choices. In the fiduciary model, there are positive obligations to assist patients to make authentically autonomous choices—that is, choices that are consistent with patients' interests, values, and moral identity.

The above distinction also illustrates the respective orientations of justice- and care-based ethics to the "right" and to the "good." The justice orientation imposes no general conception of the good on individuals; priority is to the right (universal procedural principles) over the good, however it may be construed. Conversely, the care perspective is oriented to human needs rather than to the rights of citizens *per se*; it gives priority to the good of a particular patient over the right. For example, autonomy is respected not as a matter of principle but because autonomy itself is a good that cannot be undermined if the patient's good is to be served. Absent professional caregiving relationships, what constitutes the good of particular patients cannot be known to the caregiving team.

Guided reflection. Reflection questions follow for clinicians who are committed to developing and nurturing professional caregiving relationships:

1. What value do I assign to developing and nurturing professional relationships?
2. Was the competence to establish professional relationships simply assumed in my education or was it taught with the vigor associated with intellectual and technical competencies?
3. Do I believe that caring relationships are impossible in today's culture? If yes, do I accept this and believe that it is possible to practice without developing such relationships? What are the consequences of these judgments?

4. What are my strengths and limitations in developing professional relationships, both with patients and their significant others and with colleagues? Can I identify specific communication skills that I possess that are effective in establishing and maintaining these relationships?

HUMAN DIGNITY MATTERS

In the minds of many, clinical ethics is equated with moral dilemmas about life and death of the "to remove or not to remove from the ventilator" variety. By focusing attention on the critical importance of human dignity and the respect it commands, the ethics of care restores the ethical significance of everyday choices and activities. How clinicians approach a patient; what they say or do not say; and how they look, touch, interact (or choose to not interact) are all matters that are ethically significant because of their potential to affirm or negate human dignity. This is poignantly demonstrated in the following story recounted by a woman who has struggled long with cancer.

A nurse touched me today. Well, OK, nurses touch me everyday. But not like this. This nurse *touched me*. She read my chart. She knew what procedure she had to do. But before she started thinking about *her* agenda, she asked me a simple question about events in the news. While she listened to my answer, she put her hand on my forearm. It was warm and strong and nice. She wasn't furtively feeling around to find a good vein or to count out my pulse or any other nurse thing. It was person to person touch. Not "I'm a nurse. You're a patient. Aren't you in a mess, oh, I feel your pain" touch. It was "I'm a person. You're a person. I look in your eyes and see a light. Hello!" touch. It made a huge difference. Anything she had to do to me after that was rendered tolerable by that one simple, no, profound touch.[18]

In critical care settings, the sheer invasiveness and volume of needed interventions pose a constant threat to human dignity. It is also true that the more vulnerable patients are and the more removed they are from the everyday factors that affirm their sense of worth, the more dependent they are upon the sense of worth communicated by the caregivers who are making up their world. For this reason, the ethics of care makes who we are and what we communicate to patients in the process of providing care as important an ethical issue as decisions to initiate, with-hold, or withdraw aggressive treatment. The ethics of care makes respect for human dignity a constant in each healthcare professional-patient in-teraction. It is not negotiable.

Guided reflection. Reflection questions follow for clinicians who are committed to respecting human dignity:

1. What about patients obligates me to respect their human dig-nity? Must all patients be respected equally? Are some patients more deserving of respect? Can a patient ever forfeit the right to be respected?

2. What does it mean to respect the dignity of patients? How would clinical decision making change if human dignity became the final arbiter in cases of conflict?

3. How would someone observing my practice describe specific mea-sures I take to demonstrate respect? What are my strengths and deficiencies when it comes to respecting patients? In what ways must I change (if any) if I wish to be faithful to the duty of re-specting the dignity of patients?

4. What patients most challenge my ability to care for patients re-spectfully? How do I respond to this challenge?

5. How must our unit/institution change if it is to accept the ethics of care's mandate to respect human dignity?

RESPONSIVENESS AND RESPONSIBILITY MATTER

According to physician-ethicist Ezekiel Emmanuel, the first institu-tional structure to ensure the protection of patients' welfare in the era of managed care is physicians' professionalism. He defines this as the re-dedication of physicians to the professional ideal that the welfare of pa-tients is the physician's primary goal. Sadly, he immediately notes that professionalism is not a given. Among the reasons Emmanuel cites for its insufficiency is the following: "First, as we have learned from the data that has accumulated on conflicts of commission [financial incentives to provide more services, which are inherent in the fee-for-service reim-bursement system], it [professionalism] is not a sufficiently robust value and incentive to ensure the protection of patients. Some physicians—probably a small minority, but still an important group—are willing to subvert patients' welfare for their own financial gain, and even try to rationalize this."[19] The ethics of care is critical of this sort of deficient professionalism and places a high value on caregivers' responsiveness, responsibility, and accountability.

Clinicians committed to the ethics of care hold themselves account-able for the well-being of patients entrusted to their care. Being account-able means being attentive and responsive to the healthcare needs of in-dividual patients. It means that a clinician's concern for the patient tran-scends whatever happens during a shift or rotation, and that the clinician ensures continuity of care when he or she leaves a patient. The fragmen-tation of care that exists in many critical care settings—with attending physicians, residents, and medical students changing monthly; nurses working three 12 hour shifts weekly; and changing mixes of professional and nonprofessional staff with new responsibilities—leaves many patients unable to point to any single caregiver who knows their overall situation and is capable and willing to coordinate the efforts of the healthcare team. Being responsive and responsible earns a patient's trust that "all will be well," as simple to complex healthcare needs are addressed.

When clinicians work to develop accountability, they must recog-nize that deficiencies as well as excesses of responsible caring are prob-lematic. While it is reasonable for me to hold myself accountable for securing the well-being of my patients, I can err by setting unrealistic standards of responsiveness and responsibility. Prudence is always neces-sary to balance responsible self-care with care of others. Inexperienced clinicians may feel totally responsible for effecting patient outcomes be-yond their control and become frustrated and sad when they are unable to produce the desired outcome. It is always helpful to have conversa-tions about what is reasonable to hold one another and ourselves ac-countable for.

Guided reflection. Reflection questions follow for clinicians who are committed to holding themselves and colleagues appropriately re-sponsive and responsible:

1. To what extent does my commitment to securing the human well-being of those in my care dictate my work priorities?
2. How comfortable am I in voicing unmet needs of patients to other members of the healthcare team and then working collaboratively with the appropriate parties to secure needed out-comes?
3. Do other caregivers listen when I raise concerns about a patient because of my successful track record of patient advocacy?
4. Who on our team is ultimately responsible for knowing the pa-tient and family well enough to coordinate the efforts of the entire team and to keep the team focused on the patient's goals? Who is responsible for ensuring continuity of care as patients are

transferred out of the unit? What system variables need to change for us to meet the needs of our patients?

5. In what ways must I change in order for my patients to be able to count on me to respond in a responsible way to their needs?

PARTICULARS MATTER

The care perspective rejects a theoretical indifference to the specific aims and identities of persons and broadens the notion of "what counts" in ethical analysis. This attention to particulars facilitates the task of specifying the principles to be used to resolve ethical conflict. For example, in classic dilemmas where a case turns on which of two or more competing duties takes precedence, it is helpful to know as many of the particulars of the situation as possible. When the caregiving mother of a patient dying with acquired immunodeficiency syndrome (AIDS) demands to know her son's diagnosis and the patient has requested that no one be told his diagnosis, the duty to respect confidentiality conflicts with the duty to prevent potential harm. The ethics of care focuses on the relationship between involved parties and what each owes others. Professional caregivers are directed to intervene in a way that fosters mutual respect and is responsive to the needs of both parties. Operating within an ethics of care, a clinician would attempt to understand what underlies the patient's unrelenting demand for privacy as well as what is motivating the mother's demand to know the diagnosis. Ideally, knowledge of these particulars would allow intervention to be directed to moving both parties to a successful resolution of the conflict.

The importance of this characteristic and its contributions to clinical ethics is illustrated by the current debate over defining "medical futility" so that it may be used as an objective, dispassionate standard to justify withholding or withdrawing treatment that is demanded by patients or their surrogates but believed to be medically inappropriate. The care perspective would endorse the critique of those working to define futility made by Truog, Brett, and Frader; these three physicians cite clinical heterogeneity, pluralistic values, and the evolutionary nature of social consensus as reasons why most clinical decision making on the behalf of critically ill patients defies reduction to universally applicable principles.[20] Ideally, caring relationships would not only provide a basis for identifying all the different sources of conflict regarding decisions about treatment but also facilitate their mediation—without resort to a futility policy that attempts to define futility quantitatively. A commitment on the part of caregivers to recognize and address potential sources of conflict could go a long way toward alleviating escalating conflict and the painful sense of alienation experienced by some families of critically ill patients who end up believing that no one understands their concerns. Factors contributing to futility conflicts are listed in Exhibit 3-2; these factors were identified by paying attention to particulars.

Guided reflection. Reflection questions follow for clinicians who are committed to respecting particular patient and healthcare professional variables as morally relevant factors in ethical decision making:

1. To what extent am I able to provide the "particulars" of involved participants (patients, significant others, caregivers) in ethically problematic situations? Am I sensitive to how the unique reality each of us brings to the discussion table—our respective beliefs (consciously or unconsciously held), values, life experiences, and goals—influences the group process and outcome?

2. Do I believe that we are all the same as moral agents, that what is right for one is automatically right for all? Or do I believe that there are situational factors that may influence what makes one course of action the preferable "right and good" healing action for a particular patient or family?

3. Have we as a caregiving team identified who is responsible for bringing these "particulars" to the discussion? Is this more the domain of some healthcare professions than others?

CONTEXTUAL FACTORS MATTER

A final characteristic of the ethics of care is that it calls attention to the ecology of the moral choice or act. In the ethics of care, being responsive to an ethically problematic situation entails a commitment to identifying the variables contributing to the problems as well as the forces that are making its resolution difficult. Rather than solve problems on an ad hoc basis, attention is directed to modifying the variables creating recurrent problems. Strategies to prevent and resolve ethical conflict in this model include early identification of and response to patients and caregiving teams who are "at risk" for ethical conflicts as well as the identification of ways in which the system needs to change to prevent similar types of conflict in the future. New competencies, new structures or systems of care, and new or modified policies may be needed.

Guided reflection. Questions follow for clinicians who are committed to paying attention to the ecology of the moral choice or act:

Exhibit 3-2
Factors that Have a Potential to Create Futility Conflicts

Factors that May Underlie Patients' or Surrogates' Requests for Medically Futile Care
- Faulty reasoning (such as false optimism); belief that doing the "loving" or "right" things for the patient means doing "everything that is medically possible"
- Psychological factors (such as denial, guilt)
- Unrealistic expectations (such as "modern medicine can work miracles" or "God will work a miracle if only our faith is strong enough")
- Inability to trust healthcare professionals to act in the patient's best interest
- Religious conviction that life is to be preserved at all costs
- Economic considerations (such as family depends on patient's pension, third-party payers shelter family from realistic appreciation of costs of care)
- Entitlement mentality

Factors that Predispose Clinicians to Judge a Patient's or Surrogate's Request for Treatment to Be a Request for Futile Care
- Conviction that at times aggressive care is not in the best interest of patients and their families and may even be cruel and inhumane
- Concern to preserve the moral integrity of the disciplines of medicine, nursing, and so forth
- Concern to preserve the moral integrity of individual caregivers
- Escalating healthcare costs and considerations related to justice (expensive, high-tech care should be targeted toward those it is most likely to benefit)
- Conviction that harm to identifiable third parties constitutes a justifiable limitation to the autonomy of patients and their surrogates
- Conviction that new standards of care are needed (for example, once persistent vegetative state is definitively diagnosed, life-sustaining medical therapies including artificial nutrition and hydration should be withdrawn unless there is a directive to the contrary).
- Judgment that certain patients "are not worthy" of aggressive treatment
- Belief that the benefits the patient is likely to experience from the proposed intervention do not merit the risks that caregivers must assume to provide the treatment

---

Data from C. Taylor, "Medical Futility and Nursing," *IMAGE: Journal of Nursing Scholarship*, 27, no. 3 (1995): 301.

1. What are some of the *personal* variables that I bring to discussions of ethically problematic situations that facilitate or impede problem resolution?
2. What are some of the *system* variables contributing to recurrent ethical problems in my unit? What would need to change to modify or eliminate these variables successfully? Who has the authority to initiate these changes? What resources exist to facilitate needed change? What are my obligations to secure the needed changes?

REDEFINITION OF FUNDAMENTAL MORAL SKILLS

In principle-based ethics, a fundamental moral skill is the resolution of controversy. According to Engelhardt, "Ethics is at the very least a means for resolving controversies regarding proper conduct on bases other than direct or indirect appeals to force as the fundamental basis for a resolution."[21] By way of contrast, the ethics of care emphasizes such moral skills as kindness, attentiveness, compassion, and reliability—which when used with proficiency may prevent ethical conflict and thus eliminate the need for controversy resolution. When controversy does arise, these same skills bring "a different voice" to the process of resolving the conflict. Because to date these competencies have been viewed as optional personal traits for professional caregivers, their centrality to the ethics of care asks hard questions of educators and administrators. Among the most important: Should these competencies be used as criteria for admission to the professions and for advancement within the professions?

PRINCIPLE- AND CARE-BASED
APPROACHES TO CASE ANALYSIS

Nurses in the neurosurgical stepdown unit are caring for a 32-year-old, pregnant woman who has just been found to have a pseudoaneurysm of the vertebral artery. They become concerned when the treating neurosurgeon says to the patient, "Of course you will want to abort" and begins making plans with her to schedule the abortion. The nurses know that a consulting obstetrician has written in the patient's record that it would be possible to heparinize the patient to prevent the aneurysm from rupturing during her pregnancy, without any adverse effects on the fetus. When the nurses talk with the neurosurgeon about the need to present both options to the patient so that she can make an informed decision, he shrugs their concern away and reminds them that making complex decisions about treatment is his responsibility. The nurses call an ethics consultation.

How the consulting ethicists analyze this case and how the involved caregivers see their responsibilities is very much a function of the framework used to analyze this situation. Exhibit 3-3 identifies the major differences between two popular approaches to clinical ethical case analysis, the principle-based approach and the care-based approach. The discussion below compares and contrasts the processes and outcomes of these approaches using the five principal steps of ethics workup, a common model of ethical decision making (see Exhibit 3-4). Relying solely

Exhibit 3-3
A Comparison of The Principle- and Care-Based Approaches to Ethical Analysis

Characteristic	Principle-Based Approach	Care-Based Approach
Methodology	Rational, analytic, problem-solving Principle-driven analysis Impartiality, universalizability Popularized version uses "thin" notion of the principles	Phenomenological; incorporates elements of existential, feminine, narrative, and virtue perspectives Contextual analysis oriented to human good Particulars matter When used concomitantly with principle-based approach, yields a "thick" notion of the principles
Moral Point of View	Individuals (generic rights-bearers), abstractly conceived Imposes no general conception of the good on individuals: assigns priority to the right (universal procedural principles) over the good, however it may be construed Focus on action Central question: What am I obligated to do? What is just?	Particular individuals in relationship with needs and vulnerabilities relative to us Assigns priority to the good; autonomy is respected not as a matter of principle but because autonomy itself is a good that cannot be undermined if the patient's good is to be served Focus on character as well as action Central question: How ought I to respond?
Nature of healthcare professional-patient relationship	Participants viewed as equals; emphasis on formal equality, reciprocity, individual rights Contract model	Participants often unequal in knowledge, power, resources; emphasis on interdependence and mutual obligations Fiduciary model

Fundamental moral skills	Objectivity, rationality, ability to problem solve and to negotiate compromise	Sensitivity, attentiveness, attunement, respect, compassion, empathy, caring, kindness, reliability, trustworthiness, accountability
Moral obligations of healthcare professionals	Respect patients' rights to be self-determining	Create trusting healthcare professional-patient relationship directed to securing the good of the patient
	Act so as to benefit patients and not to harm	Hold oneself and others accountable for the patient's well-being within the scope of professional responsibilities
	Distribute the benefits and burdens of healthcare equitably	Work to develop a system of care that is responsive to and effective in meeting human needs
	Act justly	Challenge the system when it compromises human well-being
	Develop and use competence in resolving ethical difference	
Potential outcomes	Tends to reduce ethics to quandaries or dilemmas	Broadens scope of ethics to include everyday matters
	May objectify and dehumanize participants in ethical dilemmas	Affirms intrinsic worth of all participants in ethical situation
	Problems solved on ad hoc basis	Focuses attention on systemic solutions that proactively address recurrent concerns
	Offers clear guides to action	Challenges caregivers to reflect on how who they are influences patient well-being and the development and resolution of ethical problems
Advantages	Compatibility with deontological and consequentialist theories	Challenges the rote application of ethical systems grounded in the principles of universalizability, impartiality, and autonomy
	Fairly specific action guides	Challenges a reductionistic-mechanistic approach to healthcare and clinical ethics, which objectifies patients

Exhibit 3-3—continued
A Comparison of The Principle- and Care-Based Approaches to Ethical Analysis

Characteristic	Principle-Based Approach	Care-Based Approach
	Relevance to bioethics and clinical ethics	Directs attention to the reality of particular patients viewed in the context of their life narratives
Limitations	Lack of unifying moral theory	Underdevelopment of caring as a concept
	Reduction of ethics to hard cases (quandary ethics)	Caring's "dark side": potential abuse of patient autonomy; imbalances in self-care and care for others
	Devaluation of everyday ethical concerns	Time- and labor-intensive
	Popularized version has led to false notion that all actions justified by a principle are equally "correct"	

Note: This exhibit incorporates some distinctions found in V.A. Sharpe, "Justice and Care: The Implications of the Kohlberg-Gilligan Debate for Medical Ethics," *Theoretical Medicine* 13, no. 4 (1992): 295-318.

on either of the two models impoverishes case analysis, and using the care-based approach to complement the principle-based approach has many advantages. Clinicians who are sensitive to the strengths and limitations of both approaches are able to craft a framework for ethical analysis that is responsive to the compelling features of each case analyzed.

STEP 1—PRESENT THE FACTS

The facts that are selected (and rejected) to present the ethical case and the verbal and nonverbal language used to communicate these facts play a significant but unappreciated role in establishing the direction of the case analysis.

Principle-based analysis. The patient is a 32-year-old, gravida2 = para 1, American Buddhist, Caucasian who is 10 weeks pregnant. Neurological symptoms led to her hospitalization and the diagnosis of a pseudoaneurysm of the vertebral artery, an artery that supplies portions of the brain that control significant functions. The consulting obstetrician wrote in the patient's record that, whereas the anticoagulant coumadin is teratogenic, heparin could be successfully used in this patient to prevent rupture of the aneurysm without any harmful effect to the fetus. Nurses expressed concern when the neurosurgeon, who did not want to take any chances with the aneurysm "blowing," told the patient, "Of course you will want to abort," and then proceeded to make the arrangements. Nurses believed that the patient was not free to elect not to abort should this be her choice.

Care-based analysis. Julie is a 32-year-old, married, American Buddhist, Caucasian woman who is pregnant with her second child. She has a three-year-old daughter at home and confided to one of the nurses with a smile and a twinkle in her eye, "I think this one is a boy." From many conversations they have had with Julie, the nurses report that she is strongly pro-life and opposed to killing any living thing. She also implicitly trusts her physician, which seems to be part of a larger pattern of respecting authority. Neurological symptoms brought Julie to the hospital where she was diagnosed with a pseudoaneurysm of the vertebral artery, a weakening in the wall of a major blood vessel that supplies a region in the brain that controls significant functions. Her neurosurgeon is eager to operate to prevent rupture of the aneurysm as the cardiovascular demands of her pregnancy increase. He has a reputation for being a superbly skilled diagnostician and healer. He thinks all the talk about "patient rights" is "a lot of bunk." "My patients do what I tell them to and are always grateful once they realize how well they are doing."

Exhibit 3-4
The Ethics Workup

The ability to work up the ethical aspects of a case is an essential part of clinical reasoning. The emphasis in the ethics workup is on a sensible progression from the facts of the case to a morally sound decision. An ethics workup (this one or a similar version) may be used by a variety of health professionals, such as physicians, nurses, and social workers. With some adjustments, it may also be used by laypersons. Using the five principal steps of the ethics workup, health professionals holding a variety of philosophical and religious positions share a basic framework for thinking about and discussing morally troubling cases.

STEP 1—PRESENT THE FACTS

It is vitally important to clarify the facts of the case in order to anchor the decision. These facts are both medical and social. For example, both an estimate of prognosis and an understanding of the patient's home situation are often relevant to an ethical decision.

- Persons involved with all their particularities: beliefs, values, interests, goals (*Who?*)
- Diagnosis, prognosis, therapeutic options, goals of current care (*What?*)
- Chronology of events, time constraints on decision (*When?*)
- Setting (*Where?*)
- Variables contributing to conflict, reasons supporting claims (*Why?*)

Nurses and social workers may be instrumental in ensuring that the patient, family, and other nonmedical health professionals understand the medical facts accurately and that the health-care team understands pertinent nonmedical information about the patient and family.

STEP 2—IDENTIFY THE ISSUE

It is necessary to identify the specific ethical issue(s) in the case. The issue may not be ethical, but rather a diagnostic problem or a simple miscommunication.

STEP 3—FRAME THE ISSUE

Some health professionals will explore the issue using only one moral approach. Others will eclectically employ a variety of approaches. But no matter what one's underlying moral orientation, the ethical issue at stake in a given case can be framed in terms of several broad areas of concern, representing aspects of the case that may be in ethical conflict. It is therefore useful, if somewhat artificial, to dissect the case apart along the lines of the following areas of concern:

1. Identify the appropriate decision makers(s).
2. Apply the criteria to be used in reaching clinical decisions.
   - *The specific biomedical or clinical good of the patient:* One should ask: What will advance the biomedical good of the patient? What are the medical options and likely outcomes?
   - *The broader goods and interests of the patient:* One should ask: What broader aspects of the patient's good (such as the patient's dignity, religious faith, other valued beliefs, relationships) and the particular good of the patient's choice are pertinent to the decision at hand?
   - *The goods and interests of other parties:* Health professionals must also be attentive to the goods and interests of other parties (such as in the distribution of resources). One should ask: What are the concerns of other parties (such as family, healthcare professionals, healthcare institution, law, society) and what differences do they make,

morally, in the decisions that need to be made about this case? In deciding about an individual case, however, these concerns should generally not be given as much importance as that afforded the good of the individual patient whom health professionals have pledged to serve.

The physician explains the medical options to the patient or surrogates and, if indicated, makes a recommendation. The patient or surrogate makes an uncoerced, informed decision. Limits to patient's/surrogate's autonomy include the bounds of rational medicine/nursing/social work, the probability of direct harm to identifiable third parties, and violation of the consciences of involved healthcare professionals. In problematic cases, the interdisciplinary team may meet to ensure consistency in their recommendations to the patient or surrogate.

3. Establish the healthcare professionals' moral/professional obligations.

   Each healthcare professional must decide what she/he owes the patient, herself/himself, the healthcare team, the healthcare institution, and other third parties. Conflicts may exist.

STEP 4—DECIDE

In clinical ethics, as in all other aspects of clinical care, a decision must be made. There is no simple formula. The answer will require clinical judgment, practical wisdom, and moral argument. Healthcare professionals must ask themselves: How should I respond? What should I do? What help do I need and where can I get it? They must analyze the data, reflect and draw a conclusion after weighing the probable consequences of each of the available options: They must be prepared to explain their decision and the moral reasons for it.

Sources of justification include:

1. The nature of the healthcare professional-patient relationship; compatibility of recommended course of action with aims of profession (internal morality of profession).

2. Approaches to ethical inquiry: principle-based ethics, virtue-based ethics, casuistry, feminist/caring/existentialist ethics, theological ethics.

3. Ethically relevant considerations:
   - Balancing benefits and harms in the care of patients
   - Disclosure, informed consent, and shared decision making
   - The norms of family life
   - The relationships between clinicians and patients
   - The professional integrity of clinicians
   - Cost-effectiveness and allocation
   - Issues of cultural and religious variation
   - Considerations of power

4. Grounding and source of ethics: philosophical (based in reason), theological (based in faith), sociocultural (based in custom)

STEP 5—CRITIQUE

Once the decision has been made, it is important to be able to critique it by considering its major objections and then either responding adequately to them or changing one's decision. The healthcare professional should also seek colleagues' input when time permits. Some cases can even be taken to an ethics committee for further reflection. Retrospective analysis is also useful in preparing for the next time such a situation is encountered.

The consulting obstetrician wrote in the patient's record that it is possible to anticoagulate pregnant patients without adverse effects on the fetus and to prevent rupture of the aneurysm by using heparin, which is not teratogenic, rather than coumadin, which is. A nurse making rounds with the neurosurgeon was surprised when he told the patient, "Of course you will want to abort so that we can get this surgery done as soon as possible," without even mentioning that there is another alternative. When she confronted the neurosurgeon after leaving the patient's room and expressed the conviction that the patient should be given the choice of whether or not to abort, the neurosurgeon shrugged off her concern. "Remember, making treatment decisions is my job, not yours. I'm the one who's ultimately responsible for what happens, and I'm not willing to take any chances with this one." Discussing her discomfort with a colleague, the nurse decided to call an ethics consultation to see if there is some way to ensure that the patient will be given all the information she needs to make an informed and voluntary decision. The nurse confided to the consulting ethicist that she has never called an ethics consultation before and feels uncertain about challenging the physician's authority, but feels even more strongly that this patient and her unborn child need an advocate.

STEP 2—IDENTIFY THE ISSUE

Principle-based analysis. Withholding of information compromises autonomy: Is the neurosurgeon justified in paternalistically depriving this woman of the opportunity to make an informed and voluntary decision about her options for treatment in light of her commitment to pregnancy and other interests? (nonmaleficene and beneficence versus autonomy).

In addition to the above issue, the care-based analysis asks: In what ways is the nurse morally obligated to advocate for the well-being of this patient? What professional response is indicated from the nurse who was attentive to this woman's predicament?

STEP 3—FRAME THE ISSUE

Identify the Appropriate Decision Maker(s). *Principle-based analysis:* Most would agree that the patient is the appropriate decision maker in this case since this woman meets the following three criteria for decision making capacity: (1) she is able to understand the information necessary to make this particular decision, (2) she is able to reason in accord with a relatively consistent set of values, and (3) she is able to communicate her preferences. Limits to patients'(or their surrogates') autonomy include the bounds of rational medicine (or nursing or social work), the probability of direct harm to identifiable third parties, and violation of the consciences of involved healthcare professionals. One could make a case using the paternalistic model of decision making that the physician is the appropriate decision maker since he has more information about, and experience with, the problem and is able to make the most technically correct decision. The obligations of caregivers differ according to which model of decision making is employed. The patient-sovereignty model (patients with intact decision-making capacity decide) is a noninterference model; using this model of decision making, the only obligations of clinicians are to provide information about options for treatment and then not to interfere with the patient's decision making. In the paternalism model, clinicians are obligated to make the best decision possible about treatment for the patient and to persuade her to comply. In this case, the patient's pattern of respecting authority may guarantee her compliance, even in the face of a decision that is repugnant to her.

Care-based analysis. According to the care-based perspective, the patient who possesses decision making capacity is the appropriate decision maker; the role of healthcare professionals is to provide not only the information she needs to make a decision but also any necessary support and assistance to ensure that the decision she makes is *right for her* (the notion of existential advocacy). The ethics of care would also direct attention to all who are affected by this decision and would seek (with the patient's permission) to include the husband in the decision making process unless this is contraindicated for special reasons.

Apply the criteria to be used to reach clinical decisions. *The specific biomedical or clinical good of the patient.* The biomedical or clinical good of the patient will be the same no matter what model of analysis one uses. In both the principle- and care-based approaches, timely surgical repair of the vertebral artery is indicated to prevent the pseudoaneurysm from rupturing, which would have potentially life-threatening consequences. Because this surgery cannot be done without lethal effects on the fetus and because the longer the pregnancy continues the greater is the mother's risk of rupture, quick abortion of the fetus is indicated with this option. Pharmacologic management of the pseudoaneurysm is also an option. Although it carries a slightly increased risk for the mother, it allows her to deliver a potentially healthy baby before undergoing surgical repair of the vertebral artery. Nontreatment would not be a medically indicated option.

The broader goods and interests of the patient. Identification of a broader sense of the goods and interests of the patient should also be the same, regardless of which method of analysis is used. However, because contextual detail and attention to particulars about the participants in the decision is a hallmark of the care-based perspective, the care-based analysis generally yields a much richer sense of what is in the patient's overall best interest.

In this case, the treating neurosurgeon is not viewing this patient as a unique individual with beliefs and values that matter. Rather, his judgment of what is in the patient's best interest is limited to what is most likely to promote the physical well-being of *anyone* similarly afflicted. What is immediately apparent is that the care-based perspective is essential if one wants a true sense of beneficence to guide decision making. Ideally, the decision about treating this woman will be mindful of her Buddhist conviction of respecting all living things and her commitment to this pregnancy. The process of challenging the neurosurgeon's decision should also be conducted in a way that does not disturb the trusting patient-physician relationship, which seems to be essential to this patient's sense of well-being. Both methods of analysis are sure to highlight the fact that depriving this woman of the opportunity to reach the decision that is right for her violates her basic dignity as a human being and her right to self-determination. The care perspective will ask the question "How does what we are proposing to do influence this woman's sense of self and dignity as a respected and unique human individual?"

The goods and interests of other parties. *Principle-based analysis*: Principle-based analysis directs attention to competing rights and might define this case in terms of the rights of the patient, her fetus, and involved caregivers. The patient's right to be self-determining, which in this case would advance the right of the fetus not to be aborted, would be weighed against the right of the neurosurgeon to practice medicine in a manner that he has found yields "the greatest good for the greatest number." Attention may also be directed to the consequences of allowing the neurosurgeon's right to practice as he chooses automatically to trump the nurse's concern to practice in the manner she deems to be morally and professionally indicated.

Care-based analysis. The care perspective rejects a model of the rights of competing individuals, each of whom is primarily dedicated to advancing his or her own interests; instead it views individuals in interdependent relationships, with moral claims on one another. A care-based analysis of this case will be directed toward effecting a solution that engages the best talents of all participants and which is responsive to their interests.

Establish the healthcare professionals' moral and professional obligations. *Principle-based analysis.* How healthcare professionals view their moral obligations to this patient will be influenced by whether autonomy or beneficence trumps as the regulating principle. If autonomy is primary, it immediately becomes clear that the neurosurgeon is obligated to provide the patient with complete information about her choices and to respect the decision she ultimately makes. The neurosurgeon has the right to offer a strong recommendation about what is in the patient's best medical interest and to explain why he believes that this is the case. Should the attending physician persist in not letting the patient know that she has options other than abortion, the involved nurse has an obligation to ensure that the patient receives this information. If the neurosurgeon elects to operate under a traditional, paternalistic model of decision making, his moral obligation is to make the decision he believes is in the patient's best interest and somehow to enlist her compliance. This will create a dilemma for the nurse and other caregivers because the U.S. legal and professional systems value (and protect) the right of competent patients to make informed and voluntary decisions.

Care-based analysis. The ethics of care obligates healthcare professionals to provide whatever support Julie and her family need to make the decision that is right for them. This entails an obligation on the part of the nurses to secure the attending physician's cooperation in discussing all of Julie's options and, if he is unwilling to do this, to go through channels and the appropriate authorities to make sure this happens. Extreme sensitivity and strong interpersonal skills will be required to do this in a manner that prevents alienation of involved parties, that is respectful of and responsive to the needs of Julie and her family, and is respectful of the attending physician. The nurse's willingness to follow through with this after being initially rebuffed by the attending physician is essential. Her following-through may also demand new competencies.

STEP 4—DECIDE

The nurses involved in this case had three basic options: (1) do nothing; view this as a physician-patient matter and continue to provide technically competent care to the patient; (2) accept the neurosurgeon's decision that abortion is in this woman's best interest and support her as she prepares for the abortion; or (3) reject the neurosurgeon's claim that he has the authority (and obligation) to make this decision and find a way to ensure that the patient is informed about her options and supported in her decision making. In using either the principle- or care-based model of analysis, one would reject options 1 and 2. Option 1 would be moral abandonment of the patient and is not consistent with professional nursing. Option 2 violates Julie's morally and legally protected right to be self-determining. Although this option may "keep the peace" on the unit, it does so at the tremendous cost of liberty; respect for the patient/family and their beliefs, values, and interests; human life; and the nurses' professional integrity. What is important is that, although in this instance the principle- and care-based approaches dictate a similar course of action, how the action is implemented may differ.

Using either principle- or care-based analysis, the decision may be justified with appeals to the nature of the healthcare professional relationship and the morality internal to the discipline, and to different sources of moral authority. These sources will differ according to the involved participants.

STEP 5—CRITIQUE

Principle-based analysis. In the principle-based critique it may suffice to determine if intervention results in the patient's receiving the information she needs to ensure an informed and voluntary decision.

Care-based analysis. Using care-based analysis, one would explore how the course of action selected and its manner of implementation affected the well-being of Julie; her family; and, secondarily, the involved healthcare professionals. One would pay attention to its effect on Julie's trust in the caregiving team. One would also explore the system variables that created this issue and their likelihood of creating similar problems in the future. If this attending physician consistently acts paternalistically in a manner that violates patients' autonomy, it will be important to note if this behavior is unique to this physician or common in the unit. A unit conference exploring these issues may be indicated as well as a workshop for nonphysician caregivers that aims to develop effective advocacy strategies. The nurses may decide that they would respond exactly the same in a similar situation in the future or that they would do some things differently.

CONCLUSION

The care perspective, jointly espoused by the healthcare team, directly confronts two of the precipitating factors of ethical conflict. By locating responsibility for securing the patient's well-being with each healthcare professional involved in the patient's care, the care perspective facilitates interdisciplinary planning and stops pitting one group of professionals against another. Thus, each caregiver is a patient advocate who ought to value collaborative planning to meet the patient's needs. The caring perspective also commits the team to view ethical reflection and discussion as an essential part of the patient's care.

NOTES

1. C. Gilligan, *In a Different Voice: Psychological Theory and Women's Development* (Cambridge, Mass.: Harvard University Press, 1982).

2. J.M. Morse et al., "Comparative Analysis of Conceptualizations and Theories of Caring," *IMAGE: Journal of Nursing Scholarship* 23, no. 2 (1991): 119-26.

3. "The Crisis of Care: Affirming and Restoring Caring Practices in the Helping Professions," ed. S.S. Phillips and P. Benner (Washington, D.C.: Georgetown University Press, 1994).

4. C. Taylor, "Nursing Ethics: The Role of Caring," *AWHONN's Clinical Issues in Perinatal and Women's Health Nursing* 4, no. 4 (1993): 152-60; C. Taylor, "Rethinking Nursing's Basic Competencies," *Journal of Nursing Care Quality* 9, no. 4 (1995): 1-13; C. Taylor, "The Morality Internal to the Practice of Nursing" (PhD. diss., Georgetown University, Graduate School of Philosophy, 1997).

5. W.T. Reich, "History of the Notion of Care," and "Historical Dimensions of an Ethic of Care in Healthcare," in *Encyclopedia of Bioethics,* rev. ed., ed. W.T. Reich (New York: MacMillan, 1995), 319-31, 331-36; N.S. Jecker and W.T. Reich, "Contemporary Ethics of Care," in *Encyclopedia of Bioethics*, rev. ed., ed. W.T. Reich (New York: MacMillan, 1995), 336-44.

6. See note 1 above.

7. V.A. Sharpe, "Justice and Care: The Implications of the Kohlberg-Gilligan Debate for Medical Ethics," *Theoretical Medicine* 13, no. 4 (1992): 295-318.

8. N. Noddings, *Caring: A Feminine Approach to Ethics and Moral Education* (Berkeley, Calif.: University of California Press, 1984).

9. S. Ruddick, *Maternal Thinking: Toward a Politics of Peace* (Boston: Beacon Press, 1989).

10. M. Mayeroff, *On Caring* (New York: Harper & Row, 1971).

11. J. Travelbee, *Interpersonal Aspects of Nursing* (Philadelphia: F.A. Davis, 1971); J.G. Paterson and L.T. Zderad, *Humanistic Nursing* (New York: National League for Nursing, 1976, 1988); J. Watson, *Nursing: The Philosophy and Science of Caring* (Boulder, Colo.: Colorado Associated University Press, 1985; first published by Little, Brown & Co., 1979); J. Watson, *Nursing: Human Science and Human Care: A Theory of Nursing* (New York: National League for Nursing, 1988); S.T. Fry, "The Role of Caring in a Theory of Nursing Ethics,"

Hypatia 4, no. 2 (1989): 88-103; S. Gadow, "Existential Advocacy: Philosophic Foundation for Nursing," in *Nursing: Images and Ideals,* ed. S.F. Spicker and S. Gadow (New York: Springer, 1980), 79-101; M. Leininger, *Caring: An Essential Human Need: Proceedings of the Three National Caring Conferences* (Thorofare, N.J.: Charles B. Slack, 1981); P. Benner and J. Wrubel, *The Primacy of Caring: Stress and Coping in Health and Illness* (Menlo Park, Calif.: Addison-Wesley, 1989); A.H. Bishop and J.R. Scudder, *Nursing: The Practice of Caring* (New York: National League for Nursing, 1991).

12. R.C. Cabot, *Adventures on the Borderlands of Ethics* (New York: Harper and Brothers, 1926); F.W. Peabody, "The Care of the Patient," *Journal of the American Medical Association* 88 (1927): 877-82; F.W. Peabody, *Doctor and Patient* (New York: MacMillan, 1930); W.A. Tisdale, "On Clinical Caring," *Pharos* 42, no. 4 (1979): 23-26; E.D. Pellegrino and D.C. Thomasma, *For the Patient's Good: The Restoration of Beneficence in Health Care* (New York: Oxford University Press, 1988).

13. S.S. Phillips and P. Benner, eds., *The Crisis of Care* (Washington, D.C.: Georgetown University Press, 1994).

14. A.C. Wicks, B.J. Spielman, and J.C. Fletcher, "Survey of Ethical Orientations and Theories," in *Introduction to Clinical Ethics,* ed. J.C. Fletcher et al. (Frederick, Md.: University Publishing Group, 1995), 245.

15. R. May, *Love and Will* (New York: W.W. Norton, 1969).

16. P. Benner, "Caring as a Way of Knowing and Not Knowing," in *The Crisis of Care,* ed. S.S. Phillips and P. Benners (Washington, D.C.: Georgetown University Press, 1994), 58.

17. I.B. Wilson and P.D. Cleary, "Linking Clinical Variables with Health-Related Quality of Life: A Conceptual Model of Patient Outcomes," *Journal of the American Medical Association* 273, no. 1 (1995): 59-65.

18. Anonymous personal communication, 1996.

19. E. Emmanuel, "Medical Ethics in the Era of Managed Care: The Need for Institutional Structures Instead of Principles for Individual Cases," *The Journal of Clinical Ethics* 6, no. 4 (Winter 1995): 338.

20. D. Truog, A.S. Brett, and J. Frader, "The Problem with Futility," *New England Journal of Medicine* 326, no. 23 (1992): 1560-64.

21. H.T. Engelhardt, Jr., *The Foundation of Bioethics* (New York: Oxford, University Press, 1986): 39.

4

Decision Making in Critical Care

Robert M. Walker

INTRODUCTION

Ethical decision making in the critical care setting can be an extraordinarily difficult process. Making good clinical decisions can be complex enough, but in the critical care setting, this complexity is increased by several factors. First, the crisis situation itself telescopes the time for decision making. Second, decisions about treating individuals who are critically ill are often more complex than other clinical decisions. Because of these two factors, there are often uncertainties regarding diagnosis, prognosis, and options for treatment. Third, patients in the critical care setting are often unable to communicate, and are thus unable to participate in decision making. In such circumstances, family members—who are themselves trying to cope with the patient's crisis—are often pressed to help with decisions—decisions that they feel ill-prepared to make. Fourth, the increased number of caregivers associated with critical care increases the likelihood of conflicting perspectives on the course of that care. On the whole, the nature and clinical context of critical care render sound ethical decision making difficult, complex, and fraught with potential for disagreement and conflict.

Consider the following cases:

1. A patient with acquired immunodeficiency syndrome (AIDS) is in the intensive care unit (ICU) for treatment of the adult respi-

ratory distress syndrome secondary to *Pneumocystis carinii* pneumonia, which is refractory to medical treatment. A discussion regarding do-not-resuscitate (DNR) status is held and the patient, still competent, consents to a DNR order. One of the nurses says that the patient should be transferred out of the unit because having DNR status is incompatible with being in the ICU.[1]

2. A patient is admitted to the ICU with 56 percent burns of the upper and lower extremities and the scrotal area. The patient refuses skin graft surgery, despite the urging of the critical care team. He understands that the physicians believe that there is a great chance of overwhelming infection and death if he does not have the surgery. The patient asks, "Don't patients have a right to refuse treatment?"

3. An 83-year-old patient with head and neck cancer that was resected five weeks ago is admitted to the ICU with aspiration pneumonia and respiratory failure. She is sedated and placed on a ventilator. She has a living will. An ICU physician requests an ethics consultation, commenting that it is inappropriate to treat such a patient in the ICU. She should be in hospice instead.[2]

4. A depressed and distraught man attempts suicide by bringing a propane tank into his bathroom, opening the valve, and lighting a match. After the explosion, he is taken by ambulance to a local burn unit. He has suffered 92 percent burns and is on a ventilator, pressors, and other forms of life support. His spouse produces a living will that was written by the patient four years earlier, and asks that the physicians not resuscitate her husband should his heart fail. The staff of the burn unit object that this would be tantamount to "completing his suicide."

These cases give a flavor for the kinds of ethical conflicts that arise in the critical care setting. How does one address the issues and answer the questions posed in these cases? Are the questions even the right ones to ask? Are there others? Have the issues at stake been properly identified? Clearly, what is needed is a consistent, principled, and practical approach to analyzing cases and reaching decisions based on that analysis. This chapter illustrates some of the complexities of the decision-making process, sketches out a model for ethical decision making, and illustrates that model with several cases.

ETHICAL PRINCIPLES

Ethical decisions in critical care, like ethical decisions elsewhere, should be based on sound ethical principles. These include beneficence, nonmaleficence, autonomy, and justice.[3] Beneficence means "doing good," or "acting so as to benefit another." Beneficence is the central ethical principle of medicine, a profession devoted to benefitting the sick by pursuing health and wholeness.[4] A necessary corollary is the principle of nonmaleficence, which is aptly summed up in the phrase, "do no harm." In modern medicine, and especially in critical care, it is sometimes difficult to ensure that benefits outweigh potential and real harms, for our efforts to help often entail risks of harm or trade-offs between harms (such as, pain and bodily invasion) and benefits (such as, cure or restoration of limited function). Achieving an acceptable balance between these two can often be challenging.

Autonomy, an ethical principle that has been given great emphasis over the past 30 years, can be considered synonymous with self-determination,[5] and was well captured in Justice Cardozo's phrase, "Every human being of adult years and sound mind has a right to determine what shall be done with his own body."[6] The principle of autonomy is at the root of most of the legal cases that have established a right to refuse unwanted medical intervention, even if it is a lifesaving or life-sustaining intervention. Beginning with the famous case of Karen Ann Quinlan[7] and continuing through the case of Nancy Cruzan,[8] (the only case about the right to refuse treatment heard by the U.S. Supreme Court),[9] court after court has affirmed a right to refuse unwanted medical intervention. Autonomy can be a particularly difficult value to uphold in the critical care setting, as many of the patients temporarily lack decision-making capacity.

The principle of autonomy is also at the root of the medical and legal doctrine of informed consent. Informed consent is a process—not a piece of paper; it is possible to get a patient to sign a consent form while failing to carry out adequately the process of informed consent. According to Jonsen, Siegler, and Winslade, informed consent has four elements: the patient must have "an ability to understand relevant information, to appreciate one's medical situation and its possible consequences, to communicate a choice, and to engage in rational deliberation about one's own values in relation to the physician's recommendations about treatment options."[10] There are important exceptions to the process of informed consent, the most notable of which is the emergency exemption to informed consent, also called "presumed consent." This is relied on when there is a medical emergency, the patient is unable to consent, and there is no one available, such as a spouse, to consent on behalf of the incapacitated patient. A second exception to informed consent, often seen in critical care units, is the treatment of patients who have attempted to commit suicide. This is exemplified in case 4 above. In such cases, treatment is given without an informed consent process. Even when the patient is able to converse, the medical effects of a suicide attempt are treated despite the patient's wishes to the contrary. For example:

A patient attempts suicide via an overdose of acetaminophen. The patient, still with suicidal ideation and intent, refuses treatment with n-acetylcysteine [an agent used to treat acetaminophen toxicity]. These wishes are ignored by the treating physician, who administers the medication over the patient's objection.

The rationale for not honoring the patient's refusal rests in the idea that an actively suicidal patient is incapable of authentically consenting to treatment. A third and rarely invoked exception to informed consent is the so-called therapeutic privilege; this is based on the idea that, in select cases, physicians who are convinced that the process of informing the patient will actually produce harm may, on those grounds, sidestep the process of informed consent. An example would be not telling a patient of his or her cancer diagnosis. For example:

A 39-year-old woman presents with acute abdominal pain. Exploratory laparotomy reveals widespread ovarian cancer with omental seeding. On rounds the next day, the surgeon comments that he is not going to tell the patient about the cancer on the grounds that telling her would "remove all hope" and thus result in an earlier death than would otherwise be the case.

This exception to informed consent, which has come under increasing criticism over the past 30 years, presupposes that information itself can be harmful, and assumes that certain patients will not be able to deal constructively with "bad news." Both of these assumptions have been challenged in the medical literature.[11] In terms of ethical principles, the concept of therapeutic privilege pits the principle of nonmaleficence against that of autonomy, and concludes that the former outweighs the latter. Today, most ethicists would conclude that the opposite is true: autonomy almost always outweighs the well-meaning but paternalistic concern that patients are better off not knowing their diagnosis. The shift is reflected in the attitudes of physicians, which have changed almost 180 degrees from emphasizing paternalism and secrecy to upholding autonomy and full disclosure.[12]

The final ethical principle is that of justice. Justice issues in clinical medicine largely center on issues of fair allocation of scarce medical resources.[13] The critical care environment can itself be considered as a scarce resource. The classic justice question regarding access to the ICU is: Who should get the last ICU bed when two patients arrive in the emergency department and both need critical care services? Another version of this conflict is the case of the arrival of a young, salvageable trauma victim who needs intensive care services when the ICU is full. What formulation of the justice principle would allow us to decide who, if anyone, should be bumped out of the unit so that the trauma victim could be accepted?[14]

An important difficulty with relying solely on ethical principles to help make decisions is that these principles can come into conflict with one another.[15] Case 2, for example, embodies a conflict between beneficence and autonomy. Unfortunately, the principles themselves do not provide a clear way to resolve such conflicts. One approach would be to seek a practical resolution that attempts to limit the degree to which any one principle is sacrificed. This calls for not only wise and careful deliberation, but also a substantial knowledge about how such value conflicts have been resolved in the past. For case 2, it would be helpful to be familiar with the following published cases:

A 73-year-old man with amyotrophic lateral sclerosis is fully conscious and competent, but ventilator dependent. He asks his doctor to discontinue the ventilator. The patient is neither suicidal nor depressed, he simply does not want to continue life on the ventilator. The case was heard in court, which ruled that a competent patient has a constitutional right to refuse unwanted medical intervention, even if it means that the patient will die.[16]

A competent, 77-year-old woman presents with a gangrenous leg, and the physicians recommend amputation. The patient refuses, indicating that she doesn't want to be a burden to her children, doesn't want to end up in a nursing home, and doesn't want to live life as an invalid. A court subsequently ruled that a competent patient can refuse lifesaving surgery.[17]

In these and many other such cases, courts have consistently given greater weight to patient autonomy than beneficence. Familiarity with this trend may help us decide what to do or not to do in case 2, where the patient refuses skin graft surgery. A general rule can thus be stated: In cases where beneficence and autonomy conflict, autonomy should be given greater weight. This kind of weighing of principles helps us to resolve conflicts between them.

In approaching problems about decisions in critical care, it is best to apply a consistent method. In most cases, people sense an ethical conflict without being able to articulate it clearly. In other cases, people focus on different facets or dimensions of an ethically complex case. What is needed is a way of usefully grouping the information one uncovers in exploring the case. Several practical approaches to clinical ethical decisions have been proposed. The approach that follows is largely based on a model proposed by Jonsen, Siegler, and Winslade.[18]

The first matter to consider is the accuracy of the perception that a case is ethically problematic. Just because one person in the critical care unit has this perception, does not mean that it is shared by all. Walker and colleagues reported in 1991 that nurses and physicians often disagree about which cases present ethical problems and, in cases where both agree there are problems, they often differ as to what the problems are.[19] Furthermore, these perceptual differences were a frequent source of interstaff conflict. The disagreements were not simply between physicians and nurses, but also between physicians and other physicians. This finding has importance in the critical care context, where so many different individuals are involved with a case, and where not all of these individuals are privy to the same information. At times, the differing perspectives regarding multifaceted cases can escalate into ethical conflicts. Thus, an essential first step in the decision making process is to isolate the source of conflict or concern, and then approach the case in a consistent way. In some instances, after analyzing the case, one discovers that the apparent conflict is not the "real" issue at all, but some other issue or issues are at stake. For example, LaPuma demonstrated that, in a number of cases, questions posed to the ethics consultation service were either misidentified conflicts or smokescreens for deeper issues.[20] Schiedermayer and colleagues later reported cases where economic issues masqueraded as ethics conflicts.[21]

A consistent and useful way of sorting out the real issues is to organize ethically relevant information into a decision making grid using the following categories: Medical indications, the patient's preferences, qual-

Exhibit 4-1
Grid to Organize Ethically Relevant Information

MEDICAL INDICATIONS (Beneficence)	PATIENT PREFERENCES (Autonomy)

• Diagnoses
• Prognosis information
• Treatment options and
  recommendations
	• Decision-making capacity?
	  YES: Informed Consent
	  NO: Proxy consent (substituted
	        judgment or best interest)

QUALITY OF LIFE (Nonmaleficence)	CONTEXTUAL FEATURES (Justice)
• Determined by patient • Determined by others	• Family members • Laws • Administrative issues • Cost of care • Just allocation of resources • Interstaff conflict • Conflicts of interest

ity of life, and contextual features (see Exhibit 4-1). Each cell in the grid is discussed below.

MEDICAL INDICATIONS

After the ethical problem, question, or conflict has been tentatively identified, the first matter is to be as clear as possible about the medical information in the case. This specifically includes information regarding the diagnoses, the prognostic assessments, and all options for treatment (including the option of no treatment). The no-treatment option and its associated prognosis are often at the center of many of the conflicts in critical care. It is important to consider these matters explicitly, rather than veiling them behind the phrase "poor prognosis." A number of disagreements may ensue from a set of cloudy clinical facts, or from different interpretations of those facts. For example:

An 87-year-old woman has "failure to thrive" after a revision of her mitral valve replacement, and is left in a debilitated condition. The patient, who had previously completed a living will, is now in a noncommunicative state. She also suffers from a lack of nutrition. All of the medical consultants on the case are convinced that the patient is terminally ill. The attending physician disagrees, saying, "I've salvaged cases like these before." He continues to press for aggressive intervention while the patient's daughter is caught in the middle, troubled over what to do.

In this case, there is disagreement over prognosis and over what can realistically be accomplished with medical intervention. This problem is best approached by convening a patient care conference so that the physicians involved can discuss the case and seek to reach a consensus about the patient's condition and prospects for recovery. Whether the conference produces consensus or merely clarifies the points of difference, either outcome is preferable to the almost intolerable situation of presenting the patient's daughter with mixed messages. In either case the daughter should be informed of the medical opinions regarding her mother. If there is consensus (that is, the attending physician comes to agree that his hope is not well founded and concurs with the consultants that pursuing aggressive intervention is unlikely to be successful), then the conflict is resolved and a palliative care plan that comports with the patient's wishes can be pursued.

If the conflict is not resolved at the conference, then the patient's daughter can be informed of this difference in perspective and decide which course of action, aggressive or palliative, best fits with her mother's previously expressed wishes. If the daughter sides with the consultants, she can attempt to find another physician to care for her mother and relieve the current attending physician from his responsibilities. If this is done in an amicable and respectful way, the relieved physician retains his integrity and his right to a moral perspective, without imposing his views on a patient who does not share them.

Until such a conference and clarification process are undertaken, the situation will become increasingly conflicted. The daughter is anguished because she is convinced that her mother is receiving care that she would never consent to. Ill will is generated among the physicians, who do not communicate among themselves personally, but learn of one another's perspectives through chart notes and the filter of the daughter's recounting. The nurses, and others involved in the case, also feel caught in a difficult situation, and want to achieve a resolution of the conflict.

THE PATIENT'S PREFERENCES

The discussion of ethical principles above demonstrates how a competent patient's preferences can be both ethically problematic and decisive. Recognizing that autonomy trumps beneficence in most cases does not mean that the physician who disagrees with the patient's decision somehow lacks moral status or agency. The physician and other caregivers are just as much moral agents as the patient. The general rule that the autonomous choice of the patient to refuse interventions outweighs the beneficent physician's desire to intervene is simply a way of recognizing that the patient has ultimate authority over what is done with and to his or her own body and person.

The moral agency of physicians and others who disagree with the patient is respected by the option of moral escape; that is, the disagreeing party is free to withdraw from the care of the patient so that care can be provided by others who do not find moral difficulty with the patient's perspective. For example, some surgeons and anesthesiologists find it morally untenable to care for Jehovah's Witness patients who need and/ or want surgery and yet refuse administration of all blood products. Others, seeing no moral difficulty in accepting the patient-imposed limitation of "no blood products," agree to perform anesthesia and surgery and refrain from giving blood products—even when it appears that the patient will exsanguinate. Similarly, in case 2, if the patient continues to refuse skin graft surgery, objecting caregivers have the option of withdrawing from the case if their conscience so leads them. The option of moral escape is a way of respecting conflicting ethical principles and of respecting the moral agency of all parties with a moral stake in the case.

Many patients requiring critical care are decisionally impaired. Some patients exhibit waxing and waning capacity; some appear incapacitated in regard to some decisions but not others; and some are completely incapacitated, either temporarily or permanently. Each case must be evaluated individually. In cases where capacity waxes and wanes, decisions that can be reached with patients during their lucid intervals, and can be shown to be consistent over time, should be considered autonomous. If the patient's capacity is temporarily impaired or lost, and it can be restored so that the patient can make his or her own decisions, then that avenue should be pursued insofar as it is practical. In critical care, many decisions must be made before capacity can be restored. Thus, clinicians must often rely on the help of a close family member or others for help with proxy decisions for the patient. The situation becomes more problematic when there are no persons available with knowledge of a now-incapacitated patient's past wishes regarding medical care.

The first step when one has a conversant patient in the ICU, is to assess the patient's decision-making capacity. The rigor with which this is done depends on the case at hand. Some patients in the unit obviously have decision-making capacity, and should be treated as such. In other cases, when capacity is in question, a more detailed assessment should follow. If it is thought that the patient's capacity may be clouded by neurologic or psychiatric illness, the appropriate consultations should be obtained. Matters become more difficult if the decisions to be reached are major, and if the time frame for the decision does not allow a clear resolution of the patient's capacity. For example, consider case 2 in more detail.

The patient consistently refused skin graft surgery, and even posed the question to the treating staff, "Don't I have a right to refuse surgery if I want to? A person has a right to refuse to be kept on a ventilator, so don't I have a right to refuse surgery?" Members of the staff had repeatedly noted in the medical chart that the patient understood that the surgery was designed to help heal his burned extremities; he also understood the proposed benefits of the surgery and the outcome should he go without skin graft surgery (he would have scarred and contracted limbs that would be of little use, and there was at least a 50 percent chance that he would become septic and die in the hospital). The staff, troubled over how to proceed in the case, requested a consultation from the hospital's ethics committee.

The ethics consultant interviewed the patient at the bedside, and found that the patient knew that everybody wanted him to have the surgery. He indicated that he preferred to take his chances without the surgery, and that he was interested in leaving the hospital. When asked about the consequences of going without surgery, the patient admitted that he knew he could die but insisted that there was also a good possibility that he would live. The patient also told the consultant that a large group of doctors came to his room and got him to sign a consent form for surgery. He added, "I got the nurse to bring the form back to me after they left and tore it up because I was coerced."

At this point it was clear to the consultant that the patient had clearly and repeatedly refused skin graft surgery. He was aware of the risks of refusing surgery and accepted them. The consultant did not stop there, but went on to ask why he didn't want surgery. The patient did not provide a reason, but instead looked at the consultant with suspicion and said, "I don't have to tell you. Why should I tell you?" The consultant said, "OK, you don't have to tell me your reasons, but there is one other thing I would like to ask. When surgeons want to do surgery, they are supposed to explain what the surgery consists of and what it is supposed to accomplish. Could you give me your understanding of what the surgeons want to do?" The patient rolled his eyes and exclaimed, "It's impossible! Simply ridiculous! It can't be done." The consultant replied, "What can't be done? Skin grafting?" The patient said, "That's right." When the consultant next offered to show the patient others on the burn ward who had undergone successful skin grafts, the patient denied that this was possible and began to become agitated. The consultant then asked, "But what do you think the surgeons think they can do?" The patient replied, "They want to put $20 bills all over my legs and they believe they'll turn into skin and I'll grow new legs, and it'll be Lincoln's Birthday." The consultant asked, "But if they really could do that, and if it really would help your legs would you want it?" The patient said, "Sure, but they can't! It's just the most ridiculous thing." At this point the ethics consultant ended the interview, convinced that he was dealing with a case of paranoid schizophrenia.

What became clear was that the patient, despite his clear and adamant refusal, failed to meet the conditions of informed refusal, because he lacked an adequate understanding of what he was refusing; he was clearly unable to reason about his choice. In this case, the surgery was necessary but not urgent. This allowed time for the patient to be evaluated by psychiatrist and started on medication to treat his schizophrenia. Fortunately, the patient had a rather quick response to the medication, such that his capacity to understand, reason, and consent were restored before the need to operate became urgent. He consented to surgery and subsequently did well. Had the situation become critical while his decision-making capacity was still impaired, the only prudent options would have been (1) to invoke the emergency exemption to informed consent or (2) to seek a proxy decision through a court order, since no family members were available to give proxy consent.

A more common situation in critical care is the case in which the patient completely and obviously lacks the capacity to make decisions. Many of the ethical problems that arise in critical care do so because of a lack of patient input and information. Permanent or temporary loss of decision making capacity poses a serious threat to patient autonomy. Some of the most difficult cases arise precisely because clinicians cannot be sure of what the patient would want done or not done. In these situations clinicians commonly turn to those most able to help understand the patient's past preferences. Usually this person is the next of kin, but it can be anyone who has had a close relationship with the patient and has information regarding the patient's values, attitudes, and previously expressed wishes regarding medical care.

The process by which substitute or proxy decisions are made is termed *substituted judgment.* The surrogate decision maker's task is to render decisions based on the incapacitated patient's previously expressed preferences. Sometimes these preferences are expressed in a living will document; however, in most cases they are statements made in the past by the patient and recalled by the surrogate and others who have shared their lives with the patient. This process is based on the principle of autonomy. One pitfall is that surrogates may not understand their role to be one of providing information and insight about what the patient would likely choose to do in the current situation; they may instead feel like they are being asked to make decisions about life and death that they are inadequately prepared for. The frequent result of misinterpreting their role is that they request that the doctors "do everything." Physicians and others who work with patients' families need to be aware of this pitfall and take active steps to circumvent it. This can be done by first explaining the proxy's role and also by emphasizing the need to work together to care for the patient in the way he or she would want to be cared for.

In cases in which there are no advance directives and no previous patient preferences can be recalled by others, a surrogate is still sought to participate in decisions, only now the decisions are made based on what is judged to be in the patient's *best interest.* In this process, the physician recommends the course of action or inaction he or she thinks is in the patient's best medical interest, and together the physician and the surrogate engage in the process of shared decision making in the best interest of the patient. The pitfall mentioned above exists to an even greater degree in this situation, for one can no longer appeal to the proxy to base decisions on the patient's preferences. Nevertheless, the physician's recommendations should in most cases be influential, and proxies should be enlisted to work with physicians, not to see themselves as the ones who decide whether their incapacitated loved one lives or dies.

The situation is especially difficult when an incapacitated, critically ill patient is in the unit, the prognosis for meaningful recovery is dismal, and there are no advance directives and no other people to serve in the proxy role. There is a need to determine whether life-sustaining interventions should be continued and whether an attempt should be made to resuscitate the patient in the event of a cardiac arrest. Although many physicians have taken it upon themselves to decide for such patients, our society has not always viewed physician beneficence as an adequate protection of the interests of vulnerable, incapacitated patients. Therefore, it is usually prudent to seek a court-appointed guardian to assist with such decisions using the best-interest standard.

CONSIDERATIONS ABOUT QUALITY OF LIFE

The above situation is one where many would raise the issue of quality of life. While it can be said that all of medicine is devoted to improving quality of life, most patients do not frame their experience with illness in such terms. Most are interested in cure, improvement, maintenance of function, and so on. The term *quality of life,* when used by medical professionals, is usually reserved for situations in which patients lack capacity and are in a severely debilitated condition, and for which medicine has little to offer in the way of benefit but still retains its potential for iatrogenic harm. It could well be said that the principle of nonmaleficence is the central principle for the quality-of-life quadrant of the decision-making grid. The central questions are: Is there any benefit to be gained by continuing what we are doing?[22] Are we not doing more harm than good here? Is it not cruelty to continue subjecting this patient to our tubes and technology? All of these are expressions of poor quality of life, and it is legitimate to be concerned about the effects of medicine on such patients.

There are actually two notions of quality of life to be addressed. The first is the patient's own assessment of his or her quality of life, while the second is an assessment of the patient's quality of life as judged by another person such as a physician, nurse, or family member. The patient's own assessment underlies, in many cases, his or her preferences for treatment at the end of life. Many patients make this kind of assessment in advance in living wills and other advance directives. For example, patients often indicate that if they are ever incapacitated and in a terminal condition, they want to refuse in advance any attempt by physicians to provide life-sustaining interventions. In other words, they judge the future prospect of that kind of life to be of such low quality that they do not desire that their life be prolonged in that condition; instead, they wish to be kept as comfortable as possible and to be allowed to die a natural death. Thus, this notion of quality of life actually belongs in the patient preferences quadrant of the decision-making grid. These are judgments that we should respect.

On the other hand, there are judgments about quality of life that we should be slow to respect and quick to suspect. These are judgments made by a person other than the patient that the patient's quality of life is so low as to warrant forgoing medical intervention. The reason we should be suspicious of such judgments is their great tendency to be biased. For example, several studies have reported that physicians tend to rate the quality of life of patients lower that the patients themselves rate it.[23] Further, one study reported that physicians' assessments of quality of life influence their decisions to withhold cardiopulmonary resuscitation (CPR) in the event of cardiac arrest.[24] Thus, we are on unsafe ground in relying solely on another person's assessment of a patient's quality of life.

This concept is dramatically illustrated in a case I participated in during my internship.

I admitted a 66-year-old diabetic to the ICU for treatment of pneumonia with respiratory failure. Over the years, this patient had lost both legs to diabetic gangrene. He was also totally blind from retinopathy and dependent on chronic hemodialysis from nephropathy. During the previous year, he had suffered from middle cerebral artery stroke with resultant hemiparesis of his dominant side. He was placed on the ventilator and sedated for comfort while he was given antibiotics and respiratory therapy. During the care of this man, I heard a number of people question the appropriateness of putting such a debilitated person in the ICU, and even overheard one of the surgeons comment that cases like this one make a powerful argument for active euthanasia.

As the patient improved, the sedation was lifted and he was extubated. After he was transferred to the floor, I had a conversation with him during a dialysis session. I asked him about his experience with illness and whether he would want us to respond in a similar way when a future crisis arrived. He said "Yes," and began to tell me that he found life precious and very much worth living. He told me that his disabilities, as difficult as they are, have actually made his life better. He cited the quality and depth of the relationship he had with his wife; she was often at his bedside, read to him, and shared her life with him. He said that he would not trade this for new eyes, limbs, and kidneys.

This phenomenon is perhaps more widespread than we think. In a study of elderly persons' preferences for CPR, investigators found that patients with disabilities actually desired CPR more often than subjects who were healthy. It seems that those who did not want resuscitation were most often the "worried well."[25] Physicians and others who participate in the care of disabled persons may also fall into that category.

The most difficult kinds of cases are those involving patients who have a poor quality of life, who are incapacitated, and for whom there is little that medicine can offer except perhaps to maintain them in their current state or in a state that is of even lower quality. Some have raised the issue of whether deploying aggressive interventions in such cases is a form of cruelty.[26] This charge, however, seems misguided to the extent that malevolent motives are absent. Nevertheless, the point is well taken that uncritically deploying all available medical technology in such cases may not be the best way to demonstrate care and concern. A palliative care plan often does a better job. However, decisions to move to a palliative mode and to withhold aggressive intervention should always be carried out after a process of shared decision making with an appropriate proxy—usually a close family member—or in some cases with a court-appointed guardian. Physicians should not take it on themselves simply to withhold standard interventions.

CONTEXTUAL FEATURES

The final cell of the decision making grid was originally called "external factors" because they were important factors that were nevertheless external to the physician-patient relationship.[27] The category is now, however, called "contextual features." The reason is that ethical dilemmas do not occur in a vacuum, nor are they limited to the doctor-patient dyad; they occur in a context that, while differing from case to case, can involve family members, legal concerns, administrative issues, concerns about cost[28] and justice, and so forth. The question is to what extent should any of these factors, or perhaps a confluence of them, be decisive in critical care decisions. In some cases, one can easily answer that they should not be decisive, whereas in other cases the answer is not so clear. Consider, for example, the following case:

A 54-year-old woman was admitted to the ICU to rule out a myocardial infarction. She had atrial fibrillation and congestive heart failure. She had an intravenous (IV) line, telemetry leads, and pulse oximeter. Her husband became angry and demanded that these "machines" be stopped since his wife had "signed a paper saying 'no machines.' "

In this case, the husband was inappropriately interfering with the patient's care. The situation was resolved by explaining that the patient's living will applies to a condition in which the patient is irreversibly incapacitated and terminally ill, and that none of these conditions yet apply. Furthermore, the patient herself, still competent, desired to continue treatment. This is a case where the conflict should not be resolved by simply and uncritically acceding to a family member's wishes.

Consider another complicated case:

A 26-year-old, indigent patient with a history of IV-drug abuse is admitted to the intensive care unit with subacute bacterial endocarditis and congestive heart failure secondary to an incompetent mitral valve. The patient, who is angry and verbally abusive, has received two mitral valve replacements in the past, and now appears in need of a third. The surgeons, however, refuse to operate, asserting that placing a third valve in this patient would constitute futile therapy and would therefore be a waste of resources. The patient, still competent, desires to have another valve operation if it will save her life.

The questions raised by this case are many. Is placing a third valve really futile? If so, what goal(s) of therapy cannot be met? Are there other goals that have not been considered? Is it just to expend resources on this patient with repeatedly self-induced illness, when others who are ill, through no fault of their own, go without adequate care? Many more questions arise, and none have easy answers.[29] However, it is hard to justify allowing a person to die when the medical indications are clear—as they are in this case—that further valve surgery is needed; when the patient wants the lifesaving surgery; and when the needed and wanted care is available. Contextual features can be complex and varied, but they should rarely if ever override clear-cut medical indications and strong patient preferences for indicated intervention.

It should be pointed out that the concept of medical futility is being used more and more in clinical medicine. One must be careful in claiming that an intervention is futile. Medical futility has been notoriously hard to define and is, in most instances, a rather subjective judgment.[30] In the above case, for example, the surgeons considered the surgery futile because the patient's IV-drug habit precluded achieving the usual goal of 10-year valve life. Yet this was not the only goal worth pursuing. The chances for a one-year valve life were assuredly better, yet this goal was not even considered. One also wonders whether other unflagged biases had entered into their assessment, such as disdain for the patient's life situation, her indigent status, and her ungrateful attitude. This possibility again reinforces the necessity of being explicit about the medical indications in the case. Only then will those involved have a chance to identify and address hidden assumptions and biases.

RESOLVING ETHICAL PROBLEMS IN THE CRITICAL CARE SETTING

This four-quadrant method of organizing information by medical indications, the patient's preferences, considerations about quality of life and contextual features represents a consistent and principled approach to clinical ethical problems in critical care. Each category or quadrant can be coupled with one of the four basic ethical principles. The process of outlining the medical indications and recommending a particular course of action is grounded in the principle of beneficence; the process of ensuring decision-making capacity and exploring patient preferences is an exemplification of the principle of autonomy; the concern about the quality of life of irreversibly incapacitated patients who are severely debilitated and beyond recovery exemplifies the principle of nonmaleficence; and the process of deciding how to allocate unit resources when medical needs outstrip them exemplifies and relies on the principle of justice. Of course, not all of the contextual features of cases are issues involving justice; they may be legal issues, administrative issues, family issues, and so forth.

The process of decision making in the critical care setting involves first clarifying the questions or issues at hand, plugging information into the four-quadrant model, and then reasoning about the data and deciding what to do. To facilitate the process of reasoning and deciding on a course of action, one should bear in mind that when autonomy and beneficence conflict, considerations involving autonomy are generally decisive, especially when the issue is one of refusing medical intervention. The extent to which one should respect an autonomous patient's demand for intervention is less clear, becoming weaker as the medical indications become less clear. Decisions to withhold treatment based on a physician's perception of the patient's quality of life must be made with great care, and almost always with the assistance of a proxy decision maker. Finally, contextual features should rarely drive decisions about what to do, with the exception being absolute scarcity of a resource (for example, the best way to allocate the last ICU bed fairly when it is needed by more than one patient).

In addition to the information presented above, it is essential that one become familiar with what Jonsen and Toulmin have called "paradigm cases" in medical ethics.[31] Once the questions have been clarified, and the case information categorized and weighed, it is immensely helpful to know how similar cases have been resolved in the past. Armed with this information, one can engage in a process of pattern matching to see how the paradigm cases of the past fit with the current case. It is rare that one will encounter an entirely new kind of case. If one finds that a case is almost an exact match with a previous case, then one will not only have precedent for handling the current case, but increased comfort and justification for one's actions. For example, a competent Jehovah's Witness trauma victim is in the ICU. She is an unmarried adult with no dependents. She is competent and expresses her refusal of all blood products. Years ago, the first of such cases caused much concern, conflict, and anguish over how to proceed. But now, such a case causes much less difficulty because it is a well-established paradigm of a competent adult's right to refuse unwanted medical intervention, even if it means that death could possibly result. Knowledge of important paradigm cases helps us to avoid reinventing the wheel every time we face an ethical conflict.

In the critical care environment, there is great opportunity for conflict over ethical issues. One reason is that so many caregivers are involved in the typical case, and another is that the decisions must often be made without the luxury of adequate time. Because ethical problems in critical care are often complex and multifaceted, there is great potential for different caregivers to focus on different aspects of the case, and thus to see the problems differently. A practical strategy in such cases is to gather the people involved around the table in a case conference; there the data regarding the case can be reviewed and clarified, and unquestioned assumptions and misperceptions can be put to rest. Such a process, while not convenient or easy, is well worth it when compared to the time and energy spent in unresolved conflict.

Of course, there is no guarantee that all ethics conflicts will be neatly resolved. Some will, but in other cases participants will at best come away with an approach or a next step. In still other cases, after the clarification process, participants will find themselves in a dilemma. Such dilemmas exist and are never comfortable, but they can at least be minimized by the above approach to ethics problems in critical care.

In sum, ethical decision making in the critical care environment is a complex process that has great potential for misunderstanding and conflict. The best way to avoid the latter is to adopt a consistent and principled approach to ethics problems in the unit. This chapter has outlined and explored a process of issue identification, data classification, principle weighing, paradigm case comparison, and conflict resolution. While such a process is difficult, it is in many cases necessary to ensure that critical care practitioners provide the best care possible amid the crises of critical illness.

NOTES

1. B. Lo et al., "Ethical Dilemmas about Intensive Care for Patients with AIDS," *Reviews of Infectious Diseases* 9 (1987): 1163-67.

2. P.E. Bellamy and R.K. Oye, "Admitting Elderly Patients to the ICU: Dilemmas and Solutions," *Geriatrics* 42 (1987): 61-63, 67-68.

3. T.L. Beauchamp and J.F. Childress, *Principles of Biomedical Ethics,* 3rd ed. (New York: Oxford University Press, 1994).

4. L.R. Kass, "The End of Medicine and the Pursuit of Health," in *Toward a More Natural Science* (New York: Free Press, 1985), 157-86.

5. J. Katz, *The Silent World of Doctor and Patient* (New York: Free Press, 1984).

6. *Schloendorff v. The Society of New York Hospital,* 211 N.Y. 125, 1914.

7. *In re Quinlan,* 70 N.J. 10 (1976); E.J. Emanuel, "A Review of the Ethical and Legal Aspects of Terminating Medical Care," *American Journal of Medicine* 84 (1988): 291-301.

8. E.J. Emanuel, "Securing Patients' Right to Refuse Medical Care: In Praise of the *Cruzan* Decision," *American Journal of Medicine* 92 (1992): 307-12.

9. *Cruzan v. Director, Missouri Department of Health,* 497 U.S. 261 (1990); 100 S. Ct. 2841 (1990).

10. A.R. Jonsen, M. Siegler, and W.J. Winslade, *Clinical Ethics* (New York: McGraw-Hill, 1992), 44.

11. See note 5 above; N.A. Cousins, "A Layman Looks at Truthtelling in Medicine," *Journal of the American Medical Association* 244 (1980): 1929.

12. D.H. Novak et al., "Changes in Physicians' Attitudes Toward Telling the Cancer Patient," *Journal of the American Medical Association* 241 (1979): 897.

13. R.M. Veatch, "The Ethics of Resource Allocation in Critical Care," *Critical Care Clinics* 2 (1986): 73-89; G.C. Graber, "Allocation of Critical Care Resources: Entitlements, Responsibilities, and Benefits," *Journal of Critical Care* 8 (1993): 128-32.

14. R.D. Truog, "Triage in the ICU," *Hastings Center Report* 22, no. 2 (1992): 13-17.

15. J.M. Luce, "Conflicts Over Ethical Principles in the Intensive Care Unit," *Critical Care Medicine* 20 (1992): 313-15.

16. *Satz v. Perlmutter,* 379 So. 2d 359 (1980).

17. *Lane v. Candura,* 376 N.E. 2d 1232 (1978).

18. See note 10 above.

19. R.M. Walker et al., "Physicians' and Nurses' Perceptions of Ethics Problems on General Medical Services," *Journal of General Internal Medicine* 6 (1991): 424-29.

20. J. La Puma, "Consultation Clinical Ethics: Issues and Questions in 27 Cases," *Western Journal of Medicine* 146 (1987): 633-37.

21. D. Schiedermayer, J. LaPuma, and S.H. Miles, "Ethics Consultations Masking Economic Dilemmas in Patient Care," *Archives of Internal Medicine* 149 (1989): 1303-05.

22. S.H. Miles, "Informed Demand for 'Non-Beneficial' Medical Treatment," *New England Journal of Medicine* 325 (1991): 512-15.

23. R.A. Pearlman and R.F. Uhlmann, "Quality of Life in Chronic Diseases: Perceptions of Elderly Patients," *Journal of Gerontology* 43 (1988): M25-30.

24. R.A. Pearlman and A. Jonsen, "The Use of Quality-of-Life Considerations in Medical Decision Making," *Journal of the American Geriatric Association* 33 (1985): 344-52.

25. R.S. Schonwetter et al., "Resuscitation Decision Making in the Elderly: The Value of Outcome Data," *Journal of General Internal Medicine* 8 (1993): 295-300.

26. S. Braithwaite and D.C. Thomasma, "New Guidelines on Foregoing Life-Sustaining Treatment in Incompetent Patients: An Anti-Cruelty Policy," *Annals of Internal Medicine* 104 (1986): 711-15.

27. M. Siegler, "Decision-Making Strategy for Clinical-Ethical Problems in Medicine," *Archives of Internal Medicine* 142 (1982): 2178-79.

28. P.N. Lanken, "Critical Care Medicine at a New Crossroads: The Intersection of Economics and Ethics in the Intensive Care Unit," *American Journal of Respiratory and Critical Care Medicine* 149 (1994): 3-5.

29. J. La Puma, C.K. Cassel, and H. Humphrey, "Ethics, Economics, and Endocarditis: The Physician's Role in Resource Allocation," *Archives of Internal Medicine* 148 (1988): 1809-11.

30. J.D. Lantos et al., "The Illusion of Futility in Clinical Practice," *American Journal of Medicine* 87 (1989): 81-84; S.J. Youngner, "Who Defines Futility?" *Journal of the American Medical Association* 260 (1988): 2094-95; L.J. Schneiderman, N.S. Jecker, and A.R. Jonsen, "Medical Futility: Its Meaning and Ethical Implications," *Annals of Internal Medicine* 112 (1990): 949-54.

31. A.R. Jonsen and S.E. Toulmin, *The Abuse of Casuistry: A History of Moral Reasoning* (Berkeley, Calif.: University of California Press, 1988).

5

Forgoing Life-Sustaining Therapies

James P. Orlowski

INTRODUCTION

One of the most difficult and angst-producing decisions and actions a physician can undertake is to forgo life-sustaining therapies. The physician and healthcare team anguish over the decision to withhold or withdraw life-support because healthcare providers see their role as one of saving or prolonging lives and view the forgoing of life-sustaining therapy as a personal affront and defeat. The patient and family often anguish over the decision because deciding to forgo life-supporting treatments usually equates with giving up the fight and accepting the inevitability of death.[1]

This chapter deals with the "how to" of forgoing life-sustaining therapies, a topic not previously handled in print. The life-sustaining therapies to be discussed include: cardiopulmonary resuscitation (CPR), admission to the intensive care unit (ICU), oxygen therapy, mechanical ventilation, dialysis, transfusions, inotropic and blood pressure support, antibiotics and other medications, surgical interventions and amputations, nutrition and hydration, burn care, and pain relief.

In this chapter, *forgoing* refers to withholding or withdrawing. *Withholding* a therapy means never starting the therapy, and *withdrawing* means stopping or terminating a therapy that has already been instituted.

DEFINITIONS AND PRINCIPLES

Life-sustaining treatment is any medical intervention, technology, procedure, or medication that forestalls the moment of death, regardless of whether the treatment affects the underlying life-threatening condition or biologic process.[2] Examples include ventilators, dialysis, CPR, acute surgical intervention, amputation, antibiotics, transfusions, nutrition, and hydration.

Discussions about forgoing life-sustaining treatments are often undertaken when death is the predictable or unavoidable result of the patient's underlying medical condition. A patient need not be terminally ill or imminently dying, however, for these discussions to take place. In fact, it is preferable that some conversations and decisions occur when the individual is still healthy and not in the process of dying, so that the patient's life values and goals can be delineated and appreciated without duress.[3]

One of the guiding principles of medicine is that the health and well-being of the individual patient is of paramount consideration. In keeping with this philosophy, there is a legitimate moral and legal presumption in favor of preserving life and providing beneficial medical care with the patient's informed consent.[4]

Clearly, however, avoiding death should not always be the preeminent goal.[5] Not all technologically possible means of prolonging life need be or should be used in every case. For the gravely ill patient and for his or her family, friends, and healthcare providers, decisions about withdrawing life-sustaining treatment may have more obvious consequences than decisions about starting a treatment.

From a medical standpoint however, it is usually better to initiate a treatment provisionally with a plan for stopping the therapy if it proves ineffective or unduly burdensome to the patient. The rationale for this approach is based on the uncertainty in medical science as to whether an individual patient may profit from a therapy, even through statistically the odds may be low. This approach is preferable to withholding a treatment altogether for fear that stopping the therapy will be impossible.[6]

When it is unclear whether the burdens or benefits are overwhelming, it is appropriate to choose on the side of life and provide the treatment. If a treatment is clearly futile in the sense that it will not achieve its physiologic objective and thus offers no benefit to the patient, there is no obligation to provide the treatment. It is both ethically and morally preferable to try a treatment and to withdraw it if it fails than not to try it at all in appropriate situations.

EXTRAORDINARY VERSUS ORDINARY

The terms *extraordinary* and *ordinary* have been used in the past to distinguish a class of treatments that might ethically be withheld or withdrawn from those treatments that must be provided. Unfortunately, these terms became a source of great confusion. People began to distinguish ordinary from extraordinary by appealing to the prevalence of a treatment or its level of technologic complexity. No treatment is intrinsically ordinary or extraordinary.[7] Instead, decisions should be based on a balancing of the potential benefits of the therapy versus the potential burdens to the patient. A clearly beneficial treatment should be provided unless the patient refuses the therapy, whereas clearly nonbeneficial or overwhelmingly burdensome therapies need not be provided.

AUTONOMY OR SELF-DETERMINATION

Patients have an ethical and legal right to control what happens to their bodies, so the decision about whether to use life-sustaining therapy should, in the final analysis, be theirs. This is often referred to as the principle of self-determination or autonomy. When a patient's request for specific therapy conflicts with the physician's judgment as to what is best for the patient, there is no obligation either to render useless care or to violate an established community standard of practice.[8] Rather, physicians should decide how much to do according to what they perceive is best for that patient.

A physician is entitled to decline to provide any treatment that he or she believes to be nonbeneficial or potentially harmful. There is, however, a distinction between treatment that a physician believes to be detrimental to a patient's health or best interest, and treatment to which a physician has a conscientious objection or personal bias. A physician must not allow the decision regarding what is in the best interest of the patient to be influenced by his or her own personal beliefs. When the patient opts for a course of action that violates the healthcare professional's personal ethical or religious convictions, the professional should discuss the conflict with the patient and, if necessary, transfer the patient's care to another professional with the patient's consent.[9]

The basic ethical principle is that competent and informed patients have the right to decide for or against therapy. A patient's decision does not need to be logical or consistent with the opinion of the majority. As long as the patient is capable of decision making, his or her decision should be respected.

CAPACITY VERSUS COMPETENCY

Proper determination of capacity is crucial to an ethical decision-making process. Caregivers have a duty to respect the wishes of a patient with decision-making capacity. Capacity differs from competence. *Competence* and *incompetence* are legal terms and are restricted generally to situations in which a formal judicial determination has been made. *Decision-making capacity* refers to a patient's functional ability to make informed healthcare decisions in accordance with the patient's personal values. The key elements[10] of decision-making capacity are as follows:

- the ability to comprehend information relevant to the decision
- the ability to deliberate about the choices in accordance with personal values and goals
- the ability to communicate either verbally or non-verbally with the caregivers

LIVING WILLS AND ADVANCE DIRECTIVES

Living wills and other advance directives such as durable powers of attorney for healthcare decisions document in writing a person's desires for treatment and terminal care or designate individuals to speak on behalf of the patient if and when the patient becomes incompetent or incapacitated. Advance directives endorse the right of a patient with decision-making capacity, or a designated surrogate for a patient who lacks capacity, to decide to forgo any life-sustaining medical treatment.

SURROGATE DECISION MAKERS

When a patient lacks decision-making capacity and the healthcare team's attempts to restore the capacity fail (for example, by rectifying reversible causes such as overmedication, pain, or dehydration) or are not possible, a surrogate needs to be identified who will be the ultimate source of consent or refusal to the healthcare team's plan of action. In identifying such an individual, the physician should first honor any surrogate the patient has chosen in advance or a court-appointed surrogate if such exists. In the absence of the aforementioned the goal is to find the person who is most involved with the patient and most knowledgeable about the patient's present and past feelings and preferences. This person may be the spouse, parent, adult son or daughter, adult brother or sister, legal guardian, or a close friend. A family member is generally the best choice, although in situations involving estranged family members, a friend or significant other may be a better choice than an emotionally distant family member.

In the absence of an available or willing surrogate, one may need to be appointed and his or her decisions reviewed by an ethics committee. Alternatively, an ethics committee, in its role as a neutral third party, may function as a surrogate. The primary function of the surrogate is to make choices as the patient would if he or she were able; this is known as the *substituted-judgment standard* of surrogate decision making.[11] In the absence of knowledge of the patient's values and wishes, one must operate on the *best-interest standard* of surrogate decision making, where one decides on a course of action based on what is presumed to be in the patient's best interest.[12]

By law and custom, parents usually act as the surrogate decision makers for their child. In the rare case where the parents' choice of treatment is considered contrary to the child's best interest, an ethics committee may be consulted. Referral to a court of law should be used only as a last resort.

THE PERSISTENT VEGETATIVE STATE AND BRAIN DEATH

The *persistent vegetative state* is a condition of prolonged unconsciousness in which patients are unaware of themselves or their environment. They exhibit no voluntary actions or behaviors, although they may exhibit periods of eyes-open wakefulness alternating with periods of sleep. This ability to demonstrate sleep/awake cycles and yet be totally unaware is the result of a functioning brainstem in the face of total loss of cerebral cortical functioning. The persistent vegetative state becomes the *permanent vegetative state* after a sufficient period of time has passed that the chances of recovery become remote (generally six months).[13]

Patients in PVS (persistent or permanent vegetative state) are generally able to breathe spontaneously and exhibit primitive reflexes (such as hand grasping, rooting, and sucking) and vegetative functions (such as swallowing and eye blinking) controlled by the brain stem, but they do not have the capacity to experience pain or suffering because of the absence of cerebral cortical functioning. Patients in PVS can survive for prolonged periods of time as long as nutrition and hydration are provided artificially.[14]

Brain death results from brain damage that is so severe and extensive that the brain ceases to function effectively and has no potential for recovery. By definition, breathing has irreversibly ceased, owing to structural damage to the brain and absence of brainstem function. Circulation is maintained, however, because of artificial ventilation. There is general agreement in the medical profession that death of the brain is an appropriate determination of death of a human being.

The concept that death can be determined based on irreversible cessation of all functions of the brain including the brain-stem is recognized through statutes or judicial decisions in all states in the United States. The model statute states that an individual is dead if he or she has sustained either irreversible cessation of circulatory and respiratory functions or irreversible cessation of the function of the entire brain (including the brain stem), with the determination of death being made in accordance with accepted medical standards. Because the individual is dead, the concepts of life-sustaining or death-prolonging therapies become immaterial. An individual who is brain dead is dead. Any and all treatments can and should be discontinued.

ETHICS COMMITTEES

Ethics committees have been established to provide consultation in difficult or complicated cases. They explore legal, medical, and ethical issues and mediate conflicts among family members or with the healthcare team. They can also help to uncover different views regarding prognosis and indications for treatment. Committee review can provide assurance that full and impartial consideration has been given to a difficult ethical decision, such as forgoing life-sustaining therapy.

A number of professional medical and ethical organizations, including the American Medical Association, the Hastings Center, the President's Commission for the Study of Ethical Problems in Medicine and Biomedical and Behavioral Research, the American College of Physicians, and the Society of Critical Care Medicine, have published statements or reports on forgoing life-sustaining or death-prolonging therapy.[15]

GUIDELINES AND SUGGESTIONS FOR WITHHOLDING OR WITHDRAWING SPECIFIC TREATMENTS

The steps in withdrawing or withholding life-sustaining or death-prolonging therapy are as follows:
1. Establish the medical facts, prognosis, the benefits and burdens of treatment, and the likely outcomes of forgoing therapy.
2. Ascertain the patient's preferences, either directly if the patient is capable, or via a surrogate if the patient is incapacitated.

3. Agree on a course of action; anticipate and discuss potential complications when possible. Agree on primacy of comfort measures, level of consciousness, pain relief, and other factors of concern to patient, family, and healthcare providers.
4. Involve all healthcare providers and patient's family or significant others in discussion and decisionmaking as much as possible.

The following specific treatments should be discussed with patients or surrogates and addressed in considerations of withholding or withdrawing life-sustaining therapies:

- CPR
- ICU admission
- oxygen therapy
- mechanical ventilation
- dialysis
- transfusion
- inotropic and blood pressure support
- antibiotics and other medications
- surgical interventions and amputations
- nutrition and hydration
- burn care
- pain relief

CARDIOPULMONARY RESUSCITATION

Cardiopulmonary resuscitation (CPR) refers to those measures used to restore ventilation and circulation in victims in whom these functions have been interrupted. These techniques represent the pinnacle of life support because they have the potential of reversing death. Resuscitation techniques have no value in the management of irreversible or terminal disease states. The purpose of CPR is to revive otherwise healthy individuals who experience a reversible catastrophe that interrupts breathing and circulation.[16]

The decision to withhold CPR is designated by the do-not-resuscitate (DNR) order.[17] The withdrawal of CPR is a decision that a physician can make when the victim has failed to respond within a reasonable time to standard and proper CPR measures; this is usually between 10 and 30 minutes when advanced cardiac life support measures have been employed and have failed to be effective. CPR can be withheld in circumstances where death is irreversible, either because of the severity of the injury or the length of time the person has been dead. Examples include decapitation, rigor mortis, dependent lividity, and decomposition.

Because of the emergency nature of CPR, a patient or surrogate should be consulted in advance whenever possible about whether to commence resuscitation in the event of cardiac or respiratory arrest. Any patient who is at increased risk for cardiopulmonary arrest should be given the opportunity to make a decision about CPR while still capable of making the decision.

Researchers have investigated the outcomes of CPR performed out of the hospital, in hospital, and in the ICU, in terms of immediate survival, survival to hospital discharge, and long-term survival.[18] Various studies have documented a 2 to 3 percent incidence of PVS after CPR.[19] The immediate and short-term survival rate for in-hospital CPR is generally only 15 to 20 percent and, in patients with metastatic cancer or New York class IV heart failure, the survival rate is nil.[20] These studies have prompted some experts to characterize in-hospital CPR as a "desperate technique that works relatively infrequently, and in many types of patients, virtually never."[21]

In the absence of a DNR order, resuscitation should be attempted and, if any doubt exists over whether a decision to forgo treatment has been properly made, treatment should be given. "Show codes," where one goes through the motions of performing CPR without any intention of performing proper or effective CPR, or "slow codes," where one purposely delays instituting proper CPR techniques in order to lessen the likelihood of success, should be avoided. Any code or resuscitation should be a full code, unless previously agreed to by the patient or surrogate.

Limited CPR refers to situations where the physician and patient agree to a partial or incomplete attempt at resuscitation in the event of a cardiopulmonary arrest.[22] For example, a patient may refuse cardiac massage or intubation but permit the administration of resuscitation drugs, defibrillation, or brief bag-and-mask ventilation. Such limits on resuscitation are appropriate in select circumstances.

At the time of cardiac and/or respiratory arrest, the healthcare professional summoned to direct the resuscitation may realize that CPR cannot restore cardiac and respiratory function, either because CPR is failing to work or because of the patient's underlying medical conditions.[23] In these cases, the professional may call off the effort and discontinue CPR.

Likewise, when a patient is receiving full but ineffective treatment for failure of other organ systems in the ICU and then develops irreversible hemodynamic or respiratory failure, it is appropriate not to institute CPR (for example, a patient is receiving maximal inotropic/pressor support with an agent like epinephrine for shock, but the shock remains refractory and continues to worsen). This situation has been referred to as an "ongoing chemical code."[24] If that patient suffers a cardiac arrest, resuscitation is not going to work because the patient's shock is already refractory to epinephrine, and epinephrine is the pharmacologic mainstay of CPR. Likewise, a patient with severe adult respiratory distress syndrome on 100 percent oxygen, who continues to deteriorate and arrests from hypoxia, will not respond to CPR since one cannot provide anything more than 100 percent oxygen.

CPR was never intended to be applied to individuals with irreversible or terminal disease states.[25] CPR has become a therapy that is applied indiscriminately to anyone who arrests, regardless of underlying disease, except where a DNR order has been appropriately recorded.[26] CPR has been characterized as the only medical therapy that can be administered without a physician's order, and instead requires a physician's order to withhold it. Clinicians are faced with the deplorable situation of instituting CPR in patients with known hopeless and terminal disease states, only because the appropriate DNR order is lacking.[27] This has created serious ethical quandaries not only for emergency room and hospitalized patients, but also for individuals with terminal illness who desire to die at home. Home care hospice services and emergency medical services (EMS) are beginning to address the best ways to handle patients with terminal illness who are outside of the medical environment and desire not to be resuscitated.

The best way to handle a cardiopulmonary arrest or impending arrest in a hopelessly and terminally ill person at home or outside of the hospital is not to call EMS. A number of states have enacted legislation that permits DNRO orders (DNR orders outside of the hospital); such orders, which instruct EMS not to resuscitate, have been signed by a physician and are prominently displayed in the home and kept with the patient wherever he or she goes.[28] Copies of these orders are often kept at the local EMS station to ensure compliance. Many individuals do not realize that once EMS has been summoned, a nonphysician cannot instruct EMS to refrain from resuscitating the victim and that producing a living will or advance directive will not stop the resuscitative efforts. EMS can only withhold or withdraw CPR in the face of a legitimate DNRO order.

Another area of conflict in the past was the issue of DNR in the operating room. For a long time, surgeons and anesthesiologists insisted that if a patient with a DNR order needed an operation, the DNR order had to be rescinded during the surgery and immediate postoperative period. The rationale was that if the patient consents to an operation, he or she consents to CPR. Proponents of this practice claimed that the normal practice of anesthesia for surgery entailed the use of many components of CPR, including intubation, ventilation, and pharmacologic agents to support blood pressure and treat arrhythmias. If one defines CPR in the operating room as external or internal cardiac massage and defibrillation, then DNR can appropriately be maintained throughout surgery and the postoperative period for patients who desire to retain their DNR status. A patient with a DNR order may require surgery for a surgical emergency unrelated to the primary disease (such as for appendicitis or a traumatic accident) or for palliative care of the primary disease. Such patients have a right to insist on keeping their DNR status if they wish during and immediately after surgery. The presumption is that, if such patients should arrest in the operating room from causes related or unrelated to their primary disease, their prognosis for meaningful, sapient recovery would be very low and that they would prefer to die under anesthesia peacefully and quickly rather than to die as expected from their primary disease.

ADMISSION TO THE INTENSIVE CARE UNIT

Patients may choose to forgo ICU admission, often as a component of forgoing life-sustaining therapy. Although it is possible to decide to forgo CPR but still desire ICU monitoring and therapy, the opposite is usually not possible. A patient who desires CPR will generally require ICU admission if CPR is successful, except perhaps in the most limited of CPR attempts.

Some combinations of patient desires to forgo life-supporting therapies may be inappropriate or inconsistent (for example, desiring CPR but refusing ICU admission, or refusing intubation and mechanical ventilation but desiring CPR). Intubation is a standard component of advanced CPR and, if CPR is successful, the patient often ends up in the ICU on a ventilator. The physician needs to clarify these inconsistencies.

The following patients are candidates for admission to ICU when it is consistent with their preferences for treatment and their goals:

- critically ill patients who require life support for organ-system failure that may be reversible or remedial

- patients with irreversible organ failure who cannot be treated appropriately in another setting
- patients at risk of life-threatening complications who require monitoring or treatment
- patients who are receiving a trial period of monitoring or treatment when there is doubt about the prognosis or the effectiveness of therapy[29]

A decision to forgo some forms of life-sustaining treatment such as CPR should not preclude other forms of treatment and admission to the ICU. The intent of ICU admission is usually to employ treatment that potentially will avoid the necessity of CPR.

Admission to an ICU should be subject to the constraints imposed by the availability of space, equipment, and personnel; the needs of patients already in the unit; and the needs of others who are also candidates for admission. The following patients generally should not be admitted to the ICU:

- patients with documented irreversible cessation of all functions of the entire brain including the brainstem (brain death) (An exception would be maintenance of organ viability for transplantation.)
- patients who have been conclusively diagnosed as irreversibly unconscious (PVS or coma)
- patients with irreversible illness who are near death (terminally ill)
- patients who, while capable of making decisions, have requested that they not receive intensive care or its equivalent (Patients are entitled to refuse admission to an ICU even when doing so puts them at risk of death.)

Patients should not be able to demand admission to an ICU. Such a demand by a patient or surrogate may be denied if admission would be medically inappropriate for the patient, detrimental to patients already in the ICU, or contrary to the admission criteria of the ICU.[30] Examples of such inappropriate admissions include a surrogate demanding ICU admission and care for a patient with brain death, or a patient demanding ICU admission for a noncritical illness.

Patients should be transferred from the ICU to another setting within the hospital or to another institution when intensive care will no longer benefit them, either because they have improved to a point where intensive care is no longer necessary or because they have deteriorated to a point where intensive care no longer offers reasonable promise of benefit. Such triage is ethically appropriate based on the principles of justice and beneficence/nonmaleficence.[31]

Although patients have a right to forgo life-sustaining treatment even when it is medically feasible or indicated, they do not have the right to demand futile or medically contraindicated therapy. With the privilege of autonomy comes certain responsibilities, not the least of which is to use medical technology appropriately and not to abuse its availability. For example, a patient with end-stage malignant cancer who has exhausted all treatment modalities can refuse experimental therapy, but he or she cannot demand ICU admission and lifesupport or cryogenic preservation in the hope of surviving until a cure is found.

A number of recent studies have examined the preferences of patients and their families for intensive care and compared them with nurses' and physicians' assessments of the value of intensive care. The assessments of neither relatives, nurses, nor physicians correlated strongly with patients' wishes or decisions.[32] These studies reported that patients believed that quality of life was a less important factor in judging the usefulness of intensive care than did their nurses. Physicians' evaluations of intensive care for patients under ideal life circumstances were strongly correlated with physicians' personal preferences for intensive care. Even family members do not decide as patients would decide. These findings raise serious questions about surrogate decision making and substituted judgment by family members, who are usually chosen as surrogates when patients are no longer capable of decision making.

OXYGEN THERAPY

Oxygen therapy is usually withheld or withdrawn as part of the overall approach to withdrawing life support in terminally ill patients, as a component of DNR, or as a component of forgoing ventilatory support.

The withholding or withdrawing of oxygen therapy can hasten death in a terminally ill patient while the provision of oxygen can prolong the dying process. Clinicians often forgo oxygen therapy in comatose or PVS patients in whom life-sustaining therapy is being withheld or withdrawn, in order not to prolong death. In conscious patients, forgoing oxygen therapy can produce agitation and anxiety, which are the symptoms of hypoxia. To counteract these adverse effects of hypoxia, clinicians often use anxiolytic agents such as diazepam or midazolam, or combination analgesic-sedatives such as morphine. These medications can be given intermittently or continuously by the intravenous route or intermittently by the oral route. It is best to provide these pharmacologic agents on a scheduled basis rather than as needed in order to control symptoms effectively without periods of inadequate symptom relief. The medications should be titrated to achieve the desired effect, namely comfort of the patient, without concern for addiction or standard dosages. The amount of medicine needed to control symptoms is the amount of medicine that should be administered. Medication guidelines are given in Exhibit 5-1.

Fortunately, hypoxia is often accompanied by hypercarbia. Although hypoxia tends to cause agitation and distress, hypercarbia is sedating and has an analgesic effect, which often overrides the hypoxic distress. Nevertheless, adequate sedation and comfort should be provided pharmacologically as necessary.

MECHANICAL VENTILATION

The withdrawal or withholding of mechanical (artificial) ventilation is perhaps one of the most agonizing decisions for physicians and one of the most stressful situations for the healthcare team. A treatment can be ethically withdrawn whenever it can be ethically withheld. If it would be appropriate not to institute mechanical ventilation under specific circumstances (patient desire or hopelessness of situation), then it is ethically appropriate to withdraw mechanical ventilation under the same circumstances. But from a sociologic and psychologic standpoint, taking away life-sustaining mechanical ventilation or failing to institute it, and watching a patient struggle to breath, creates tremendous stress for the

Exhibit 5-1
Analgesia and Sedation of Patients Foregoing Life-Support

Drug	Route	Initial Starting Dose	Maximum Dose
Analgesics			
Morphine	IV, IM	0.1 mg/kg/hr	None
Fentanyl	IV, Oral	1-2 mg/kg/hr	Whatever is necessary
Hydromorphine	Oral, PR, IM, IV	0.1 mg/kg q 2 hr	None
Methadone	Oral	0.1 mg/kg q 4h	Whatever is necessary
Roxanol	Oral	.2 - .4 mg/kg q 3-4h	Whatever is necessary
Codeine	Oral	1 mg/kg q 3-4h	Whatever is necessary
Sedatives			
Midazolam	IV, PO	0.1 mg/kg	--
Lorazepam	IV, PO	0.05 mg/kg	--
Diazepam	IV, PO	0.2 mg/kg	--

healthcare team. The knowledge of what it must be like to die from respiratory failure adds to the duress of allowing a patient to die from forgoing mechanical ventilation. Fortunately, there is a great deal that the healthcare team can do to provide comfort and ease the death of the patient. In fact, once a decision to forgo life-sustaining therapy has been made, it is the team's responsibility to make sure the patient does not suffer.

It is not appropriate to remove a ventilator-dependent patient from a ventilator without the permission of the patient or surrogate, or to pretend to use the ventilator properly while intentionally using it inadequately.[33] If oxygen concentration or minute ventilation (tidal volume multiplied by respiratory rate) is decreased, the intent of withdrawing therapy should be stated. The responsible healthcare professional should not ask other healthcare personnel to carry out a decision that he or she would not personally carry out.

When a patient or his or her proxy decides to forgo ventilation, it is ethically acceptable to sedate the patient if necessary to ensure comfort. Supplemental oxygen can be used to relieve dyspnea caused by hypoxemia, with the understanding that oxygen may prolong the dying process. If relieving the patient's dyspnea or other discomfort requires sedation to the point of unconsciousness, it is ethically acceptable to do so with the approval of the patient or surrogate.

A combination of an analgesic and an anxiolytic is typically used when forgoing mechanical ventilation in patients. Physicians often prescribe a morphine drip and a midazolam drip intravenously in combination. The morphine drip is started at 0.02 to 0.04 mg/kg/hr and the midazolam drip at 0.02 to 0.04 mg/kg/hr, and both are titrated to ensure the patient's comfort. If the patient has already been on analgesic or sedative medications, those dosages can be used as guidance.

As a rule of thumb, a continuous drip intravenously is a better method of providing analgesia and sedation than intermittent parenteral or oral medications in the patient where mechanical ventilation is being forgone. The patient may prefer oral medication if alert, rather than have an intravenous line started, but oral medications are slower to act, more unpredictable, and much more difficult to titrate to achieve the desired effect. Continuous infusion is preferred to intermittent bolus administration because the desired degree of sedation and analgesia can be obtained with minimal side effects; bolus medication doses sufficient to control symptoms and prevent suffering often produce respiratory depression, apnea, and hypotension, which may hasten or even contribute to death.

The ethical principle of "double effect" states that, if one's intent in administering sedative and analgesic medications is to provide patient comfort but side effects of the medications hasten or contribute to the patient's death, such hastening is acceptable as long as one's primary intent is not to hasten or cause death. If one can use medications to provide comfort that do not hasten death or use medications in such a way that comfort is provided with minimal adverse side effects, then that method is ethically preferable.

Providing comfort and preventing suffering often require the use of medicines that may hasten or contribute to the patient's death and, therefore, may cross the line from comfort measures to assisted suicide or euthanasia. Although this line is becoming increasingly blurred with greater acceptance of physician-assisted suicide and euthanasia, it is safe to say that as long as one's intent is to provide comfort and prevent suffering, it is ethically acceptable to use these medications in whatever dose is necessary to achieve the patient's comfort. The question of whether death is theoretically or actually hastened is probably irrelevant in the terminally ill patient.

There are a number of techniques for discontinuing mechanical ventilation when the intent is to forgo life-sustaining therapy. To some extent, these techniques can be thought of as a continuum from the minimally intrusive or invasive to the maximally intrusive technique of simply shutting off the ventilator and extubating the patient.

In the most critically ill patient, where maximal oxygen and positive end-expiratory pressure (PEEP) therapy are being employed to support life (for example, in adult respiratory distress syndrome), simply discontinuing PEEP therapy may be all that is needed to engineer the death of the patient. Obviously, the patient should have DNR status and receive comfort measures as necessary. Discontinuing PEEP therapy may result in rapid hypoxia and death even while mechanical ventilation and oxygen therapy are maintained. The next step might be to withdraw medically supplied oxygen therapy while still providing mechanical ventilation, by turning the oxygen level down to that of normal room air. Again, in the most critically ill patients, this minimally invasive maneuver may produce rapid hypoxia and death.

The next step might be to wean the patient from mechanical ventilation with sedation and analgesia if necessary, by decreasing tidal volume and/or rate (minute ventilation) and allowing carbon dioxide to build up in the blood. As stated earlier, hypercarbia can be sedating and produce an analgesia effect. One may reach a level of reduced mechanical ventilatory support that is incompatible with life in the particular patient without needing to discontinue mechanical ventilation completely.

An alternative approach is simply to discontinue the ventilator and, if desired, extubate the patient. This is the maximally invasive approach to discontinuing life support, but it is also the quickest, simplest, and most effective. The healthcare team provides appropriate sedation and analgesia before discontinuing mechanical ventilation and extubating, and then titrates those medicines as needed after extubation. The author's approach is to allow the family to be in the room throughout this time, and then to have the healthcare team leave the room, draw the curtains or close the door, and allow the family to be alone with the patient as long as they wish. The patient is monitored remotely for heart rate and respirations, with the in-room monitor shut off. If it is likely that the patient may need additional medications, a nurse or doctor may stay in the room with the family to titrate the medicines. If the need for additional medication is unlikely or unnecessary, the family is instructed to call the nurse or doctor if the patient seems uncomfortable or is struggling. The family is then notified respectfully when the remote monitor shows that death has occurred.

In pediatric patients, the author typically extubates the child and then places the child in the parents' laps, who are sitting comfortably next to the bedside. The parents are allowed to hold the child without the encumbrances of tubes and machines during the dying process, and for as long afterwards as they wish.

One area of controversy in discontinuing mechanical ventilation is whether neuromuscular blockades should be discontinued or reversed before removing the ventilator. If the patient is pharmacologically paralyzed when mechanical ventilation is discontinued, this condition guarantees that the patient will not be able to breathe. In the author's opinion, this approach crosses the line to euthanasia. Some authors have argued that if the intent and expected outcome of discontinuing mechanical ventilation is death, then using or maintaining neuromuscular blockade and paralysis is both quicker and more humane. However, this reasoning has many faults. First of all, one never knows with absolute certainty whether or how quickly a patient will die once mechanical ventilation is discontinued. Patients can continue to breathe for hours or days after ventilation is stopped, even though all of the experts predict a rapid demise. For example, Karen Ann Quinlan was predicted to die once mechanical ventilation was discontinued, but she lived for seven more years. Second, the use of neuromuscular blockade prevents assessment of the patient's comfort. A paralyzed patient may look completely peaceful and at rest but be suffering immensely from the inability to breathe. It is recommended that clinicians ensure that neuromuscular blockade is no longer present before discontinuing mechanical ventilation.

Conscious and competent patients may decline to be weaned from mechanical ventilation and may wish simply to be disconnected from the ventilator as part of the decision to forgo any and all life-sustaining treatment. In such a case, it is permissible to disconnect the ventilator without weaning.[34] Careful attention should be given to supplemental oxygen, sedation, and analgesia as needed. Only the rare patient desires to remain conscious during ensuing respiratory failure and, fortunately, carbon dioxide narcosis usually produces sedation and unconsciousness.

There is no necessity to continue to ventilate a patient who is brain dead, despite the requests or insistence of the family. The only exception would be to maintain organ viability for transplantation or to provide a reasonable opportunity for emotional acceptance of death. Otherwise, a patient who has fulfilled the criteria for brain death can and should be disconnected from life support.

DIALYSIS

It has become increasingly common for competent patients to decide to forgo dialysis.[35] Often these patients have decided that their quality of life is unacceptable on dialysis, and their opportunities for transplantation are remote or nonexistent. Surrogates also seem to have an easier time forgoing dialysis than forgoing other life-sustaining treatments in incompetent patients, probably because dialysis is viewed as an extreme form of medical technology that need not be employed in patients whose prognosis or quality of life is poor.

An essential part of the discussion of whether to forgo dialysis concerns the patient's transplantation options and the possibility of recovery of renal function. In order to make an informed decision about forgoing dialysis in either acute or chronic renal failure, the patient or surrogate must receive information about whether the renal failure can reverse, what the possibilities are for transplantation, and the implications of long-term dialysis and/or transplantation.

Because dialysis is often supervised most directly by personnel other than the physician, it is important that all such personnel participate in the evaluation process. It is important to explore with patients already on dialysis why they wish to stop the treatment. It may be that their discomfort can be ameliorated without stopping the treatment entirely.

Another important aspect of the discussion should be the question of where death will occur when the decision has been made to forgo dialysis. Often patients wish to die in the hospital where supportive and palliative care are readily available. If the patient wishes to die at home, the healthcare professional should inform the patient and caregivers of the risks and burdens, as well as the benefits. The patient's preference concerning the place of death should ordinarily prevail, as long as adequate care can be arranged.

The uremic effects of forgoing dialysis are often merciful; uremia from renal failure usually produces coma so that the patient does not suffer. Hyperkalemia, when present, often results in a rapid and painless death. In patients in whom death from uremia is not rapid and painless, the use of intravenous morphine or oral Robaxin (a muscle relaxant) along with parenteral or enteral midazolam can provide the necessary comfort. Cimetidine is useful for counteracting the pruritus of uremia.

Withdrawing dialysis once a patient has experienced the therapy is generally preferable to withholding it, although the ultimate decision rests with the patient. As a rule of thumb, trying a therapy, and then withdrawing it if it proves to be unduly burdensome to the patient, is preferable to never trying the therapy. However, in some situations such as multiple organ system failure, supporting a single organ system with a therapy such as dialysis is unreasonable, even though healthcare professionals have the technical capability to do so.

One study of forgoing dialysis lends support to the concept that families and physicians can decide in a manner similar to patients. This study reported no difference in decisions about treatment and the factors that govern those decisions, between 66 competent patients who decided to forgo dialysis and 66 incompetent patients for whom families and physicians decided to forgo dialysis. In addition, this study reported no important differences between the 17 incompetent patients for whom families decided to terminate dialysis and the 47 incompetent patients for whom physicians decided.[36]

A number of caveats are important in any situation where a patient desires to forgo life-sustaining therapy, but they are especially important in the patient with renal failure who decides to withdraw from dialysis. First, it is necessary to confirm, usually by psychiatric evaluation, that the patient is competent to make the decision. Various chemical imbalances and toxicities from renal failure and lack of dialysis can create organic brain syndromes that could alter the patient's capability to decide rationally. Second, it is important to explore the reasons behind the decision to stop treatment. Discomforts or depression can be ameliorated without resorting to a permanent solution to a temporary problem. Third, it is important that all healthcare providers, ancillary personnel, and family members participate in some phase of the discussion. Although the ultimate decision rests with the patient, other caregivers may have important observations and data to contribute, and many individuals will be affected to varying degrees by the patient's decision. All have a right to be heard, even though none has the right to overrule a competent patient's decision.

TRANSFUSION

Among the treatments a patient may choose to forgo is the administration of blood and blood products, including whole blood, red blood cells, platelets, white cells, plasma, and albumin[37]. This refusal arises most frequently on religious grounds, typically asserted by a Jehovah's Witness. An individual's freedom to act in accord with personal religious values is one aspect of autonomy, and the right of Jehovah's Witnesses to refuse blood should be recognized. However, as with nonreligious aspects of autonomy, the right of self-determination is not absolute. Exceptions include situations in which parents make decisions for a child or when the patient is pregnant or has dependent children. These exceptions exist because the right to forgo treatment may sometimes be restricted on the grounds that it will cause harm to specific others. Patients who are not Jehovah's Witnesses may also refuse blood and blood products.

The decision to refuse blood transfusion may occur at almost any time—in advance of any need for blood, when serious bleeding is expected but has not yet occurred, when bleeding is present but there is time to go through the entire decision-making process, or when treatment for bleeding has begun and the question is whether to continue.

All patients should receive treatment for bleeding in an emergency except when the patient, while capable of making decisions, has given direction refusing blood and blood products under all circumstances.

In the past, patients who refused blood or blood products did so almost exclusively on religious grounds, but in this time of the acquired immunodeficiency syndrome (AIDS) crisis, more and more patients are refusing blood transfusions out of fear of contracting this deadly disease. This situation creates a difficult dilemma for healthcare professionals. On the one hand a patient has the right to refuse any treatment; on the other hand, if the decision is based on misconceptions and irrational fears, the refusal may not be based on truly informed dissent. There is greater ethical and legal support for forgoing transfusions because of religious beliefs than for accepting a request to forgo transfusions from someone other than the patient when the basis for that decision is questionable or ill-informed. As in all situations involving forgoing life-supporting treatment, if questions exist about the validity or appropriateness of a decision in an emergency situation where the patient is incapable of clarifying or reaffirming his or her stance, it is better to err on the side of life and provide treatment, pending clarification.

The withholding or withdrawing of blood and blood products can be very stressful for the healthcare team, especially when the immediate consequence of forgoing this treatment will be death. Physicians and nurses in the ICU are used to concrete actions that aim to save a life or avert death. To stand by and watch a patient bleed to death is antithetical to the goals of critical care medicine. Fortunately, death from anemia is not usually terribly uncomfortable for the patient, as long as the bleeding site is not painful. Progressive, severe anemia, although causing tachycardia and tachypnea, results in unconsciousness or reduced consciousness. However, failure to clot can produce discomfort for patients, and disseminated bleeding can make breathing, swallowing, and bodily functions uncomfortable. Sedatives and analgesics should be administered to the bleeding patient when necessary.

There are a limited number of alternatives available for patients who refuse blood but will permit blood substitutes when faced with life-threatening anemia or blood loss. Blood substitutes such as the perfluoro chemical emulsions have not been proven effective in life-threatening bleeding or anemia. New hemoglobin substitutes such as stroma-free hemoglobin appear promising but are derived from blood products. Blood salvage and retransfusion is an option in only severely restricted circumstances and is usually not feasible in the typical acute ICU case. In patients with slow bleeding or chronic anemia, various options are available to individuals who refuse blood transfusions, including erythropoietin and intravenous iron infusions. These therapies, however, require seven to 10 days to produce a noticeable effect and therefore are not effective in the typical, critically ill ICU patient.

Blood and blood-product transfusions can be forgone by patients or families as part of withdrawing or withholding death-prolonging procedures, or by physicians when the transfusions prove futile and will not attain the physiologic goals.

INOTROPIC AND BLOOD PRESSURE SUPPORT

At times, patients receive inotropes (drugs to increase the pumping power of the heart) or vasopressors (drugs to increase blood pressure) for diseases such as shock, circulatory failure, or heart failure. Examples of these drugs include dopamine, dobutamine, amrinone, epinephrine, and norepinephrine; these drugs are often administered as continuous intravenous infusions. Some of these drugs are also employed in the pharmacologic armamentarium of CPR. In severe cases of shock, refractory circulatory failure, or heart failure, the doses employed as a continuous infusion may approach or even exceed the doses used in CPR. Such situations have been referred to as "ongoing chemical codes" in the ICU. These situations carry a very poor prognosis and, if cardiac arrest should occur despite these heroic efforts, CPR is highly unlikely to be successful. In such situations, it is appropriate to withhold CPR despite the lack of a properly executed DNR order, because of its futility.

Patients or surrogates may also choose to withhold or withdraw inotropes and/or vasopressors as part of forgoing death-prolonging therapies. Patients in shock or circulatory failure would generally not be competent to make such a decision themselves, but patients in heart failure (such as patients on dobutamine awaiting heart transplantation) could be capable of such decision making. Patients in shock or circulatory failure would be unconscious in all likelihood and would not suffer from forgoing these medications; however, appropriate efforts to ensure comfort would still be indicated. When conscious patients elect to forgo drugs such as dobutamine, healthcare professionals should pay careful attention to provide comfort measures including analgesia, sedation, and anxiolysis.

Because the half-life of these drugs by continuous infusion is relatively short (minutes), the drugs can usually be shut off without a necessity for weaning. If the drugs are producing any pharmacologic effect, their discontinuation will have fairly immediate effects. A word of caution is that sometimes discontinuing the drug results in improvement in the patient's blood pressure rather than the expected precipitous drop in blood pressure. This phenomenon only serves to reemphasize the folly in predicting to family members a rapid demise after the drug is discontinued.

ANTIBIOTICS AND OTHER MEDICATIONS

Patients or surrogates may also elect to discontinue other medications such as antibiotics and antiarrhythmics that may play a role in prolonging the patient's life or delaying death. When a decision has been made to forgo life-sustaining therapies, discontinuing these other drugs may be ethically and financially appropriate. Medications are expensive; if they are not contributing to the patient's comfort, they can and should be forgone. The only exception would be a situation in which discontinuing the medication might pose a risk to others (such as discontinuing an antibiotic for a contagious infectious disease).

Discontinuing an antiarrhythmic (a drug to counteract heart arrhythmias or abnormal heart rhythms) might be decided as part of a decision against CPR and for DNR status. Death from arrhythmia is usually quick and painless for the victim.

For years, pneumonia and other pulmonary infections were known as the "old man's friend," because dying of pneumonia with its attendant hypoxia and hypercarbia was believed to be rather painless. Before antibiotics, most elderly patients died peacefully of pneumonia. Thus, when a decision has been made to forgo life-sustaining therapies, forgoing antibiotics in the face of pneumonia or sepsis is not cruel and may, in fact, be humane. Nevertheless, when such a decision is made, the provision of comfort measures including analgesia and anxiolysis is preferable.

SURGICAL INTERVENTIONS AND AMPUTATIONS

Patients and surrogates may also choose to forgo surgical interventions including amputations as part of the decision to forgo life-sustaining therapies.

In *How We Die*, Sherwin Nuland recounts the story of Hazel Welch, a 92-year-old nursing home resident with crippling arthritis. She fell and was brought to the hospital, where evaluation revealed a perforated bowel. She refused indicated surgery, saying she had lived on this planet "quite long enough, young man." Nuland was incredulous and told her that her chances of successful surgery were one in three, compared to certain death without it. When he returned later in the day, she relented, stating "I'll do it, but only because I trust you." The operation did not go as easily as anticipated, and the patient experienced multiple postoperative complications. More than a week later, when Miss Welch could speak, she reproached Nuland for operating. She died of a massive stroke two weeks later.[38]

Nuland states that he realized that he was wrong to have insisted on the surgery. "Had I the chance to relive this episode . . . I would listen more to the patient and ask her less to listen to me." But then he goes on to state that he probably would not have acted differently, because not to operate would have risked the scorn of his peers:

It is in such matters that ethicists and moralists run aground when they try to judge the actions of bedside doctors, because they cannot see the trenches from their own distant viewing point. The code of the profession of surgery demands that no patient as salvageable as Miss Welch be allowed to die if a straightforward operation can save her, and we who would break that fundamental rule, no matter the humanness of our motive, do so at our own peril. Viewed by a surgeon, mine was strictly a clinical decision, and ethics should not have been a consideration.[39]

It is hoped that this book, *Ethics in Critical Care Medicine*, will help to change these attitudes. The ethics of a healthcare professional's decisions are as important as the technical aspects, and a procedure should not be undertaken just because it is technically feasible. One should also consider the ethical aspects of the procedure. What does the patient want? What are the risks and benefits? What are the chances that the patient will be helped by the procedure? Should the procedure be done in light of the patient's age, health status, and reluctance?

A decision to forgo surgery usually requires increased emphasis on comfort measures and pain control. It may also require decisions concerning antibiotics and other medications. Patients in serious condition who forgo surgery are often unconscious, and unconsciousness often blunts suffering. However, adequate pain management and comfort measures should be ensured.

NUTRITION AND HYDRATION

Medical procedures for supplying nutrition and hydration treat malnutrition and dehydration; they may or may not relieve the hunger and thirst that can occur. Conversely, hunger and thirst can be treated without necessarily employing medical nutrition and hydration techniques. For instance, dehydrated patients may have their thirst relieved by having their lips and mouth moistened with ice chips or lubricants.

Patients in their last days before death may spontaneously reduce their intake without experiencing hunger or thirst. In fact, dehydration may offer benefits for certain dying patients. Dehydration can reduce secretions and excretions, thus decreasing breathing problems, vomiting, and incontinence. Dehydration can also produce a sedative effect on the brain, making dying more tolerable.

The decision to forgo nutrition and hydration is one of the most difficult decisions because of the association of nutrition and hydration with basic human needs and caring. Individual cases should be decided by weighing potential benefits with the burdens to the individual of the technology needed to provide artificial nutrition and intravenous hydration. The artificial provision of nutrition and hydration is a form of medical treatment and may be forgone when requested by a patient.[40] Patients may also refuse to eat and drink. Clinicians have observed that this may not be an unpleasant way to die. Surrogates can refuse artificial nutrition and hydration but cannot refuse oral feeding and fluids if the patient will eat and drink willingly.

Forgoing nutrition and hydration is one of the most heavily debated issues in medical care and medical ethics at present. Clearly a competent patient has the right to forgo nutrition and hydration and its artificial provision as part of wishes to forgo life-sustaining and death-delaying therapies. What is contested is whether others such as family members or physicians can make the decision to withdraw or withhold the artificial provision of nutrition and hydration from incompetent patients when the patient's desires are unknown or uncertain.[41]

Various states have enacted laws regarding living wills and durable powers of attorney for healthcare that specifically exclude the refusal or discontinuation of nutrition and hydration unless provision of nutrition and hydration would shorten the patient's life, could not be assimilated, or would not provide comfort, or unless lack of hydration and nutrition would not result in death by dehydration or malnutrition. The official stance of the American Medical Association and the position taken by the President's Commission and the Hasting's Center are that the artificial provision of nutrition and hydration—that is, other than eating and drinking by mouth—is a medical therapy and can be withheld or withdrawn when it is no longer a benefit or when the burdens exceed the benefits.[42]

A decision to withdraw or withhold nutrition and hydration requires special attention to comfort measures and the provision of pain and symptom management.

BURN CARE

Burn patients differ from many other patients in the ICU because, in the early stages after injury, burn patients are often alert and capable of decision making despite the severity of their injuries. Such patients should be presented with the facts and options and permitted to forgo therapy if that is their wish.

Studies on patients with massive third-degree burns with low survival odds report that these patients often forgo aggressive treatment and opt for comfort measures only. Of 24 patients diagnosed on admission to have severity of injury without precedent for survival, 21 chose nonheroic medical care.[43]

Opting for only comfort measures allows the treatment team to concentrate all of their efforts on providing pain relief and comfort with the realization that the patient will not survive the injuries.

PAIN RELIEF

Pain relief is the most important aspect of providing humane care to dying individuals. Although the majority of dying patients do not feel substantial pain, most fear the possibility of pain—perhaps more than death itself.

Because the primary goal of compassionately caring for dying patients is to relieve their pain and suffering unless the patient chooses otherwise, measures involving substantial risk may be considered, although they might not be undertaken to relieve the discomfort of patients with a reasonable chance of survival. Examples of such measures include large doses of analgesics, percutaneous cordotomy, or neurolytic blocks.

The proper and adequate use of analgesics, especially narcotics, is critically important to alleviate pain for patients who are dying. Concerns about addiction or physical dependence are irrelevant to the dying patient. Likewise, psychological dependence on narcotics is most often the result of undermedication rather than overmedication. Patients are less likely to become psychologically dependent when narcotic agents are given on a prophylactic or anticipatory schedule to prevent pain, rather than in response to a request after pain is experienced.

The healthcare professional should ordinarily seek to give sufficient medication to relieve pain while allowing the patient to remain as mentally alert as the patient wishes. The continuous intravenous infusion of narcotics is appropriate therapy to alleviate pain and suffering in a dying patient, even to the point of unconsciousness with the consent of the patient or surrogate, and even though alleviation of the pain and suffering may hasten death.

Even in unconscious patients, it is recommended that healthcare professionals administer an appropriate dose of analgesics when withdrawing life-prolonging therapies, to ensure that the patient is not suffering or feeling pain. Pain relief and control is an important aspect of intensive care, and its provision in adequate doses or measures becomes paramount when a decision has been reached to forgo life-sustaining or death-prolonging therapies.[44] When medicine can no longer cure, it has a duty to comfort.

Although most dying patients probably do not feel substantial pain, it is better to err on the side of comfort and provide adequate analgesia. The continuous infusion of narcotics is appropriate therapy to alleviate pain and suffering in the dying patient.

Exhibit 5-1 lists the appropriate doses, routes of administration, and maximum doses for common analgesics and sedatives employed in the ICU and used when forgoing life-sustaining therapies. Note that there are no maximum doses for any of these drugs; one uses the dose necessary to achieve the desired goal of alleviation of pain and suffering.

NOTES

1. M.J. Edwards and S.W. Tolle, "Disconnecting a Ventilator at the Request of a Patient Who Knows He Will Then Die: The Doctor's Anguish," *Annals of Internal Medicine* 117 (1992): 254-56

2. Hastings Center, *Guidelines on the Termination of Life-Sustaining Treatment and the Care of the Dying* (Briarcliff Manor, N.Y.: Hastings Center, 1987), 1-69; President's Commission for the Study of Ethical Problems in Medicine and Biomedical and Behavioral Research, *Deciding to Forgo Life-Sustaining Treatment—A Report on the Ethical, Medical, and Legal Issues in Treatment Decisions* (Washington, D.C.: U.S. Government Printing Office, 1983).

3. Hastings Center, "Guidelines on the Termination," see note 2 above.

4. Ibid.

5. See note 2 above.

6. Hastings Center, "Guidelines on the Termination," see note 2 above.

7. Ibid.

8. See note 2 above.

9. Ibid.

10. Ibid.

11. Ibid.

12. American College of Physicians, "American College of Physicians Ethics Manual. Part 2: The Physician and Society; Research; Life-Sustaining Treatment; Other Issues," *Annals of Internal Medicine* 111 (1989): 327-35.

13. The Multi-Society Task Force on PVS, "Medical Aspects of the Persistent Vegetative State (Part I)," *New England Journal of Medicine* 330 (1994): 1499-508; The Multi-Society Task Force on PVS, "Medical Aspects of the Persistent Vegetative State (Part II)," *New England Journal of Medicine* 330 (1994): 1572-79.

14. Ibid.

15. American Medical Association, Council on Scientific Affairs and Coun-

cil on Ethical and Judicial Affairs, "Persistent Vegetative State and the Decision to Withdraw or Withhold Life Support," *Journal of the American Medical Association* 263 (1990): 426-30; Task Force on Ethics of the Society of Critical Care Medicine, "Consensus Report on the Ethics of Forgoing Life-Sustaining Treatment in the Critically Ill," *Critical Care Medicine* 18 (1990): 1435-39; see note 2 above.

16. "Standards and Guidelines for Cardiopulmonary Resuscitation (CPR) and Emergency Cardiac Care (ECC)," *Journal of the American Medical Association* 255 (1986): 2979-89.

17. P.A. Jonsson, M. McNamee, and E.W. Campion, "The 'Do Not Resuscitate' Order," *Archives of Internal Medicine* 148 (1988): 2373-75.

18. L.J. Blackhall, "Must We Always Use CPR?" *New England Journal of Medicine* 317 (1987): 1281-82.; G.E. Taffet, T.A. Teasdale, and R.J. Luchi, "In-Hospital Cardiopulmonary Resuscitation," *Journal of the American Medical Association* 260 (1988): 2069-72.

19. S. Bedell et al., "Survival after Cardiopulmonary Resuscitation in the Hospital," *New England Journal of Medicine* 309 (1983): 569-76.

20. See note 18 above.

21. Blackhall, "Must We Always Use CPR?" see note 18 above.

22. J. Wilson and D. Pugh, "Limited Cardiopulmonary Resuscitation: The Ethics of Partial Codes," *Quarterly Review Bulletin* 14 (January 1988): 4-8.

23. See notes 16 and 18 above.

24. S. Stern and J.P. Orlowski, "DNR or CPR: The Choice is Ours," *Critical Care Medicine* 20 (1992): 1263-72.

25. See note 16 above.

26. Blackhall, "Must We Always Use CPR?" see note 18 above.

27. Ibid.

28. R.J. Ayres, "Current Controversies in Prehospital Resuscitation of the Terminally Ill Patient," *Prehospital and Disaster Medicine* 5 (1990): 49-58.

29. Hastings Center, "Guidelines on the Termination," see note 2 above.

30. Ibid.

31. Ibid.

32. M. Danis et al., "A Comparison of Patient, Family, and Nurse Evaluation of the Usefulness of Intensive Care," *Critical Care Medicine* 15 (1987): 138-43; M. Danis et al., " A Comparison of Patient, Family, and Physician Assessments of the Value of Medical Intensive Care," *Critical Care Medicine* 16 (1988): 594-600; M. Danis et al., "Patients' and Families' Preferences for Medical Intensive Care," *Journal of the American Medical Association* 260 (1988): 797-802.

33. L.J. Schneiderman and R.G. Spragg, "Ethical Decisions in Discontinuing Mechanical Ventilation," *New England Journal of Medicine* 318 (1988): 984-88.

34. Ibid.

35. J.E. Munoz-Silva and C.M. Kjellstrand, "Withdrawing Life Support,

Do Families and Physicinas Decide as Patients Do?" *Nephron* 48 (1988): 201-05; D.C. Lowance, P.A. Singer, and M. Siegler, "Withdrawal from Dialysis: An Ethical Perspective," *Kidney International* 34 (1988): 124-35.

36. Munoz-Silva and Kjellstrand, "Withdrawing Life Support," see note 35 above.

37. J.M. Luce and T.A. Raffin, "Withholding and Withdrawal of Life Support from Critically Ill Patients," *Chest* 94 (1988): 621-26.

38. S.B. Nuland, *How We Die: Reflections on Life's Final Chapter* (New York: Alfred A. Knopf, 1994).

39. Ibid., 253.

40. R. Steinbrook and B. Lo, "Artificial Feeding—Solid Ground, Not Slippery Slope," *New England Journal of Medicine* 318 (1988): 286-90; see note 2 above.

41. Ibid.

42. See notes 2 and 15 above.

43. S.H. Imbus and B.E. Zawacki, "Autonomy for Burn Patients When Survival Is Unprecedented," *New England Journal of Medicine* 297 (1977): 308-11; S.H. Imbus and B.E. Zawacki, "Encouraging Dialogue and Autonomy in the Burn Intensive Care Unit," *Critical Care Clinics* 2 (1986): 53-60.

44. W.C. Wilson et al., "Ordering and Administration of Sedatives and Analgesics During the Withholding and Withdrawal of Life Support from Critically Ill Patients," *Journal of the American Medical Association* 267 (1992): 949-53.

6

Pain Management in the ICU

Serena J. Fox

*We must all die. But that I can save him from days of torture,
that is what I feel as my great and ever new privilege. Pain is a more
terrible lord of mankind than even death itself.*
—Albert Schweitzer

INTRODUCTION

There is no ethical debate surrounding the responsibility of the physician to alleviate pain, even when cure of the underlying disease is elusive or death is imminent. From antiquity to the present, pain has been addressed by physicians and its physiologic role acknowledged. In a series of lectures delivered at Yale University in 1913, William Osler traced the origin of medicine to "the primal sympathy of man with man . . . the desire to help those in sorrow, need, and sickness," and quoted the medical historian Payne as saying that the basis of medicine is "sympathy and the desire to help others . . . whatever is done with this end must be called medicine."[1]

The Greek physician Galen made the following observation in the first or second century A.D.: "If we could check the cause of pain, we would not only be able to overcome the symptoms but really treat the illness itself. If . . . we are unable to counteract the dyscrasia of the humors, at least we should be in a position to alleviate the intensity of pain." He went on to observe that it is "impossible to transmit the impression of pain by teaching, since it is only known to those who have experienced it."[2] Physicians who have been dealing with patients' pain for years are often extremely surprised when they experience visceral pain themselves.

It is the privilege of the modern intensive care practitioner to intervene in acute and life-threatening illnesses or accidents, and it is the healthcare professional's responsibility to use an expanded armamentarium of pharmacologic knowledge and technical ability to treat pain. No intensive care unit (ICU) patient need experience unrelieved, prolonged, or uncontrolled pain. However, high percentages of medical and postoperative patients do not receive adequate pain management, even in the ICU.

This chapter presents guidelines for the management of pain, anxiety, and agitation in the ICU setting, which are intended as a prototype for treatment. The nuances of drug choice, dosing, and delivery have been outlined in great detail elsewhere.[3] The chapter then offers a definition of pain and discusses three areas of ethical concern regarding pain control in the ICU: (1) inadequate management of acute pain, despite seemingly appropriate orders; (2) pain control during withdrawal of life support, especially mechanical ventilation; and (3) pain control at the end of life.

GUIDELINES FOR THE MANAGEMENT OF PAIN, ANXIETY, AND AGITATION

The goals of acute pain management are "(1) to provide for the emotional and psychological well-being of the patient and his or her family (patient satisfaction), (2) to provide superior pain relief with a minimum of side effects, (3) to restore or maintain preoperative physiologic function, and (4) to minimize postoperative complications and thereby shorten the duration of the ICU or hospital stay."[4]

Systemic (intravenous) opioid analgesics, morphine, and analogues remain the mainstay of treatment. Sedatives and neuromuscular blocking agents (NMB or paralytics), when indicated, are used in combination with analgesics. In 1995, the Society of Critical Care Medicine published guidelines for analgesia and sedation[5] and practice parameters for sustained neuromuscular blockade[6] in the critically ill adult patient who requires prolonged therapy. These guidelines, which are summarized below, were compiled by a task force of more than 40 experts in disciplines related to the use of analgesic and sedative agents in the ICU.

Conclusions: A consensus of experts provided six recommendations with supporting data for intravenous analgesia and sedation in the ICU setting: (a) morphine sulfate is the preferred analgesic agent for critically ill patients; (b) fentanyl is the preferred analgesic agent for critically ill patients with hemodynamic instability, for patients manifesting symptoms of histamine release with morphine, or morphine allergy; (c) hydromorphone can serve as an acceptable alternative to morphine; (d) midazolam or propofol are preferred agents only for the short-term (< 24 hrs.) treatment of anxiety in the critically ill adult; (e) lorazepam is the preferred agent for the prolonged treatment of anxiety in the critically ill adult; (f) haloperidol is the preferred agent for the treatment of delirium in the critically ill adult. This executive summary *selectively* presents supporting information and is not intended as a substitute for the complete document.[7]

Conclusions: A consensus of experts provided three recommendations with supporting data for achieving sustained neuromuscular blockade in critically ill patients: (a) pancuronium bromide is the preferred neuromuscular blocking agent for most critically ill patients; (b) vecuronium is the preferred neuromuscular blocking agent for those patients with cardiac disease or hemodynamic instability in whom tachyphylaxis may be deleterious; (c) patients receiving neuromuscular blocking agents should be appropriately assessed for the degree of blockade that is being sustained. This executive summary *selectively* presents supporting information and is not intended as a substitute for the complete document.[8]

In the executive summaries, the members of the task force define *analgesia* as the absence of sensibility to pain or noxious stimuli and *neuromuscular blockade* as the chemical interruption of neuromuscular transmission resulting in skeletal muscle weakness or paralysis. The clinically significant physiologic responses to pain that need to be prevented in critically ill patients include tachycardia, increased myocardial oxygen consumption, hypercoagulability, immunosuppression, and persistent catabolism (that is, the neuroendocrine stress response).[9]

Other modalities for pain control exist when prolonged, continuous analgesia and sedation are not indicated. These include patient-controlled delivery, central neural blockade, transcutaneous electrical nerve stimulation, and regional nerve-blocking techniques.

PAIN MANAGEMENT TECHNIQUES

ANALGESIA

Indications for analgesia with opiates include pain from pathologic processes and pain from diagnostic or therapeutic procedures. Risks of opiates include sedation, respiratory depression, constipation, urinary retention, nausea, and confusion. Opioid analgesics exhibit little if any amnestic properties.

NEUROMUSCULAR BLOCKADE

Indications for neuromuscular blockade include facilitation of mechanical ventilation, safe transport from the operating room to the ICU, certain procedures, prevention of intracranial pressure "spikes," prevention of bodily injury, facilitation of adequate oxygenation and ventilation in status epilepticus, decrease of metabolic demands during shivering or muscle rigidity, prevention of lactic acidosis in neuromuscular poisoning, tetanus, and neuroleptic malignant syndrome. Complications of prolonged paralysis include deep vein thrombosis, corneal ulcers, nerve compression syndromes, and muscle atrophy. Neuromuscular blocking agents are devoid of any amnestic, analgesic, or sedative properties. Always use these agents concurrently with appropriate sedatives or analgesics. Administration of sedation does not guarantee absence of patient awareness.

Two scientifically unverified complications of sustained paralysis are described often enough in the medical literature to deserve special reference. First, a nondepolarizing neuromuscular blocking agent should always be used to reestablish neuromuscular blockade when a nondepolarizing agent was used initially because the administration of depolarizing agents in this circumstance have been associated with exaggerated hyperkalemia.[10] Second, sustained neuromuscular blockade has been temporally and anecdotally associated with prolonged skeletal muscle weakness and/or paralysis.[11] Note, however, that the connection to neuromuscular blockade agents is based on histopathological findings that are difficult to distinguish from the myopathies and axonal polyneuropathies primarily associated with critical illness.[12]

Agents that are not recommended include tubocurarine (curare), atracurium, metocurine, and doxacurium.

Monitoring consists of constant surveillance, one-on-one nursing, frequent assessment by physical exam, laboratory testing, and maintaining a specific clinical end point to avoid undesirable accumulation of drug and/or active metabolites. Direct observation for ventilatory efforts does not ensure avoidance of toxic levels of a drug.

Peripheral nerve stimulation using train-of-four stimulation ("twitch monitoring") is the most widely used method in the operating room for quantifying the degree of neuromuscular blockade. In this test, an electrode connected to a peripheral nerve stimulator is placed over an easily observable peripheral nerve such an the ulnar nerve at the wrist. Four supra maximal electrical stimuli of 2 Hz are delivered .05 seconds apart. Four "twitches" can be observed when greater than 70 percent of the acetylcholine receptors are occupied. The ratio of the height of the fourth block to the first block is used to quantitate the degree of blockade. When the fourth twitch response is abolished, a 75 percent block exists. When the third and second are abolished, the blockade is 80 percent and 90 percent, respectively. When all four responses are absent, a 100 percent or complete block exists. The degree of blockade can be controlled by monitoring and documenting the train-of-four (number of twitches) and titrating the agent in use. Massive peripheral edema; peripheral nerve injury; or trauma, burns, or infections at the skin site may invalidate the test. Although the equipment needed to perform train-of-four peripheral stimulation is inexpensive, readily available, easy to use, and well-tolerated by patients, this monitoring device is not widely used in ICU practice.[13] There is a clear consensus among experts that peripheral nerve stimulation should be used to guide sustained neuromuscular blockade in the ICU.

PATIENT-CONTROLLED ANALGESIA

Patient-controlled analgesia (PCA) was introduced in 1984 as an alternative to conventional pain management. The use of PCA has resulted in better pain relief with higher patient satisfaction, more sustained levels of analgesic potency, less sedation, lower patient anxiety levels, lower or equivalent total amount of drug administered, fewer side effects, improved pulmonary function, fewer postoperative complications, and shortened hospital stay. It is standard of care for selected trauma, cancer, and general postoperative patients, and for patients following thoracic, obstetric, and orthopedic surgery.

An analgesic is delivered via a pump with a preset bolus dose and maximum hourly dose. The bolus dose may be superimposed on a background continuous infusion rate. A bolus dose is generally delivered when the patient pushes a button. A "lockout interval," in which no drug is delivered, even if the patient uses the system, prevents continuous dosing by the patient. A variety of commercially available devices accomplish this and provide documentation and security features.

The use of PCA is more likely to result in adequate, individualized dosing, with less fluctuation in analgesic levels. Side effects were estimated at approximately 0.7 percent in an analysis of 1,122 postoperative patients.[14]

The potential complications of PCA are those complications expected from narcotics. The most serious, respiratory depression, occurs with the same frequency as seen with other routes of narcotic administration. Patients who become ly sedated usually fall asleep and stop self-administering narcotics. This situation is more likely to occur in a small subset of patients with a continuous background infusion (such as patients with low pain tolerance) or in a monitored setting (such as the critical care setting).

Background infusion can improve the effectiveness of analgesia within 4 hours of treatment.[15] Ketorolac, a nonnarcotic, intravenous (IV) analgesic related to non-steroidal anti-inflationary (NSAID) drugs, may decrease total dose of PCA. Ketorolac is administered around the clock and concurrently with the PCA.

Although PCA has not been studied rigorously, this pain-management technique is excellent for cooperative, alert patients (such as postpartum, intermediate care, and conscious postoperative patients admitted to the ICU for "routine monitoring").

CENTRAL NEURAL BLOCKADE

Central neural blockade involves delivery of analgesics or anesthetics to the epidural, spinal, or intrathecal space. Epidural anesthesia is the most widely used of these techniques and has important applications to pain management in the ICU.

The use of epidural anesthesia was described as early as 1901. The use of postoperative intrathecal local anesthetics (bolus doses) was reported in 1949. Morphine was first used in the epidural space in 1979. With the development of continuous infusion and newer opioid derivatives, and the combination of opiates with local anesthetics, the technique has become more flexible. The ability to control pain without general sedation is of great benefit to selected groups of ICU patients.

Excellent pain relief can be achieved with epidural analgesia, especially in thoracic and abdominal procedures and with chest injuries.

Obstetrical patients and some patients with pulmonary disease are also excellent candidates. The use of epidural analgesia at cervical spine sites is associated with more complications than sites lower down the spinal column.

With the development of highly lipophilic drugs that are absorbed by epidural fat, there is less absorption by the central nervous system, hence less sedation. A combination of opioid and local anesthetic is commonly used. Patients who are awake can be weaned more rapidly from the ventilator, clear secretions better, and ambulate sooner than sedated patients. In addition it is easier to evaluate their mental status.

Risks of epidural anesthesia include technical complications during catheter placement, infection, spinal cord injury, bleeding, and medication side effects. Urinary retention and pruritus are common. Respiratory depression can occur up to 12 hours after opioid instillation. Hypotension, motor blockade, and dorsal root postganglionic neural blockade can also occur. The catheters are frequently placed and managed by a pain management team or anesthesiologist.

Epidural catheter placement is absolutely contraindicated in patients with bleeding disorders, local infections, elevated intracranial pressure, local trauma, anesthetic allergy, or inability to cooperate with catheter placement. It is relatively contraindicated in systemic sepsis, preexisting neurologic dysfunction, hypovolemia, some chronic obstructive pulmonary diseases, anatomical abnormalities, and some immune disorders.

Researchers who compare selective epidural anesthesia with systemic analgesics and local anesthetics report that epidural anesthesia results in superior analgesic effect, improved clinical outcomes with fewer postoperative complications, reduced length of stay in the ICU and in the hospital, and decreased morbidity and mortality.[16]

TRANSCUTANEOUS ELECTRICAL NERVE STIMULATION

Transcutaneous electrical nerve stimulation (TENS) is a form of afferent stimulation often called neuromodulation. The use of electricity to fight pain has been traced to antiquity. People who suffered from headache, gout, and other complaints were instructed to walk over tropical fish and electric eels buried in wet sand. The success of this treatment was questionable.

The technique has been modified since then. In 1965, the authors of the spinal-gate-control theory of pain hypothesized that stimulation of certain nerve fibers could impede pain signals moving through a "gate" region of the spinal cord, thus blocking them. Today, devices that do this are useful in a limited group of patients. These devices are noninvasive, noninjurious (of tissue), and relatively benign. In patients without a history of narcotic use these devices can decrease the amount of narcotics needed for acute pain. This technique is ineffective in patients who have used narcotics for longer than two months. Because it does not cause respiratory depression and sedation, TENS is an option for patients who have undergone thoracotomy or for patients with broken ribs.

Complications mostly arise as skin reactions at the electrode sites. Care must be taken in the region of the carotid artery bifurcation and over the skull in epileptics. Tolerance may develop over an extended period of time. TENS is contraindicated in first-trimester pregnancy and in patients who have demand pacemakers. It is of limited use in the elderly and in patients who are sedated or too impaired to manipulate the device. The role of TENS for critically ill patients has not been fully defined.

REGIONAL NERVE-BLOCKING TECHNIQUES

Many techniques for instilling anesthetics locally exist to manage isolated injuries. These include regional blockade, local infiltration, IV regional blockade (e.g. for manipulation of limb fractures), peripheral nerve block, intercostal nerve block, and intrapleural blockade.

SPECIAL SITUATIONS

Burns and multiple trauma represent special situations in which regimens of around-the-clock opiates plus ketamine anesthesia for procedures and bolus IV analgesia and sedation may need to be delivered. Patients with multisystem organ dysfunction are at high risk for being undertreated; these patients require regimens tailored to pharmacokinetics and altered metabolism. Pain management for patients with head injury and central nervous system pathology represents a challenge, especially when the blood-brain barrier has been disrupted, because an opioid-induced increase in arterial carbon dioxide tension can cause increased intracranial pressure. This risk must be balanced by the need to control agitation, ventilation, oxygenation, and catabolism. Short-acting agents that can periodically be stopped to allow evaluation of mental status can greatly assist in the care of these patients. Patients with central nervous system pathology who cannot communicate *must* be presumptively treated for pain and anxiety.

SUMMARY

Management of pain, anxiety, and agitation in the ICU is receiving more attention. This is due to increasing awareness of the physiologic consequences of acute pain and the evidence that many patients, including adult and pediatric postoperative patients, are vastly undertreated. A tremendous increase in knowledge about the physiology of pain; increased knowledge about the mechanisms of action of analgesics, sedatives, paralytics, and anesthetics; and the development of sophisticated delivery systems allow physicians to control pain effectively. Therapy consists of intravenous opioid analgesics; sedatives; and, in select cases, neuromuscular blockers administered at appropriate intervals or as a continuous drip. Intramuscular injection has no role in the ICU. Detailed knowledge of pharmacokinetics and drug interactions is necessary to decide on the effective drug, dose, and dose interval. Careful monitoring for clinical signs of pain or anxiety and for drug side effects is essential. Patients who cannot communicate must be treated presumptively. Sedatives are not analgesics. Neuromuscular blocking agents are neither analgesics nor anxiolytics; patients on continuous infusion of these agents require monitoring with a peripheral nerve stimulator. Selective techniques for regional pain control as well as patient-controlled devices should be considered for selected awake patients. Although not required, a pain management team is often beneficial.

DEFINITIONS

As might be expected in the high-technology environment of the ICU, most clinical guidelines are directed toward the treatment of acute pain. It is important to realize that untreated, acute pain can evolve into a chronic pain syndrome, and that patients who have been in the ICU for a prolonged course may also develop chronic pain, anxiety, and psychosis. Patients who have been on continuous drips for weeks often require weaning over an extended period. Withdrawal symptoms from nicotine, alcohol, and drugs also figure prominently in the assessment of and need for sedation, analgesia, and specific antidotes. The ICU patient may also have a history of chronic pain, psychiatric disorder, or substance abuse. A multidisciplinary orientation is warranted in pain management for the long-term ICU patient and may involve behavioral techniques and emotional support not routine in ICU activities.

ACUTE PAIN

Bonica defines *acute pain* as "a complex constellation of unpleasant sensory, perceptual, and emotional experiences and certain autonomic, psychologic, emotional, and behavioral responses . . . provoked by noxious stimulation produced by injury and/or disease of skin, deep somatic structures or viscera, or abnormal function of muscle or viscera that does not produce actual tissue damage."[17] Acute pain serves a biologic function of warning, fight or flight response, and limitation of movement.

By the time the patient has been stabilized in the ICU, many of these compensatory mechanisms have been addressed and hemodynamic stability has been achieved. The relief of acute pain then serves to mitigate the undesirable physiological burden that continued pain poses. It is useful to subdivide acute pain into three categories: (1) *background*—existing during rest or inactivity, (2) *acute response*—present during movement such as coughing or activity, and (3) *breakthrough*—occurring after seemingly adequate analgesia; may serve to alert the clinician to a new problem or exacerbation of an ongoing process.

CHRONIC PAIN

Bonica defines *chronic pain* as "pain that persists a month beyond the usual course of an acute disease or a reasonable time for an injury to heal or that is associated with a chronic pathologic process that causes continuous pain or pain that recurs at intervals for months or years."[18] He notes that many patients with chronic pain do not show the characteristic stress responses typically apparent in acute pain. He states that chronic, persistent pain never has a biologic function, but is a "malefic force that often imposes severe emotional, physical, economic, and social stresses on the patient and on the family, and is one of the most costly health problems for society."[19] That is, acute pain is a symptom; chronic pain (the pain itself) is a disease.

SUFFERING

Suffering has been defined as a state of severe distress associated with events that threaten the intactness of a person and may or may not be associated with pain. Although healthcare providers recognize that it is their responsibility to provide appropriate analgesia after trauma, the requirement to modify stress and mental discomfort is more controversial. Therapy is difficult to titrate because of the lack of clear end points.[20] An inexcusable example of iatrogenic "suffering" in the ICU is when clinicians inappropriately use a neuromuscular blocking agent to control agitation and movement without adequate analgesia and hypnosis. Lasting psychological trauma can result.

WITHDRAWAL SYMPTOMS

Patients with a history of substance abuse or preexisting psychiatric illness may have exaggerated responses to pain and require supranormal doses of medication to achieve an adequate result. Adjunct therapy with nicotine patches, antipsychotics, and psychosocial support as well as high doses of narcotics and sedatives may be necessary.

The ICU is not the place to subject patients to detoxification or to teach patients a lesson. Going "cold turkey" from substances such as alcohol or benzodiazepines can be fatal. Careful weaning of drips and judicious use of medications like methadone can be crucial. It is important to explain to the patient and the family why these medications are being used, since there is stigma in both the general and medical public associated with the use of certain substances. Chemical rather than physical restraints should be used whenever possible.

Adequate pain relief during critical illness does not lead to drug dependency and is a vital and integral part of recovery.[21] Healthcare professionals, especially physicians, tend to ignore the problem of drug abuse and addiction.[22] Lack of education and a fear of addiction make it more comfortable to treat the medical sequelae of addiction than the addiction itself. Low tolerance for the personality of the addict may contribute to this discomfort, despite scientific evidence that genetics may play a significant predisposing factor in addiction.

Abuse of drugs can exist independently from addiction and dependence, and is more common than either. Multiple drug use is common and may necessitate multiple withdrawals. Substance abusers are at high risk for trauma and winding up in the ICU. It is important for clinicians to overcome biases and maintain a high index of suspicion so that they can recognize and diagnose symptoms of withdrawal. Physical exam and toxicology screens assist the clinician if the patient's medical history is not immediately available. Specific antagonists should be considered.

If the decision is made to treat the patient for withdrawal, this is usually accomplished by a weaning schedule that reduces the dose of drug by 10 percent over approximately 10 days. The most common mistake is to increase the interval between doses of medication, often going beyond the duration of action of the drug. This error results in repeated withdrawal symptoms with only partial relief. Clinicians who prescribe drugs to treat withdrawal symptoms must have knowledge of pharmacokinetics; it is important for the prescriber to understand cross-tolerance and cross-dependence, as well as the appropriate dosage, interval, and schedule. Sudden cessation of alcohol and sedative hypnotics can be life-threatening. Unless the patient arrives in withdrawal, acute withdrawal should be anticipated and prevented from occurring in the hospital setting.

Treatment of intoxication and withdrawal and their medical sequelae is not a definitive treatment for addiction. Patients with addictions need referral for long-term treatment.

AGITATION

A large portion of ICU patients become agitated or disoriented at some point in their ICU stay. It is important to relieve agitation which, in itself, is associated with increased mortality and morbidity, while searching for an etiology. Agitation is frequently the result of physiologic decompensation; it can also result from sleep deprivation, loss of sensory cues, and rapid weaning or abrupt discontinuation of analgesia and sedation. Agitation can, but does not always, signify pain.

Acute brain dysfunction without apparent physiologic cause is frequently called "ICU psychosis." It usually manifests as agitation, but can also present as withdrawal (a catatonic-like state). Agitation can be physically harmful to the patient and also mentally distressing. Patients are often aware that they are hallucinating or that something is wrong but cannot control their fear. Psychotropic drugs are beneficial and warranted in this situation. In the case of advanced pregnancy, short-acting agents such as vecuronium and midazolam, as well as haloperidol and methadone, have been used successfully.

A MULTIDISCIPLINARY APPROACH

Pain control in the ICU is a challenge that requires a multidisciplinary approach. For acute pain, clinicians must administer rapid analgesia, sedation, and possibly neuromuscular blockade when indicated. Concurrently, they must monitor for symptoms of breakthrough pain, pay attention to pharmacokinetic detail, be familiar with treating preexisting or ICU-induced withdrawal symptoms, and monitor for and treat acute disorientation. Finally, it is within the realm of the intensive care physician to address suffering as well as pain.

Consider the following case:

A 41-year-old woman who was 21 weeks pregnant was admitted to the ICU in acute respiratory failure secondary to community-acquired pneumonia with adult respiratory distress syndrome. She had a history of severe sciatica with the pregnancy and smoked. She was hemodynamically unstable and required right heart monitoring and an arterial line. She was treated with fentanyl and midazolam via continuous infusion and IV bolus vecuronium to control severe agitation and allow permissive hypercapnia and elevated positive endexpiratory pressure. She improved over the following week and was maintained on a fentanyl patch (she had a documented morphine allergy) and IV lorazepam, as well as a nicotine patch. She had an acute exacerbation of respiratory failure during the second week, requiring open-lung biopsy and tracheotomy. She was put back on continuous sedation/analgesia and neuromuscular blocking agents. The patient improved with therapy but became disoriented and hallucinated during weaning from the IV drips. She was started on methadone and haloperidol, from which she was gradually weaned with much improvement in sensorium. She was discharged after one month on no medications for pain or anxiety. The fetus appeared to be growing normally. On follow-up one month after discharge, the patient had no recollection of pain and only remembered the last four or five days of her ICU stay. Her husband, however, remembered every minute.

The technology and pharmacology to relieve pain are widely available. Fear and anxiety related to pain influence the physician-patient relationship, and relief of pain is associated with great improvement in patients' complaints. Pain is commonly the reason that a person seeks the help of a physician in the first place. It is an important symptom and can lead to chronic complexes if not addressed.[23] The responsibility of physicians to relieve pain, regardless of whether they can influence the underlying disease, is universally accepted. The existence of inadequate pain control in many settings is disturbing and intolerable.[24]

AREAS OF ETHICAL CONCERN

INADEQUATE MANAGEMENT OF ACUTE PAIN

The advanced monitoring and life-support available in the ICU might suggest that inadequate pain relief would not occur often. However, it does. The following case describes a patient whose pain is not adequately managed despite seemingly appropriate orders:

A 76-year-old man with heart failure, atrial arrhythmias, and known occlusion of two out of four coronary vein grafts is admitted to the ICU with acute pancreatitis. The patient, who is chronically anticoagulated and whose level of anticoagulation is elevated above the therapeutic range due to acute liver congestion, is treated with intravenous fluid, antiemetics, and meperidine administered intramuscularly, as needed. He can take nothing by mouth. When this patient's son comes to visit, he notices that his father is grimacing, pale, has a rapid heart rate, and can barely speak. When the son suggests calling the nurse, the patient refuses, stating that the injections hurt more than his abdomen. The son asks his sister, an intensive care practitioner, whether anything is available to make their father more comfortable. The head nurse states that she prefers that her nurses do not give any pain medications by intravenous push for fear of complications. When PCA morphine or some form of IV analgesia is demanded, the head nurse is only too glad to arrange for the former. The patient's cardiologist thinks the PCA is great and asks the patient's daughter the next morning how it works. The patient, meanwhile, is resting comfortably.

Traditionally, especially in the postoperative setting, pain medication is given on demand by intramuscular injection at set intervals. In one study, Marks and Sacher documented that 73 percent of medical inpatients experienced moderate to severe distress despite orders for as needed (prn) analgesics.[25] A study of surgical patients reported that 75 percent experienced moderate to severe distress.[26] Underdosing occurred because of no adjustment in dose for weight, increased pain frequency, or previous response, and was compounded by physicians' fear of addiction and respiratory depression. Nursing choices reflected similar concerns. A conviction that complete pain relief is not necessary prevailed.

In one ICU, 5 to 10 percent of physicians and nurses advocated use of pancuronium (a neuromuscular blocking agent) for analgesia and 50 to 70 percent advocated its use for anxiety. Patients receiving this treatment are often critically ill, intubated, and on mechanical ventilation. Not only are they in pain, but they cannot communicate verbally. After they are given pancuronium, they are suddenly and terrifyingly paralyzed while awake.[27]

Equally horrifying is the finding that the bias against treating postoperative pain is exaggerated in pediatrics because of a misconception that children do not experience pain in the same way as adults. Shecter has documented inadequate pain relief for children with burns and children who have undergone circumcision and diagnostic procedures, reporting that "some were not treated at all."[28]

If, indeed, "the ineffectiveness of prn intramuscular opioids should be intuitive,"[29] why is this method of pain management inadequate and how is it perpetuated? Intermittent, intramuscular narcotic dosing can trap the patient in a cycle of recurrent pain and inadequate relief, exacerbated by delays in drug delivery and pain at the site of injection. A typical scenario finds a patient in sufficient pain to call a nurse, who then needs to evaluate the situation and decide to medicate. Both the patient and the nurse may be delayed for various reasons. If an order is in place, the nurse must obtain the drug and document its use. If the dose is too small, the cycle recurs; if it is too large, excess sedation occurs and the patient later awakens in pain. This scenario is assuming that the interval at which the drug is ordered and the means by which the patient is assessed for pain is accurate and appropriate. A pattern of peaks and troughs occurs, with periods of pain interspersed with too little or too much medication.

Factors responsible for inadequate pain control include underestimation of effective dose range, overestimation of duration of action, exaggerated fear of addiction, inadequate amount of narcotic prescribed, and an inadequate amount of narcotic given (when nursing discretion is allowed). Other issues include poor assessment of pain despite clear indications and appropriate orders. Common reasons for undertreating include inadequate knowledge of drug pharmacology; failure to titrate standard prescriptions to the individual; lack of appreciation for the importance of pain control; difficulty in pain assessment due to muscle relaxants, poor technique, or lack of standardized tests or scales; concerns about clinically significant side effects or risk of addiction; and failure to administer prescribed medications, because priority is assigned to other elements of care.[30]

In a 1995 study of the use of sedatives and analgesics in a surgical unit, morphine was the most commonly prescribed drug for pain and sedation. The dose administered was considerably less than the maximal dosage allowed by the physician. In addition, 90 percent of the orders were written on an as-needed basis. An increased number of sedative doses were administered between midnight and 4 a.m. Standard protocols and sedation scores were not used. Patients received 23 different drugs with an average of 1.9 drugs per patient. Trauma patients reported that they often felt that they had been treated for pain inadequately, although most of the physicians and nurses caring for them thought they were delivering adequate relief of pain. Approximately 80 percent of physicians and 40 percent of nurses endorsed use of diazepam (a muscle relaxant) for analgesia.[31]

Another study designed to describe dimensions of the pain experience in the ICU analyzed responses of 24 ICU patients. Of the respondents, 63 percent rated their pain as moderate to severe in intensity. The cardiac surgery patients reported a lack of total relief. They also described difficulties in communicating and nonpharmacologic methods that helped. The authors of the study note that pain research studies almost always exclude patients who are critically ill.[32]

In the ICU, patients with dysfunction of multiple major organ systems can be undertreated due to fear of worsening the clinical picture or precipitating side effects. Knowledge of pharmacokinetics is essential for treating such patients (for example, in the patient with renal failure, the clinician would choose a short-acting analgesic not excreted by the kidney). Patients with head injury present another challenging subgroup. It must be assumed that the head-injured patient requires analgesia especially in the situation of trauma. However, sedation can lead to increased carbon dioxide tension and perhaps elevated intracranial pressure, and sedation can make mental status examinations difficult. Again, short-acting drugs delivered by continuous infusion can be of great value. The patient can be awakened periodically, assessed, and quickly resedated.

One must also assume that a patient in the ICU who has been there for a while and no longer requires analgesics will require them on a short-term basis after undergoing a procedure (for example, a patient with chronic obstructive pulmonary disease who goes to the operating room for a tracheostomy and requires short-term post-operative mechanical ventilation). After several weeks in an ICU, the relief of pain and agitation may be more a matter of restoring eyeglasses and hearing aids, mobilizing joints with physical therapy, administering nonnarcotic analgesics, assessing for decreased vital sign measurements during sleep, and allowing liberal family visits—rather than administering narcotics. In addition it is also easy and important to medicate for pain during routine procedures such as central line placement in the awake patient.

In an era of minimizing costs, the ICU or a procedure room with monitoring equipment can be used for conscious sedation in patients who are very scared of simple procedures. Consider, for example, the following case:

A 41-year-old woman with a history of prolonged nausea and vomiting due to postoperative ileus was referred to the intensive care clinician for central line placement for total parenteral nutrition. The patient was diaphoretic and anxious and said that she would refuse the line unless she could be "put out." The patient was evaluated and reassured that this was fine. She was transferred to the ICU for monitoring during conscious sedation with fentanyl and midazolam and local administration of lidocaine. A subclavian catheter was placed without complication. The patient was sent back to the floor when she was fully awake. She was relieved and thankful.

Adequate pain control is the responsibility of the physician—on both medical and ethical grounds. According to Hess, "For the critically ill patient in an ICU, intramuscular use of narcotics seems totally unwarranted given the fact that almost every patient will have adequate intravenous access. Intermittent medication . . . provided by the nurse on patient request today seems ancient and out of place within the critical care practice."[33] This statement does not necessarily imply that intravenous administration of narcotics is the only acceptable way to control pain. Transcutaneous (transdermal) delivery systems (such as fentanyl patch) or intravenous nonnarcotic analgesics (such as ketorolac) can be used judiciously for some patients.

If a patient's pain cannot be controlled on the floor, he or she should be admitted to a monitored setting and supported (for example, with airway protection). Severe pain has physiologic consequences that limit recovery. As always, the risks of intervention, including analgesic and sedative regimens, must be weighed against the benefits, in order to cause the least harm to the patient. It is not acceptable to accomplish medical goals until they can be achieved with reasonable comfort. There may be time pressure to do this too quickly at the patient's expense. Clinical judgment is necessary to differentiate pain from anxiety, delirium, or withdrawal so that each may be treated accordingly.

PAIN CONTROL DURING WITHDRAWAL OF LIFE SUPPORT OR AT THE END OF LIFE

The high-tech environment of the ICU may present itself as a panacia to patients and physicians alike. What happens when intensive care "fails" or succeeds well enough to maintain life, but not living? Two events that arise in the intensive care setting deserve mention because they are sited so frequently and present such a challenge to staff who are trained in aggressive, acute care medicine: (1) withdrawal of mechanical ventilation (with or without extubation) and (2) the dying process (with or without withdrawal of inotropic or other support).

When "everything" has been done, one more task awaits the practitioner of the art of medicine—the choreography of a dignified death, as devoid of suffering as possible for the patient, the patient's loved ones, and the patient's caretakers. This task requires time; a modicum of privacy; openness to cultural rituals; and the commitment of the intensive care practitioner not to abandon the patient, the family, or the nurse and other healthcare professionals who have been involved in caring for a patient. Physical presence within reach of the bedside is respectful and responsible, and perhaps most difficult, emotionally, for the physician.

Although an ethics consultation is often not necessary in the ICU, it may facilitate the decision-making process and provide support. The multicultural and multidisciplinary composition of most consultation teams may enhance communication, especially where withdrawal of therapy is being considered.[34]

The amount of medication necessary to ensure comfort is not an issue. The intent is always to expedite comfort and dignity and diminish suffering. In many situations, "death" or impending death is what brought the patient to the unit in the first place, and the patient has arrived in a transitional, artificially maintained state of being. Death in an ICU does not have the implications of sudden collapse at the shopping mall, yet it may be nearly impossible to forgo acute, extraordinary resuscitative measures in the face of dying. Clinicians should remember that adequate treatment of pain supersedes life-threatening side effects (the "double effect").

In a study of 79 patients from whom life support was withdrawn, investigators concluded that large doses of sedatives and analgesics were ordered mostly to relieve pain and suffering during the withholding and withdrawal of life support and that death was not hastened by the medications.[35]

In 1989, 85 percent of deaths in the United States occurred in the hospital. Approximately 70 percent of these deaths followed a decision to withhold or withdraw life-sustaining therapy.[36] According to the *Medical Ethics Advisor*, "Suffering while dying must become a bad outcome in the healthcare system. Our society needs to create a vision for living well while dying."[37] Physicians must and do assist patients under their care in withdrawing unwanted mechanical and chemical support and must do so in a humane fashion.

The observation in the Study to Understand Prognosis and Preferences for Outcomes and Risks of Treatment (SUPPORT)(n = 9,105) that "substantial shortcomings" exist in care of seriously ill adults is sobering and calls into question how well physicians take care of the seriously ill. Of conscious adults who died in the hospital, 50 percent reported moderate to severe pain; 38 percent of patients who died spent at least 10 days in an ICU; only 47 percent of physicians knew when CPR was not desired; 46 percent of do-not-resuscitate (DNR) orders were written within two days of death; and intervention aimed at enhancing communication did not appear to change established practice or reduce use of hospital resources.[38]

Withdrawal of support does not necessarily mean the patient will die, but it is to be expected that a dying patient may die more quickly off of life support, with or without pain medication and sedation. It is unwarranted for such a patient to suffer. By the same token, a patient who appears comfortable or does not want to be groggy may not need medication. Examples of life-sustaining therapies that do not typically cause distress when withdrawn are cardiac bypass, dialysis, temporary pacing, antibiotics, and blood products.

Withdrawal of mechanical ventilation is a special category because of the emotional impact of cessation of breathing and the necessity to decrease respiratory drive in order to suppress feelings of dyspnea. Clear orders should be written that give the nurse at the bedside specific end points for giving medication and permit the nurse to use judgment in timing of the doses. Optimally, the physician remains at the bedside. Careful documentation of the rationale for medication is kept. Respiratory devices such as nasal continuous positive airway pressure should be used when indicated, for comfort, even if mechanical ventilation is refused or withdrawn. The use of neuromuscular blockers in the setting of withdrawal of mechanical ventilation is controversial and may make assessment of discomfort too difficult to warrant their use.

According to DeVita, "The goal of ventilator withdrawal is to remove unwanted or nonbeneficial therapy while guaranteeing patient comfort and dignity. In the United States, it is unlawful to cause patient death, although death remains the expected outcome of removing ventilatory support."[39] Fear of "killing" the patient and the threat of legal investigation results in reluctance on the part of the physician to order large doses of medication, even when it is agreed that the therapy being provided is not of benefit to the patient. Ambiguity is inherent in the concept of "double effect." Stated bluntly, guaranteeing comfort and dignity implies giving the amount of medication necessary. In the case of withdrawal of mechanical ventilation, enough medication to provide for the patient's comfort by suppressing dyspnea may hasten death.

Consider the following cases:

An 84-year-old practicing dentist is admitted to the ICU after failed angioplasty and coronary artery bypass grafting. His course is complicated by his return to the operating room for bleeding and cardiac tamponade, cardiogenic shock, nonoliguric renal failure, pneumonia, and hemispheric cerebrovascular accident (CVA). The patient's wife and daughters clearly state that the patient would not want prolonged life support if he could not return to an independent life. They are especially concerned that he has stated that he would not want to be on a breathing machine. The patient is gradually weaned from the ventilator over 24 hours. Orders for IV morphine and lorazepam are written. The patient is stabilized over the next week and transfers from the ICU to the floor. Several weeks later, he is transferred to a rehabilitation facility. He has significant neurologic sequelae following the CVA. A DNR order in case of acute deterioration is in place. The patient and the family have expressed satisfaction with what took place.

An 84-year-old woman with pulmonary edema is admitted to the ICU 24 hours after elective surgery. She has been up and walking while on the floor and has been fully independent prior to admission. Her course was complicated by aspiration pneumonia, disseminated intravascular coagulation, allergic dermatitis due to an antibiotic, respiratory failure requiring mechanical ventilation, and persistent pulmonary edema. Several days after her arrival in the ICU, a DNR order was written at the request of her family, in case of sudden cardiac arrest. She improves over the next two weeks to the point where tracheotomy was indicated. Two days after the procedure, the patient suffers an acute myocardial infarction with cardiogenic shock. When the family is informed that the patient's likelihood of surviving the event is very low, they requested that she be allowed to die. Her son, daughter-in-law, and four sisters gathered at the bedside. The patient was extubated and all inotropes stopped. She was given morphine sulfate intravenously by continuous drip and bolus, and lorazepam intravenously to maintain comfort and decrease dyspnea. The physician remained at the nurses' station and periodically entered the room to assess the patient and talk to the family. A chaplain was available. The patient died two hours after extubation. Several members of the family stated that when they died, they hoped it was quietly with their family around and thanked the ICU team.

As the responsibility to provide pain relief and dignity at the end of life becomes more widely accepted and the "mechanics" to do so readily available, the decision-making process, itself, is being scrutinized. The public has heightened the awareness of the medical community to these issues by calling for more control in end-of-life decisions, especially in the highly charged debate surrounding physician-assisted suicide and euthanasia. This debate is often linked to effectiveness of pain management during terminal illness and dying. The Patient Self-Determination Act (PDSA) (1991) that requires that each patient admitted to a hospital be asked whether or not he or she has an advanced directive, was an effort to address these questions en masse.

In a follow-up study of seriously ill patients, undertaken to assess the effectiveness of written advance directives [ADs], particularly after promotion of ADs by the PSDA, and enhanced by SUPPORT interventions [n = 9,105], Teno et al. concluded that ADs did not significantly augment physician communication or decision making about resuscitation. PSDA and SUPPORT interventions increased documentation of ADs, but not their effect. "Current practice patterns indicate that increasing the frequency of ADs is unlikely to be a substantial element in improving care of seriously ill patients. Future work to improve decision-making should focus upon improving the current pattern of practice through better communication and more comprehensive advance care planning."[40]

Sullivan studied 48 patients currently living with pain from metastatic cancer to analyze the impact of a potential future state of severe unrelieved pain on their end-of-life decisions. Although 73 percent of the group were found to have inadequate pain relief, "interest in hastening death in the possible circumstance of severe unrelieved pain failed to correlate to present pain. . . . It is therefore possible that present pain and the abstract concept of future pain are so different that one does not influence the appraisal of the other. . . . The prominent role played by symptoms and dysfunctions associated with pain further supports the hypothesis that patients fear a constellation of symptoms and dysfunctions surrounding severe pain and not just the spectra of pain itself."[41] In this sample, over 90 percent felt that all persons with terminal illness should have the right to refuse any and all medical treatment and to receive extra pain medication even if it would hasten death. Current psychological symptoms of depression did not correlate significantly with interest in hastening death. Fewer than 25 percent felt that the impossibility of a cure would make pain intolerable, but constant exhaustion (42 percent), no satisfying sleep (46 percent), or no control over pain (47 percent) would. An even larger group cited pain accompanied by inability to concentrate, confinement to bed, or constant nausea as intolerable. It becomes crucial for the care provider to know what constellation of symptoms and values helps define what the patient sees as intolerable pain.[42] "Palliative care must reach beyond pain management to address other sources of suffering, including impact of pain on valued functions. . . ."[43] The following case report offers insight into the use of the ICU for control of pain and suffering during withdrawal of mechanical ventilation and into the decision-making process:

> A 77-year-old male, HD, who was legally blind, but relatively independent, fell and sustained a fracture of C-2 with spinal cord compression, quadriplegia, and apnea. The family reported the patient's previously stated wishes for no aggressive life-sustaining therapies in the event of a catastrophic illness. The patient communicated, nonverbally, his wish to have ventilator support withdrawn. The staff were unwilling to honor his request, because they thought an expert spinal cord evaluation was necessary to validate the poor prognosis, and they feared that withdrawal of the ventilator could not be done in a conscious, apneic patient without causing distress. Therefore, he was transferred to an urban, level-one trauma center, where the poor prognosis, including ventilator dependence was confirmed.

With the support of his family, HD requested withdrawal of the ventilator. All agreed that he had full decision-making capability. He received a "shot of whiskey," private time with his family, and sacraments from a Catholic priest. Weaning was done slowly to allow hypercarbia, with its narcotizing effects, to occur, and measurement of brain activity. He was monitored using bispectral index (BIS) to follow cerebral function, end-tidal CO_2, vital signs, and fascial muscle activity for signs of distress. Sedation and analgesia were administered as needed with the help of the monitoring devices. The ventilator was turned off when the BIS showed minimal brain activity. Death occurred five minutes later. The family prayed, talked to him, and stroked his face during weaning. On-going discussions of ethical principles were held with concerned staff.[44]

Technology and ICU care were introduced to allow closer monitoring of HD's response to ventilator withdrawal, because his spinal cord injury eliminated much of his ability to show distress. This contrasts the usual reduction of technological intervention during withdrawal of life-sustaining therapy. "The patient's motive was that the quality of his remaining life would be insufficient. Our rationale was that he was facing a poor prognosis and was making a capable, informed decision to refuse treatment: therefore, we were respecting his autonomous rights. His previous statements had relevance, because they supported the contemporaneous decision and provided us with evidence of consistency between HD's current wishes and his earlier wishes when the situation was hypothetical."[45]

This case report corroborates the general findings of the Society of Critical Care Medicine pertaining to ethical, legal, and clinical aspects of withholding and withdrawing. The conclusion is summarized below:

> "Most ICU physicians consider withholding and withdrawal ethically similar and appropriate processes, . . . they consider patient and surrogate wishes paramount in deciding to forgo treatment, but place these wishes in the context of their own assessment of prognosis, and . . . concerns about cost or distributive justice are not important in decision-making."[46]

The study goes on to note that limiting therapy is frequently initiated by patients or families, but that physicians will sometimes impose limitations, unilaterally; withdrawal occurs more frequently than withholding in the ICU; mechanical ventilation and vasopressors are the interventions most frequently withdrawn; gradual withdrawal of ventilation is preferred over rapid extubation; analgesics and sedatives are usually provided during the withdrawal period, although undermedication for pain still needs to be addressed.

The evolution of pain control, then, becomes part of an ethic of caring that includes, but is not encompassed by, physiology, technology, abstract ethical principles, and patient rights. In a pilot study investigating what kind of ethical problems nurses face in clinical situations and what process they use in deciding to take action, Leners and Beardslee found pervasive references to suffering and pain in all data analyzed. "The researchers found . . . an overarching theme: suffering and ethical caring: incompatible entities."[47] Study participants (six staff nurses, including ICU) were "adamant that clients and families should experience as little suffering and pain as possible. Being ethical meant minimizing or eliminating the possibility of pain and suffering in the event of a poor prognosis."[48]

The researchers found that nurses rarely used a "moral voice of justice," but instead used a "moral voice of caring"—understanding themselves and patients through empathy and the "do unto others" adage. They noted that although nurses spend more time with patients than physicians do, their voices may not be heard, even though many ethical dilemmas involve interaction between them. More and more, the medical literature, both physician- and nurse-oriented, is focusing on a multidisciplinary approach and enhanced communication and education in the management of pain and the orchestration of "a good death."

CONCLUSION

In conclusion, it is the ethical and medical responsibility of the intensive care practitioner to treat and relieve pain. The mainstays of therapy for acute pain are intravenous narcotic analgesia; sedation; and, when indicated, neuromuscular blockade. Morphine, lorazepam, and pancuronium are recommended for most situations. Fentanyl, midazolam, and vecuronium can be used when short-acting agents are indicated and for hemodynamic instability. Sedation and analgesia must always accompany paralysis.

Special consideration is warranted in difficult cases such as multisystem organ failure, burns, and closed-head injury. The appropriate medications can achieve good control and amnesia in most if not all ICU patients.

Alert patients can be evaluated for PCA and epidural or regional analgesia. In the case of long-term admission, disorientation and withdrawal symptoms must also be addressed. Slow, purposeful weaning from drips may be necessary. Chemical rather than mechanical restraints for severe agitation are preferred. Transdermal and nonnarcotic analgesics may have a role, as do anesthetic agents such as ketamine and propofol.

For the dying patient who no longer needs intensive care but is not in the "comfort-measures-only" category reserved for hospice patients, the ICU team can provide expertise and direction. A collaborative effort by the ICU staff and the ethics committee at the University Hospital at Stony Brook to develop a new service, acute palliative care, is one such example. The group developed a mission statement, admission and exclusion criteria, a therapeutic plan, and policies and procedure regarding transfer to and from acute palliative care.[49]

Adequate pain control and preservation of dignity and comfort during dying or withdrawal of mechanical or chemical life support are required, despite the risk that medications used for this purpose may hasten death. Hippocrates wrote that the role of medicine is "to do away with the sufferings of the sick, to lessen the violence of their diseases, and to refuse to treat those who are overmastered by their disease, realizing that in such cases, medicine is powerless."[50] Today our goal remains the same. We just have more tools at our disposal and a proportionately greater responsibility to use them well.

NOTES

1. W. Osler, *The Evolution of Modern Medicine: A Series of Lectures Delivered at Yale University on the Silliman Foundation, April 1913* (New Haven, Conn.: Yale University Press, 1921), 6.

2. R.E. Sergil, *Galen on Sense Perception* (Basel, Switzerland: Karger, 1970), 184-90.

3. W.C. Shoemaker et al., *Textbook of Critical Care,* 3rd ed. (Philadelphia: W.B. Saunders, 1995); J.M. Fakhry, T. Dogra, and R. Fischer, "Pain Management in Critically Ill Patients: Patient Controlled Analgesia, Epidural Analgesia, and Transcutaneous Nerve Stimulation," in *Critical Care: State of the Art,* ed. R.W. Taylor and W.C. Shoemaker (Anaheim, Calif.: Society of Critical Care Medicine, 1995), 402; Acute Pain Management Guideline Panel, *Acute Pain Management: Operative or Medical Procedures and Trauma Clinical Practice Guideline* (Rockville, Md.: Agency for Health Care Policy and Research, Public Health Service, U.S. Department of Health and Human Services, 1992), AHCPR pub. no. 92-0032.

4. C.A. Hess, "Acute Pain in the Intensive Care Units," in *Textbook of Critical Care,* 3rd ed., ed. W.C. Shoemaker et al. (Philadelphia: W.B. Saunders, 1995), 1492.

5. B.A. Shapiro et al., "Practice Parameters for Intravenous Analgesia and Sedation for Adult Patients in the Intensive Care Unit: An Executive Summary," *Critical Care Medicine* 23 (1995): 1596-600.

6. B.A. Shapiro et al., "Practice Parameters for Sustained Neuromuscular Blockade in the Adult Critically Ill Patient: An Executive Summary," *Critical Care Medicine* 23 (1995): 1601-05.

7. Ibid., 1596.

8. Ibid., 1601.

9. K.S. Lewis et al., "Effect of Analgesic Treatment in the Physiological Consequences of Acute Pain," *American Journal of Hospital Pharmacy* 51 (1994): 1139-54.

10. J.A.J. Martyn et al., "Up-and-Down-Regulation of Skeletal Muscle Acetylcholine Receptors," *Anesthesiology* 76 (1992): 822-43.

11. V. Tegredo et al., "Persistent Paralysis in Critically Ill Patients after Long-Term Administration of Vecuronium," *New England Journal of Medicine* 327 (1995): 524-28.

12. C.F. Bolton, "The Polyneuropathy of Critical Illness," *Intensive Care Medicine* 9 (1994): 132-38.

13. H.T. Klessig et al., "A National Survey on the Practice Patterns of An-

esthesiologists and Intensivists in the Use of Muscle Relaxants," *Critical Care Medicine* 20 (1992): 1341-45.

14. B.M. Fleming and D.W. Coombs, "A Survey of Complications Documented in a Quality Control Analysis of Patient-Controlled Analgesia in the Postoperative Patient," *Journal of Pain Symptom Management* 7 (1992) 463.

15. E.P. McCoy, G. Furness, and P.M. Wright, "Patient Controlled Analgesia with and without Background Infusion: Analgesia Assessed Using the Demand: Delivery Ratio," *Anesthesia* 48 (1993): 256.

16. M.P. Yeager, D.G. Glass, and R.K. Neff, "Epidural Anesthesia and Analgesia in High-Risk Surgical Patients," *Anesthesiology* 66 (1987): 729; R.M. Sorensen and N.L. Pace, "Mortality and Morbidity of Regional versus General Anesthesia: A Meta-Analysis," *Anesthesiology* 75 (1991): A1053; K. Tulman et al., "Effects of Epidural Anesthesia and Analgesia on Coagulation and Outcome After Major Vascular Surgery," *Anesthesia and Analgesia* 73 (1991): 696.

17. J.J. Bonica, *The Management of Pain,* 2nd ed. (Philadelphia: Lea & Febiger, 1990), 1: 19.

18. Ibid., 19.

19. Ibid., 19.

20. P.D. Lamb and T.J. Gallagher, "Sedatives and Muscle Relaxants in the Intensive Care Unit," in *Textbook of Critical Care,* 3rd ed., ed. W.C. Shoemaker et al. (Philadelphia: W.B. Saunders, 1995), 1163.

21. See note 4 above.

22. S.H. Schnoll, "Drug Abuse, Overdose, and Withdrawal Syndromes," in *Textbook of Critical Care,* 3rd ed., ed. W.C. Shoemaker et al. (Philadelphia: W.B. Saunders, 1995), 1176.

23. Fakhry et al., "Pain Management in Critically Ill Patients," see note 3 above.

24. P.M. Marks and E.J. Sacher, "Undertreatment of Medical Inpatients with Narcotic Analgesics," *Annals of Internal Medicine* 78 (1973): 173; D.S. Stevens and W.T. Edwards, "Management of Pain in Intensive Care Setting," *Anesthesiology Clinics of North America* 10 (1992): 395; R.H. Wolman and J.H. Shapiro, "Pain Management in the Critically Ill," in *Critical Care: State of the Art,* ed. R.W. Taylor and W.C. Shoemaker (Anaheim, Calif.: Society of Critical Care Medicine, 1991), 1: 417-76; M. Tittle and J.C. McMillan, "Pain and Pain Related Side Effects in an ICU and on a Surgical Unit: Nurses Management," *American Journal of Critical Care* 3 (1994): 25.

25. Ibid.

26. F.L. Cohen, "Post Surgical Pain Relief: Patients' Status and Nurses' Medication Choices," *Pain* 37 (1980): 315, as cited in Hess, "Acute Pain in the Intensive Care Units," see note 4 above.

27. K.A. Loper et al., "Paralyzed with Pain: Need for Education," *Pain* 37 (1989): 315-19.

28. N.L. Shecter, "The Undertreatment of Pain in Children: An Overview," *Pediatric Clinics of North America* 36 (1989): 781-94.

29. See note 4 above, p. 1487.

30. Fakhry et al., "Pain Management in Critically Ill Patients," see note 3 above.

31. J.F. Dasta, T.M. Fuhrman, and R.N. McCandles, "Issues in Pharmacology: Use of Sedatives and Analgesics in a Surgical Intensive Care Unit: A Follow-Up and Commentary," *Heart and Lung* (January/February 1995): 76-78.

32. K.A. Pontillo, "Pain Experience of Intensive Care Unit Patients," *Heart and Lung* 19, no. 5, part 1 (September 1990): 526-33.

33. See note 4 above.

34. D.F. Kelly and M.D. Hoyt, "Ethics Consultation," *Medical Ethics* 12, no. 1 (1996): 66.

35. W.C. Wilson et al., "Ordering and Administering Sedatives and Analgesics During the Withholding and Withdrawal of Life Support from Critically Ill Patients," *Journal of the American Medical Association* 267 (1992): 949-53.

36. M.A. DeVita and A. Grenvic, "Foregoing Life-Sustaining Therapy in Intensive Care," in *Textbook of Critical Care*, 3rd ed., ed. W.C. Shoemaker et al. (Philadelphia: W.B. Saunders, 1995), 1802-08.

37. "Providers Persist in Search for 'Good Health'," *Medical Ethics Advisor* 12, no. 1 (1996): 1.

38. The SUPPORT Principal Investigators, "A Controlled Trial to Improve Care for Seriously Ill Hospitalized Patients: The Study to Understand Prognosis and Preferences for Outcomes and Risks of Treatments (SUPPORT)," *Journal of the American Medical Association* 274 (1995): 1591-98.

39. See note 36 above, p. 1804.

40. J. Teno et al., "Advance Directives for Seriously Ill Hospitalized Patients: Effectiveness with the Patient Self-Determination Act and the SUPPORT Intervention," *Journal of the American Geriatric Society* 45 (1997): 500.

41. M. Sullivan et al., "Pain and the Choice to Hasten Death in Patients with Painful Metastatic Cancer," *Journal of Palliative Care* 13, no. 3 (1997): 25.

42. Ibid., 23.

43. Ibid., 27.

44. M.L. Campbell et al., "Case Report: Integrating Technology with Compassionate Care: Withdrawal of Ventilation in a Conscious Patient with Apnea," *American Journal of Critical Care* 7, no. 2 (March 1998): 85-89.

45. Ibid., 87.

46. J.M. Luce, "Withholding and Withdrawal of Life Support: Ethical, Legal, and Clinical Aspects," *New Horizons—Ethical Issues in Critical Care* 5, no. 1 (February 1997): 36.

47. D. Leners and N. Beardslee, "Suffering and Ethical Caring: Incompatible Entities," *Nursing Ethics* 4, no. 5 (1997): 368.

48. Ibid., 368.

49. "Should You Offer a Bridge of Acute Palliative Care?" *Medical Ethics Advisor* 12, no. 1 (1996): 6.

50. Hippocrates, *The Art*, as cited in Devita and Grenvic, "Foregoing Life-Sustaining Therapy," see note 36 above.

7

Scoring Systems in the ICU: Outcome Predictors for Ethically Responsible Resource Utilization

William T. McGee and Daniel Teres

INTRODUCTION

Severity of illness measures using derangements in acute physiology or the presence of acute and chronic clinical conditions are widely utilized. Comparisons among health systems can be performed by evaluating severity-adjusted mortality, outcome, and cost. Long-term functional outcome is a more useful parameter than hospital mortality. For large numbers of patients, severity measures are helpful when evaluating quality of care. Present severity measures cannot be used for individual patient treatment decisions, particularly those decisions related to withdrawal of support.

There is no societal consensus on what appropriate end-of-life care should be. On an individual level, cost-benefit analysis is not helpful as the economic consequences of treatment are not experienced directly. The principle of justice is not routinely considered for resource allocation in the United States health system and, therefore, is not helpful for treatment decisions in the intensive care unit. Autonomy, beneficence, and nonmaleficence are the paramount considerations for ethical treatment of ICU patients. Futility could be useful for therapeutic decision making but the definition of futility remains ambiguous. The ethical application of scoring systems can define high-performance ICU and health systems by evaluating severity-adjusted outcomes against other competitors; ultimately this will improve quality of care for all patients.

GILGUNN V. MASSACHUSETTS GENERAL HOSPITAL

Joan Gilgunn sued the Massachusetts General Hospital and two physicians who had cared for her mother, Catherine Gilgunn, alleging negligent infliction of emotional distress on the basis of a do-not-resuscitate (DNR) order.[1] She sued for emotional distress and argued that the physicians and the hospital were bound to honor her request for cardiopulmonary resuscitation (CPR) for her mother. Specifically, the issue was writing and carrying out a DNR order against her stated wish, without seeking prior court approval. Gilgunn argued that the defendants violated their duty of care by not attempting resuscitation. The defense argued that CPR would have been futile and harmful and that the physicians had followed well-established standards of medical practice and the hospital's institutional procedures.

In order to determine the merits of the plaintiff's claim of negligent infliction of emotional distress, the jury was first required to determine if the medical treatment of the mother was negligent. Medical negligence would be a prerequisite to any emotional distress claim advanced by the daughter. The judge instructed the jury: "The State's interest in pursuing life is high when human life can be saved and where the inflictions are curable, but wanes when the inflictions are incurable."[2] He further instructed the jury that they must "balance" the patient's preference against the medical judgment to withdraw treatment in the context not of whether her life might be extended, but for how long and at what cost. The jury fund that Catherine Gilgunn would have wanted medical care extended, but they also found that it would have been futile and of no medical benefit; therefore, there was no negligence. The doctors and hospital were found not guilty.

This case was tried in the Suffolk Superior Court in Massachusetts. If New York State's DNR Law[3] had been applied to this case, a different outcome would have been likely. The New York law considers CPR to be futile if, according to the best medical judgment, it would be "unsuccessful in restoring cardiac and respiratory function or if the patient would experience repeated arrest in a short period of time before death occurs."[4] This narrow definition of futility would encompass only a few cases and certainly not Catherine Gilgunn's.

The *Gilgunn* case illustrates some of the problems to be anticipated if scoring systems are employed to determine the use of resources in the intensive care unit (ICU). Society is simply not ready and case law is still evolving and may be contradictory. Catherine Gilgunn was in a vegetative state and receiving mechanical ventilation in the ICU. The debate in the case focused solely on the DNR order. This patient had already been hospitalized for a considerable time and had consumed multiple resources prior to the DNR decision. At what point did her care become futile?

Catherine Gilgunn was 71 years old when she entered the hospital on 7 June 1989 for the repair of a fractured hip. She had multiple severe, chronic medical problems. Previously, she had undergone surgery for breast cancer, and she had diabetes mellitus and peripheral vascular disease. As a consequence of her vascular disease, she had experienced a prior stroke and a myocardial infarction resulting in congestive heart failure. During her June 1989 admission for the fractured hip, she developed status epilepticus, which was very difficult to control; ultimately her condition deteriorated to a persistent vegetative state. The patient continued to receive intensive care, and she had numerous complications typical of the chronically critically ill. She received the highest level and most expensive care that can be delivered in a hospital for approximately two months. The medical team was deeply troubled by their continued treatment of the patient to no positive end. The hospital's optimum care committee believed that CPR was "medically contraindicated, inhumane, and unethical and therefore not a genuine therapeutic option."[5] The care team's opinion was that by providing the current level of care, they were already mistreating the patient. The daughter's motivation for insisting on a level of care that the entire care team—nurses, social workers, dietitians, students, doctors, and the optimum care committee—found to be inhumane and unethical is unclear.

It is potentially disabling to the care team to put caregivers, who have devoted their life's work to taking care of critically ill patients, in a position where their moral and ethical values are severely undermined and their cumulative knowledge is ignored. Healthcare providers should never be forced to provide what they consider to be inhumane treatment. The philosophies of others who have no clinical basis to understand the medical and nursing care of the critically ill should not dictate how healthcare professionals perform their work. If nonmedical outcomes are determined by society (not academics) to be philosophically and ethically important, then this type of care should be allowed to continue in a setting where healing is not a primary goal. Continuation of aggressive medical treatment in an ICU to no positive medical outcome is the real tragedy of the *Gilgunn* case.

Many of the questions about resource utilization in the ICU have been based on the assumption that it is appropriate to limit care when the probability of mortality appears high. However, the *Gilgunn* case and New York State law illustrate the diversity of opinion regarding futility. It is potentially more fruitful to identify those patients who traditionally have been placed in ICUs who could be managed in a less intensive setting. Scoring systems could help to accomplish this task.

The futility of resuscitation in the *Gilgunn* case appears apparent, even though it may not meet the standards set by New York State. However, focusing on resuscitation is far removed from looking at decisions about treatment in the ICU early during a patient's critical illness. Nonetheless, the court decision was interpreted as a major victory for doctors and hospitals. This case only emphasizes the difficulties that would be encountered in attempting to base ICU resource utilization on scoring systems. If doctors can be sued in court for refusing to provide what they regard to be futile medical care, we are a long way from making do-not-treat decisions based on models that estimate probability of mortality (at best, such models can say there is a 5 to 10 percent chance of doing well, the converse of a 90 to 95 percent probability of mortality). In the case of Catherine Gilgunn, the patient's predicted mortality may not have been, but her functional outcome would have been vegetative. This case illustrates that functional outcome data are much more useful than predictors of mortality probability. The jury in the *Gilgunn* case considered this issue in reaching its decision.

What are the potential liabilities for physicians who limit care? The jury must consider the necessary four elements of negligence (duty, breach, causation, and harm/injury) in determining a negligence claim, and all four elements must be present. In cases of medical negligence, the proper standard is whether the physician has exercised the degree of care and skill of the average qualified practitioner, taking into account the advances in the profession.[6] The finding of neglegence may be based on an omission or action and requires thoughtlessness, inattention, or other lack of concern involving the omission or action. When applied to the *Gilgunn* case, this language made it difficult for the jury to find negligence, considering the efforts and documentation made by the physicians and the hospital. A recent study reports that many ICU physicians act similarly to the physicians caring for Catherine Gilgunn in withholding or withdrawing care, with possibly less thought and consensus than occurred in her case.[7]

Any discussion of resource limitation for triage in the ICU must be firmly based on the principles of medical ethics. This chapter examines how these principles relate to the specific models that have been developed. The current clinical uses of these models may be simply to determine the characteristics and identity high-quality ICUs. The use of scoring systems for resource allocation in intensive care has the potential to facilitate better judgments in the care of ICU patients. To realize this potential, organizations must apply these models intelligently while respecting their limitations. In addition, the ethical application of these models must be explored.

Simply stated, ethics consists of making judgments. Any judgment requires certain criteria for the decision. How one decides to use resources in the ICU will be based on how one views the efficacy of that intervention. If efficacy is defined simply as survival, these mortality probability models will help us to determine triage and resource allocation for ICU patients. However, survival without function is generally not desirable. Few patients would define efficacy this way. Applying these models ethically must always respect this limitation.

ETHICAL PRINCIPLES

The toughest ethical problems involve a dilemma—a conflict of principles in which only one may be chosen. These principles are reviewed below and applied to the use of scoring systems.

AUTONOMY

Much has been said about the principle of autonomy, which states that individuals should be the ones to make decisions involving their own welfare. Patients who make decisions at the end of life need accurate information; patients' confidence in that accuracy can allow them to make better decisions. Good information and good data are critical for good decision making. However, a patient's judgment incorporates many other aspects of his or her personality into a decision. In the *Gilgunn* case, because of the incapacitated condition of the patient, it was impossible to apply this principle. The jury decided that the patient would have wanted care, but that this care would not have been beneficial. It is unknown whether the jury would have made a similar decision if the patient had been competent.

For patients without decision-making capacity, courts have generally sided with the decisions of proxies. In the *Wanglie* case,[8] the physician asked if a third party could be appointed conservator in lieu of the husband. Helga Wanglie was a vegetative patient on mechanical ventilatory support in an ICU. She had been in a vegetative state for months as a result of several strokes. There was no hope of recovery of higher-brain function, although the patient could survive on a ventilator. It was her husband's wish, based on his religious convictions that his wife be sustained on mechanical ventilation, a treatment that the physicians considered futile. The Minnesota judge concurred that the patient's spouse of 53 years should be appointed her conservator. The court's decision, which affirmed Mr. Wanglie as the appropriate decision maker, allowed his wife to have care continued. This case illustrates that the probability of mortality may play an important but not necessarily overriding role in any individual decision.

BENEFICENCE

The principle of beneficence may not be significantly affected by the use of scoring systems in the ICU. This patient-centered principle states that the doctor ought to do what is in the best interest of the patient. Insofar as this principle relies upon making a judgment, good information enhances judgment. It is quite clear, however, that the interpretation of best interest is based upon individual judgment and thus it can vary. This principle gives the doctor considerable leeway in deciding how to treat patients. It is not uncommon for residents (physicians-in-training) unfamiliar with intensive care to believe that many ICU interventions are either painful or injurious to patients and that some patients might be better off left alone. In retrospect, this is undeniably true for the patients who die despite aggressive, invasive, and uncomfortable treatments. However, Elpem and colleagues report that it is not common for patients who survive a critical illness after aggressive interventions to complain or to believe that such interventions were not in their best interest.[9]

Leaving this type of decision solely to the doctor places undue emphasis on the doctor's opinions and moral beliefs and is seen as paternalistic. Therefore, when there is uncertainty about diagnosis or prognosis, most doctors err on the side of overtreatment for the minority of critically ill patients who may respond to therapy. The surviving patients are likely to be very grateful that treatment was offered to them.

NONMALEFICENCE

The principle of nonmaleficence, or not doing harm, at first seems easy to describe; however, this principle is subject to judgments that are impossible to classify as either right or wrong. Healthcare providers would like to believe that it is extremely rare that intentional harm occurs during routine therapy, but this may be an inescapable conclusion for a sick ICU patient who ultimately has a bad outcome. How easily can the healthcare team say that they did no harm if the patient did not improve and the treatment was painful or uncomfortable? In these instances, a frank discussion and the incorporation of the patient's or surrogate's understanding of the relative benefits and burdens of any treatment can offer guidelines for decisions about treatment. Insofar as prediction models may help in determining the potential benefit, they may provide patients and families with information that may help them make decisions.

JUSTICE

The principle of justice, which states that medical resources should be distributed fairly, may have many implications for social welfare; however, it has little practical meaning in 1999 for a patient who has already entered the medical care system. The players involved in decisions about treatment arguably have little ability to determine how medical resources will be distributed. For example, saving dollars by not treating the hopelessly ill will not result in increased resources for nutrition programs in the inner city. If the patient has insurance, it is unlikely that any money saved will be spent on medical resources for other patients; any money saved is likely to be returned to the insurance company to be distributed to the shareholders or executives. Although it is appealing to think that each dollar spent on healthcare can be allocated in a way to provide the greatest benefit for that dollar, this approach does not occur in American medicine.

Triage systems are designed to provide the most efficient use of scarce resources. Given the abundance of hospital beds in the U.S. healthcare system, it is unusual for triage decisions to be a regular part of daily medical practice, except in large, urban hospitals or during a temporary increase in census. In fact, an ever-increasing percentage of hospital beds are now designated as intensive care, special care, or step-down or progressive ICU beds. With overcapacity, there is little incentive on anyone's part to deny even marginal care.

Stephen Schroeder, president of the Robert Wood Johnson Foundation, comments on the U.S. healthcare system after spending a year studying European medical care.[10] He states that it is unlikely that medical care savings will stay in the healthcare sector and be used to expand services for the uninsured; it is more likely that these savings will contribute to profits, dividends, executive salaries, and so forth. He also comments that European hospitals have fewer ICUs, fewer ICU patients, and significantly fewer dying patients in the ICU. In the European medical system, it is rational to apply triage. Fewer dying patients in ICUs implies more efficient triage and resource utilization. Hospital-based healthcare—and, specifically, intensive care and ICU beds—cannot be considered a scarce resource in the United States. There is little incentive on the part of hospitals, physicians, or patients to limit care, as the principle of justice arguably does not apply to medical care and treatment in the United States.

The *Gilgunn* case may represent a conflict between the principles of autonomy (the presumed wishes of the patient or her proxy) and justice (whether medical resources are being distributed fairly when care is determined to be futile). This case may represent a paradigm shift in the way similar cases will be handled in the future. This type of decision making might become more straightforward if our society expected that resources not used in the care of a particular patient might be distributed to provide the greatest good for the greatest number of people.

Prior landmark cases such as *Baby K,* which appear to choose autonomy over justice, are actually very narrowly focused on the language but perhaps not the intent of the law.[11] Baby K, an anencephalic infant born without a cerebral cortex, was resuscitated on numerous occasions at the mother's request against medical judgment. The hospital asked the court if it was obliged to provide "inappropriate" medical treatment. The U.S. Court of Appeals in a two-to-one decision examined the Emergency Medical Treatment and Active Labor Act and upheld the district court finding, which determined that the emergency department is obligated to provide emergency treatment whenever it is requested.[12] The district court specifically stated that the statute made no provision for futile or inappropriate care but further determined that because breathing could be restored care was not futile. George Annas eloquently argues that "defining appropriate medical care will be removed from physicians altogether if they cannot get and then adhere to standards for medical practice."[13] Letting the courts apply the law to those cases that are legally but perhaps not medically appropriate only confuses these issues. One of the three judges who heard the case of *Baby K* interpreted these same facts very differently from the other judges.

In the *Wanglie* case, the courts only decided who should be the conservator for Helga Wanglie. In going to court, the hospital and the physicians had hoped for a more encompassing decision regarding the issue of futility. The court ruled that the conservator for the patient should be her husband and did not address the fact that he wanted medical treatment continued even though the medical team considered it futile. Thus the court did not consider the important issue of futility.[14]

This type of decision making might become more straightforward if our society expected that resources not used in the care of a particular patient might then be redistributed to provide the greatest good for the greatest number of people. The Oregon Basic Health Services Act, with its idea of a fixed budget for healthcare, embraces the principle of justice and a cost-utility analysis of health services.[15]

FUTILITY

The most important aspect of the *Gilgunn* case is the concept of futility. The definition of this concept has changed over time. According to Reiser and colleagues, "Whenever the illness is too strong for the available remedies, the physician surely must not expect that it can be overcome by medicine. To attempt futile treatment is to display an ignorance that is aligned to madness."[16] "For those whose lives are always in a state of inner sickness," Asclepius, the Greek god of medicine, did not attempt to prescribe a regimen and make their life a prolonged misery. He asserted, "A life with preoccupation of illness and neglect of work is not worth living."[17] The judge in the *Gilgunn* case evoked these same sentiments.[18]

To provide proper medical care for patients, physicians should avoid providing medical care that is ly burdensome, especially if it has no possible benefit. The dichotomy of issues surrounding futility is illustrated by the difference between the New York statute[19] that calls for obtaining a beating heart as a medical goal and the *Gilgunn* decision that considers quality of life when defining medical futility. The *Gilgunn* jury further implied that the application of specific medical technology, in this case mechanical ventilation and CPR, was not appropriate to sustain the patient's quality of life.

MEDICAL FUTILITY

This section examines the idea of futility and then applies several ICU mortality models to see if they can help determine futility (see Exhibit 7-1). In discussions of *medical futility*, the common definition is based on a 99 percent predicted risk of dying. Should aggressive, high-cost care be provided to patients with a 1 percent chance of survival? No current ICU prediction model is close to the 99 percent accuracy level. Schneiderman and colleagues state that a treatment should be considered futile only if, after treating 100 consecutive patients, there are no survivors.[20] If this can be demonstrated, then the model can be applied to the next 100 patients. The current general ICU models, which do not use confidence intervals, are simply not good enough to be applied to individual patients based on Schneiderman's definition of medical futility.

Life or death is not the parameter that most families and patients are interested in when attempting to make judgments about quality of life. There is a need for functional outcome data—a measure of quality of life that can be reported to patients and their families in a way that has meaning for them. To date, a functional outcome model has been developed for use with nontraumatic coma.[21] Such a model has more potential than a futility model to affect the rational use of resources in the ICU. Medical futility is only clear in extreme cases; a decapitated patient as a result of trauma need not be resuscitated. Almost anything else is much less clear, as the case of *Baby K* illustrates. Furthermore, there is little agreement about who should be making decisions regarding futile medical care. Most court decisions and common teaching in medical ethics em-

---

Exhibit 7-1
General Models for Probability of Mortality

- APACHE II/III
- Mortality Probability Model (MPM) II
- Simplified Acute Physiology Score (SAPS) II
- Study to Understand Prognoses and Preferences for Outcomes and Risks of Treatment (SUPPORT)

---

phasize the wishes of the family when the patient is unable to make decisions, which may not lead to the outcome desired by the medical team. There are also data suggesting that some physicians make unilateral decisions about the futility of treatment.[22]

FUTILITY AND SEVERITY MODELS

Futility, especially considering the certainty we would like to have when making this judgment, cannot be defined adequately with existing models. These difficult decisions involve many value judgments on the part of the patient, family, physicians, and other interested members of the community. All of these parties, in some way or another, pay for healthcare costs. Although patient autonomy is currently a dominant principle in ethical decision making in the United States, this is not the trend everywhere. American society is made up of individuals from diverse cultural backgrounds. Cultural differences in viewing the doctor-patient relationship are probably not well represented by all ethicists.[23]

The concept of futility is an appealing one for clinicians who are asked to provide an intervention that is clearly futile or to continue to provide care that is not expected to be of any benefit. Unfortunately, there is no consensus—nor will there be—concerning this definition. This problem could be partially resolved by searching for a uniform standard of useful life or by developing a new definition of brain death that focuses on higher cortical function rather than brain-stem activity. Both of these approaches, however, look for a simple solution to a very complex problem and seek to obviate difficult clinical decision making. Family and patient discussions are absolutely necessary in cases involving the issue of futility.

The large volume of literature on futility underscores the fact we are a long way from reaching consensus on a definition for futility.[24] Despite this, hospital ethics committees across the United States are developing futility guidelines. An alternate approach that uses severity-of-illness models to identify potentially ineffective care is discussed later in this chapter.

FUTILITY AND VALUE JUDGMENTS

It is quite clear that no patient would want a treatment that is "futile," but the questions is—futile according to what standard? As Waisel and Truog point out, the definition of futility always will involve some value judgment on the part of the physician.[25] They argue that the existing severity models will not help us with this issue. They emphasize that when physicians impose their values regarding whether CPR is indicated, they are not respecting the patient's autonomy and may not be considering the benefit of this intervention from the patient's viewpoint. Their extreme position in analyzing the policies for unilateral DNR at four different hospitals focuses strictly on physiologic futility. For example, "CPR is futile only if it is impossible to do cardiac massage and ventilation. As long as circulation and gas exchange are occurring, CPR is not futile, even if no one expects improvement in the patient's condition."[26] This defines *medical futility*—no expected benefit from the treatment. These authors offer this definition as having the least possible risk for proposed value judgments. What opinion would they offer if bypass surgery or other interventions were offered to those who could not benefit? Do they propose that all interventions should always be offered or attempted?

Physicians, whose art is healing and whose responsibility is to the patient, should not be dissuaded by these ideas. Physicians' values, however, necessarily enter any therapeutic decision. Tomlinson and Brody point out that values enter into the most mundane of decisions such as not offering antibiotics for patients with a viral syndrome.[27] Any assertions that particular treatments are good or bad are based on probabilities, not certainties. Physicians look at the benefits versus the burdens of any treatment, and physicians' values play a significant role in all treatment decisions. The practice of medicine could not occur without value judgments. These authors argue that any definition of "physiologic futility will not provide the value free sanctuary that the Hastings Center Task Force[28] thinks they will."[29] They argue that even resuscitation that does not restore the heartbeat potentially has other values to the patient or family who are functioning under a spiritual imperative never to give up. Physicians' and families' value judgments cannot be removed from decisions about medical care. Similarly, futility cannot be defined outside of these value judgments. Thus, it appears that there is no simple resolution to this complicated issue, and that the only approach is to arrive at a consensus opinion with the patient and the family. This practice occurs daily in ICUs all over the country.

FUTILITY AND POLICY DECISIONS

Alternatively, a public policy decision can be made that certain types of care will not be offered for reasons of probability, cost-effectiveness, quality of life, scarcity of resources, or any other reason that can publicly be agreed upon. Unless we develop a national policy, physicians, patients, and families will continue to make clinical decisions based on consensus. It is hoped that probability models might help, by providing patients and families with the best information regarding the expected mortality outcome and the expected functional status and quality of life.

PROBABILITY MODELS

ICU severity-of-illness or probability models have improved substantially over the past 10 years. These advances include emphasis on a probability rather than a physiology score and end points that go beyond prediction of hospital mortality (such as six-month mortality and two-month functional disability). In addition, specialized models have been developed (such as cardiac surgery models).[30] General ICU severity-of-illness models are gaining acceptance, particularly the APACHE system, the Simplified Acute Physiology Score (SAPS), the Mortality Probability Model (MPM), and the Study to Understand Prognosis and Preferences for Outcomes and Risks of Treatment (SUPPORT). These models are based on a large sample size (MPM, SAPS, and APACHE are based on 20,000 patients) and a high level of discrimination, high level of calibration, and high standards for validation. In a comparison of the MPM, SAPS, and APACHE, independent investigators reported that the new versions of the models are better than the old ones and that the three models are comparable with regard to discrimination and calibration.[31]

APACHE

APACHE III, introduced in 1991, is a score based on 12 physiologic variables in addition to age and seven chronic health conditions. To convert this score to a probability of hospital mortality, one also must know the specific disease category (one of a possible 78 categories) precipitating the admission, the surgical status, and where the patient was admitted from—either the Emergency Ward, hospital ward, or operating room. The values recorded are the worst values obtained in a 24-hour period. Conversion of this score to a probability of hospital mortality is accomplished with individual logistic regression equations for each of the 78 nonspecific diagnostic categories and for the nine patient origins. The use of these scores has been criticized for a number of reasons. The scores potentially have the best clinical utility for patients with either low or high probabilities of survival; the likelihood of using them as a surrogate for futility or as a basis for rationing healthcare resources is unlikely at the present time. The scores are not highly correlated with outcomes for some patient populations, including surgical patients and patients with sepsis, acquired immunodeficiency syndrome (AIDS), and *Pneumocystis carinii* pneumonia.[32] The use of such a scoring system is likely to have little applicability to individual patients.

The APACHE system has the most widespread use of any of the probability models. This tool can serve as a useful adjunct to help physicians, patients, and families make decisions independently. The score provides more standardization and better data than subjective estimates and thus can help with judgments about treatment.[33]

The data generated from the APACHE III data base can be graphically represented at the bedside showing a probability of ICU mortality followed by a probability of in-hospital mortality. This type of visual display may have a significant effect on families who are reluctant to agree to withdraw care. However, the daily probability value is not as valid as the initial admission 24-hour value (see Exhibit 7-2). The APACHE III system is a complicated, labor-intensive, and costly system. Other systems have been developed that are simpler to use and less expensive without any significant variation in accuracy.

SIMPLIFIED ACUTE PHYSIOLOGY SCORE II (SAPS II)

The SAPS II model[34] is another tool that predicts the probability of hospital mortality. The SAPS score is based on the patient's physiology, chronic health conditions, and age. SAPS, like APACHE, is treatment dependent. The worst scores obtained over a 24-hour period are converted into a probability of hospital mortality. A patient with a clinically suspected or graphically estimated high-mortality physiology score, if treated less aggressively within the first 24 hours, may create a self-fulfilling prophecy. Alternatively, many of us can recall situations in

---

Exhibit 7-2
Daily Probability Models

- APACHE III (more than 7 days)
- MPM II (up to 72 hours)
- Potentially ineffective care (day 5)
- SUPPORT (day 3)

which patients with poor physiology scores (because of acute severe illness) survive when treated, despite a high probability of mortality. Any patient that is expected to die but then survives because of intensive care is a strong motivator for those of us who work in the ICU. On the other hand, many patients have low physiology scores (such as isolated neurologic injuries) and have a terrible prognosis in terms of functional recovery. Functional outcome may convey much greater meaning to patients and families who are dealing with these complex issues.

MORTALITY PROBABILITY MODEL II (MPM II)

The Mortality Probability Model II produces a direct probability. This system is based on 19,000 patients from 139 ICUs. It provides a probability of hospital mortality at the time of ICU admission as well as a distinct probability model at 24 hours.[35]

There are significant advantages to having a treatment-independent model available at ICU admission. Such a model could be used for resource allocation. However, this model was based on patients who were admitted to the ICU. A treatment-independent parameter that provides clear information is likely to be more applicable across the wide variety of ICUs in the United States.

MPM has no physiology score component and requires minimal laboratory testing. No single precipitating diagnosis is needed, obviating the difficulties that may be inherent in selecting a diagnosis when the patient has multiple competing problems. The MPM II meets high standards for discrimination and calibration using goodness-of-fit testing.

SUPPORT

The SUPPORT models are available on day three of admission for a variety of conditions with an estimated six-month mortality of 50 percent. They are considered general models but are not specific to the ICU.[36] See Exhibit 7-3 for additional potential applications of probability models.[37]

USING PROBABILITY MODELS

At the present time, are there any individual patient applications for these models? It may be argued that objective prognostic information should be part of every patient's medical evaluation. It is recognized that a physician has a responsibility when offering various treatment options to make a prognosis and to estimate the likely effects of any recommendation. These types of estimates are commonly done for many surgical and medical procedures. The probability ranges that are used are typically broad and depend on the particular physician's assessment of his or her own experience along with what he or she may know from other sources. This type of data is routinely given to patients to help them make a decision. The scoring systems can be used in a similar way to help patients and their families make decisions. Fear about using these systems stems from the concern that patients who have been classified as having a high likelihood of dying may survive with good ICU care. No probability estimate would eliminate this fear. This is a primary reason that these systems can only be used as an adjunct for individual patient applications.

Because of the predominance of third-party payments in the United States, cost-benefit analysis from an individual patient's standpoint is always largely skewed toward benefit, as monetary costs to patients are typically minimal. With no apparent economic consideration in the majority of cases, these decisions become relatively simple from the patient's and family's point of view. This phenomenon helps to explain why a European would say, "We really admire the sophistication of American medicine, but you don't know when to stop."[38] There is little reason to stop. Cost does not enter into medical or ethical decision making in the United States. Furthermore, under our present reimbursement system, there is little incentive for the physician to broach these issues. If the physician cannot say with certainty that the patient will die and the physician will be paid for taking care of the patient as long as he or she lives, the ethical imperative mandates that continued therapy is reasonable and the economic analysis implies that it is beneficial to the physician. Simplistic analysis of benefits and burdens highlights the difficulties that are perceived to be occurring in U.S. medicine. When the evidence from the outside world is so conflicting as to whether we should

---

Exhibit 7-3
Potential Individual Patient Applications of ICU Probability Models

---

- Admission
- Discharge
- Triage (comparative entitlement)
- Limitation of care
- Futility determination
- Potentially ineffective care

---

use our own particular value judgments when taking care of patients, the issue for the physician can be further simplified when dealing with complicated cases. Engaging in complicated, often lengthy discussions with the patient or family concerning difficult decisions about treatment at the end of life when we are admonished to ignore our own value systems quickly becomes an exercise in futility for the physician. If physicians attempt to push their own values on patients or the families they are viewed as paternalistic. Finally, with no recourse to the principle of justice (that is, the physician's role is not seen as providing the greatest benefit for the greatest number of people) and with relatively little pressure on the majority of hospital beds, these complicated decisions can be made rather simply. This is why the effort put forth by the physicians in the *Gilgunn* case may be viewed as heroic. It would have been much easier simply to maintain the patient on the ventilator.

The conflicting ethical principles differ in managed care. In a fully integrated healthcare system, the principle of justice may become significant. At the present time, society is ambivalent regarding the level of care at the end of life. Arguably, physicians are in the best position to know what is medically reasonable. However, there is no consensus on whether or how physicians should use their medical knowledge or value systems.

TRIAGE (COMPARATIVE ENTITLEMENT)

Triage is a complex process that identifies who should be admitted to an ICU to displace another patient already in the ICU. A shortage of beds in the ICU is a common situation. Can severity models assist in these patient comparisons?

ICU models are not well refined for patients who are late into the ICU course. The daily APACHE probability system can produce probability of mortality based on data generated up to seven days following ICU admission. The daily MPM system is validated to 72 hours, but neither APACHE or MPM would be applicable for use with individuals or for entitlement comparisons. Daily probability models need to be further developed, refined, validated, and compared with patients in the emergency room or the recovery room. A model to calculate the probability of mortality prior to ICU admission is not available, so the severity-of-illness scores can not be used explicitly for triage purposes.

The Ethics Committee of the Society of Critical Care Medicine has issued a consensus statement on the triage of critically ill patients.[39] During times when the ICU is operating in a triage mode, these guidelines provide a framework for distributing the available resources efficiently and equitably. The general principles guiding ethical decision making are incorporated in these guidelines.

1. The provider should advocate for patients. The triage person should have broad experience in the evaluation of patients for determination of the need for critical care. Potential conflicts may arise when the triage person has also been designated as the patient's medical care provider. Further conflicts may arise in the managed care environment where gatekeepers may have a monetary incentive to limit care. Treatment denial in this setting might occur more frequently when the benefits are difficult to quantify.

2. Collaboration should occur amongst the providers in an attempt to develop the most efficient treatment plan.

3. Care cannot be restricted in an arbitrary manner. When decisions are made to limit care or to prioritize patients in a triage mode, explicit policies should be written that provide guidelines for how triage decisions will be carried out. For those patients triaged out of ICU a specific plan for alternative care is necessary.

4. The medical benefits anticipated from critical care should be well defined. Patients who are not expected to benefit from ICU care should not be placed in the intensive care unit.[40]

Following these guidelines will ensure that these important issues have been fully considered. Adherence to the guidelines will reasonably ensure that triage is equitable when it occurs. Regardless of the staffing model employed in the ICU (that is, "closed," with all patients falling under the direct care of the intensive care staff, or "open," where the primary care is delivered by the patient's primary attending physician), the institution should designate a person to assume the position of triage officer for those times when triage is necessary. In a truly equitable system, patients already residing in the ICU should have no special privileges over those considered for admission. The goal of triage is to provide the greatest benefit for the greatest number of patients.

Using the ethical principle of justice has the greatest potential to allow healthcare providers to make decisions in a way that benefits the greatest number of patients at the lowest cost. Benefitting society with the greatest value from healthcare expenditures is a desirable goal. For the reasons outlined above, this will probably not occur in the United States in the foreseeable future, and scoring systems are not likely to play a major role.

INDIVIDUAL PATIENT APPLICATIONS

One concern about using models for individual patients is the interpretation of probability. These probabilities reflect an estimate of hospital mortality. A 50 percent probability of dying means that one-half of similar patients will die. What is not answered is which 50 percent of patients will die. This difficulty does not preclude using this probability as part of the information presented to the patient and family. It merely highlights the problem of trying to apply this measure to individuals. Probabilities, along with information concerning functional outcome and the patient's values, should influence clinical decision making, but probabilities should not directly determine decisions.

The use of a scoring system for individual patients should conform to the principles of medical ethics. Does it support the principle of autonomy? Allowing the patient to use this information as part of the overall decision-making process preserves autonomy. Does it uphold the Hippocratic principle to do no harm or the ethical principle of nonmaleficence? There is no evidence that for many patients using this type of data is harmful. However, caution must be applied when dealing with patients from ethnic and cultural minorities. Current opinions largely reflect the white, American male's view of ethical decision making. These viewpoints may not encompass large segments of our population. Reporting a high probability of mortality or encouraging patient autonomy may be seen as maleficent to certain cultures.[41]

Is the use of scoring systems in the best interest of the patient? If used as part of the overall data base that the patient has to consider, a probability score should provide the patient with an idea of how similarly ill patients are expected to do in a given circumstance. The scoring systems are likely to be more accurate than an individual physician's prediction of the outcome.[42] Explaining the consequences of ongoing intensive care versus other forms of care helps the patient to make a decision about what to expect and about how care might be provided.

The use of the fourth ethical principle, justice, has already been explained. Although justice is frequently discussed in American medicine, this principle plays a minor role.

OTHER USES OF PROGNOSTIC SCORING SYSTEMS

QUALITY IMPROVEMENT

Prognostic scoring systems could be used for internal quality improvement. There are several examples of a baseline data set using observed versus expected outcomes for the ICU as a whole or for a given patient population within the ICU. Depending on the results of the study or other quality monitors, new protocols may be instituted to address particular problems that are identified. The institution could then repeat these studies to see if outcomes improve (see Exhibit 7-4).

PERFORMANCE COMPARISON

The most important and most appropriate use of ICU severity models is comparison of one ICU to another. By collecting data (including admission variables) on 200 or 300 consecutive ICU patients, it is possible to calculate a standardized mortality risk that can be compared to a referent group of hospitals. If the observed hospital mortality for an ICU is similar to the predicted mortality, then the ICU is performing in a comparable way to those hospitals in the reference data base. Note that the referent data base usually includes teaching hospitals with full-time ICU directors. Comparisons must be made to ICUs with similar case mixes.[43]

In addition, these measurements could be used for external reporting to the Joint Commission on Accreditation of Healthcare Organizations or to state departments of health. Several states—including New York, Pennsylvania, and Iowa—have standardized state-mandated reporting, particularly for cardiac surgery. Is it ethical to publish the rankings of cardiac surgeons' performance? Are these data reliable enough to present to the public?

The public does have a right to know about the performance of hospitals and physicians. Although some may criticize the use of cardiac surgery report cards, it is ethical to provide this information.[44] Self-reporting, on the other hand, would not be acceptable. The state systems audit a percentage of records to ensure accuracy.

The performance of a particular ICU can also be compared to what is considered an outstanding ICU. Applying the same scoring system,

---

Exhibit 7-4
Potential Group Applications of Scoring Systems

- Quality improvement
- Comparison of ICU performance
- Risk stratification
- Comparison of health systems
- Comparison of physicians' performance
- Economic credentialing

one could determine if the ICU in question is above or below the reference group. Applying these models could indicate whether an institution's quality-improvement activities are actually working. There are potentially important problems with either of these uses. Data collection must be accurate. Data collectors must be well trained and consistent. This may be difficult to accomplish across hospitals. If the APACHE III system is being used, it is critical to make sure that there is agreement among admitting diagnoses. Similarly, some of the assessments may be clouded for patients who are being treated with drugs. In interpreting coma, the data collector would have to decide what Glasgow Coma Scale points should be given to a heavily sedated patient or a patient on neuromuscular blockers. If a particular ICU's patient mix or practice setting differs from those of the reference group, performance scores may differ.

It is important to calibrate these models periodically to see if calibration has changed or the instrument has drifted.[45] Old data may not reflect use of new technologies that have been introduced to the ICU. Ultimately, data become obsolete and new models must be adapted. Physicians may interpret the importance of selected end points differently; some may focus on ultimate outcome and mortality, while others emphasize functional outcome. These functional models have not yet been developed.

EARLY DISCHARGE OF LOW-RISK PATIENTS

Can severity models help with cost containment? These models have potentially great ability to help us understand how to use ICU resources. Helping to determine the best use of ICU resources may be the most reasonable application. One could argue that patients with low physiology scores or low probability of mortality do not need the intensive monitoring of the ICU. A combination of systems can identify patients who are at low risk for mortality or ICU morbidity and be safely discharged from the ICU based on a low probability of dying (using APACHE, MPM, or SAPS), a low physiology score (using APACHE or SAPS), and a low therapeutic measure (using the Therapeutic Intervention Scoring System).[46] Some patients who are traditionally treated in ICUs (such as patients with major vascular surgery, coronary artery disease, or thoracotomy) might be better cared for less expensively in a less acute setting if they are routinely predicted to have a low probability of mortality.

The routine placement of certain categories of patients in the ICU may not be based on resource utilization or severity of illness. Using an outcome model would add clarity to these determinations, and emphasizing resource utilization may redirect many of these patients to step-down units or the ward. In large, busy ICUs, very few low-risk patients are even admitted to the unit. However, in many nonteaching ICUs that do not require close screening of admissions by a qualified critical care physician, physicians admit their patients as they wish and low-risk patients occupy ICU beds. In such ICUs, use of an ICU severity system would be ethical and would help to contain costs.

Physicians' judgment is still important. A patient with severe, multiple-vessel coronary artery disease and a heart rate of 120 following surgery has minimal derangement of acute physiology but a likely probability of a poor outcome. The present models, if used incorrectly, could result in ICUs turning away such a patient. A more appropriate application of these models may be resource allocation for the hospital as a whole—such as determining whether the number of ICU beds is appropriate for the case mix of a particular hospital—rather than for individual patient assignments.

MANAGED CARE

These models could also be used in today's healthcare environment of managed competition. Outcome studies could possibly be used by managed-care organizations or hospital marketing departments to identify high-performance ICUs. A high-performance ICU may not be a low-cost ICU, however. The ability to look at cost per outcome may have a much greater impact in a competitive situation.

REPORT CARDS

Should data from these scoring systems be made available to the public? The Health Care Financing Administration (HCFA) publishes mortality rates for Medicare patients treated in U.S. hospitals. Initially, HCFA did not adjust for severity of illness, which led to widespread criticism of these studies despite their enthusiastic reception in the press. More recently, HCFA has added information about comorbid conditions. The ICU severity measures are more advanced than the HCFA model. Caution is appropriate when using report cards, because more research is necessary to identify the impact of patient mix, transportability of models into different settings, and the stability and longevity of models over time. Mortality studies must be performed carefully and interpreted cautiously. Although the public has a right to know, the data must be accurate. Other outcome parameters such as cost effectiveness, patient satisfaction, respect for autonomy, and functional recovery may become more important than mortality rates.

Mortality probability is influenced by the percentage of patients who are allowed to die without receiving care or whose care changes to palliative care. Some ICUs may be more proactive than others in obtaining DNR orders. The physicians may spend more time with the family and discuss these issues in more detail (such as in the case of patients with a reasonable probability of survival but expected low functional recovery). Other ICUs may treat these patients more aggressively and prolong their lives. The problems associated with comparing data from ICUs with these two philosophies are obvious. Probability models may be misapplied in other ways such as defining what patients go into what specific categories.

STAFFING PATTERNS

Can these models be used to estimate staffing patterns or collaborative practice patterns? The association between physiology scores for mortality probability and the intensity of bedside therapeutic care is not strong. Further, the intensity of care is not adequately incorporated into the therapy-based models such as the Therapeutic Intervention Scoring System.[47]

PHYSICIANS' REPORT CARDS

Can these severity measures be used to compare the performance of individual physicians with local or national standards? It is difficult to compare the performance of individual physicians in today's team-oriented ICU, with its heterogeneous patient population, multiple consultants, and varying levels of physician expertise or full-time staffing. The composition of the team is likely to differ from patient to patient and may change for long-term patients. Studies of individual physicians are best focused on high-volume procedures in which the surgical technique is highly associated with outcome (such as cardiac surgery, aortic aneurysm repair, and carotid artery surgery). Risk adjustments for these cases would require special modifications of these models. Other aspects of care may be independent of the individual surgeon; these include perioperative assessment, anesthesia techniques and practices, and postoperative care. General severity models by themselves have little application in such areas of care.

Because it is not appropriate to use these models as absolute performance indicators for individual physicians, specific ICUs, and specific institutions, regulating agencies or managed-care organizations should not attempt to adopt this methodology for licensing, practice-privilege requirements, or economic credentialing.

PATIENT DECISION MAKING

How should patients and families be told their estimated probability of survival? These models have only been validated for use at certain, specific times. Any other use of the models involves speculation. The MPM II has been validated for use at ICU admission. At 24 hours after ICU admission, the MPM II, SAPS II, and APACHE III have been validated. These models have not been validated for use outside of these times. It would be inappropriate and misleading to place great emphasis on what a model predicts until it has been validated. Further, because of the wide spectrum of diseases included in the clinical terms used in these models, the clinician must interpret the estimated probability for any individual patient, possibly adding confusion. The SUPPORT model does allow for a physician's estimate at day three and may be complementary to the statistical model.

Can patients use these data to make intelligent choices about physicians or hospitals? In an emergency situation, this may not be practical. The risks of transferring a patient from one hospital to another because it has a "high-performance ICU" may far outweigh any potential benefits. Physician-specific data may be best applied toward physicians from the same specialty working in the same hospital. There is little justification for using these models to compare physicians at different hospitals.

INSURANCE CONTRACTS

Should insurance plans use severity measures to determine coverage? Should they pay only when there is an expected health gain? In the present environment, this would be unethical. There does not seem to be any clamoring from insurance companies to do this. However, if one went to a single-payer system or if one looks at the Oregon Health Plan, this type of contracting with individuals may ultimately make sense. If medical resources are seen as limited and finite, then it can be argued that certain procedures should be favored over others. Techniques are becoming available to make these types of determinations, such as cost per quality-adjusted-life-years.[48] These models can be used to make decisions for optimal allocation of dollars. Let us suppose a patient is in the ICU with an increasing probability of mortality that rises from 20 percent on day one to 90 percent on day seven. These statistics could be incorporated into the insurance provider's reimbursement decision (that is, once the mortality probability reaches a certain level, care is determined to be of marginal benefit). The insurance provider may have a clause in the contract stating that it will not provide marginal care defined in this way. A model could affect resource use across a state. Oregon is attempting this type of contracting with its Medicaid population. Everyone knows that certain services will not be covered by the carrier if certain definitions of ineffective care are met. These definitions are based on the expected cost-benefit ratio. Better models incorporating some type of functional outcome other than survival will be important to implement cost-allocation systems more fully.

FUTURE USES OF SCORING SYSTEMS

Robert Wachter and John Luce present two scenarios regarding the future use of scoring systems. In the first vision:

> As the ICU has become a symbol of the financial excesses and possibly misguided prioritization of modern medicine, the ICU director has emerged as a potential source of improved efficiency and resource allocation in some people's minds. This "ideal" director is seen as a physician armed with APACHE III or some other software that can predict with ease and precision who will live and who will die. It is unclear in this vision exactly how the director uses this information, but the assumption is that many patients will not be allowed either to enter the ICU or linger there. Whether patients or their families agree with this process—indeed, whether they are involved in it at all—is unclear.[49]

In another vision:

> The ICU director is replaced by a gatekeeper who is even further removed from the patient, if not the ICU. This gatekeeper might be a utilization review nurse who visits the unit occasionally to tell a physician whom to discharge in keeping with hospital policy. Alternatively, it might be the even more distant representative of a third party payor who determines whether the physician or the hospital will be reimbursed for their services by, for example, Medicare. Both

technicians base their decisions on a variety of group statistics including those provided by prognostic scoring systems.[50]

In managed care, is it ethical to apply population statistics to individual patients?

HEALTHCARE REVOLUTION

Although many argue that the above scenarios seem far-fetched, the U.S. healthcare scene is changing rapidly. There is a growing emphasis on patient autonomy just as cost concerns come to the fore, but it is not impossible to imagine a scenario where contracts exclude expensive care for diseases with high probabilities of mortality. The ethical imperative to "do everything possible" for the patient may be replaced by the imperative to "do what is reasonable." Defining a term such as *reasonable* will prove problematic; the definition must reflect the patient's own value system and not strictly a probabilistic model. Wachter and Luce argue that these scoring systems will inevitably be developed and that they will ultimately have a greater effect on healthcare.[51]

MEDIA VERSION OF SEVERITY MODELS

A recent article in *Forbes* highlights the increasing importance of prognostic scoring systems.[52] The APACHE system is now a business, APACHE Medical Systems. Because the corporate model is necessarily profit driven, clinicians and institutions must exercise caution. A salesperson for the company, especially if not versed in statistics, might overestimate the performance of this product. In addition, the hospital purchasing agent may request a trial of the product and become excited if the data appear positive. The marketing department for the hospital now may develop tremendous enthusiasm for using these data to sell the quality of the hospital and its doctors to the public. Higher levels of public scrutiny and statistical confidence must be employed when evaluating the claims of a profit-oriented corporate entity.

DECISION MAKING AT THE END OF LIFE

Can the APACHE III system, which describes daily probabilities to seven days, be used to make decisions at the end of life? For patients who have a predicted mortality risk of 90 percent or higher any time during the seven-day period, the observed hospital mortality was 90 percent. One might think that repeated measures of high-mortality probability would be more accurate than simply the high probability at admission. Regardless, one would expect 10 percent of the patients to survive if the predicted mortality is 90 percent. However, among the few survivors, the long-term function may not be very good. It may be ethical to use daily probabilities as an adjunct to clinical decision making, but the models cannot be the driving force.

DECISIONS ABOUT ADMISSION TO THE ICU

It would be unethical to use prognostic scoring systems to deny admission. APACHE and SAPS require 24 hours of observation and treatment in order to calculate the probability. The MPM does have a presentation model, but the developers of MPM do not recommend its use to deny admission. MPM was based on patients who were admitted to the ICU, so it would be inappropriate to calculate MPM and use this as a basis for denying admission.

THE EFFECTS OF OUTCOME PREDICTORS ON PATIENT CARE

Does providing daily probabilities of mortality and estimates of dysfunction alter patient choice or patient care? Although there are anecdotal examples of physicians using readily available ICU probabilities, SUPPORT provides the best analysis of this issue. The SUPPORT investigators looked at nine high-mortality disease groups (such as acute respiratory failure, multiorgan failure and sepsis, nontraumatic coma, and multiorgan failure and malignancy) that had a 50 percent expected mortality at six months.[53] The study was conducted at five high-quality teaching hospitals. The first phase of the SUPPORT DNR study evaluated 4,301 patients. The study, which was used to develop the SUPPORT models, documented poor communication between physicians, patients, and surrogates regarding decision making at the end of life. The second phase of the study was important because of unique interventions related to ICU severity modeling. There were 2,152 control patients and 2,652 patients who underwent two unique interventions:

- Physicians received daily estimates of six-month survival and two-month functional disability probabilities.
- A special nurse was assigned to the patients in the intervention group with multiple contacts among patient, family, attending physician, and staff. The goals of these contacts were to update the patient's preferences for DNR orders and life support; to

explain outcomes to the medical staff, family, and patient; to pay attention to pain control; to facilitate advance-care planning; and most importantly to increase the level of communication between the patient and the physician of record (the cornerstone of ethical medical decision making).

However, despite the presentation of daily probabilities and increased communication, there was no reduced use of hospital resources for the patients in the intervention group. Poor communication or physicians' misunderstanding of the patients' preferences occurred in 80 percent of the cases. A large percentage of conscious patients who ultimately died in the hospital reported moderate to severe pain half the time. A low percentage of patients discussed CPR preferences with their physicians, despite the expected six-month mortality of 50 percent.

In summary, daily ICU probabilities did not improve the care or patient outcomes in high-quality teaching hospitals. Explanations about why these two interventions had such little impact remain speculative.

IDENTIFICATION OF POTENTIALLY INEFFECTIVE CARE

The term *potentially ineffective care* does not have the same ethical limitations as the term *futility.* Another use of severity models, related to end-of-life decision making and broader than futility guidelines, is the use of sustained high probabilities of mortality to identify patients with poor outcomes and high resource use (possibly 10 percent of ICU patients). By using decision-tree analysis, Esserman and colleagues determined that, over five days, if the initial probability times the fifth-day probability exceeded 0.36, then the patient's prognosis was very poor despite aggressive ICU care.[54] Perhaps on day six the hospital ethics committee can serve as a neutral negotiating body between the patient/surrogate and the medical team to decide whether to continue aggressive care or switch to comfort care.

SHIFT TO FUNCTIONAL OUTCOME

One of the limitations of ICU severity models is the emphasis upon mortality. For example, in cardiac-surgery patients, the overall mortality is only 3 percent; however, these patients have a high risk of stroke, respiratory failure, renal failure, and prolonged ICU care. A better measure to help cardiac patients make decisions would be prediction of functional outcome. There is no doubt that the next generation of cardiac surgery models will present risk stratification based on functional outcome in addition to mortality prediction.

The same limitation is evident for ICU patients. It would be far preferable to have models that present functional outcome. One recent example is based on data from a subset of 596 SUPPORT patients regarding functional outcome from nontraumatic coma.[55] The diagnostic categories included postcardiac arrest, cerebral infarction, and cerebral hemorrhage. The overall two-month mortality rate was 70 percent, and the logistic-regression model identified five risk factors—abnormal brain-stem response, absent verbal response, absent response to pain, renal failure with creatinine greater than 1.5 milligrams per deciliter, and age of 70 years or more. With three of these factors present, the mortality was 90 percent. By itself, this mortality rate would not be high enough to act upon, especially considering that the lower limit of the confidence interval was only 84 percent. However, the confidence interval is much tighter when the outcome measure is two-month severe-disability rate rather than two-month mortality. For patients with absent response to pain or abnormal brain-stem response, the prediction of severe disability, performed on day three in the ICU, was 97 percent, with a confidence interval of 95 to 99 percent. The next generation of severity models will emphasize functional disability and the use of confidence intervals.

PATIENT INTERPRETATION

It is doubtful that functional models will have an impact on resource utilization. A recent study of nursing home residents reported that a majority of residents (89 percent) would prefer hospitalization (and presumably critical care) in the event of serious illness, and 60 percent would want CPR in the event of sudden cardiac arrest. Only 15 percent actually changed their CPR preferences after being given a survival probability of 5 percent. In addition, 70 percent of patients believed that important medical decisions should be made by their physicians.[56]

Although ICU scoring systems represent a step forward in quantifying outcomes objectively, this is rarely the only information patients are looking for. Ultimately, a new paradigm for making decisions about healthcare at the end of life and a more realistic cost-benefit analysis where individuals have a financial stake will be required to change substantially the amount of care that patients receive at the end of life.

CONCLUSION

ICU severity models are important tools to help with clinical decision making for *groups* of ICU patients. However, for most individual applications, the severity models should not be the driving force behind decisions about treatment, and the unqualified use of these systems for individual applications would be unethical.

ACKNOWLEDGMENTS

We would like to thank Suzanne Allen for her invaluable help in preparing this manuscript. We also would like to thank Noreen McCarron, JD, RN, for aiding us with the interpretation of the legal issues in the various cases we reviewed.

NOTES

1. *Gilgunn v. Massachusetts General Hospital,* No. 92-4820, Suffolk Co., Mass., Super. Ct. (April 1995).

2. J. Ellement, "Jury Sides with Doctors on Ending Woman's Life Support," *Boston Globe,* 22 April 1995, p. 18.

3. New York Public Health Law, Article 29-B, 2960-78.

4. Ibid.

5. A.M. Capron, "Abandoning a Waning Life," *Hastings Center Report* 25, no. 4 (July-August 1995): 24-26.

6. *Brune v. Belinkoff,* 354 Mass. 102, 109 (1968).

7. D.A. Asch, J. Hansen-Flaschen, and P.N. Lanken, "Decisions to Limit or Continue Life-Sustaining Treatment by Critical Care Physicians in the United States: Conflicts between Physicians' Practices and Patients' Wishes," *American Journal of Respiratory Critical Care Medicine* 151 (1995): 288-92.

8. M. Angell, "The Case of Helga Wanglie: A New Kind of 'Right To Die' Case," *New England Journal of Medicine* 325 (1991): 511-12; S.H. Miles, "Informed Demand for 'Non-Beneficial' Medical Treatment," *New England Journal of Medicine* 325 (1991): 512-15.

9. E.H. Elpem et al., "Patients' Preferences for Intensive Care," *Critical Care Medicine* 20, no. 1 (1992): 43-47.

10. S.A. Schroeder, "Cost Containment in U.S. Healthcare," *Academic Medicine* 70 (1995): 861-66.

11. G.J. Annas, "Asking the Courts to Set the Standard of Emergency Care— The Case of Baby K," *New England Journal of Medicine* 330 (1994): 1542-45.

12. *In re Baby K,* 832 K Supp. 1022 (E.D. Va. 1993); *In re Baby K,* 16 F. 3d 590 (4th Cir. 1994).

13. See note 11 above, p. 1545.

14. See note 8 above.

15. Oregon Health Services Commission, *Prioritization of Health Services* (Salem, Ore: 1991).

16. S.J. Reiser, A.J. Dyck, and W.J. Curran, eds., *Ethics in Medicine: Histori-*

cal Perspectives and Contemporary Concerns (Cambridge, Mass.: Massachusetts Institute of Technology Press, 1977), 6-7.

17. Plato, *Republic,* trans. G.M.A. Grube (Indianapolis: Hackett, 1981), 76-77.

18. See note 2 above.

19. See note 3 above.

20. L.J. Schneiderman, N.S. Jecker, and A.R. Jonsen, "Medical Futility: Its Meaning and Ethical Implications," *Annals of Internal Medicine* 112, no. 2 (1990): 949-54.

21. M.B. Hamel, "Identification of Comatose Patients at High Risk for Death or Severe Disability," *Journal of the American Medical Association* 273 (1995): 1842-48.

22. See note 7 above.

23. L.J. Blackhall et al., "Ethnicity and Attitudes toward Patient Autonomy," *Journal of the American Medical Association* 274 (1995): 820-25.

24. D. Waisel and R. Truog, "Cardiopulmonary Resuscitation Not Indicated Order: Futility Revisited," *Annals of Internal Medicine* 122 (1995): 304-08; J.D. Lantos et al., "The Illusion of Futility in Clinical Practice," *American Journal of Medicine* 87 (1989): 81-84; S.J. Youngner, "Who Defines Futility?" *Journal of the American Medical Association* 260 (1988): 2094-95; T. Tomlinson and H. Brody, "Futility and Ethics of Resuscitation," *Journal of the American Medical Association* 264, no. 10 (1990): 1276-80; see note 5 above.

25. Waisel and Truog, see note 24 above.

26. Ibid., 306.

27. Tomlinson and Brody, "Futility and Ethics of Resuscitation," see note 24 above.

28. Hastings Center, *Guidelines on the termination of Life-Sustaining Treatment and the Care of the Dying* (New York: Hastings Center, 1987).

29. Tomlinson and Brody, "Futility and Ethics of Resuscitation," see note 24 above, p. 1278.

30. For more details on severity-of-illness models, see D. Teres, J.S. Avrunin, and S. Lemeshow, "Severity of Illness Modeling," in *Intensive Care Medicine* 2nd ed., ed. J.M. Rippe (Boston: Little, Brown and Company, 1991), 1953-62.

31. K. Castella et al., "Mortality Prediction Models in Intensive Care: Acute Physiology and Chronic Health Evaluation II and Mortality Prediction Model Compared," *Critical Care Medicine* 19 (1991): 191-97.

32. J.R. Le Gall et al., and ICU Scoring Group, "Customized Probability Models for Early Sepsis in Adult Intensive Care Patients," *Journal of the American Medical Association* 273 (1995): 644-50; R.L. Smith, S.M. Levine, and M.L. Lewis, "Prognosis of Patients with AIDS Requiring Intensive Care," *Chest* 96 (1989): 857; J.M. Civetta, "The Clinical Limitations of ICU Scoring Systems," in *Problems in Critical Care,* ed. J.C. Farmer, R.R. Kirby, and R.W. Taylor (Philadelphia, PA: J.B. Lippincott, 1989), 3:681-95.

33. J.A. Kruse, M.C. Thill-Baharozian, and R.W. Carlson, "Comparison of

Clinical Assessment with APACHE II for Predicting Mortality Risk in Patients Admitted to a Medical Intensive Care Unit," *Journal of the American Medical Association* 260 (1988): 1739-42; H.S. Perkins, A.R. Jonsen, and W.V. Epstein, "Providers as Predictors: Using Outcome Predictions in Intensive Care," *Critical Care Medicine* 14 (1986): 105-10; D.K. McClich and S.H. Powell, "How Well Can Physicians Estimate Mortality in a Medical Intensive Care Unit," *Medical Decision Making* 9 (1989): 125-32; W.A. Knaus, D.P. Wagner, and J. Lynn, "Short Term Mortality Predictions for Critically Ill Hospitalized Adults: Science and Ethics," *Science* 254 (1991): 389-93.

34. I.R. Le Gall, S. Lemeshow, and F. Saulnier, "A New Simplified Acute Physiology Score (SAPS II) Based on a European/North American Multicenter Study," *Journal of the American Medical Association* 270, no. 124 (1993): 2957-63.

35. S. Lemeshow et al., "Refining Intensive Care Unit Outcome Prediction by Using Changing Probabilities of Mortality," *Critical Care Medicine* 16 (1988): 470-77; S. Lemeshow et al., "Mortality Probability Models (MPM II) Based on an International Cohort of Intensive Care Unit Patients," *Journal of the American Medical Association* 270, no. 20 (1993): 2478-86.

36. The SUPPORT Principal Investigators, "A Controlled Trial to Improve Care for Seriously Ill Hospitalized Patients: The Study to Understand Prognoses and Preferences for Outcomes and Risks of Treatments (SUPPORT)," *Journal of the American Medical Association* 274, no. 20 (1995): 1591-98; W.A. Knaus et al., "The SUPPORT Prognostic Model: Objective Estimates of Survival for Seriously Ill Hospitalized Adults," *Annals of Internal Medicine* 122 (1995): 191-203.

37. J.R. LeGall et al., "A Simplified Acute Physiology Score for ICU Patients," *Critical Care Medicine* 12 (1984): 975-77; W.A. Knaus et al., "The APACHE III Prognostic System: Risk Prediction of Hospital Mortality for Critically Ill Hospitalized Adults," *Chest* 100 (1991): 1619-36; W.A. Knaus et al., "APACHE II: A Severity of Disease Classification System," *Critical Care Medicine* 13 (1985): 818-29; see note 34 above.

38. See note 10 above, p. 862.

39. Society of Critical Care Medicine Ethics Committee, "Consensus Statement on the Triage of Critically Ill Patients," *Journal of the American Medical Association* 271 (1994): 1200-03.

40. Ibid., 1200.

41. See note 23 above.

42. See note 33 above.

43. R.L. Murphy-Filkins et al., "Effect of Changing Patient Mix on the Performance of an ICU Severity Model," *Critical Care Medicine* 24 (1996): 1968-73; D. Teres and S. Lemeshow, "Why Severity Models Should Be Used with Caution," *Critical Care Clinic* 10, no. 1 (1994): 93-110.

44. J. Green, "Report Cards on Cardiac Surgeons," *New England Journal of Medicine* 333, no. 14 (1995): 938-c.

45. J.R. LeGall et al., and ICU Scoring Group, "Customized Probability Models for Early Sepsis in Adult Intensive Care Patients," *Journal of the American Medical Association* 273, no. 8 (1995): 644-50; see note 43 above.

46. D.J. Cullen et al., "Therapeutic Intervention Scoring System," *Critical Care Medicine* 2 (1974): 57-60.

47. Ibid.

48. T.M. Gill and A.R. Feinstein, "A Critical Appraisal of the Quality of Quality-of-Life Measurements," *Journal of the American Medical Association* 272, no. 8 (1994): 619-26; M.A. Rie, "Healthcare Reform and Cost Containment," in *Intensive Care Medicine*, 3rd ed., J.M. Rippe, et al., ed., (Boston: Little Brown and Company, 1996), 2:2576-88.

49. R.M. Wachter and J.M. Luce, "The Ethical Appropriateness of Using Prognostic Scoring Systems in Clinical Management," *Critical Care Clinics* 10, no. 1 (1994): 229.

50. Ibid., 239.

51. Ibid.

52. S. Oliver, "What are my Chances, Doc?" *Forbes*, 31 July 1995, 136-37.

53. See note 36 above.

54. L. Esserman, J. Belkora, and L. Lenert, "Potentially Ineffective Care: A New Outcome to Assess the Limits of Critical Care," *Journal of the American Medical Association* 274, no. 19 (1995): 1544-51.

55. See note 21 above.

56. L.A. O'Brien et al., "Nursing Home Residents' Preferences for Life-Sustaining Treatments," *Journal of the American Medical Association* 274 (1995): 1775-79.

8

Ethics in Critical Care Research

Christopher W. Johnson

INTRODUCTION

Advances in technology and medical knowledge in the past three decades have allowed modern intensive care units (ICU) and healthcare providers to monitor life's physiologic processes throughout the course of a critical illness. Beginning with basic arrhythmia monitoring in the 1960s, the technology of the ICU has expanded rapidly. Invasive and noninvasive methods now exist to continuously monitor a patient's electrocardiogram in 12 leads, arterial blood pressure, intracardiac and intrapulmonary pressures, electroencephalogram, and a variety of other physiologic parameters involving virtually every organ system. This ability to monitor and manipulate a patient's physiology has led to advances in the care of the critically ill and has allowed patients who once would have succumbed to sepsis, shock, or organ failure to survive and recover.[1]

Within the setting of the ICU lies great potential for research. Development and testing of pharmaceuticals, medical technologies, and procedures contribute to improvements in morbidity and mortality, the enhanced comfort of patients, decreased length of stay, and lower costs in the care of the critically ill. Critical care research may also help to determine which patients will benefit from ICU interventions and to identify patients for whom advanced technologies will only prolong the dying process. The institution of inappropriate, untested, or unproven therapies can exacerbate the pace of an illness and violate the basic tenet of medical ethics—above all, do no harm.

Despite the significant potential of research in critical care, use of critically ill patients for medical research warrants caution. By virtue of the severity of their illnesses and the often rapid pace of their disease processes, these patients are among the most vulnerable of research subjects, and therefore deserve greater protection than the normal volunteer. Although earlier critical accounts of human experimentation exist, it was the atrocities committed by Nazi physicians during the Second World War that prompted modern concern for the protection of research subjects. The *Nuremberg Code,* developed by the Nuremberg military tribunals during their trial of the Nazi physician-researchers, established standards for judging the outrages committed in the name of science by Nazi physicians and scientists.[2] In 1964 the World Medical Association produced the *Declaration of Helsinki,* which developed the theory of consent beyond the *Nuremberg Code's* requirement that "the voluntary consent of the human subject is absolutely essential." The *Declaration of Helsinki* recognized the legitimacy of proxy consent for research involving children and persons with cognitive impairment.[3]

BASIC REQUIREMENTS OF RESEARCH

The Nazi atrocities, together with circumstances in the United States, such as the Tuskegee Syphilis Study, the Willowbrook Hepatitis Experiments, and the Jewish Chronic Disease Hospital case helped provide the impetus for the development of federal regulation, "Protection of Human Subjects," in the *U.S. Code of Federal Regulations (CFR).*[4]

The federal regulations apply to any facility that receives federal funding for research, and they are used as basic guidelines by most institutions. For approval of research with human subjects, the regulations require that the risks to patients are minimized, that the risks are reasonable in relation to anticipated benefits, and that informed consent is sought from each prospective patient or the patient's legally authorized representative.[5]

INFORMED CONSENT

Central to the federal regulations is the concept that research participants have a right to self-determination, and that individuals who are unable to assert their self-determination deserve protection. A research subject therefore must be adequately informed before participating in any research project. Informed consent requires that the subject is fully informed, that the subject comprehends the information, and that the consent is voluntary.[6]

Information must be presented to subjects in a way that they can understand, if their consent is to be truly informed. In informing subjects, researchers must state clearly that the subjects will be involved in research; they must describe the purpose of the research, and its duration, methods, and potential risks and benefits; and they must provide a person to answer any questions the subjects may have. Information should also be provided concerning confidentiality of medical records and the subject's right to withdraw from the study at any time without penalty.[7] One standard for evaluating the amount and type of information a patient should receive is determined according to a patient-oriented or "reasonable-volunteer" standard—that is, the information that a reasonable patient objectively needs to hear from a researcher to make informed and intelligent decisions regarding participation in the proposed research.[8]

The researcher is obligated to confirm that the patient has a sufficient understanding of all pertinent research information, particularly the potential risks involved. The scope of this obligation increases commensurate with the degree of possible risk to the patient. The patient's participation in the research project must also be without coercion or undue influence.

The process of informed consent must be fully documented, and a consent form should be signed by the subject. The consent form should include all protocol information; it should document that the subject has read and understood the information and is entering the study voluntarily. The researcher always holds final responsibility for assessing the adequacy of the informed consent.

In addition to obtaining an informed consent, the researcher should always discuss a proxy directive (such as a durable power of attorney for healthcare) with the patient and encourage its execution. This instrument enables the patient to designate another person to act on his or her behalf should the patient become incapable of making healthcare decisions.[9]

If the patient is incapacitated[10] and therefore unable to execute a proxy directive, someone should be designated to protect the patient's rights and welfare. The person designated should be someone authorized either by statute or legal proceeding. This legal representative or surrogate has the authority to make healthcare decisions and, presumably, research decisions on behalf of the prospective subject. In this situation, the researcher's obligation to obtain consent is transferred from the patient to the patient's surrogate. The surrogate must render decisions consistent with the patient's wishes, if known. If the patient's wishes are unknown, the surrogate should make decisions consistent with the patient's best interest. Controversy exists over whether surrogates can or should give consent for research. Iserson and Mahowald contend that "because of the urgency of evaluation and treatment, as well as the usual absence of a suitable surrogate, it is impossible to obtain substitute consent in most acute care situations."[11] Notwithstanding these concerns, the surrogate remains one of the best and potentially most important safeguards for the patient's protection—particularly in the research setting.

ALTERNATIVE APPROACHES TO INFORMED CONSENT

The continuum of ICU care frequently extends from a patient's hospital admission through discharge planning; thus, acute care research[12] is often a part of critical care research. When patients present with life-threatening illnesses that require prompt lifesaving measures, enrolling these patients in acute care research studies can be ethically and legally difficult. Often these subjects are incapacitated and without available surrogates. Several approaches have been suggested for the timely enrollment of nonconsensual subjects in emergency situations: the medical emergency consent exception, deferred consent, and prospective consent. Central to all these approaches is the concept that acute care research studies are necessary and valid, and that an alternative to traditional informed consent is required for such research to proceed.

Medical emergency consent exception. Some ethicists argue that nonconsensual research in an emergency setting is justified by the medical emergency consent exception.[13] The medical emergency consent exception refers to crises in which an individual patient is at imminent risk of significant injury, decline, or death if treatment is withheld or postponed. If the need to obtain consent would result in a delay, and this delay might result in substantial harm to the patient; and no evidence exists that the person would refuse the treatment, the law relieves the physician of the obligation to obtain informed consent.[14] Increasingly, ethicists have cited this doctrine—sometimes in conjunction with other criteria such as institutional review board (IRB) oversight—as the basis for proceeding with acute care research (such as cardiac and brain resuscitation research).[15]

An extension of the emergency consent exception for research purposes is troublesome. The statutory and common law exceptions to consent in medical emergencies are for therapeutic purposes. Accordingly, the procedures employed pursuant to this exception should be therapeutic and intended for the patient's benefit. The distinction between therapy and research should not be blurred; although therapy and research often occur together, the goals of the intervention and roles of the physician are quite different. An additional concern is that this approach fails to attempt to obtain a surrogate or ombudsman for the patient, even when circumstances might allow. Further, although consent to treatment is often said to be "implied" in an emergency, based on a reasonable-person standard,[16] it is unlikely that a reasonable person in a life-threatening condition would gratuitously undergo the added burden of participation in a research protocol—particularly if the research is nontherapeutic and the risk is greater than minimal.

Deferred consent. The notion of deferred consent was developed as an extension of the medical emergency consent exception. Deferred consent is a process whereby consent is not obtained prior to a patient's entry into a research study. The patient is immediately enrolled in the research protocol upon presentation, and the patient's participation in the research is later discussed with the patient or patient's surrogate after the research has been initiated and, in some cases, completed.[17] According to Miller, this approach is problematic because "one cannot consent meaningfully to something that has already happened. Consent implies the possibility of refusal. How can one refuse to participate in some activity that has taken place before one knew about it?"[18] Deferred consent cannot reasonably be considered consent; rather, it is a process seeking validation and ratification for that which has already occurred.

Prospective consent. For protocols involving diseases that require repeated acute interventions (such as diabetes, congestive heart failure, asthma, and sickle-cell disease), prospective consent is another approach for nonconsensual emergency research. Here the researcher has the opportunity to enroll patients with decision-making capacity in a study, to explain and discuss the protocol with them, and to obtain their consent for enrollment for any subsequent presentations, including when the patient may be incapacitated and unable to reconfirm consent.[19] Although prospective consent may, in limited circumstances and with selected populations, be a valid consent method for critical care research, there are some problems. Some ethicists have raised valid concerns about the ability of healthcare providers to obtain fully informed consent from critically ill patients.[20] Concerns regarding the validity of informed consent are increased in the ICU; patients are often in a critical physiologic state and are less likely to comprehend or deliberate about such decisions.[21] The fact that the ICU can be overwhelming to patients, the urgency with which decisions must sometimes be made, and the often sudden and unanticipated onset of the illness all add to difficulties in obtaining informed consent. Also problematic is the timeliness of the consent; it is unclear whether a person can adequately consent to a research intervention that may not occur for days, months, or even longer. Finally, prospective consent cannot cover unanticipated events.[22]

WAIVER OF CONSENT

Given the legal and ethical problems of the proposed alternatives to informed consent, healthcare providers' inability to obtain consent in many settings, and the necessity of critical care research, one must consider the possibility of waiving the requirement for consent in research. In doing this, the researcher is ultimately confronted with the fundamental ethical problem in critical care research: the conflict between the autonomy and welfare of the individual patient and the need for such research.

Some assistance with this dilemma is provided by federal regulation, which allow for a waiver of the consent requirement where: (1) the research involves no more than minimal risk to the subjects; (2) the waiver or alteration will not adversely affect the rights and welfare of the subjects; (3) the research could not practicably be carried out without the waiver or alteration; and (4) whenever appropriate, additional information is provided to the subjects after participation.[23]

The federal regulation defines *minimal risk* as follows: "The probability and magnitude of harm or discomfort anticipated in the research are not greater in and of themselves than those ordinarily encountered in daily life or during the performance of routine physical or psychological examinations or tests."[24] Although this definition has caused some confusion, it is intended to apply to those risks the research subject may encounter on a daily basis. In earlier drafts of these regulations, the definition for minimal risk made reference to the "daily lives of healthy people." The phrase "healthy people" was deleted from the final text because it would have unnecessarily imposed a standard on research involving ill people that would severely restrict a range of beneficial research and could have had the effect of stifling advances in therapeutic intervention.[25] Accordingly, for persons with severe health problems (such as patients in the ICU), it could be entirely appropriate to use invasive procedures that carry major risks but are intended to benefit the subject, or have at least as favorable a risk-benefit ratio as alternative procedures during research protocols designed for minimal risk.[26]

Waiver of the consent requirement also requires that the rights and welfare of the subject will not be adversely affected. Patients' rights, respect for persons, patients' autonomy, and informed consent are high priorities in research ethics. However, when consent is not possible at all, this ethical requirement must be examined to determine whether it is appropriate and reasonable. Federal regulation fails to offer specifics for assessing this important criterion. The determination of whether patients' rights are adequately protected is probably best made by the IRBs, strictly on a case-by-case basis. Researchers, together with IRBs, should determine whether the welfare of patients will be adversely affected. These determinations require strict IRB review of the protocol, and may require concurrent IRB review of the research, particularly in situations where a patient is incapacitated and no surrogate is available.

The third condition for waiving the consent requirement—that the research could not be practically carried out without a waiver—is easily met in an ICU, where patients frequently are incapacitated or have fluctuating capacity, and consent by a surrogate is not always practical. Finally, there is no difficulty providing information to subjects or their surrogates after participation, where appropriate.

In response to growing concerns over the ability to conduct high quality research in emergency circumstances, the U.S. Secretary of Health and Human Services in October of 1996 announced a waiver of the applicability of the federal regulations requirement for obtaining and documenting informed consent for a strictly limited class of research. For human subjects who are in need of emergency therapy and for whom—because of their medical condition and the unavailability of legally authorized representatives of the subjects—no legally effective informed consent can be obtained, the requirement for obtaining and documenting informed consent from each human subject (or his or her legally authorized representative) prior to initiation of research may be waived, if the waiver of informed consent is approved by an IRB and strictly limited conditions are met (see Exhibit 8-1).

The regulations and incorporated safeguards are only as good as the researchers and the institutions that implement them. An even greater safeguard than informed consent "is the presence of an informed, able, conscientious, compassionate, responsible investigator."[27] Accordingly, the greatest reliance ought to be a reliance on the professional integrity of the individual physician.[28] This statement is illustrated by the fact

Exhibit 8-1
Emergency Research Consent Waiver

Pursuant to Section 46.101(i), the Secretary, HHS, has waived the general requirements for informed consent at 45 CFR 46.116(a) and (b) and 46.408, to be referred to as the "Emergency Research Consent Waiver" for a class of research consisting of activities, each of which have met the following strictly limited conditions detailed under *either* (a) or (b) below:

- **(a) Research subject to FDA regulation**
  The IRB responsible for the review, approval, and continuing review of the research activity has approved both the activity and a waiver of informed consent and found and documented:
- (1) That the research activity *is subject* to regulations codified by the Food and Drug Administration (FDA) (see **Federal Register**, vol. 61, pp. 51498-51531) at Title 21 CFR Part 50 and will be carried out under an FDA investigational new drug application (IND) or an FDA investigational device exemption (IDE), the application for which has clearly identified the protocols that would include subjects who are unable to consent, and
- (2) That the requirements for exception from informed consent for emergency research detailed in **21 CFR Section 50.24** have been met relative to those protocols, **or**
- **(b) Research not subject to FDA regulation**
  The IRB responsible for the review, approval, and continuing review of the research has approved both the research and a waiver of informed consent and has (i) found and documented that the research *is not subject* to regulations codified by the FDA at 21 CFR Part 50, and (ii) found and documented and reported to the OPRR that the following conditions have been met relative to the research:
- (1) The human subjects are in a life-threatening situation, available treatments are unproven or unsatisfactory, and the collection of valid scientific evidence, which may include evidence obtained through randomized placebo-controlled investigations, is necessary to determine the safety and effectiveness of particular interventions.
- (2) Obtaining informed consent is not feasible because:
  - (i) the subjects will not be able to give their informed consent as a result of their medical condition;
  - (ii) the intervention involved in the research must be administered before consent from the subjects' legally authorized representatives is feasible; and
  - (iii) there is no reasonable way to identify prospectively the individuals likely to become eligible for participation in the research.
- (3) Participation in the research holds out the prospect of direct benefit to the subjects because:
  - (i) subjects are facing a life-threatening situation that necessitates intervention;
  - (ii) appropriate animal and other preclinical studies have been conducted, and the information derived from those studies and related evidence support the potential for the intervention to provide a direct benefit to the individual subjects; and
  - (iii) risks associated with the research are reasonable in relation to what is known about the therapy, if any, and what is known about the risks and benefits of the proposed intervention or activity.

- (4) The research could not practicably be carried out without the waiver.
- (5) The proposed research protocol defined the length of the potential therapeutic window based on scientific evidence, and the investigator has committed to attempting to contact a legally authorized representative for each subject within that window of time and, if feasible, to asking the legally authorized representative contacted for consent within that window rather than proceeding without consent. The investigator will summarize efforts made to contact representatives and make this information available to the IRB at the time of continuing review.
- (6) The IRB has reviewed and approved informed consent procedures and an informed consent document in accord with Sections 46.116 and 46.117 of 45 CFR Part 46. These procedures and the informed consent document are to be used with subjects or their legally authorized representatives in situations where use of such procedures and documents is feasible. The IRB has reviewed and approved procedures and information to be used when providing an opportunity for a family member to object to a subject's participation in the research consistent with paragraph (b)(7)(v) of this waiver.
- (7) Additional protections of the rights and welfare of the subjects will be provided, including, at least:
    - (i) consultation (including, where appropriate, consultation carried out by the IRB) with representatives of the communities in which the research will be conducted and from which the subjects will be drawn;
    - (ii) public disclosure to the communities in which the research will be conducted and from which the subjects will be drawn, prior to initiation of the research, of plans for the research and its risks and expected benefits;
    - (iii) public disclosure of sufficient information following completion of the research to apprise the community and researchers of the study, including the demographic characteristics of the research population, and its results;
    - (iv) establishment of an independent data monitoring committee to exercise oversight of the research and;
    - (v) if obtained informed consent is not feasible and a legally authorized representative is not reasonably available, the investigator has committed, if feasible, to attempting to contact within the therapeutic window the subject's family member who is not a legally authorized representative, and asking whether he or she objects to the subject's participation in the research. The investigator will summarize efforts made to contact family members and make this information available to the IRB at the time of continuing review.

In addition, the IRB is responsible for ensuring that procedures are in place to inform, at the earliest feasible opportunity, each subject, or if the subject remains incapacitated, a legally authorized representative of the subject, or if such a representative is not reasonably available, a family member, of the subject's inclusion in the research, the details of the research and other information contained in the informed consent document. The IRB shall also ensure that there is a procedure to inform the subject, or if the subject remains incapacitated, a legally authorized representative of the subject, or if such a representative is not reasonably available, a family member, that he or she may discontinue the subject's participation at any time without penalty or loss of benefits to which the subject is otherwise entitled. If a legally authorized representative or family member is told about the research and the subject's condition improves, the subject is also to be informed as soon as feasible. If a subject is entered into research with a waived consent and the subject dies before a legally authorized representative or family member can be contacted, information about the research is to be provided to the subject's legally authorized representative or family member, if feasible.

For the purpose of this waiver "family member" means any one of the following legally competent persons: spouses; parents; children (including adopted children); brothers; sisters; and spouses of brothers and sisters; and any individual related by blood or affinity whose close association with the subject is the equivalent of a family relationship.

Source: the website < http://www.nih.gov/grants/oprr/hsdc97-01.htm >, "Emergency Research Consent Waiver," *Federal Register* 61, sec. 46.101(i), 51531-51533.

---

that, in 1931, Germany published strict regulations governing human experimentation and the use of innovative therapies in medicine, which were legally binding throughout the period of Nazi abuses of internees of concentration camps, prior to the development of the *Nuremberg Code.* These guidelines, which were issued by the Reich's Health Department, stated that human experimentation was impermissible without consent.[29] Ironically, no other nation appears to have had in place such moral and legally advanced regulations during this period. Although the *Nuremberg Code* is widely assumed to be the first major document in the history of research ethics, Reich's 1931 regulations are comparable in scope to those provided by the *Nuremberg Code* itself.

INSTITUTIONAL REVIEW BOARDS

MISSION

Federal regulations require that research with human subjects in applicable facilities must be reviewed, approved, and subject to continuing review by an IRB.[30] The mission of an IRB is to protect research subjects, rigorously assess the overall merits of a study, and act as an agent of an institution. The task of determining whether there is any "adverse affect on the rights and welfare" of a subject, as required by the consent waiver, is also the responsibility of the IRB. In critical care research, where there is an increased likelihood that patients are or will become incapacitated, an IRB and a researcher are held to a higher standard to ensure that a study has merit and is based on solid preliminary data. Incapacitated, critically ill patients should be viewed as part of a protected research group, just as children are. For such protected groups, there is an obligation to have more stringent research protections.

COMPOSITION

The composition of an IRB that reviews critical care protocols is crucial for ensuring the validity of a research study. It is preferable to have a standing, multidisciplinary committee that includes representatives from medicine, nursing, pharmacy, social services, the clergy, the legal profession, and an institution's administration as well as lay members. An IRB should also include persons primarily concerned with bioethics and critical care medicine. When presented with a research proposal, an IRB must be capable of addressing medical and scientific issues, overall research design, exclusion and inclusion criteria, burdens and benefits, and validity of the proposed study.

In certain circumstances, an IRB should concurrently review the research and the results obtained to ensure that no harm is being done to the enrolled patients. An IRB should do this, for example, when incapacitated patients without surrogates are enrolled in studies involving more than minimal risks. An IRB may be responsible for actively monitoring ongoing studies; depending on the design of the study, an IRB may require a limited initial enrollment with interim data analysis and a reevaluation prior to a full study. An IRB may also require researchers to submit scheduled oral or written progress reports.

PROTOCOL REQUIREMENTS

Critical care research protocols submitted to an IRB should state clear research objectives and include a specific section addressing ethical issues, the proposed method of consent, and criteria for continuation or early termination of the research protocol. A protocol should describe the anticipated degree of incapacity of the subjects during the study. With each protocol, the investigator must justify the study and clearly define the goals, which should have some significance for critical care. Critical care research should be limited to the study of critical care illnesses and should be performed only if the research could not reasonably be done on adult subjects who are not critically ill.

An IRB may properly require that proposed protocols have adequate preexisting data indicating that outcomes are expected to be as good or better than those with conventional therapy. This requirement does not preclude innovative research therapies, but rather requires a substantial body of preceding experimental data that indicates potential benefit from the experimental therapy.[31] The preliminary studies on which the research protocol is based (such as pilot studies or animal studies) should be comprehensive so as to avoid harm that might occur to subjects by a premature or needlessly hazardous experiment.[32]

In addition to its role in protecting patients in research studies, an IRB functions as an agent of the research facility, with a corresponding duty to protect the facility's interests. Although federal regulation provides some legal protection if it is adhered to, this protection is not absolute. The regulations do not preempt applicable federal, state, or local laws and would likely yield to conflicting constitutional provisions (particularly those regarding privacy rights and liberty interests), existing statutes, or common law where more stringent requirements or protections are provided. Where a state has stricter research standards than those in federal regulation and these state standards are not followed, some would argue that federal regulation does not sufficiently protect the patient's statutory, common law, or constitutional rights; thus, violating state standards can expose researchers and their facility to possible liability.[33] An IRB and individual researchers should be aware of all applicable laws and proceed with caution.

Federal regulation does not preclude a physician from providing emergency medical care consistent with existing federal, state, or local law. Although experimental and innovative emergency interventions are often employed in critical care medicine, significant departures from standard or accepted practice do not in themselves constitute research. Accordingly, federal regulation does not apply to such departures. The fact that a procedure is experimental does not mean that it is automatically "research." Research constitutes an activity designed to test a hypothesis, permit conclusions to be drawn, and thereby develop or contribute to generalizable knowledge. Therapy, on the other hand, is designed to benefit a particular patient.[34]

CONDUCTING CRITICAL CARE RESEARCH: A SUGGESTED APPROACH

PATIENTS WITH DECISION-MAKING CAPACITY

For patients with decision-making capacity, the research team must ensure adequate protection of patients while it provides a workable mechanism so that appropriate research can proceed. The capacitated patient should always be encouraged, and in certain circumstances required, to execute a proxy directive for healthcare decisions. Research involving minimal risk should proceed after the informed-consent process has been completed.

Research with greater than minimal risk but potential benefit to a patient should proceed only after a patient has completed the informed consent process and after a staff member has discussed and encouraged the patient to execute a proxy directive. An IRB should be notified promptly of a patient's enrollment because of the risk to the patient. For research with greater than minimal risk without potential benefit to the patient, an ethics consultation should be a required portion of the informed consent process. The purpose of the consultation is to ensure that the patient has decision-making capacity and understands the protocol, the risks involved, and the lack of direct benefit to the patient. Execution of a proxy directive should be required, and an IRB should be notified promptly of a patient's enrollment (see Exhibit 8-2).

INCAPACITATED PATIENTS

For research involving incapacitated patients, a researcher has a responsibility to ensure that adequate protective mechanisms are in place, and an institution must require and ensure that these mechanisms are adhered to strictly. A researcher should periodically reconfirm a subject's lack of capacity.

In studies involving minimal risk, enrollment of an incapacitated patient should be allowed by consent of a legal surrogate; without consent of a legal surrogate, enrollment should be allowed with concurrent IRB review to protect the patient's rights and welfare.

The initial enrollment of an incapacitated patient into a study with greater than minimal risk but potential benefit to the patient should be allowed by consent of a legal surrogate. Additional protection is required in studies involving higher risks to patients or when patients are severely impaired. In such cases, a patient should be assigned a court-appointed guardian, within 24 to 72 hours. The process for enrolling patients into critical care research should allow the time to assign a court-appointed guardian. If no legal surrogate is available, a patient should not be enrolled into a research protocol. This policy does not preclude therapy, including experimental therapy, in emergency circumstances.

Enrollment of an incapacitated patient into studies that involve greater than minimal risk with no direct benefit to the patient should be allowed only by consent of a court-appointed guardian. In such cases, an ethics consultation should be a required portion of the informed consent process, to ensure that a court-appointed guardian understands the protocol, the risks involved, and the lack of direct benefit to the patient, and to ensure that enrollment of a patient is consistent with the best understanding of what the patient's desires would have been. The enrollment of incapacitated patients into studies with greater than minimal risk and no direct benefit to the patient, if authorized by a court-appointed guardian with appropriate safeguards, recognizes in many cases the altruism of individuals who may have communicated directly or indirectly their desire to potentially benefit others. In no circumstance should research involving greater than minimal risk with no direct benefit to the patient be performed without approval of a court-appointed guardian (see Exhibit 8-2).

CONCLUSION

The practice of critical care medicine has advanced dramatically during the past few decades. Further advances in the care of critically ill patients will depend, in part, on critical care researchers' ability to conduct well-designed studies on these patients. The future of critical care research will depend not only on the issues of science and medicine, but also on the ethical, economic, and legal issues that researchers must confront.

The federal regulation governing research with human subjects currently provides guidance for many aspects of critical care research, but it is not comprehensive. The formulation of alternatives to informed consent—such as deferred consent, prospective consent, and extensions of the emergency consent doctrine—are attempts to justify the pursuit of important and necessary nonconsensual research in critically ill patients. The absence of clear guidelines for this special research population creates two problems. First, these subjects may be exposed to risk by a premature or needlessly hazardous experiment in projects that do not receive thorough review. Second, there may be an unwillingness to engage in research in the face of general federal regulation and state laws that are unclear and perhaps prohibitory, since no special provisions are made to protect these subjects for whom direct or surrogate consent cannot be obtained.[35] The medical emergency consent exception does help in addressing some of these concerns over obtaining and documenting informed consent.

Medical researches' ability to conduct sound research, enroll patients, and obtain financial support to perform research depends in part on maintaining the public trust. Although the current regulations allow a

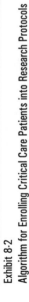

Exhibit 8-2
Algorithm for Enrolling Critical Care Patients into Research Protocols

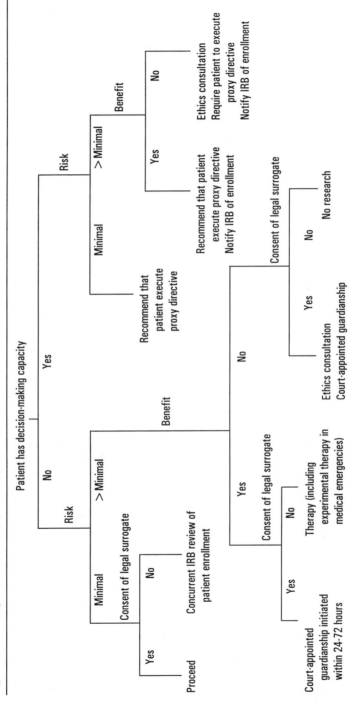

Note: This algorithm was derived in part from the National Institutes of Health Clinical Center's policy for consent process for research with impaired human subjects.

great deal of research on the critically ill to go forward, continuing to address the issues of consent in this specific population of patients and further developing clear and concise standards for conducting nonconsensual research in the critically ill is necessary. We must strive to develop guidelines that are not so burdensome as to discourage sound, much needed research; at the same time, we must enhance the protection of critically ill research subjects.

NOTES

1. J.M. Rippe et al., ed., *Intensive Care Medicine* (Boston: Little, Brown and Co., 1991).

2. R.J. Levine, "New International Guidelines for Research Involving Human Subjects," *Annals of Internal Medicine* 119 (1993): 339-41.

3. Ibid.

4. U.S. Department of Health and Human Services, "Protection of Human Subjects," 45 *CFR* 46 (1978; 1 October 1995).

5. Ibid., sec. 111.

6. National Commission for the Protection of Human Subjects of Biomedical and Behavioral Research, *The Belmont Report: Ethical Principles and Guidelines for the Protection of Human Subjects of Research* (Washington, D.C.: U.S. Government Printing Office, 1978), DHEW Publication no. 78-0012.

7. See note 4 above, sec. 116 (a).

8. See note 6 above.

9. Hastings Center, *Guidelines on the Termination of Life-Sustaining Treatment and the Care of the Dying* (Bloomington: Indiana University Press, 1987).

10. The term *incapacitated* is used here to mean "lacking decisional capacity" and is roughly equivalent to the legal usage of the term *incompetent.*

11. K.V. Iserson and M.B. Mahowald, "Acute Care Research: Is It Ethical?" *Critical Care Medicine* 20 (1992): 1032-37.

12. Some authors distinguish *acute care patients* as those critical care patients who have suffered unexpected events that carry a high probability of mortality or serious morbidity unless immediate intervention is provided. They separate these from the broader category of *critical care patients,* which they refer to as a wide variety of patients, most of whom are very ill, but not currently in a medical crisis.

13. A. Meisel, "The Exceptions to the Informed Consent Doctrine: Striking a Balance Between Competing Values in Medical Decisionmaking," *Wisconsin Law Review* 1979 (1979): 413-88.

14. R. Faden and T.L. Beauchamp, *A History and Theory of Informed Consent* (New York: Oxford University Press, 1986).

15. N.S. Abramson, A. Meisel, and P. Safar, "Deferred Consent: A New Approach for Resuscitation Research on Comatose Patients," *Journal of the*

American Medical Association 255 (1986): 2466-71; B.L. Miller, "Philosophical, Ethical, and Legal Aspects of Resuscitation Medicine: I. Deferred Consent and Justification of Resuscitation Research," *Critical Care Medicine* 16 (1988): 1059-62; see note 11 above.

16. See note 14 above.

17. W.H. Spivey et al. "Informed Consent for Biomedical Research in Acute Care Medicine," *Annals of Emergency Medicine* 20 (November 1991): 1251-65.

18. Miller, "Philosophical, Ethical, and Legal Aspects," see note 15 above.

19. W.H. Spivey, "Informed Consent for Clinical Research in the Emergency Department," *Annals of Emergency Medicine* 18 (July 1989): 766-71.

20. R.M. Veatch, "Abandoning Informed Consent," *Hastings Center Report* 25, no. 2 (1995): 5-12; see note 11 above.

21. See note 14 above.

22. See note 19 above.

23. See note 4 above; sec 116 (d).

24. Ibid., sec. 102 (i).

25. See note 17 above.

26. Ibid.

27. H.K. Beecher, *Research and the Individual: Human Studies* (Boston: Little, Brown and Co. 1970), 289-90.

28. R.J. Levine, "Clinical Trials and Physicians as Double Agents," *Yale Journal of Biology and Medicine* 65 (1992): 65-74.

29. H.M. Sass, "Reichsrundschreiben 1931: Pre-Nuremberg German Regulations Concerning New Therapy and Human Experimentation," *Journal of Medicine and Philosophy* 8 (1983): 99-111.

30. See note 4 above, sec. 103.

31. A. Petros et al., "Effect of Nitric Oxide Synthase Inhibitors on Hypotension in Patients with Septic Shock," *Lancet* 338 (1991): 1557-58.

32. *Ethical and Legal Considerations of Patient Care: Durable Power of Attorney for CC Protocols* (Bethesda, Md.: National Institutes of Health, The Warren G. Magnuson Clinical Center, 1987), 41.

33. See note 17 above.

34. See note 6 above.

35. President's Commission for the Study of Ethical Problems in Medicine and Biomedical and Behavioral Research, *Implementing Human Research Regulations: Second Biennial Report on the Adequacy and Uniformity of Federal Rules and Policies, and of their Implementation, for the Protection of Human Subjects* (Washington, D.C.: U.S. Government Printing Office, March 1983), 192-94.

9

Defining Death in the ICU: Implications for Morality and Organ Transplantation

Henry Silverman

Death . . . is such a simple natural event that, like birth, it does not require an exact determination of its elements.
—Friedrich Carl von Savigny, 1840

A woman declared brain-dead about four months into her pregnancy gave birth to a premature, but healthy, baby girl. Twenty minutes later, doctors removed her from life-support machines and she died.
—*New York Times,* November 16, 1997

INTRODUCTION

Today, there is a great deal of confusion surrounding the determination of death. In contrast, determining death in the nineteenth century was simple, and thus it was unnecessary to formulate a concept of death. Although modern technology has given us greater power to control the timing of death, it has also generated confusion over the once simple concepts of life and death and over whether an individual is alive or dead. The confusion surrounding the concept of brain death has generated profound ethical dilemmas involving the determination of death and candidacy for organ transplantation.

Conceptual clarity about how death is defined is essential for several reasons. First, a clear concept of death is needed to develop medically precise tests to determine the state of death. Second, a moral issue is present in the sense that, just as it is wrong to treat a living person as dead, it is morally wrong to treat a dead person as alive. Third, confusion surrounding the concept of brain death may contribute to the discomfort of physicians who must pronounce brain-dead patients as dead and explain this concept to families. Finally, the supply of organs for transplantation depends on philosophically clear concepts of death, because organ procurement is contingent on a determination of death and on society's trust of the medical profession in determining that a patient is actually dead and that death was not surreptitiously hastened.

The public and medical debate on death and brain death, however, lacks consensus on the following issues: (1) the concept of death itself, (2) concrete medical tests for the determination of brain death, (3) cogent arguments for why brain death should be equated with death of the individual, (4) whether public policy should require or merely permit death to be pronounced on the basis of any one concept of death, and (5) whether organs should be procured only from patients who are dead. Adequate responses to these issues can be made only after a careful consideration of a philosophical concept of death combined with an ethical analysis of issues surrounding organ procurement and transplantation.

CONCEPT, CRITERIA, AND CLINICAL TESTS OF DEATH

A distinction needs to be made between a concept of death (or the "condition" of being dead) and recognized criteria and tests for diagnosing death, because the latter can only be derived logically from the former. Indeed, according to the philosopher Christopher Pallis, "Criteria of death . . . must be related to some overall concept of what death means. The tests we carry out and the decisions we make should be logically derived from the explicit conceptual and philosophical premises. . . . Technical data can never answer purely conceptual questions."[1]

Determining criteria and defining medical tests (stethoscopes, electroencephalograms, angiograms, and so forth) to assess whether death has occurred are a matter of medical and physiologic knowledge and, as such, are appropriately interpreted by medical experts. But, answering the question, "What is death?" or defining a concept of death to determine whether a person in a particular condition should be called dead is a philosophical issue and should be formulated on the basis of philosophical argument.[2]

A starting point in the exploration of the concept of death is a purely formal definition of the term *death,* which may take the following form: "Death means a complete change of the status of a living entity characterized by the irreversible loss of those characteristics that are essentially significant to it."[3] To give content to this formal analysis of death as it relates to a human being, characteristics that are essential to humanness need to be defined. To ask what is essentially significant to a human being is a philosophical question based on ethical values and cultural points of view, rather than inferred from scientific facts.

After clarifying a concept or definition of what it means to die, operational criteria are needed to determine whether death has occurred. Essentially, criteria are anatomical loci associated with physiologic functions that are essential to humanness, as previously defined conceptually. Finally, specific medical tests are required to determine whether a specific criterion has been satisfied. Alternative and competing concepts of death, along with their associated criteria and tests, are listed in Exhibit 9-1.[4]

TRADITIONAL CONCEPT, CRITERION, AND TESTS OF DEATH

The predominant traditional concept of death focused not on the heart and lungs, *per se,* but on the flow of "vital fluids" (the breath and the blood). The nature of a human being was seen as related to this vital

---

Exhibit 9-1
Alternate Concepts of Death

Definition	Criterion	Tests
Permanent cessation of the flow of vital body fluids	Irreversible loss of heart and lung functions	No pulse or respiratory effects
Permanent cessation of the integrative functioning of the organism as a whole	Irreversible loss of all brain functions	No responsiveness or voluntary movements, no brain-stem reflexes
Permanent loss of consciousness and cognition	Irreversible loss of those higher brain areas responsible for consciousness and social interaction	No effective test at this time

activity of fluid flow, which humans share with other animals. According to this view, the human organism, like other living organisms, dies when there is an irreversible cessation of the flow of these fluids.[5] Since it was clear that cessation of spontaneous breathing and heartbeat would quickly produce the cessation of vital fluid flow (and, hence, the cessation of all vital functions, including brain functioning), the cessation of spontaneous respiration and circulation was considered the operational criterion for the presence of death.

Medical tests to determine cessation of heart-lung function in a person who fell unconscious consisted of feeling for the pulse, listening for breathing, holding a mirror before the nose to test for condensation, and assessing whether the pupils were fixed. For centuries, however, people had little confidence in these clinical tests. Indeed, in response to the fear of premature burial, cabinetmakers developed coffins with elaborate escape mechanisms and speaking tubes to the world above, mortuaries employed guards to monitor the newly dead for signs of life, and legislatures passed laws requiring a delay before burial.[6]

Physicians were also concerned with the accurate determination of death and actively sought to develop competence in the determination of death.[7] The invention of the stethoscope in the mid-nineteenth century enabled physicians to detect heartbeat with enhanced sensitivity. The twentieth century brought even more sophisticated technological means to determine death, particularly the electrocardiograph. Hence, as knowledge and practical skills increased, physicians and the public had more confidence that death could be diagnosed reliably by using tests assessing cardiopulmonary function.

CIRCUMSTANCES THAT FOSTERED A BRAIN-ORIENTED CONCEPT OF DEATH

References to brain death date at least to the earliest part of the twentieth century. In 1902, Harvey Cushing described a condition in which, with swelling from an intracranial tumor, a patient's spontaneous respiration ceased but his heart was kept beating with artificial respiratory assistance for 23 hours.[8] With advances in ventilator technology in the 1950s, there was more widespread clinical recognition of brain death (or "respiratory brain" as the condition was initially named) by clinicians who described autolysis or liquefaction of the brain after prolonged ventilation of comatose patients. This phenomenon itself was pathologically explored in 1959 by Mollaret and Goulon,[9] who observed patients with massive brain damage maintained on a ventilator with complete unresponsivity, lack of spontaneous respiration, flaccidity, altered thermal regulation, absence of mesencephalic reflexes, and progressive circulatory collapse. They called this condition *coma depassé,* (a state beyond coma), but specifically declined to say at what point they thought death had occurred.

Scientists began to question the validity of the cessation of vital fluid flow as a concept of death as modern technology brought to light the possibility that some parts (tissues) and/or functions of the body may be essential and others not essential for life. In earlier times, because the death of all vital organs occurred at approximately the same time, society did not have to consider how to describe a person if the brain ceased to function but the heart and lungs did not. Essentially, one did not have to determine *the* essential quality of human life, because the failure of the heart and lungs produced the cessation of *all* vital bodily functions. Hence, *a* concept of death was never made explicit, because doing so was unnecessary.

But now that circulation and breathing can be maintained mechanically, it is possible for an individual to exist despite the permanent cessation of all brain function. Such patients seem to straddle the line between life and death, as they have some characteristics associated with living (such as a beating heart, breathing, urine production, food metabolism, and the presence of warm/moist skin) and conditions associated with being dead (such as unresponsiveness to the environment). Whether such patients are dead or alive depends on a more explicit concept of death. Indeed, the existence of such cases compels us to look more closely into the essential meaning of death that was implicit in our previous, traditional understanding of death. Specifically, when medical intervention is responsible for a patient's circulation and breathing, the compelling questions is whether some function or functions of the brain (criterion) may be used to determine death and whether there are other methods (tests) to diagnose death.

Efforts, however, to "redefine" death and to develop neurologic criteria to predict which ventilated, comatose patients had brain death remained quiescent and obscure. Rothman argues that redefining death was unnecessary for the following reason: "Doctors, inside the closed world of the intensive care units, turned off the machines when they believed the patient's death was imminent and irreversible. . . . The intensive care units were a private domain, whatever the formal definition of death, and doctors exercised their discretion."[10]

However, the success of transplantation procedures in the 1960s forced a public consideration of the validity of brain death as a criterion (or standard) of death. When advances in transplantation technology (such as immunosuppressive therapy) outpaced the supply of available organs, patients on ventilators whose brain function had ceased but whose hearts continued to beat were identified as a potential source for organs. Previously, organs had come from two sources: living donors and dead donors (non-heart-beating cadavers). The use of living donors was problematic because of concerns about potential coercion of donors and commercialization of organ donation, and the use of dead donors presented problems of organ viability due to warm ischemia time (organ injury caused by lack of oxygen). Furthermore, livers and hearts cannot be procured from living donors because, unlike the kidneys, these organs are not paired. Consequently, liver and heart transplantation depended on either improved cadaver organ preservation techniques or new sources of heartbeating organ donors (such as patients whose brains had ceased to function).

Considering heartbeating patients whose brain function had ceased as organ donors prompted questions about the "true" nature of death (and life) and raised the issue of whether it is ethical to procure organs from patients with beating hearts. The unanswered question was, "does the death of a patient depend upon the premise of a non-beating heart?" The use of heartbeating donors also raised the issue of a potential conflict of interest within the medical profession involving the termination of care for one patient (the potential donor) so that another might live (the recipient). Indeed, although the transplantation "successes" in the late 1960s led to widespread optimism about conquering heart and liver disease, it also fueled a growing public uneasiness with taking organs from donors who were not yet dead based on traditional tests. To avoid public controversy, transplantation surgeons avoided declaring potential organ donors dead based on neurologic criteria.[11]

It was in this climate that the Ad Hoc Committee of the Harvard Medical School to Examine the Definition of Brain Death (Harvard Committee) was convened in 1968 with a goal to quell "the controversy in obtaining organs for transplantation" by defining new criteria to replace "obsolete criteria," (that is, cardiopulmonary criteria previously used for defining death). In its report, this committee endorsed "irreversible coma" as a new criterion for determining death. Subsequently, it listed the following guidelines consisting of clinical and laboratory tests by which a determination of irreversible coma or brain death could be made:[12]

- unreceptivity and unresponsitivity (total unawareness to externally applied stimuli and complete unresponsiveness)
- lack of spontaneous movements and ability to breathe spontaneously (total absence of spontaneous breathing may be established by turning off the ventilator for three minutes and observing for any spontaneous breaths)
- absence of reflexes (pupillary reflexes, oculocephalic and oculovestibular reflexes, corneal reflex, pharyngeal reflexes, spinal reflexes) and no evidence of postural activity (decerebrate)
- lack of cortical activity as measured by an electroencephalogram (EEG) (a flat or isoelectric EEG)

The committee stated that the presence of a flat EEG provides confirmatory data, and when an EEG is available it should be used. Furthermore, "all of the above tests shall be repeated at least 24 hours later with no change," in order to "obtain evidence of the irreversibility of the condition."[13] Finally, "the validity of such data as indications of irreversible cerebral damage depends on the exclusion of two conditions [that could mimic brain death]: hypothermia (temperature below 90°F) or central nervous system depressants, such as barbiturates."[14] Because the intent of the Harvard Committee was to diagnose irreversible "diffuse disease," this set of tests is considered a determination of whole-brain death or *irreversible* loss of *all* brain functions.

After its publication, the Harvard Committee's report sparked criticism and galvanized a diffuse public discussion. Several philosophers, theologians, and others voiced opposition to the concept of brain death. They argued that equating brain-death with the death of an individual was not the result of philosophical inquiry; instead, the concept of brain death was developed to "achieve practical ends" (obtaining organs for transplantation).[15]

Despite this opposition and the lack of a philosophical concept explaining why a person with irreversible loss of all brain functions should be considered dead, the brain-death criterion for determining death adapted by the Harvard Committee eventually received widespread support. In the same year as its publication, the criterion of brain death was approved by the American Bar Association and the American Medical Association.[16] In 1970, Kansas was the first state to adopt brain death as a criterion for death.[17] Today, all 50 states have statutes endorsing brain death as a criterion for the determination of death.[18] Furthermore, religious groups as well as other countries have supported the concept of brain death as a criterion for death of the individual.[19] For more than a decade, the brain death criterion of death has been the foundation of public policy related to the issue of organ donation.

Several factors account for the acceptance of brain death as a criterion for determining death without a corresponding, widely accepted concept explaining exactly why patients with irreversible loss of all brain functions should be considered dead. First, irreversible loss of all brain functions was thought to be easy to diagnose clinically in adults; thus, it seemed to offer, like the cardiopulmonary criterion, clear means for separating the living from the dead. Second, once the diagnosis is evident, so too is the prognosis; patients whose brains are dead suffer somatic death within a short period of time. Finally, the utilitarian appeal of organ transplantation has greatly contributed to the acceptance of brain death; individuals who are brain dead have served as an excellent source of kidneys and are the only source of hearts and livers.[20]

Despite its general acceptance in the practice of medicine, concerns still persist, however, regarding the coherency of the concept of brain death. Specifically, there are concerns regarding the validity of the clinical tests in determining the "permanent cessation of all brain functions," as well as doubts regarding the philosophical basis for equating death of the whole brain with death of the individual. The following sections discuss these sources of the incoherency of the whole-brain death concept.

VALIDITY OF CLINICAL TESTS TO
DETERMINE WHOLE-BRAIN DEATH

The criterion for satisfying the definition of brain death is the "irreversible loss of all brain function." Any tests defined for evaluating when this criterion has been satisfied must, therefore, be shown that it defines a state of "irreversible loss of all brain function." Several validating concepts have been used to certify whether the satisfaction of any set of clinical tests indicated whole-brain death.[21]

Some general comments deserve mention before looking specifically at how certain sets of clinical tests have been validated. First, the selection of specific clinical tests to determine a state of irreversible loss of all brain functions will vary depending on the validating concept used, thus adding to the complexity of establishing guidelines for the diagnosis of brain death. Second, that several validating principles have been used indicates that different investigators have embraced different medical opinions on the physiologic evidence required to show that irreversible loss of brain function exists. Such diversity probably also represents a difference of opinion on the level of certainty required to demonstrate that a state of affairs represents the "truth." That is, how much certainty is needed to show that an individual person has irreversible loss of all brain functions. Differences in levels of certainty represent a difference in balancing two types of errors; the error of treating dead individuals as if they were alive versus the error of treating the alive as if they were dead. Which type of error is chosen to be minimized in selecting a set of clinical tests represents a moral, as opposed to a medical, judgment. Finally, as will be shown, evidence regarding the validity of the chosen set of clinical tests to diagnose a state of brain death has either been soft or not even presented.

One validating concept used to show that a certain set of clinical tests predicts brain death involves the demonstration of widespread brain necrosis at autopsy; presumably, there could then be no return to function. This approach has two difficulties: the first is deciding the minimal changes that constitute brain death pathologically and the second is making certain that such changes do not represent post-mortem changes: that is, degeneration that has occurred between the time of cardiac standstill and fixation of tissues. Another validating method entails the demonstration of no evidence of any brainstem or cortical activity and that such patients would inevitably, within a short period of time, suffer somatic death via cardiac arrest despite any possible treatment. Presumably, the requirement of subsequent somatic death was necessary to show that brain function was irreversibly lost. Problems with this validating principle include: (1) determining what is an appropriate "short period of time," whether days, weeks, or months; (2) failure of survival may depend on contemporary therapeutic modalities; and more importantly (3) this approach confuses a prognosis with a diagnosis, as demonstration of somatic death within a certain interval to time could be used only to support the claim that people meeting the selected tests will soon be dead, not that such people are presently dead. Other validating concepts entailed either the demonstration of a "flat" electroencephalogram or an imaging study showing no intracranial filling (for example, arteriogram or nuclear medicine blood flow study) as sufficient findings in themselves to establish the diagnosis.

Concerning the clinical tests endorsed by the Harvard Committee report, a major criticism was that it did not present any scientific evidence that the tests accurately measured irreversible brain death. Subsequent to the publication of the Harvard report, morphologic evidence of widespread destruction of the brain was used to validate the Harvard tests.[22] For example, Richardson found that the brains of 128 patients meeting the Harvard tests showed extensive destruction changes.[23] However, in a larger series of autopsy studies, fulfillment of the Harvard tests was not always associated with the presence of widespread brain destruction.[24] Indeed, the exact nature and distribution of such morphologic lesions in the brain were shown to be dependent on the etiology and on the interval between fulfillment of the Harvard tests and pathologic examination. Subsequently, it was felt that the existence of widespread destruction may not be necessary to show the impossibility of return to brain function and, hence, not necessary to validate the clinical diagnosis of brain death. Accordingly, pathologic validation was thought to be too stringent and unreliable.

However, a concern surfaced that the Harvard tests themselves were too strict; that is, the use of such tests described patients as being alive when such patients should be declared as being brain dead. Accordingly, support grew for the use of less restrictive tests; that is, tests that would be more inclusive than the Harvard tests yet be "completely accurate" in diagnosing brain death clinically. For example, the National Institute of Neurological and Communicative Disorders and Stroke (NINDS) published in 1977 the results of a multihospital, cooperative study that determined which sets of tests assessing a clinical state of absent brain activity were associated with cardiovascular collapse within three months and, hence, indicative of irreversible failure of all brain functions.[25] The resulting tests consisted of the following: coma with cerebral unresponsivity, apnea (no effort to override the ventilator for 15 minutes), dilated pupils (to exclude patients with drug intoxication other than those with glutethimide or scopolamine intoxications), absent brain stem reflexes, and a flat EEG. The investigators proposed that all of these conditions must be present for 30 minutes at least six hours following the onset of coma and apnea. The group also proposed that if one of these tests is met imprecisely or cannot be tested, then demonstration of absence of cerebral blood flow could be used as a confirmatory measure. Of the initial 503 patients who were initially screened (those with deep coma without spontaneous respiration), 189 patients met these clinical tests, whereas only 19 met the Harvard tests. Noteworthy differences between the clinical tests defined by the NINDS collaborative study and the Harvard tests include the shorter observation interval required (six hours versus 24 hours), the different definition of apnea, the irrelevance of spinal reflexes to the diagnosis, and the introduction of a blood-flow test as a confirmatory procedure.

In 1981, in an effort to establish uniform guidelines for the diagnosis of brain death, the President's Commission for the Study of Ethical Problems in Medicine and Biomedical and Behavioral Research (President's Commission) proposed tests that include the standard condition of deep coma, the absence of brain stem functions, and a 10-minute period of apneic oxygenation (assuming that the carbon dioxide pressure would be greater than 60 mm Hg after this interval). They recommended that the proximate cause of coma must exclude the following potentially reversible conditions: sedation, hypothermia, neuromuscular blockade, and shock. Moreover, they recommended that the required period of observation of cessation of brain function (six, 12, or 24 hours) should depend upon the tests done and the underlying etiologies of the neurologic dysfunction. For example, only six hours is required if documentation of cessation is achieved by clinical examination (coma and brain-stem reflexes) and confirmatory EEG or test for absent cerebral blood flow. In the absence of confirmatory tests and when an irreversible condition is well-established, observation for at least 12 hours is recommended. In the presence of anoxic brain damage, observation for 24 hours is recommended, but this period may be reduced if an EEG shows electrocerebral silence in a patient without the presence of a reversible condition, or if a test shows cessation of cerebral blood flow even in the presence of a reversible condition. Unfortunately, the President's Commission provided no evidence that their tests accurately identified patients who have irreversibly lost all brain functions.[26]

A 1984 study reported a wide variation in the practice of neurologists and neurosurgeons in declaring brain death, despite the President's Commission's attempts to establish uniform guidelines.[27] For example, 44 percent thought that the hypothermia exclusion was unnecessary; 29 percent thought that one flat EEG was necessary, while 36 percent thought that two flat EEGs were necessary; and approximately equal numbers chose each of three observation intervals (0 to 12, 12 to 24, and 24 hours).

Variation between practices in different countries has also been observed. For example, in Britain the EEG is not considered a critical part of the declaration of brain death (mainly due to the acceptance that absence of brain-stem reflexes signifies not only damage to the brain stem itself but also represents a reliable sign of profound damage to other intracranial structures), and the diagnosis of brain death can only be made on establishing a definite abnormality in structure (thus patients in coma from an unknown cause are not declared brain dead).[28]

In contrast, the absence of intracranial blood flow by angiographic or isotopic techniques has become central to the diagnosis of brain death in several European countries. Many consider this test by itself to be diagnostic of brain death.[29] Indeed, the absence of intracranial blood flow over a 10-to-15 minute interval is uniformly associated with subsequent necrosis and liquefaction of the brain.[30] The absence of blood flow is believed to be the result of cerebral swelling, caused either by extensive trauma or hypoxia from inadequate cerebral blood flow, which raises the intracranial pressure above the perfusion pressure; this causes obstruction to circulation and subsequent global destruction of the brain. This test was developed in the context of evaluation of intracranial circulation several hours after injury (more than six hours, as this was approximately the time required to stabilize the patient for transport and perform of the test); thus, it is not known whether this test is adequate if it is applied during the first several hours following injury.

The most recent guidelines for the determination of brain death developed by the American Academy of Neurology (see Exhibit 9-2), which define brain death as the irreversible loss of the clinical function of the brain, also reflect the fragile consensus on the tests required for the diagnosis of brain death.[31] The consensus group refers to their statement only as "guidelines" instead of the more restrictive term "standards." Indeed, the consensus group defined "guidelines" as "recommendations for patient management that may identify a particular strategy and that reflect 'moderate clinical certainty'," whereas the group defined "standards" as "generally accepted principles for patient management that reflect a high degree of clinical certainty."

A lack of consensus is also present regarding the diagnosis of death in newborns and young children. This lack of consensus results from difficulties involved with clinical assessment and from the widely held belief that the brains of children under the age of five may be more resistant than adult brains to anoxia and more likely to recover substantial functions even after exhibiting unresponsiveness for long time periods. This perception, however, is controversial and lacks convincing clinical documentations.[32] The guidelines established in 1987 by the Task Force for the Determination of Brain Death in Children (see Exhibit 9-3) differ from guidelines for adults in regard to the required duration of observation and the need for confirmatory tests, such as flat EEGs.[33] However, investigators have reported variation in practices for determining brain death in children,[34] and competing sets of tests have been recommended.[35]

The concerns with the reliability of the various validating principles used to determine whether a set of tests fulfills the criterion of brain death (that is, irreversible loss of all brain functions) is given credence by

---

Exhibit 9-2
Parameters for Determining Brain Death in Adults

Overview

Brain death is defined as the irreversible loss of the clinical function of the brain, including the brain stem.

Diagnosis Criteria for Clinical Diagnosis of Brain Death

A. Brain death is the absence of clinical brain function when the proximate cause is known and demonstrably irreversible.
    1. Clinical or neuroimaging evidence of an acute central nervous system catastrophe that is compatible with the clinical diagnosis of brain death
    2. Exclusion of complicating medical conditions that may confound clinical assessment (no severe electrolyte, acid-base, or endocrine disturbance)
    3. No drug intoxication or poisoning
    4. Core temperature $\geq$ 90°F
B. The three cardinal findings in brain death
    1. Coma or unresponsiveness: no cerebral motor response to pain in all extremities
    2. Absence of the following brain-stem reflexes: pupillary, oculocephalic, oculovestibular, corneal, pharyngeal, and tracheal
    3. Apnea: no respiratory movements when the pCO_2 is $\geq$ 60 mm Hg or there has been a 20 mm Hg increase over baseline
C. Confirmatory tests are recommended when existing conditions may interfere with the clinical diagnosis, such as severe facial trauma, preexisting pupillary abnormalities, or toxic levels of relevant drugs (sedatives, tricyclic antidepressants, anticholinergics, antiepileptic drugs, etc.).
D. A repeat clinical evaluation six hours later is recommended, but this interval is arbitrary.
E. The following confirmatory tests are listed in the order of the most sensitive test first.
    1. Conventional angiography
    2. Electroencephalography
    3. Transcranial Doppler ultrasonography
    4. Technetium 99m hexamethylpropyleneamineoxime brain scan
    5. Somatosensory-evoked potentials

Source: Report of the Quality Standards Subcommittee of the American Academy of Neurology, "Practice Parameters for Determining Brain Death in Adults," (summary statement) *Neurology* 45 (1995): 1012-14.

the observation that many individuals who fulfill a set of clinical tests for brain death do not have "permanent cessation of functioning of the entire brain." Indeed, many of these individuals have persistence of certain types of brain functions. Three areas of persistent functioning have been demonstrated: (1) cortical functioning, as shown by significant nonisoelectric EEGs; (2) brain-stem functioning, as demonstrated by evoked responses; and (3) neurohormonal regulation, as shown by anterior and posterior pituitary function.[36] The inconsistency in the tests-criterion relationship has provided one source for the confusion surrounding the concept of brain death.

Exhibit 9-3
Guidelines for the Determination of Brain Death in Children

Historical Criteria
    Determination of the proximate cause of coma.[1]
Physical Examination Criteria
    Coexisting coma and apnea[2]
    Absence of brain-stem function
    Absence of hypothermia or hypotension
    Flaccid tone or absence of spontaneous or induced movements (except spinal cord events)
    Consistent examination findings thoughout observation and testing periods
Observation Periods and Laboratory Testing
    7 days to 2 months: two clinical examinations and apnea tests and two
        electroencephalograms 48 hours apart
    2 days to 12 months: two clinical examinations and apnea tests and two
        electroencephalograms at least 24 hours apart[3]
    < 12 months: two clinical examinations and apnea tests 12 hours apart[4]

NOTES
1.   Absence of remediable or reversible conditions: toxins, drugs (sedatives, hypnotics, paralytics), metabolic disorders, surgically correctable conditions, hypotension, and hypothermia.
2.   Apnea test using standardized methods.
3.   Repeat examination and electroencephalogram obviated by absence of flow on cerebral radionuclide angiography.
4.   If hypoxic-ischemic encephalopathy is suspected, the observation period should be extended to 24 hours. Laboratory testing is not required if there is absence of a remediable or reversible condition.
Source: Task Force on Brain Death in Children, "Guidelines for the Determination of Brain Death in Children," *Pediatrics* 80 (1987): 298-99.

PHILOSOPHICAL ARGUMENTS
JUSTIFYING THE CONCEPT OF BRAIN DEATH

The other source of confusion for the concept of brain death involves the problematic nature of the philosophical arguments put forth to explain why brain death should be equated with the death of an individual. Interestingly, public acceptance of the brain death concept preceded any such philosophical defense. Indeed, an important criticism of the Harvard report was that it merely presumed a concept of death and advanced no arguments to justify why brain death should represent human death.

It was not until several years after the publication of the Harvard Committee's report that several theorists provided a conceptual framework for equating brain death with human death.[37] These theorists embraced the concept that persons who have lost all brain functions are dead because there is irreversible cessation of the "integrated functioning of the organism as a whole." The phrase "organism as a whole" refers not to the "whole organism" (that is, the sum of its tissue and organ parts), but rather to the total list of integrating mechanisms possessed by the body that coordinate the organ subsystems to permit the organism to thrive, eat, breathe, and reproduce successfully. According to Bernat and colleagues: "The organism no longer functioning as a whole is merely a collection of independent subsystems, the continued functioning of each of which is no longer meaningful."[38] In other words, the body's capacity for integrating its functions is seen as the significant indication of human life. Furthermore, it is not the death of the brain itself that is critical, but the irreversible loss of the functions normally carried out by the brain.

This concept rests on the distinction between the life or functioning of individual bodily cells and life of a human being who is able to think, perceive, respond, and regulate and integrate bodily functions. Humans are more than the flowing of fluids or the collection of cells and isolated organ systems. A person with brain death is essentially a collection of live organs, whereas a human organism with intact brain functions is able to function "as a whole." In short, the biologically live human body of a patient with brain death is not a living human being. The distinction made between isolated cells and integrated functioning explains why death is declared despite the continued growth of hair and nails for several days after the presence of other unequivocal signs of death.

The concept of the brain's role in integrating the functions of the organism as justifying a whole-brain criterion for death received support from the President's Commission in 1981.[39] Furthermore, in an attempt to give credibility to the concept of brain death, the President's Commission and others[40] advanced the argument that the introduction of neurological criteria to assess functional wholeness was not introducing a new concept of death; they argued that the use of neurological criteria captured the traditional meaning and concept of death and, hence, simply supplemented the traditional cardiopulmonary criteria. They argued that the traditional heart-lung tests for death had always been reported as ways of testing for absence of integrating capacity of the brain. They argued that the move from a heart-lung to a whole-brain definition of death does not represent a change in the concept of death, but rather a shift to the use of more direct and sophisticated measures (neurological criteria) for the traditional concept of death. Hence, whenever the traditional heart-lung tests are used, they are used as effective surrogates for neurological tests (that is, loss of heartbeat and respiration are indirect signs that brain function has been irreversibly destroyed). This is a reasonable inference, especially if sufficient time has passed for the brain to die as well. Hence, in the absence of artificial support, instead of using more complex tests for brain death (such as apnea testing), the use of heart-lung criteria can be considered a shortcut for determining death.

Although this claim is logically sound, it is not consistent with previous usage.[41] For example, for centuries no one spoke of death being based on neurological functions; instead, people associated death with loss of capacity for the flow of vital fluids. In fact, a significant minority of people today (including some physicians) believe that persons with fluid flow capacity but no brain function are alive.[42]

The concept of brain death also contradicts current usage, as states' statutes defining death permit the use of either cardiopulmonary or brain-oriented criteria for the determination of death. For example, the Uniform Determination of Death Act, advanced by the President's Commission in 1981, specifies two alternate criteria for determining death. It reads as follows: "An individual who has sustained either (1) irreversible cessation of circulatory and respiratory functions, or (2) irreversible cessation of all functions of the entire brain, including the brain stem, is dead. A determination of death must be made in accordance with accepted medical standards."[43]

Essentially, this statement recognizes not one, but two, criteria for the determination of death, specifically, one based on cardiopulmonary function and the other based on whole-brain function. According to Bernat and colleagues, a statute of death that would be more conceptually agreeable to a brain-death concept would contain only one criterion (or standard) of death (thus making clear that death is a single phenomenon) and set or sets of tests needed to determine when the criterion has been fulfilled. Their proposed statute would read as follows: "An individual who has sustained irreversible cessation of all functions of the entire brain, including the brainstem, is dead: (a) In the absence of artificial means of cardiopulmonary support, death (the irreversible cessation of all brain functions) may be determined by the prolonged absence of spontaneous circulatory and respiratory functions; (b) In the presence of artificial means of cardiopulmonary support, death (the irreversible cessation of all brain functions) must be determined by tests of brain functions."[44]

Another troublesome concern with the concept of whole-brain death is the use of tests that, when fulfilled, only approximate the criterion of whole-brain death. Indeed, as mentioned above, many individuals who fulfill clinical tests for brain death do not have "cessation of functions of the entire brain." This inconsistency in the tests-criterion relationship creates a clinical situation that contradicts the concept of "whole-brain" death itself. Specifically, if patients are declared dead by the available inexact tests for "whole-brain" death, some patients will still have brains that maintain the integrating functioning of the whole organism, as exemplified by the ability of physicians to maintain the somatic existence of pregnant women until the fetus reaches viability. Such a situation conflicts with the proposed concept of death as the loss of the integrative function of the organism as a whole. Indeed, one of the validating principles for the tests of brain death and, hence, a central ethical justification for the concept of brain death was that an organism without a functioning brain would rapidly disintegrate and thus experience somatic death within a short period of time. That such "rapid" disintegration may not occur for some individuals declared dead by tests for whole-brain death seriously undermines the concept of brain death.

In an attempt to reconcile the existence of persistent brain functioning with the concept of brain death, whole-brain theorists have recently opined that the entire brain need not be entirely dead for the individual as a whole to be dead.[45] Indeed, in response to the above-mentioned concern that the clinical tests for whole-brain death only approximate the brain-death criterion, James Bernat claims that the existence of residual functioning of "nests of brain cells" does not contradict the concept of whole-brain death, as such continued functioning does not "contribute significantly to the functioning of the organism as a whole."[46] Subsequently, Bernat has modified the definition of death to "the permanent cessation of the *critical* functions of the organism as a whole" and, accordingly, has modified the criterion of death to "the irreversible cessation of all clinical functions of the entire brain."[47] In essence, an evaluative judgment is now being made about which brain functions do or do not contribute significantly to the functioning of the organism "as a whole." Such evaluations are based on different philosophical assessments of which functions are essential to human life. Unfortunately, such evaluations challenge the integrity of the whole-brain concept of death.[48]

Due to the inconsistencies between the tests and the criterion for determining whole-brain death and the lack of conceptual clarity with the concept itself, some have concluded that the concept is fundamentally flawed and that it represents only a "superficial and fragile consensus."[49] Accordingly, it is not surprising that confusion has been associated with its use. For example, the persistent use of the term *brain death* rather than *death* indicates some ambiguity and confusion about its meaning and implications. Indeed, the term fails to distinguish between the biological claim that the brain is dead and the social, legal, and moral claim that the individual as a whole is dead because the brain is dead.[50] Thus, the use of the term *brain death* may promote confusion with families concerning why a patient is being pronounced dead (see Exhibit 9-4). Furthermore, the news media as well as health professionals regularly report that patients who have been declared brain dead later "die" when "life-support" measures are removed.[51] Finally, Youngner and colleagues reported evidence of conceptual confusion within the medical profession; in response to hypothetical cases, 58 percent of physicians and nurses did not use a coherent concept of death consistently, and one-third embraced a higher-brain rather than a whole-brain concept of death to explain why a brain-dead patient was dead.[52]

Exhibit 9-4
Using the Term "Brain Death" with Families

Use of the term "brain death" is ambiguous as it does not mean to everyone the death of the person "as a whole" based on a neurologic criterion of death. It could be construed as just the death of particular cells and other tissues in the brain, rather than the failure of functions of the brain that are responsible for the functioning of the person as a whole. It is more likely that the former concept is conveyed to lay individuals when clinicians use the term "brain death." Hence, to avoid giving the impression that only the brain has died, clinicians, when communicating to families, should say that a patient has been declared "dead" and that the determination was based on neurological tests. If a family objects to the use of a neurologic criterion of death (for example, Orthodox Jews), then death should only be determined by cardiopulmonary tests.

ALTERNATIVES TO THE WHOLE-BRAIN FORMULATION OF DEATH

Due to the concerns with the whole-brain concept of death, several scholars have expressed the opinion that functions of the lower brain stem do not contribute to the essential nature of humans and have argued for a "higher-brain" concept of death that focuses on the loss of cognitive functions.[53] These commentators argue that the capacity for integrating one's self with the social environment through consciousness is considered the essential characteristic of human life. Under this concept, the total and irreversible loss of all higher-brain functions is considered the real attribute of death. Proponents of this view use the purposely ambiguous term *higher-brain function* instead of cerebral brain death because (1) not all areas of the cerebral cortex are relevant to consciousness and cognition, and (2) more importantly, this phrase emphasizes that the key philosophical issue is which brain functions, rather than which anatomical areas, are important.[54]

Advocates of the higher-brain concept of death have suggested several specific mental and social functions as ultimately significant to human life. One candidate is the capacity for consciousness and cognition.[55] Another is the capacity for memory, reasoning, and other higher-brain functions.[56] A third possibility rests on the notion of personal identity. Green and Wikler are proponents of this third view: "A given person ceases to exist with the destruction of whatever processes there are which normally underlie that persons's psychological continuity and connectedness."[57] Supporters of this view argue that the mere continuation of biological activity in the body is irrelevant to the determination of death, because after the brain has ceased functioning the body is no longer identical with the person. A fourth view is that death is "the irreversible loss of the embodied capacity for social interaction."[58]

There are several criticisms of the higher-brain definition of death. First, deciding which higher-brain functions contribute significantly to life is fraught with the same subjectivism as is deciding which lower-brain functions are significant to "functioning of the organism as a whole." Furthermore, the higher-brain formulation of death is vulnerable to a slippery-slope course that would eventually consider persons with only marginal consciousness (such as persons with advanced senile dementia) as lacking significant function and, hence, defined as dead.[59]

Another criticism against a higher-brain formulation of death is that medical science is unable to measure precisely the irreversible loss of these higher functions based on current neurophysiological techniques. But, proponents of the higher-brain formulation of death contend that, even if we cannot presently measure accurately the loss of key higher functions such as consciousness, this failure is irrelevant to the question of whether it represents the proper conception of what it means to be dead.[60] This inability to measure would have a bearing only on the clinical implementation of the higher-brain definition, not the validity of the concept itself. Indeed, several defenders of the higher-brain definition of death concede that it may be most practical to base policy on the current clinical tests for brain death because: (1) a consensus on which higher-brain functions are significant to the living human person has not been reached; and (2) only with these tests can one be certain that there is loss of higher-brain functions. However, the proponents of a higher-brain criterion of death emphasize that such an overdetermination should neither deny the possibility that some day we will be able to measure the loss of higher functions accurately enough to use the measures clinically nor discourage the careful examination of which brain functions are the essential qualities of human life.

Alternatively, other commentators have recently argued that the entire concept of brain death is fundamentally flawed, regardless of the parts of the brain involved and, hence, that society should return to the traditional criterion of death requiring permanent cessation of circulation and breathing.[61] Indeed, instead of arguing for a higher-brain concept of death based on the contention that lower-brain functions do not contribute significantly to the "functioning of the organism as a whole," one could argue that the brain functions that still persist in individuals who are clinically brain dead can be considered essential characteristics of human life. Although it is not difficult to accept an abstract distinction between the life of individual cells from the life of the organism as a whole, it is not intuitive, however, that the whole body of a *clinically* brain-dead person is a mere colossal "cell-culture" that is biologically dead. As argued by Josef Seifert:

> How can one claim that a body that can still be fed intravenously and accepts nourishment is dead? How can one claim that an organism as a whole is dead when most of its organs function completely or partially? How can one justifiably call someone dead who actively produces procreative cells? How is a mother dead who can carry her child to term? The dynamic self-generation of the organism through regeneration, growth, metabolism, and procreation is the most central of the exclusive marks of a living being. But all or some of the basic marks of this dynamic self-generation are preserved in the brain dead patients.[62]

Hence, there is not a philosophical consensus that persons declared dead based on neurologic criteria are dead.

The disagreement among the different definitions or concepts of death results from different opinions about the relevance of various functions to human life. Any isolation of biological functions considered to be significant represents an evaluative, arbitrary choice. The moment of death is not solely a medical judgement (as thought by the Harvard Committee) and cannot be discovered by an empirical process. Instead, it is dependent upon values and beliefs. Indeed, several cultural traditions (such as Jewish, Japanese, and Native American) do not accept any neurologic grounds for the diagnosis of death.[63] Even within the medical profession, a small but persistent minority of physicians hold this view.[64]

The mere fact that the moment of death is arbitrary and can be different for different cultures and societies makes clear that death—rather than being an indisputable and unequivocal threshold event—is a process that occurs on a continuum of declining life; this process is manifested by the sequential death of organ systems, individual organs, and ultimately separate cells—each declining on a somewhat independent trajectory.[65] Each of the three contending definitions of death under the threshold model (cardiopulmonary, whole brain, and higher-brain) corresponds to a different point on this continuum. Understanding death as a process makes clear that, with each definition of death, there is "obvious residual life of one degree or another." The reality of residual life underscores the realization that any formulation of death that presupposes a sharp line between life and death, although convenient for certain societal functions (such as burial, payment of life-insurance policies, and organ procurement) is biologically artificial and socially constructed.

The recognition that death is an evaluative judgment points out the difficulty in any selection of criteria in a pluralistic world. The task for society, therefore, is to develop a public policy that recognizes and values the differences in opinion regarding concepts of death. One approach proposed by Linda Emanuel is to define a "bounded zone" definition of death within which individuals are permitted to choose a concept of death that conforms most closely to their religious and philosophical convictions.[66] Emanuel's proposal entails adopting the cardiorespiratory criterion as the "lower bound" for determining death that would apply to all cases, but would allow individuals to endorse a concept of death based on neurological dysfunction up to the level of the permanent vegetative state, the "higher bound." Adoption of such a bounded zone would also establish a range of morally permissible behaviors, from burial to organ donation. Rather than trying to create a single, theoretically satisfactory criterion of death, a bounded approach is able to handle and respect differences in moral positions among people. Hence, any disagreements that individuals may have concerning when a person is dead will be attributed to differences among legitimate values, provided the positions taken on the concept of death fall within the defined zone. This approach is similar to that taken on the abortion issue; society recognizes that people hold different beliefs concerning when life begins and, accordingly, permits a range of morally permissible behaviors. If different conceptions of the beginning of life are tolerated, it makes sense that a similar approach should be adopted for the end of life.

New Jersey provides an example of legislative tolerance for diversity; the state adopted a law with a conscience clause that permits patients or their surrogates to object to a neurologic diagnosis of death if such a declaration would violate their personal religious beliefs.[67] Obviously, more work is needed to craft a statute that would allow a higher-brain concept of death, but initial proposals have been suggested.[68]

THE MORAL STATUS OF ORGAN DONATION: WHEN SHOULD IT BE PERMITTED?

The recognition of the arbitrary nature of any definition of death accentuates the concern that previous efforts to endorse whole-brain death as the criterion of death were a gross attempt to move the line between life and death to satisfy the utilitarian concerns of organ transplantation. Indeed, the promulgation of whole-brain death as a criterion of death enabled society to increase the donor pool without crossing the moral prohibition against killing as it related to organ transplantation, that is, without violating the dead-donor rule. This dead-donor rule, which entails that patients must not be killed by organ retrieval or must not be killed so that their organs can be taken, describes an unwritten, uncodified standard that has guided organ procurement in the United States since the late 1960s in order to reassure society that severely compromised patients would be protected from harms that might result from overzealous quests to satisfy the utilitarian appeal of organ transplants.[69] However, how protective is the dead-donor rule if the definition of death and the criterion for determining it can be tampered with and then "thrust" upon society? Furthermore, even if an attempt to "redefine" death actually represents no change in the conception of death, a perception that the line between life and death has been redrawn may foster suspicion and fear of the procurement process and decrease people's willingness to donate organs.

Recent protocols to obtain organs from non-heart-beating donors (NHBDs) also raise concerns with changing the criterion used to determine death.[70] Such protocols, spurred by the recent shortage of organs, detail the process of a scheduled organ procurement following the discontinuation of life support in patients who are either cognitively intact with an intolerable quality of life, or in patients who are severely and terminally brain injured who have failed to develop the full clinical syndrome of brain death. For example, according to the protocol at the University of Pittsburgh,[71] if a patient or a family requests organ donation following and separate from the decision to withdraw life support, the patient is taken to the operating room where life support is withdrawn. The patient is then monitored for the development of cardiac arrest, which is expected to occur, as these patients have been maintained on artificial ventilation or on circulatory assistance. The patient is declared dead based on the criterion of irreversible cessation of cardiac and pulmonary function, which is considered satisfied when the following tests have been fulfilled: (1) the patient is apneic, (2) the patient is unresponsive to verbal stimuli, and (3) there has been two minutes of ventricular fibrillation, asystole, or electromechanical dissociation. Organs are procured only if cardiac arrest occurs a short time after withdrawal of life support in order to minimize organ ischemia, an issue that originally limited the previous usefulness of organs obtained from NHBDs. If cardiac arrest does not occur within an appropriate time interval (for example, two hours), a determination can be made to cancel organ procurement.

One of the major issues generated by NHBD protocols involves the determination of the time of death; specifically, what should be the time interval between the detection of cardiac arrest and the declaration of death? The appropriate time interval is crucial in NHBD organ procurement to prevent premature determination of death. However, this goal is in tension with the goal of obtaining viable organs for transplant, as the viability of organs decreases as the time interval increases.

All NHBD protocols equate the time of death with the "irreversible" cessation of circulatory and respiratory functions. However, equating the time of death with a state of "irreversible" cardiopulmonary function is problematic for two reasons. First, protocols and practices in the United States and other countries vary significantly in defining what should be the appropriate period of observation after the cessation of cardiopulmonary function to ensure a state of "irreversibility" of cardiopulmonary function. For example, this time interval is two minutes for the Pittsburgh protocol, whereas others prescribe intervals of one, two, or five minutes, some do not require any elapsed time, and some leave the definition to the attending.[72] Such variability stems from a lack of consensus on whether the point of "irreversibility" should be defined by when the heart lacks the capacity to autoresuscitate or when cardiac function cannot be reversed with resuscitative measures, as well as to the lack of scientific data examining the probability of autoresuscitation after cardiac arrest. The existence of variable time intervals engenders the concern that the criterion of death is being manipulated to maximize the chances for organ procurement at the expense of ensuing that organs are not being prematurely removed from patients who are still alive.

Another concern with determining death at the point of "irreversibility" of cardiopulmonary function is that under a whole-brain criterion of death, it is not at all certain that patients are dead within the first few minutes after cessation of cardiopulmonary function, as it probably takes significantly longer than a few minutes to ensure the development of irreversible brain damage.[73]

A recent Institute of Medicine report recommends a time interval of five minutes to ensure the irreversibility of cardiac autoresuscitation, a time interval based on "expert information and advice from its senior special experts."[74] In addressing the issue of the irreversibility of cardiac and pulmonary functions, the Institute of Medicine report opined that because resuscitative measures after the onset of cardiac arrest have been refused, either by the patient or the surrogates, the issue of irreversibility of cardiac and pulmonary function only hinges on the probability of the heart to autoresuscitate and not on the likelihood of the reversibility of cardiac function from the implementation of resuscitative measures. It is interesting to note that the five-minute interval recommended by the Institute of Medicine report was apparently only based on the time thought to be needed to ensure that the probability of cardiac reversibility was "vanishingly small," and not on any concerns that such a time interval supported a determination of death based on a whole-brain criterion of death. The report did note that "although . . . not relevant to a determination of death, the interval of absent circulation recommended here will . . . produce irreversible brain damage."[75]

Rather then endorse procedures and protocols that appear to be manipulating the definition of death, others maintain that an alternative approach to fulfill the needs of organ transplantation would be to abandon the dead-donor rule and replace it with a process that is governed and constrained by a rigorous consent process.[76] The task is now conceived as the need to arrive at a societal consensus regarding the definition of who is and is not eligible to be a donor, rather than who is and is not dead. Such a process of organ procurement would have to be legitimated as a form of justified killing. Subsequently, patients who are ventilator-dependent or who are imminently and irreversibly dying can give consent for organ removal before they are dead. Similarly, surrogates could give consent for organ donation for patients who are permanently and irreversibly unconscious. Recently, Robert Truog recommended that society should uncouple the link between organ donation and brain death by adopting a policy of organ donation based on the principles of consent and nonmaleficence.[77] Consequently, the concept of brain death would become obsolete and society could then revert back to the traditional approach to determining death, that is, the cardiorespiratory standard. Subsequently, the long-standing debate over fundamental inconsistencies in the concept of brain death would be resolved. However, many commentators are concerned about the effects on our moral character of treating individuals as replaceable body parts.[78] Whether society ultimately embraces the moral acceptability of intentionally ending lives for the good of other lives may prove to be as difficult as defining death.

Alternatively, it is instructive to see how the previously described attempt to define a bounded zone of death would apply to organ transplantation.[79] Such an approach would appeal to a more inclusive range of moral positions that people actually hold without requiring distortions of language or concept and would engender less distrust. Adoption of a bounded zone of death that includes cardiopulmonary, whole-brain, and higher-brain death would make organ donation permissible from patients declared dead with any of these criteria. Although a concept of death may be thought to be determined by the utilitarian appeal of organ donation, it may very well be determined by the type of moral value assigned to the residual life left in the person who has "died."[80] For example, the value of residual life in a person declared dead based on a higher-brain concept of death could lie in the person's status as a potential donor. Arguably, another individual may see the residual life of such a person as having moral value that commands attempts to preserve it. Although conflicting positions and views will occur, the goal is to permit a good approximation to the range of moral positions and intuitions that people have about concepts of death. Such an approach would respect the pluralistic makeup of the society within which we live.

NOTES

1. C. Pallis, "Whole Brain Death Reconsidered: Physiological Facts and Philosophy," *Journal of Medical Ethics* 9 (1983): 32-37.

2. K. Gervais, *Redefining Death* (New Haven, Conn.: Yale University Press, 1986); R.M. Veatch, *Death, Dying, and the Biological Revolution: Our Last Quest for Responsibility,* 2nd ed. (New Haven, Conn.: Yale University Press, 1989); J. Seifert, "Is 'Brain Death' Actually Death?" *Monist* 76 (1993): 175-202.

3. Veatch, *Death, Dying,* see note 2 above, p. 17.

4. A. Halevy and B. Brody, "Brain Death: Reconciling Definitions, Criteria, and Tests," *Annals of Internal Medicine* 119 (1993): 519-25.

5. J.D. Arnold, T.F. Zimmerman, and D.C. Martin, "Public Attitudes and the Diagnosis of Death," *Journal of the American Medical Association* 206 (1968): 1949-55.

6. Ibid.

7. President's Commission for the Study of Ethical Problems in Medicine and Biomedical and Behavioral Research, *Defining Death: Medical, Legal and Ethical Issues in the Determination of Death* (Washington, D.C.: U.S. Government Printing Office, 1981).

8. H. Cushing, "Some Experimental and Clinical Observations Concerning States of Increased Intracranial Tension," *American Journal of Medical Sciences* 124 (1902): 375-400.

9. P. Mollaret and M. Goulon, "Le Coma Depasse (Memoire Preliminaire)," *Revue Neurologique* (Paris) 101 (1959): 3-15.

10. D.J. Rothman, *Strangers at the Bedside: A History of How Law and Bioethics Transformed Medical Decision Making* (New York: Basic Books, 1991), 160.

11. T. Starzl et al., "Orthotopic Homotransplantation of the Human Liver," *Annals of Surgery* 168 (1967): 392-415; C. Barnard, "Reflections on the First Heart Transplant," *South African Medical Journal* 72 (1967): 19-20.

12. Ad Hoc Committee of the Harvard Medical School to Examine the Definition of Brain Death, "A Definition of Irreversible Coma," *Journal of the American Medical Association* 205 (1968): 337-40.

13. Ibid., 338 and 340.

14. Ibid., 338.

15. H. Jonas, "Against the Stream: Comments on the Definition and Redefinition of Death," in *Philosophical Essays: From Ancient Creed to Technological*

Man, ed. H. Jonas (Englewood Cliffs, N.J.: Prentice Hall, 1974), 132-40; H. van Till-d'Anulnis de Bourouill, "Diagnosis of Death in Comatose Patients under Resuscitation Treatment: A Critical Review of the Harvard Report," *American Journal of Law & Medicine* 2 (1976): 1-41; C. Perry, "Applying the Harvard Criteria," *Journal of Medicine and Philosophy* 4 (1979): 232-33.

16. M.A. DeVita, J.V. Snyder, and A. Grenvik, "History of Organ Donation by Patients with Cardiac Death," *Kennedy Institute of Ethics Journal* 2 (1993): 113-29.

17. W.J. Curran, "The Brain-Death Concept: Judicial Acceptance in Massachusetts," *New England Journal of Medicine* 298 (1978): 1008-09.

18. A.M. Capron and F.H. Cate, "Death and Organ Transplantation," in *Treatise on Health Care Law,* ed. M. MacDonald et al. (Conklin, N.Y.: Matthew Bender, 1991).

19. F.J. Veith et al., "Brain Death: I. A Status Report of Medical and Ethical Considerations," *Journal of the American Medical Association* 238 (1977): 1651-55; see note 16 above.

20. S.J. Youngner et al., " 'Brain Death' and Organ Retrieval: A Cross-Sectional Survey of Knowledge and Concepts Among Health Professionals," *Journal of the American Medical Association* 261 (1989): 2205-10.

21. P.M. Black, "Brain Death," *New England Journal of Medicine* 299 (1978): 338-44, 393-401.

22. R.D. Adams and M. Jequier, "The Brain Death Syndrome: Hypoxemic Panencephalopathy," *Schweizerche Medizinische Wochenscrift: Journal Suisse de Medecine* (Basel, Switzerland) 99 (1969): 65-73; Task Force on Death and Dying of the Institute of Society, Ethics and the Life Sciences, "Refinements in Criteria for the Determination of Death: An Appraisal," *Journal of the American Medical Association* 221 (1972): 48-53; J.F. Alderete et al., "Irreversible Coma: A Clinical, Electroencephalo-graphic and Neuropathological Study," *Transactions of the American Neurology Association* 93 (1968): 16-20; A.E. Walker, E.L. Diamond, and J. Moseley, "The Neuropathological Findings in Irreversible Coma: A Critique of the 'Respirator Brain'," *Journal of Neuropathology and Experimental Neurology* 34 (1975): 295-323.

23. Task Force on Death and Dying, "Refinements in Criteria," see note 22 above.

24. Walker, Diamond, and Moseley, "The Neuropathological Findings," see note 22 above.

25. A.E. Walker, E.L. Diamond, and J.L. Moseley, "An Appraisal of the Criteria of Cerebral Death: A Summary Statement," *Journal of the American Medical Association* 237 (1977): 982-86.

26. "Guidelines for the Determination of Death: Report of the Medical Consultants on the Diagnosis of Death to the President's Commission for the Study of Ethical Problems in Medicine and Biomedical and Behavioral Research," *Journal of the American Medical Association* 246 (1981): 2184-86.

27. P.M. Black and N.T. Zervas, "Declaration of Brain Death in

Neurosurgical and Neurological Practice," *Neurosurgery* 15 (1984): 170-74.

28. See note 21 above.

29. J. Korein, "Radioisotopic Bolus Technique as a Test to Detect Circulatory Deficit Associated with Cerebral Death: 142 Studies on 80 Patients Demonstrating the Bedside Use of an Innocuous IV Procedure as an Adjunct in the Diagnosis of Cerebral Death," *Circulation* 51 (1975): 924-939; see note 21 above.

30. T. Breitz et al., "Aortocranial and Carntis Angiography in Determination of Brain Death," *Neuroradiology* 5 (1973): 13-19.

31. E.F.M. Wijdicks, "Practice Parameters for Determining Brain Death in Adults," *Neurology* 45 (1995): 1003-11; Report of the Quality Standards Subcommittee of the American Academy of Neurology, "Practice Parameters for Determining Brain Death in Adults," (summary statement) *Neurology* 45 (1995): 1012-14..

32. J.A. Schwartz, J. Baxter, and D.R. Brill, "Diagnosis of Brain Death in Children by Radionuclide Cerebral Imaging," *Pediatrics* 73 (1984): 14-18; S.L. Moshe and L.A. Alverez, "Diagnosis of Brain Death in Children," *Journal of Clinical Neurophysiology* 3 (1986): 239-49.

33. Task Force on Brain Death in Children, "Guidelines for the Determination of Brain Death in Children," *Pediatrics* 80 (1987): 298-99.

34. R.E. Mejia and M.M. Pollack, "Variability in Brain Death Determination Practices in Children," *Journal of the American Medical Association* 274 (1995): 550-53.

35. Ad Hoc Committee on Brain Death, The Children's Hospital, Boston, "Determination of Death," *Journal of Pediatrics* 1 (1987): 1015-19; J.M. Freeman and P.C. Ferry, "New Brain Death Guidelines in Children: Further Confusion," *Pediatrics* 81 (1988): 301-03.

36. See note 4 above.

37. J.L. Bernat, C.M. Culver, and B. Gert, "On the Definition and Criterion of Death," *Annals of Internal Medicine* 94 (1981): 389-94; J.L. Bernat, "How Much of the Brain Must Die in Brain Death?" *The Journal of Clinical Ethics* 3, no. 1 (Spring 1992): 21-26; Veith et al., "Brain Death," see note 19 above.

38. Bernat, "How Much of the Brain Must Die," see note 37 above, p. 22.

39. See note 7 above.

40. A.M. Capron and L.R. Kass, "A Statutory Definition of the Standards for Determining Human Death: An Appraisal and a Proposal," *University of Pennsylvania Law Review* 121 (1972): 87-118; Bernat, Culver, and Gert, "On the Definition," see note 36 above.

41. Veatch, *Death, Dying,* see note 2 above.

42. P.A. Byrne, S. O'Reilly, and P.M. Quay, "Brain Death—An Opposing Viewpoint," *Journal of the American Medical Association* 242 (1979): 1985-90; see note 20 above.

43. See note 7 above.

44. J.L. Bernat, C.M. Culver, and B. Gert, "Defining Death in Theory and Practice," *Hastings Center Report* 12, no. 1 (1982): 5-9, 8.

45. J.L. Bernat, "A Defense of the Whole-Brain Concept of Death," *Hasting Center Report* 28, no. 2 (1998): 14-23; Bernat, "How Much of the Brain Must Die," see note 37 above.

46. Bernat, "How Much of the Brain Must Die," see note 37 above, p. 25.

47. Bernat, "A Defense of the Whole-Brain Concept," see note 45 above.

48. R.M. Veatch, "The Impending Collapse of the Whole-Brain Definition of Death," *Hastings Center Report* 23 (1993): 18-24.

49. S.J. Youngner, "Defining Death: A Superficial and Fragile Consensus," *Archives of Neurology* 49 (1992): 570-72.

50. See note 48 above.

51. S.J. Youngner et al., "Psychosocial and Ethical Implications of Organ Retrieval," *New England Journal of Medicine* 313 (1985): 321-24.

52. See note 20 above.

53. S.J. Youngner and E.T. Bartlett, "Human Death and High Technology: The Failure of the Whole-Brain Formulations," *Annals of Internal Medicine* 99 (1983): 2520-58; see notes 20 and 47 above.

54. See note 48 above.

55. Youngner and Bartlett, "Human Death," see note 53 above.

56. H.T. Engelhardt, "Defining Death: A Philosophical Problem for Medicine and Law," *Annual Review of Respiratory Disease* 112 (1975): 587-90.

57. M. Green and D. Wikler, "Brain Death and Personal Identity," *Philosophy and Public Affairs* 9 (1980): 105-33.

58. Veatch, *Death, Dying,* see note 2 above.

59. Bernat, "How Much of the Brain Must Die," see note 37 above.

60. See notes 48 and 53.

61. R.D. Troug, "Is It Time to Abandon Brain Death?" *Hastings Center Report* 27, no. 1 (1997): 29-37; R.M. Taylor, "Re-Examining the Definition and Criterion of Death," *Seminars in Neurology* 17 (1997): 265-70.

62. Seifert, " 'Is 'Brain Death' Actually Death?" see note 2 above, p. 189.

63. U.S. Congress, Office of Technology Assessment, *Life-Sustaining Technology and the Elderly* (Washington, DC: U.S. Government Printing Office, 1987).

64. See notes 20 and 42 above.

65. R.S. Morrison, "Death: Process or Event?" *Science* 173 (1971): 694-98; L.L. Emanuel, "Reexamining Death: The Asymptotic Model and Bounded Zone Definition," *Hastings Center Report* 25, no. 4 (1995): 27-35.

66. Emanuel, "Reexamining Death," see note 63 above.

67. R.S. Olick, "Brain Death, Religious Freedom, and Public Policy: New Jersey's Landmark Legislative Initiative," *Kennedy Institute of Ethics Journal* 1 (1991): 275-88.

68. See notes 4 and 65 above.

69. R.M. Arnold and S.J. Youngner, "The Dead Donor Rule: Should We Stretch It, Bend It, or Abandon It?" *Kennedy Institute of Ethics Journal* 3 (1993): 263-78.

70. S.J. Youngner and R.M. Arnold, "Ethical, Psychosocial, and Public Policy

Implications of Procuring Organs from Non-Heart-Beating Cadaver Donors," *Journal of the American Medical Association* 269 (1993): 2769-74.

71. University of Pennsylvania Medical Center Policy and Procedure Manual, "Management of Terminally Ill Patients Who May Become Organ Donors After Death," *Kennedy Institute of Ethics Journal* 3 (1993): A1-A15.

72. Institute of Medicine, *Non-Heart-Beating Organ Transplantation: Medical and Ethical Issues in Procurement* (Washington, D.C.: National Academy Press, 1997).

73. J. Lynn, "Are the Patients Who Become Organ Donors Under the Pittsburgh Protocol for 'Non-Heart-Beating Donors' Really Dead?" *Kennedy Institute of Ethics Journal* 3 (1993): 167-78; Troug, "Is It Time?" see note 61 above; Bernat, "A Defense of the Whole-Brain Concept," see note 45 above.

74. See note 72 above, p. 59.

75. Ibid.; P. Safar, "Resuscitation of the Ischemic Brain," in *Textbook of Neuroanesthesia: With Neurosurgical and Neuroscience Perspectives,* ed. M.S. Albin (New York: McGraw-Hill, 1997).

76. See note 69 above; Troug, "Is It Time?" see note 61 above.

77. See note 61 above.

78. R.C. Fox, " 'An Ignoble Form of Cannibalism': Reflections on the Pittsburgh Protocol for Procuring Organs from Non-Heart-Beating Cadavers," *Kennedy Institute of Ethics Journal* 3 (1993): 231-39; P. Ramsey, *The Patient As Person: Explorations in Medical Ethics* (New Haven: Yale University Press, 1970).

79. Emanuel, "Reexamining Death," see note 63 above.

80. Ibid.

10

The ICU as Holy Ground

Russell B. Connors, Jr.

Moses . . . came to Horeb, the mountain of God. There an angel of the Lord appeared to him in flaming fire out of a bush. As he looked on, he was surprised to see that the bush, though on fire, was not consumed. So Moses decided, "I must go over to look at this remarkable sight, and see why the bush is not burned."... God called to him from the bush, "Moses! Moses!" He answered, "Here I am." God said, "Come no nearer! Remove the sandals from your feet, for the place where you stand is holy ground. I am the God of your father," he continued, "the God of Abraham, the God of Isaac, and the God of Jacob." Moses hid his face, for he was afraid to look at God.

—Exodus 3:1-6 *New American Bible*

"The surgery went well: four bypasses," Dr. Anderson said in the hurried minute we had with him. "Her heart is strong, so there is reason to be optimistic. But of course surgery of this kind is quite a trauma to the body, especially hard on someone your mother's age; the next 48 hours are critical." With that, he was off. Some time later the nurse emerged from behind the ICU doors. "If you like you can see her now," she said. Then she asked, "Have you ever seen someone in an intensive care unit?" I answered, "Yes, several times," while my sister responded, "Never." She tried to prepare us, describing in some detail the sedation, the tubes, the ventilator, as well as Mom's body temperature and skin color. We took in what we could. Minutes later, as the automatic doors of the ICU closed behind us, we had the feeling of being in a place where we didn't belong. We were open-eyed and silent, somewhere between awed and terrified by the power of the place. I recall beeps and buzzes, but no human sounds. And then Mom: what was lying in the bed was limp and lifeless, as if some sort of controlled violence had been perpetrated against it. It did not seem like a person, much less our mother. Her color was ashen gray, and she seemed at death's door; perhaps she was. My sister sobbed. I was overwhelmed—frightened, numb, and other things I can't name. We didn't stay long.

INTRODUCTION

As the title of this chapter states, and as these two scenes suggest, the intensive care unit (ICU) may be imaged as holy ground. The image is both instructive and fruitful. It is *instructive* in that it provides an opportunity for reflecting on the kinds of places where "the holy" and where "God" may be experienced in our culture; it is *fruitful* in that such imaging yields valuable insights relative to the type of response and the kind of behavior appropriate for those who regularly tread upon such turf.

The chapter is in two parts. The first part attempts to unpack what it means to suggest that the ICU may be holy ground. It discusses three concepts—the holy (named by many, though certainly not all, as God), limit experience, and sacred space—and examines two phenomena regularly experienced in the ICU that warrant the image of holy ground—vulnerability and mortality. The second part of the chapter discusses some of the implications of this imagery. If the ICU is the kind of place where human vulnerability and mortality are regularly "part of the turf," then what kind of personal skills—virtues, really—ought to characterize those who find themselves ministering (to stay with religious language) in the ICU? The proposal here is that such people ought to be especially good at two things: reverencing life (physically, interpersonally, and ethically) and dealing with death.

THE ICU AS HOLY GROUND: THE IMAGE

THREE CONCEPTS

To argue that the ICU may be imagined as holy ground requires an elaboration on the image itself, and then an explanation of why the ICU may be such a place. The first task calls for a discussion of three important and interrelated concepts: "the holy," "limit experience," and sacred space.

"*The holy.*" Rudolf Otto's classic discussion of this concept in *The Idea of the Holy* is the place to begin.[1] Although Otto's discussion was directed toward the *idea* of "the holy," what Otto had in mind is more an *experience* than a concept. At the beginning of his book, Otto invited his readers to direct their minds "to a moment of deeply-felt religious experience. . . . Whoever cannot do this, whoever knows no such moments . . . is requested to read no farther."[2] Readers of this more humble enterprise are invited similarly to connect what follows with their own experience of "the holy."

For Otto, religious experience is the experience of the holy or, as he describes it, "*mysterium tremendum et fascinans.*" The holy is *mysterium* in that it is mysterious, "hidden and esoteric" (it defies words);[3] it is *tremendum* in that it is an experience of terrifying awe and ultimate anxiety; and it is *fascinans* in that it is an experience so attracting, so exhilarating, as to move one beyond oneself and beyond words. To *experience the holy* is to experience mystery, which is to experience a dimension of reality that is capable of evoking a response of ultimate wonder and awe and/or ultimate terror and dread.[4] The following may help to illustrate this concept.

A group of travelers approach the rim of the Grand Canyon. They have seen the pictures and listened to the descriptions of friends. Now they see; they experience; a spontaneous, reverent silence overtakes them all. The expansiveness is so awesome that they know they will never take it all in. For some, the experience is *theistic,* and they name the grandeur of the place as a mighty work of God: "Bless the Lord, my soul. Lord my God, how great you are. . . . You fixed the earth on its foundations, unshakable forever and ever" (Psalm 104:1,5). For others, the ex-

---

Exhibit 10-1
ICU as Holy Ground

- The holy mysterium
- Experiential limit situation
- Sacred space of vulnerability and mortality
- Reverencing life
- Dealing with death

perience may not be theistic but is no less religious in that it involves ultimate wonder and awe. The response of this latter group, whether silent or verbal, is equally religious in nature. This is what led John Haught (drawing on Otto's insights) to define religion (some theistic, some not) as simply the "discernment of and response to mystery."[5]

But mystery comes in other places and at other times: at the grave of a child; at the loss of a loved one; at the horror of war; at the assassination of a world peacemaker; or as one leaves the Holocaust Museum with a friend, wandering through the streets of Washington, D.C., in silence, wondering how such horrors could have happened, terrorized by the thought that they could happen again. In these moments, the theist might turn to God, either in plea—"Deliver us, O Lord"—or perhaps in anguish—"Where were you, where are you, O God? What kind of God are you?" With just as much anguish, a religious but non-theistic[6] person may respond with silence or a scream. In either case, the experience is religious in nature because it involves *ultimate terror and dread.*

The "limit experience." To know that one is standing on holy ground is obviously no trivial matter. It is not about having a good or a bad day. Rather, to experience *mysterium tremendum et fascinans* is to stand in a place—literally or figuratively—where one is pushed to the limit of one's experience. In the following passage from *Blessed Rage for Order,* David Tracy describes what he calls "limit situations." In this context, he says well what limit experience entails:

> The concept limit-situation is a familiar one in the existentialist philosophy and theology of the very recent past. Fundamentally, the concept refers to those human situations wherein a human being ineluctably finds manifest a certain ultimate limit or horizon to his or her existence. The concept itself is mediated by "showing" the implications of certain crucial positive and negative experiential limit-situations. More exactly, limit-situations refer to two basic kinds of existential situation: either those "boundary" situations of guilt, anxiety, sickness, and the recognition of death as one's own destiny, or those situations called "ecstatic experiences"—intense joy, love, reassurance, creation.[7]

Limit experience, then, is about *ultimate* wonder and awe and/or *ultimate* terror and dread. Among the ways such experience manifests human limitation is in regard to language. Words inevitably fall short of capturing such experiences; what is affirmed about these experiences—

sometimes in some of the world's greatest literature (from Shakespeare's love sonnets, on one end of the spectrum, to Elie Wiesel's horrifying Holocaust story, *Night*,[8] on the other)—is true by way of analogy. The effort to describe such experiences is valuable; they are not completely "unshareable." Nevertheless, as Moses knew on the mountaintop in the presence of God, silence is never an inappropriate response.[9]

One further comment about limit experience is important. As the quotation from Tracy exemplifies, limit experiences are most frequently described as either positive or negative; usually they come in the form of ecstasy or horror. True enough. But I wish to assert what is perhaps a more elusive and subtle twofold truth (and I appeal to the reader's experience for verification): some events and places are capable of eliciting *both* ecstasy *and* horror, and sometimes they happen together. For example, some have stood at the rim of the Grand Canyon, overcome by the grandeur of the place, and at the very same time moved to anguish by the awareness of the sacrilege done to creation elsewhere. And some have stood near the casket of a loved one, perhaps a child, anguished over life's unfairness and futility, and yet, in some magnificently mysterious way, touched by the graciousness of life, made manifest in the tearful and loving embraces of friends. Thus, some experiences, some places, are capable of eliciting a response of both ultimate wonder and awe and ultimate terror and dread; sometimes they happen together. The intensive care unit is such a place.

Sacred space. Perhaps more than any one else, Mircea Eliade is associated with the notion of sacred space.[10] He has shown that in virtually all religions, certain times and spaces are considered to be sacred, in the literal sense of that word, apart from "ordinary" times and spaces, not only for special rituals but also so that "the holy"/mystery/God can be made manifest. (Although the image of sacred space is of primary interest here, it should not be missed that time and events such as birth, growth, sickness, and death—times and events that have become medical events in our culture—are almost inevitably considered to be sacred times.)

Sacred space sometimes is in the form of natural wonders—from the Grand Canyon, to the mountaintop (a biblically important place), to one's own meadow that few others seem to know about. Sometimes sacred space is a shrine built by human hands: the mosque, the temple, the most grandiose of cathedrals, or the simplest of community prayer rooms. The sacredness of a space may have a great deal to do with the fact that the religious community of which one is a part considers it to be sacred; the communally constructed sacred meaning of a space is part of the phenomenon. Even so, the communally constructed sacred meaning of a space is not arbitrary.[11] There is a reason why the snow-capped mountain peak and the Cathedral of Chartres are sacred for so many people. Such places can move one to ultimacy; they can push the limits of our experience of beauty and of finitude. They can, in other words, move us to mystery and elicit from us a response that is nothing but religious. Invoking an idea from Catholic theology (although far from exclusively so), it is the principle of *sacramentality* that suggests that we human beings encounter mystery, we experience God, in and through concrete human experience.[12] In and through times and spaces—some of them magnificent, some of them dreadful—"the holy"/mystery/God can be disclosed.

The word *can* is important. There is nothing automatic about, no necessary connection between, a space and religious experience. Although specific words and deeds or times and spaces can be mediators of mystery, and although mystery is always experienced in some mediated manner, "the holy" mystery/God is not imposed upon us in some necessary fashion. Without the "spirit in the heart" of the hearer[13]—a heart that must be open and receptive, disposed to receive mystery as a kind of gift—the voice of mystery will not be heard. Whether it is the Grand Canyon or the child's grave, whether it is the sanctuary of the church or the ICU of the modern hospital, "the holy"/mystery/God *may* be experienced in a variety of sacred spaces. However, it is not automatic. Those who regularly tread on the turf of such holy places know that they do not manufacture mystery, but neither should they run from it. Reverent response—that is what we seek.

THE TERRAIN OF THE ICU: HOLY GROUND

If sacred space is the kind of space in which limit experience tends to occur, and if it is a space in which "the holy"/mystery/God is often made manifest, then the ICU is such a space. Put differently, the ICU may be considered to be holy ground.

What is it about the ICU that makes it the kind of ground that may be experienced as holy? Vulnerability and mortality. Other things happen in the ICU, to be sure, but vulnerability and mortality are two of the most common and yet deepest experiences of many patients and loved ones in the ICU setting; this is why the ICU is a place where one might be on the lookout for wonder and awe and/or terror and dread.

Before moving to a discussion of vulnerability and mortality, it is important to ask, "Whose vulnerability? Whose mortality?" The best answer is, "anyone who treads on such turf: patients, loved ones, and healthcare professionals." The remainder of the first part of this chapter focuses on the experiences of vulnerability and mortality of patients and their loved ones—those who come to ICUs occasionally, in what are usually difficult and trying times. The second part of the chapter focuses on the experiences of healthcare professionals—who, hopefully, are not immune from vulnerability and mortality themselves—and explores what the implications of the ICU's "holiness" might be for such "ministers."

Vulnerability. It may be instructive to discuss three different dimensions of the vulnerability of patients and loved ones in the ICU: physical, relational, and ethical. In each way, vulnerability is a potential doorway to "the holy."

The ICU scene depicted at the opening of this chapter captures something of the terror of seeing a loved one lying limp and seemingly lifeless in an ICU bed. If it is true that at times many of us suffer from the illusion of being indestructible, then such ICU experiences can reintroduce us, coldly and cruelly, to our frailty and vulnerability. To the extent that Merleau-Ponty was right in reminding us of the embodied nature of humans—that in large measure we *are* our bodies[14]—then to that extent the experience of physical vulnerability, our own or that of others', can occasion the "holy" experience of ultimate terror and dread.

Although mortality is related to the experience of physical frailty and vulnerability, vulnerability and mortality are distinct. To know our own vulnerability or, more difficult perhaps, the physical frailty or vulnerability of a child,[15] is to learn again that we can hurt, that sometimes it is in our very bodiliness that we suffer. Who does not know this? But sometimes—and the ICU is the kind of place where this can happen—the experience of pain, physical frailty, and vulnerability can move one to ask some of life's hardest questions: "Why must this be so?" "Why must there be this hurt?" "Why must our child suffer?" "What kind of world is this, and what kind of power, or God, is it that does not make it different?" Not only are these hard questions, but they are religious questions; those who ask them and hear them stand on holy ground.

A related but distinct type of vulnerability is relational in nature. The son and daughter standing open-eyed and silent at the edge of the ICU bed experienced this type of vulnerability: "I recall beeps and buzzes, but no human sounds. And then Mom: what was lying in the bed was limp and lifeless, as if some sort of controlled violence had been perpetrated against it. It did not seem like a person, much less our mother."

What this scene suggests is that the ICU can sometimes be a place in which vulnerability appears in the form of relational disconnection. Whether experienced by the patient or the patient's loved ones or both, physical illness—often the type that leads one to the ICU—can bring with it the loss of what may well be humankind's greatest treasure, the ability to be in meaningful and loving relationship with others. Years ago, Richard A. McCormick considered the "potential for human relationship" so important that he was willing to consider it the decisive quality-of-life criterion for determining appropriate medical treatment in many situations.[16] What is the point? The kind of critical illness that takes a patient to the ICU—very often in a condition that makes significant human communication or conscious interpersonal relationship impossible—can occasion a profound experience of human vulnerability.[17] For the son and daughter in the opening scene, Mom seemed reduced to an "it," and the reduction was ushering in a most disturbing religious question: "Is our relationship with Mom over?"

A third type of vulnerability that may lurk about in the ICU is ethical in nature. This is related to the interpersonal dimension of vulnerability just described and, like the other types of vulnerability, this can be a doorway to religious experience. As this book attests, the ICU is sometimes a setting in which medical-moral questions about life and death must be addressed and answered. Whether one's ethical framework is grounded first and foremost in some notion of the principle of respect for patient autonomy,[18] or whether one's approach begins with some account of the principle of beneficence (or "beneficence-in-trust"[19]), most all would agree that appropriate ethical decisions at life's edges are best made when they take sufficient account of the values and wishes of the patient concerning medical treatment and quality of life.

The ICU is often the kind of place that makes connection with the patient's values and wishes difficult. This may be the case, first and most obviously, because of the frequency with which ICU patients' medical condition leaves them without decision-making capacity. As a result, it is necessary to rely upon advance directives or surrogate decision makers. As experienced ICU health professionals attest, the surrogate decision makers' own vulnerability is a difficulty to contend with in attempting to make decisions about medical treatment that are genuinely in the patient's best interest (that is, reflective of the patient's values and wishes).

Other chapters in this volume provide a detailed discussion of medical-moral decision making in the ICU. The focus here is religious, and the point is that ICU medical-moral questions may give rise to religious questions. To respect patient autonomy is to respect patients as persons, and to respect others as persons is, in religious terms, to recognize and revere the dignity and sacredness of persons.[20] In the ICU setting, where knowledge of and attention to the patient's moral values and wishes are sometimes blurred and where treatment decisions may thereby be made that do not respect the patient as person, nothing less than the moral and religious dignity and sacredness of the person is in danger of being compromised. Vulnerability—it has many faces. The point here is that the ICU may sometimes be a setting in which vulnerability has a decidedly ethical dimension.

Mortality. In a most worthwhile essay in *On Moral Medicine,* William F. May discusses, with his usual insight, the religious significance of death. He begins with the following assertion: "Theologians of the secular persuasion may be right when they attempt to free the gospel from its earlier, uncritical ties with religion, but they are wrong when they assume that religion is dead. While religions, in the sense of official historical traditions, may indeed have entered a period of decline, the experience of the sacred is still very much with us. Nowhere is this more apparent than in the contemporary experience of death."[21]

May has it right. Whatever one may think of the state of organized religion, religious experience—that is, the discernment of and response to ultimate wonder and awe and/or ultimate terror and dread—is part of the fabric of human existence. And he is also right that perhaps no phenomenon is more capable of moving us to religious experience, nothing more "holy" in this sense, than death. Accordingly, any "space" in which we tend to become aware not only that we are vulnerable, but also that we and our loved ones are vulnerable in an *ultimate* sense—any space in which death is in the air—is a "sacred space." The ICU of the modern hospital is such a space.

There is something both paradoxical and elusive about the ICU and human mortality. On one hand, at least at first glance, the ICU seems to be a place of human power and control. Through an amazing assortment of high-tech interventions, it is possible to "keep someone alive" in ways unthinkable a few decades ago. ICU successes at "holding death at bay" in this manner can give the impression of enormous power, power over life and death itself. But with all that, the ICU is a place where death is in the air, where patients are often in a condition of precarious vulnerability (ultimate vulnerability), and where patients' loved ones can literally see the possibility of death or ultimate vulnerability in a way that may be all too unusual in our culture. And so, in an elusive and paradoxical way, the ICU, seemingly a place of power, is at the same time a place of humility, a place where we human beings may be *invited* to come to terms with all that we are, and with all that we are not. We are not ultimately invulnerable. We are mortal.

It is worth commenting on the word *invited* used above. Recall Tracy's description of limit situations: "those human situations wherein a human being ineluctably finds manifest ultimate limit or horizon to his or her existence."[22] Something is *made manifest to us* in limit situations. Those whose spirits are open and attentive (as Otto suggested) may be invited by the ICU to recognize the horizon of human life. The image of horizon is significant.[23] On one hand, the horizon serves as the outer limit of our field of vision; beyond it we cannot now see. But on the other hand, the horizon is in some more elusive way a point of departure, a point where imagination and hope begin. How often is it the case in human experience that an ending turns out to be a beginning? How often is it (as previous examples have suggested) that a moment of terror and dread can occasion an experience of consolation, love, wonder, and awe? And how often is it that an encounter with mortality—our own and/or our loved one's—can occasion a hint of hope that we can move on, even from death?

The holy invitation that may be issued from the ICU is often a clarion call that our human life has an ending but, much more subtly, a whisper or hint that we may also look for new beginnings. The limit experience of human mortality, the reminder of the horizon of human life—so frequent in the ICU setting—can involve both ultimate terror and dread and ultimate wonder and awe at the very same time. Isn't it a good thing, and isn't it what we need, when those who tread on such turf with any regularity—ICU healthcare professionals—happen to be people who are sensitive to the fact that both endings and beginnings are part of the holy ground upon which they walk and work?

THE ICU AS HOLY GROUND: THE IMPLICATIONS

The story about Moses' encounter with God with which this chapter began portrays in a paradigmatic way that the experience of "the holy"/mystery/God is not a matter of human initiative, but of human response.[24] Moses' experience of *mysterium tremendum et fascinans* elicits from him not only an "internal" response of wonder and awe and/or terror and dread, but also two other types of responses: silence and reverence. Aware that he is on holy ground, Moses is first brought to silence and then, in obedience to the word addressed to him, he removes his sandals in a gesture of humility and reverence.

Perhaps it seems like a long way from Mount Horeb to the modern hospital's ICU; but this is not so. To the extent that it is warranted to imagine the ICU as holy ground, it is appropriate to reflect on the responses—both internal, attitudinal responses, as well as responses of word/silence and gesture—that may be fitting for those whose life's work regularly takes them to this sacred space. In other words, the image of the ICU as holy ground has implications for the kind of attitudes and dispositions as well as for the kinds of words and deeds that we might hope to find with regularity in those whose professional lives take them to this place.[25]

In view of the experiences of vulnerability and mortality that the ICU occasions with some regularity, ICU health professionals ought to be particularly good at two things: reverencing life and dealing with death. And in regard to both, the response of ICU health professionals, not unlike the response of Moses, might well include strong doses of silence, humility, and reverence.

REVERENCING LIFE

If the ICU is a setting in which human vulnerability—physical, relational, and ethical—is manifest frequently, then it is important that it also be a setting in which reverence for human life is equally manifest. In a recent publication from the Catholic Health Association (CHA), the authors describe well how technological interventions in contemporary medicine can, at their worst, lead to depersonalization. The antidote, they suggest, has a great deal to do with the ability of healthcare professionals to focus on "the primacy of the person":

The threat of depersonalization makes guarding against the pressure of technological domination so critical for the appropriate care of the dying. Our reliance upon technology can too easily become a substitute for the healing touch of human interpersonal relationships. For example, physicians can now diagnose and prescribe medicine on the basis of data provided by machines, which means, in some instances, they never have to see or touch the patient. Also, machines often come between the caregiver and the patient so that the patient no longer feels like an independent person, but rather, an extension of the machine. In such a setting, a patient can easily lose the sense of personal identity, dignity, independence and control over the direction of his or her life. . . . Healthcare professionals whose identities have been fashioned out of a ministry of person-to-person healing must be made aware of the risk of depersonalizing care for the dying. The availability of technology can too easily reduce healing to fixing. Fixing treats bodies as interconnected parts, while healing treats the person holistically as a multidimensional being with physical, emotional, intellectual, social and spiritual needs.[26]

With this passage as a springboard, two reflections on "reverencing human life" in the ICU seem appropriate. First, technology itself is not an ICU problem. Technology may very well be part of the "the holy"; it may move one to wonder and awe. The problem is *technological domination*. This term refers to not only "the technological imperative" ("because we *can*, we *should*"),[27] but also the fact that technological interventions may unwittingly become the dominant mode of ICU intervention, obliterating the patient as person, and blinding healthcare professionals to the personal and spiritual vulnerability of the patient and the patient's loved ones. One can only respond reverently to what one recognizes as "the holy."[28] Such is the danger of technological domination: blindness to the patient and patient's loved ones as persons, and thereby the inability to respond in a way that reverences their vulnerability and sanctity and that reverences the holy wonder and awe and/or terror and dread that they may be experiencing.

Second, if the ability of health professionals to "reverence human life" in the ICU is anything other than a slogan, then it means something seemingly simple: the ability to touch. In this context—of personal, relational, and perhaps ethical vulnerability—the ability to touch means the ability to enter into the personal, relational, ethical world of the patient and the patient's loved ones.

But such "entering," of course, is not simple at all. It requires the ability to be as concerned about comforting and healing as about fixing and curing. For health professionals to be good at this would mean being good at everything from physical touches that are tender and caring, to the ability to listen to and care about the worry and anxiety of patients and loved ones, to a steadfast commitment to respecting the values and wishes of patients as much as they are known, to reverencing the relational and spiritual welfare of patients as much as their bodily organ systems. Is this possible? No doubt we all know terrible horror stories in which something far from all of this has taken place. But we probably know other stories as well, stories in which an ICU physician or nurse keenly recognized and responded in a way that was nothing short of reverent.

Often ICU health professionals know better than most others that wonder and awe and/or terror and dread are part of the turf they tread. That is as it should be. The initiation of those who aspire to practice medicine in such a place should entail hearing not only the horror stories, but "the holy stories" as well.

DEALING WITH DEATH

In the presence of the physical, relational, and ethical vulnerability that may be made manifest in the ICU, an appropriate response is reverencing life; in the presence of the ultimate vulnerability—mortality—an appropriate response of healthcare professionals is the ability to deal with death in a way that is both truthful and compassionate. Dedication to truth and commitment to compassion are ways ICU health professionals can facilitate an experience of mortality (whether death occurs or not—the terror/dread of death is sufficient) that may be genuinely "holy."

The following passage from Sherwin B. Nuland's best-selling *How We Die: Reflections on Life's Final Chapter* is instructive:

> I have written this book to demythologize the process of dying. My intention is not to depict it as a horror-filled sequence of painful and disgusting degradations, but to present it in its biological and clinical reality, as seen by those who are witnesses to it and felt by those who experience it. Only by a frank discussion of the very details of dying can we best deal with those aspects that frighten us most. It is by knowing the truth and being prepared for it that we rid ourselves of that fear of the *terra incognita* of death that leads to self-deception and disillusions.[29]

Nuland may not be saying something new—Elizabeth Kubler-Ross has been saying similar things for some time[30]—but he is surely saying something important and he is saying it well. It is by knowing the truth, the truth about death, that we can best deal with it.

The importance of this ability to face death for ICU healthcare professionals is not because most patients who come to the ICU die; in fact, they do not. But what does happen with great regularity in the ICU is an experience of ultimate vulnerability (mortality) on the part of patients and loved ones, and this is the reason an experience of ultimate wonder and awe and/or ultimate terror and dread may also be close at hand.

To the extent that Kubler-Ross, Nuland, and so many others are right in suggesting that ours is a death-denying culture, then it is also right that an appreciation of the spiritual dimension of death—with all its features, *tremendum et fascinans*—is likewise missed. How important it is, then, for ICU health professionals to be sensitive to the fact that ultimate questions concerning death are regularly part of their work environment, and what a grace it is when they find appropriate ways to name the reality of death as a possibility.

Nuland's discussion of the details of death is presented in a straight forward way that does little frightening but a great deal of liberating. Like Nuland, healthcare professionals do a great service—not only medically, but spiritually—when they are able to tell the truth about the realities of the patient's condition, to discuss the realistic possibilities of beneficial treatments along with the burdens of those treatments, and to respond to the questions and concerns of patients and loved ones with candor.

Sometimes the truth may be that there is plenty of reason to be hopeful about a patient's recovery. In such time, the truth delivered by physicians may set the patient and his or her loved ones free from a fear and dread that may be disproportionate to the situation. At other times, the truth may be that there is little hope of recovery and that death is close at hand. In those times, healthcare professionals do well to be convinced that death is not the worst thing that can happen. Illusion, false hope, denial of reality, abandonment to overly burdensome and ultimately futile treatment because the truth has not been spoken—these are the real enemies. When the truth about human mortality is offered to patients and loved ones, what is facilitated is nothing less than an experience of "the holy"; in such situations, "the holy" is made manifest to us not out of illusion and denial, but out of real, human experience, especially when that experience concerns life's limits.

But dedication to the truth is not enough. What is needed in the presence of the ultimate terror and dread that an experience of mortality may occasion is compassion. To be good at dealing with death, ICU healthcare professionals need to be good at responding with compassion to the experiences of fear and anxiety—indeed, terror and dread—of patients and their loved ones.

Others have written well about compassion.[31] It requires attentiveness to another's difficult situation; it requires a willingness to enter into that situation in some real way; and it requires the ability to respond—perhaps in gesture, sometimes in word, frequently in silence.

Recalling some of the insights of the Catholic Health Association's statement above, the temptation of the ICU may sometimes be to attend more to fixing and curing than to healing and caring. This temptation may be particularly strong when death is in the air, when efforts at fixing and curing have run their course. Compassionate presence with patients and loved ones is called for, especially in those times. If healthcare professionals are not always able to fix or to cure medically, their response cannot be to fix or cure spiritually. Compassionate presence is not about taking away fear or suffering or death. In fact, it is about being with others in the midst of those things.

And what is required of those persons who would attempt to be with others in fear and anxiety, terror and dread? Humility and silence. Both of those qualities take us back to Moses' mountaintop experience. In the presence of "the holy," whether in the form of ultimate wonder and awe and/or ultimate terror and dread, Moses' best response was his humble removal of sandals and his silence in the face of ultimate mystery. As Stanley Hauerwas has eloquently argued in *Naming the Silences: God, Medicine and the Problem of Suffering,* in the face of the mystery associated with suffering, we are at our best not when we attempt to give explanations, not when we attempt to take it all away, but when we are able to be with one another in humility and in silence.[32] Nothing is more compassionate; nothing is more reverent. Hauerwas argues that if, in the face of suffering, there is any hope of moving on (and I add, if, in the presence of ultimate terror and dread, there is any hope of transformation to ultimate wonder and awe), that hope has everything to do with the compassionate presence of others. The healthcare professionals who tread so regularly on the holy ground of the ICU may often be the instruments through which such amazing graces and transformations take place.

NOTES

1. R. Otto, *The Idea of the Holy* (London: Oxford University Press, 1923).

2. Ibid., 8.

3. Ibid., 13.

4. This definition, although my own, has been drawn from the insights of J.F. Haughty in *What Is Religion? An Introduction* (Mahwah, N.J.: Paulist Press, 1990). Chapter 10, "Mystery" (pp. 158-70), is a particularly clear exposition of the concepts of mystery, the holy, and religion.

5. Ibid., 159.

6. Note that *nontheistic* does not mean *atheistic.* The latter term indicates a conviction of the non-existence of God. *Nontheistic* simply refers to religious experience that does not move one to a theistic affirmation, either because the individual involved is skeptical about God's existence and/or relevance or simply because the particular religious experience in question did not move *in this instance* to a theistic affirmation.

7. D. Tracy, *Blessed Rage for Order: The New Pluralism in Theology* (New York: Seabury Press, 1978), 105. Tracy's discussion of limit experience throughout this book (but especially in Chapter 5, "The Religious Dimension of Common Human Experience and Language") is the richest and most helpful presentation of the concept. Along the way he refers the reader to the works of many others who have probed this important concept, including Otto, Schleiermacher, Tillich, Weber, Durkheim, Berger, Jaspers, and Maslow.

8. E. Wiesel, *Night* (New York: Bantam Books, 1960).

9. For excellent treatment of the role of analogy in language about mystery generally and about God specifically, see E.A. Johnson, *She Who Is: The Mystery of God in Feminist Theological Discourse* (New York: Crossroad, 1993), see especially pp. 113-17.

10. M. Eliade, *The Sacred and the Profane: The Nature of Religion* (New York: Harcourt, Brace, 1959). See also C.F. Crews, *Ultimate Questions: A Theological Primer* (Mahwah, N.J.: Paulist Press, 1986), 90-95.

11. Otto, "Means of Expression of the Numinous," in *Idea of the Holy*, see note 1 above, pp. 60-71.

12. R.P. McBrien, *Catholicism,* new ed. (New York: Harper Collins, 1994), 8-12.

13. See note 1 above, p. 61.

14. Drawing on Merleau-Ponty's insights, James B. Nelson provides an excellent discussion of bodiliness and religious experience in the context of developing a "sexual theology." See J.B. Nelson, *Embodiment* (Minneapolis, Minn.: Augsburg, 1978), 19-36. See also W.S. Sahakian, "Merleau-Ponty," in *History of Philosophy* (New York: Barnes & Noble, 1978), 339-41.

15. Stanley Hauerwas argues convincingly that, as far as the religious significance of suffering is concerned, "the hardest case" is the suffering of children. See S. Hauerwas, *Naming the Silences: God, Medicine, and the Problem of Suffering* (Grand Rapids, Mich.: Eerdmans, 1990).

16. R.A. McCormick, "Questions in Bioethics" in *Notes on Moral Theology, 1965-1980* (Washington, D.C.: University Press of America, 1981), 565.

17. J.B. Nelson and J.A. Smith Rohricht, *Human Medicine: Ethical Perspectives on Today's Medical Issues* (Minneapolis, Minn.: Augsburg, 1984), 21.

18. T.L. Beauchamp and J.F. Childress, *Principles of Biomedical Ethics,* 3rd ed. (New York: Oxford University Press, 1989), 67-119.

19. E.D. Pellegrino and D.C. Thomasma, *For the Patient's Good: The Restoration of Beneficence in Health Care* (New York: Oxford University Press, 1988),

51-58.

20. Paul Ramsey's classic, *The Patient as Person*, makes the point I am attempting to make here with obviously far greater sophistication (New Haven, Conn.: Yale University Press, 1970). See also many of the articles in the volume edited by S.E. Lammers and A. Verhey, *On Moral Medicine: Theological Perspectives in Medical Ethics* (Grand Rapids, Mich,: Eerdmans, 1987); particularly helpful on the religious dimension of respect for persons is D.C. Thomasma, "The Basis of Medicine and Religion: Respect for Persons," *Hospital Progress* 60 (September 1979): 54-57 and 90.

21. W.F. May, "The Sacral Power of Death in Contemporary Experience," in *On Moral Medicine*, ed. Lammers and Verhey, see note 20 above, p. 175.

22. See note 7 above.

23. For a discussion of the concept of horizon and various types of conversion see B. Lonergan, *Method in Theology* (New York: Seabury Press, 1972), pp. 235 and forward. For insights about the way limit experience can disclose the finitude of our horizons as well as point toward "certain fundamental structures of our existence beyond" them, see D. Tracy, *Blessed Rage for Order*, note 7 above, pp. 92 and forward.

24. For an excellent exposition of the "responsive" nature of life, especially the moral life, see H.R. Niebuhr, *The Responsible Self* (New York: Harper & Row, 1963). Niebuhr suggests that two of the most important questions to be asked in all moral situations are "What is going on here?" and "What is a fitting response?" Discernment becomes the key, most important event in such a view of the moral life.

25. The emphasis here on the importance of attitudes and dispositions as well as the responses of word and deed is part of the important effort to retrieve "virtue ethics" in recent years. For a Roman Catholic perspective on this, see J. Porter, *The Recovery of Virtue* (Louisville, Ky.: Westminster/John Knox Press, 1990); and W.C. Spohn, "The Return of Virtue Ethics," *Theological Studies* 53, no. 1 (March 1992): 60-75. Among Protestant ethicists no one has emphasized the significance of virtue more consistently and passionately than Stanley Hauerwas. See S. Hauerwas, *Vision and Virtue* (Notre Dame, Ind.: Fides, 1974); S. Hauerwas, *A Community of Character* (Notre Dame, Ind.: University of Notre Dame Press, 1981).

26. The Catholic Health Association, *Care of the Dying: A Catholic Perspective* (St. Louis, Mo.: Catholic Health Association, 1993), 9-10.

27. Many have written about "the technological imperative." See, for example, note 26 above, pp. 8-9; R.A. McCormick, "If I Had Ten Things to Share with Physicians," in *The Critical Calling: Reflections on Moral Dilemmas Since Vatican II* (Washington, D.C.: Georgetown University Press, 1989), 353-54; E.D. Pellegrino and D.C. Thomasma, *For the Patient's Good: The Restoration of the Beneficence in Health Care* (New York: Oxford University Press, 1988), 92-93.

28. Two works of "Christian moral philosophy" that emphasize the way recognition sets the parameters for moral response are H.R. Niebuhr, *The Re-*

sponsible Self, see note 24 above; and E. McDonagh, *Gift and Call: Towards a Christian Theology of Morality* (St. Meinrad, Ind.: Abbey Press, 1975).

29. S.B. Nuland, *How We Die: Reflections on Life's Final Chapter* (New York: Alfred A. Knopf, 1993), xvii.

30. I have in mind Kubler-Ross's forceful and effective naming of the denial of death as the first reality that must be dealt with if one is to move well though the stages of death as she describes them. E. Kubler-Ross, *On Death and Dying* (New York: Macmillan Publishing, 1969).

31. See D.P. McNeill, D.A. Morrison, and H.J.M. Nouwen, *Compassion: A Reflection on the Christian Moral Life* (New York: Image Books, 1983); and N. Wolterstorff, *Lament for a Son* (Grand Rapids, Mich.: Eerdmans, 1987). Much of the literature on the ethics of care provides a foundation for the role of compassion in healthcare. See A.V. Campbell, "Caring and Being Cared For," in *On Moral Medicine,* see note 20 above; and for a fine overview of the ethics of care in light of the work of Carol Gilligan and other feminist writers, see C.S.W. Crysdale, "Gilligan and the Ethics of Care: An Update," *Religious Studies Review,* 20, no. 1 (January 1994): 21-28.

32. See note 15 above.

11

Coma Confusion in Critical Care

Ronald E. Cranford

INTRODUCTION

Critical care medicine has witnessed a new generation of neurologic syndromes—unique neurologic conditions that did not exist (or existed rarely) prior to the advent of modern medical technology (see Exhibit 11-1) These conditions have given rise to some relatively new ethical and legal dilemmas. In order to be able to resolve these ethical and legal problems, one must understand the medical facts surrounding these neurologic syndromes and their similarities and differences. Because these conditions are of relatively recent vintage, there is still confusion and misunderstanding about their terminology and precise boundaries. This chapter discusses the important medical facts related to these conditions and illustrates how understanding the medical and neurologic facts can help to address ethical dilemmas.

CASES

The two cases that follow are examples of the types of ethical dilemmas generated by neurologic syndromes. The first type of case, which involves a family's demands to stop treatment, commonly occurs in a critical care setting. The second type of case, which involves a family's

Exhibit 11-1
Neurological Syndromes

	Brain Death	Permanent Vegetative State	Locked In Syndrome	Dementia
Basic definition (functional)	Irreversible loss of all brain functions, both cerebral hemisphere and brain stem.	Irreversible loss of all neo-cortical functions; brain stem functions intact.	Irreversible loss of motor functions to a severe degree.	Irreversible loss of neocortical functions to a variable degree.
Clinical syndrome	Deepest possible coma; no brain stem functions; apnea (total respirator dependence).	Awake, but unaware, eyes-open unconsciousness; sleep/wake cycles present; respirator independence.	Severe paralysis with preservation of relatively normal consciousness.	Impairment of neocortical functions; varies in severity from mild to profound.
Anatomic substrate	Destruction of entire brain—both cerebral hemisphere and brain stem.	Varies, but most commonly extensive destruction of of neocortex (hypoxic-ischemic encephalopathy) or subcortical white matter (head trauma).	Varies, often extensive bain stem destruction with preservation of arousal system.	Varies, but usually destruction of neocortex to a variable degree (Alzheimer's disease) or subcortical white matter (multi-infarct dementia)
Onset and course (temporal profile)	Sudden onset; syndrome well-defined within hours.	Sudden onset, secondary to hypoxic-ischemic insult or acute head trauma.	Usually sudden onset (brain stem stroke or head injury) or slow onset and gradually	Gradual onset of progressive neurologic deterioration over 5-10 years.

Prognosis for survival (cardio-respiratory)	Usually only hours to days (even with maximal treatment).	Usually long-term, years or even decades.	Varies by cause, but long-term survival possible, years, or even decades; progressive over months to years (primary motor neuron disease).	Varies by cause, but long-term survival possible, years or even decades.
Time when prognosis for recovery of neurologic functions can be determined with a high degree of certainty	Within hours.	Varies by cause; in hypoxic-ischemic encephalopathy usually 1-3 months; in head trauma, usually 6-12 months.	Varies by cause; usually several months.	With gradually increasing of neocortical functions, certainty increases as disease progresses (months to years).
Degree of physical or psychologic suffering	None.	None.	Varies; may be extremely severe because consciousness intact.	Varies; less suffering with increasing impairment of neocortical functions.
Correlation with laboratory studies	Essentially 100% correlation with EEG and blood flow studies to the brain.	Good correlation with CAT or MRI; excellent correlation with PET; fair correlation with EEG.	Good correlation with CAT or MRI.	Fair to poor correlation with CAT, MRI, PET and EEG until advanced

demands to continue treatment, occurs more commonly in a chronic care facility.

CASE 1

A middle-aged patient has been admitted to a critical care unit after incurring severe head trauma as a result of a motor vehicle accident. The patient is comatose with relatively preserved brain-stem reflexes. The initial computed tomography (CT) scan shows scattered subcortical hemorrhages and diffuse cerebral edema.

From the onset of hospitalization, the immediate family has expressed strong feelings that this patient would never have wanted to live in a severely disabled state. The family insists that, if there is any significant chance that the patient may be left neurologically impaired, all treatment should be stopped now and the patient should be allowed to die. They believe that this plan is entirely consistent with what the patient would have wanted, were he able to express his own views.

Because the prognosis for recovery of neurologic functions is probably poor but somewhat uncertain at this early stage, the healthcare professionals in the critical care unit are extremely uncomfortable with this demand by the family, even if it may be consistent with the wishes of the patient.

CASE 2

A middle-aged female experienced a cardiac arrest, secondary to long-standing, severe coronary artery disease. The patient was comatose for about 20 days before her condition evolved into a vegetative state, secondary to hypoxic-ischemic encephalopathy. Six months have passed, and the patient has not recovered consciousness. Even though the family has been told repeatedly that the prognosis for recovery is extraordinarily poor, her husband and children strongly believe that she will recover and do well. The family has noted on numerous occasions that, after the patient began to open her eyes from the initial coma, she has "looked" at them at various times. She also "watches" television and grimaces when she is undergoing physical therapy for the beginning contractures in her arms and legs. This loving, caring family spends a great deal of time at the bedside. The more that physicians caring for the patient have articulated a poor prognosis to the family, the more insistent the family is that she will get better eventually, even if it takes years.

COMA

One of the most common sources of confusion in the critical care setting has been confusion about the differences between two unconscious states—coma and the vegetative state. Coma describes an acute neurologic condition manifested by an eyes-closed unconsciousness. The unconsciousness is secondary to an impairment of the *level* of consciousness (arousal) secondary to dysfunction of the reticular activating system in the brain-stem and thalamus, as opposed to a decreased *content* of consciousness (awareness), such as dysfunction of the cerebral cortex in dementia. Coma has various causes, but two of the most common are traumatic injuries to the brain and nontraumatic injuries such as lack of oxygen or blood after an acute cardiac or respiratory arrest (such as hypoxic-ischemic encephalopathy). Whatever the causes, coma usually lasts hours or days, rarely weeks or months, and the common question raised in a critical care setting is how aggressive should healthcare providers be in the face of an apparently poor prognosis for coma.

The major problem with any coma in an acute care setting is that the prognosis for recovery of neurologic functions—and for life itself—may vary tremendously depending on the depth of coma, the underlying etiology, the age of the patient, and other medical complications. For example, patients in a coma from hypoxic-ischemic encephalopathy generally do poorly if the coma lasts longer than three days and very poorly if it lasts longer than seven days. On the other hand, patients in a coma from a traumatic brain injury may do well, even after several days or longer in a coma. Often patients do poorly not necessarily because of the etiology of the coma itself, but because of underlying medical complications that may arise as a result of their age and associated medical problems.

Patients in a coma rarely remain that way for more than a few days or weeks. Patients in a deep coma may develop brain death, or often die in the early stages secondary to autonomic and hypothalamic instability. If death does not occur in the early stages, patients may improve to the point of regaining consciousness with gradual return of cognitive functions. Or their condition may evolve in two to four weeks into an eyes-open unconsciousness. Cases of prolonged coma—where the coma itself lasts more than a few weeks—are uncommon, but they do occur. These cases usually occur from shearing injuries to the brain-stem after head trauma and also after severe hemorrhagic or nonhemorrhagic brain-stem strokes.

VEGETATIVE STATE

In contrast to the eyes-closed unconsciousness of coma, the vegetative state is an eyes-open unconsciousness. These patients are best described as awake, but unaware. Sleep-wake cycles are present, and brainstem functions are generally intact. These patients have roving eye movements that do not track or pursue objects in the environment in any consistent, reproducible fashion. Since the original description of the vegetative state by Plum and Jennett in 1972,[1] a great deal of literature has accumulated on this syndrome, including a definitive report from the Multisociety Task Force on the Persistent Vegetative State (PVS Task Force), published in 1994,[2] and guidelines developed by the Royal College of Physicians of London in 1996.[3]

The exact incidence of the vegetative state is not known, but the PVS Task Force estimated there were approximately 14,000 to 35,000 children and adults in the United States in this condition.

Guidelines have been developed by numerous groups establishing, among other things, the prognosis for the recovery of neurologic functions for patients in a vegetative state. The prognosis for neurologic recovery varies according to two major factors: the etiology of the underlying brain injury and the age of the patient. Patients in a vegetative state from hypoxic-ischemic injuries, in all age groups, do extremely poorly after three months (often after one month), and the chances of any meaningful recovery of cognitive functions after three months is extremely remote. With traumatic brain injuries, however, the prognosis is more variable, and patients in a posttraumatic vegetative state may show significant recovery of cognitive functions after six months or even a year. The chances for meaningful recovery between six and 12 months is greater in children than in adults. But good recovery after 12 months in a traumatic vegetative state, in either children or adults, is extraordinarily rare. Those patients who have recovered after 12 months have almost invariably been left with severe or profound neurologic disability. So-called miracle recoveries reported in the medical and lay literature have been either poorly documented or the patients were left with motor and cognitive abnormalities.

BRAIN DEATH

Brain death is a form of coma in which the prognosis can be established with an extraordinarily high degree of certainty, usually within hours or days of the original injury. Thus, this condition is the major exception to the rule that a high degree of certainty cannot be achieved in the first few days after coma. The reason for the certainty about the prognosis is because of the unique pathophysiology that occurs in most cases of brain death. Whatever the underlying etiology of the brain injury—whether traumatic, hypoxic-ischemic, or otherwise—a common sequence of events occurs that leads to brain death. This sequence includes the development of severe cerebral edema (brain swelling) secondary to the original injury, which in turn results in an extremely high intracranial pressure. The intracranial pressure is so high in brain death that it exceeds the systolic blood pressure, resulting in a subsequent loss of blood flow to the brain, both in the cerebral hemispheres and in the brain-stem, with subsequent infarction of the entire brain. This sequence of events occurs usually within a matter of hours after the original injury, and thus the diagnosis of brain death can be readily made in this time frame by knowledgeable and experienced clinicians. The diagnosis of brain death in neonates and young children is more problematic but can be established in many cases.

With the widespread acceptance of brain death as a medical syndrome by healthcare professionals and the legalization of brain death as a form of death by case law or statute in all 50 states, the major ethical dilemma is not whether the patient is allowed to die, but when the patient is dead. Furthermore, explicit guidelines on the criteria for brain death have been developed by a variety of organizations.[4]

LOCKED-IN SYNDROME

The locked-in syndrome describes patients who are severely motor impaired to the point of appearing unconscious, but whose content of consciousness is either normal or fairly normal. In other words, these patients have a severe impairment of the motor system, but functions of the cerebral cortex are relatively intact. This syndrome occurs under a variety of circumstances; it occurs most commonly in the context of an acute brain-stem stroke where the motor system through the brain-stem

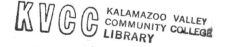

is extensively impaired, but consciousness is still intact. In addition, the condition of patients suffering severe head injuries may evolve from a vegetative state into a severe paralysis, but with normal cognitive functions; these patients should be carefully monitored for signs of increasing cognition.

Even though patients with the locked-in syndrome may have normal consciousness, they are so severely motor impaired that it may take a great deal of time and effort to establish a reliable means of communication. This is usually done through eye movements, and computer systems may be established with eye movements to allow communication with the patient. Patients who are severely paralyzed from a variety of neurologic mechanisms may gradually improve over a period of weeks, months, or occasionally even years. It is extremely important to keep this in mind when assessing permanency of the condition.

DEMENTIA

The most common condition for a decreased content of cognitive functions caused by impairment of the cerebral cortex is Alzheimer's disease, a progressive degenerative disease occurring in the elderly. However, patients with acute injuries to the brain may also experience dementia that ranges anywhere from minimal to profound dementia. The condition of patients with severe, acute head trauma may evolve from a comatose state into either a vegetative state, locked-in syndrome, or a combination of severe motor and cognitive impairment.

In some cases, it is difficult to distinguish between cognitive and motor impairment when the patient is extremely paralyzed. It is difficult to communicate with the patient and know how much consciousness is actually present. This neurologic condition of a combined dementia and paralysis is becoming more common because of medical advances; however, the actual incidence of this syndrome after acute brain injuries cannot be readily ascertained, nor is there any commonly accepted term used to describe this combination of decreased cognitive and motor functions. A new syndrome recently advocated by rehabilitation and neurological specialists is the "minimally conscious state." This condition describes patients who may be evolving out of the vegetative state into some minimal degree of awareness, with or without motor impairment. Any sign of conscious behavior is an important finding in patients who have been in a vegetative state, and so this minimally conscious state may be a first indication that the patient will show continued improvement and possibly regain meaningful functions. Some patients may regain minimal consciousness and remain at this level for the rest of their lives, in which case one has to wonder whether being profoundly disabled and aware of one's condition is not worse than being in a vegetative state.

TEMPORAL PROFILE AND IRREVERSIBILITY

In all of the neurologic syndromes described above, two critical features are the temporal profile and irreversibility. As described in the PVS Task Force report, patients may enter the vegetative state through either (1) an acute injury to the brain; (2) a chronic, slowly progressive degenerative process; or (3) a developmental anomaly present at the time of birth.[5] In patients with an acute injury, such as traumatic brain injuries or hypoxic-ischemic encephalopathy, the initial coma from two to four weeks is followed by evolution into the vegetative state. In a degenerative process such as Alzheimer's disease, the temporal profile is one of a progressive, downhill loss of cerebral cortical functions over a period of five to 10 years, culminating in a state of profound dementia and sometimes deteriorating into a vegetative state. Infants with anencephaly exemplify a congenital anomaly present at the time of birth, and this is a developmental form of the vegetative state. These different temporal profiles also apply to the other neurologic syndromes with acute, degenerative, and developmental forms of dementia and the locked-in syndrome.

Irreversibility is closely tied to the pathophysiology and temporal profile of the underlying neurologic condition. The term *permanent* was defined by the PVS Task Force to mean an irreversible vegetative state when the irreversibility of the condition can be diagnosed with an extremely high degree of certainty (that is, after three months with hypoxic-ischemic injuries and after six months to a year with traumatic head injuries).[6] In the past, there has been a great deal of confusion generated by the use of the terms *persistent, chronic,* and *permanent.* Originally, Plum and Jennett used the term *persistent vegetative state* to describe patients in a vegetative state for a long period of time but who have the potential for recovery of cognitive functions.[7] As defined by the PVS Task Force, *persistent* means being in a vegetative state for at least one month after the original injury; it no longer means "permanent."[8] The new guidelines developed by the Royal College of Physicians of London use the term *chronic* rather than persistent; they use the term *permanent* to mean "irreversible."[9]

CERTAINTY OF PROGNOSIS

Critical care specialists commonly face dilemmas with comatose patients, but rarely with patients in a vegetative state. As noted previously, it usually takes two to four weeks for the patient's condition to evolve from a comatose condition into a vegetative state. In extremely rare cases, a patient's condition may rapidly evolve from an eyes-closed unconsciousness to an eyes-open unconsciousness within a few days. The common questions asked in the early stages are "What is the prognosis for recovery in coma?" and "How aggressively should we be in treating the patient?" It is important to distinguish clearly between coma and the vegetative state because, as a general rule, the degree of certainty of neurologic recovery for comatose patients is much less in the early days than for those in a vegetative state. Thus, withholding or withdrawing treatment from a comatose patient is usually more problematic than it is for patients in a vegetative state, primarily because of the uncertainty of the prognosis—especially in the cases of head trauma. Critical care specialists do not want to start treatment in patients with a poor prognosis, but the degree of certainty for patients in an acute comatose condition is often less than one would want to make a definitive decision to stop treatment. The degree of certainty necessary to make definitive decisions to forgo treatment may not be achieved for a matter of days, weeks, or even months, long after the patient has left the critical care unit.

WITHHOLDING VERSUS WITHDRAWING TREATMENT

Some critical care specialists are tempted to avoid an ethical dilemma by never starting treatment rather than withdrawing treatment later. It may be emotionally easier not to start a treatment than to withdraw the same treatment later. But, in terms of neurologic prognosis and the degree of certainty of this prognosis, it may be far more preferable to decide on an aggressive course of action early and then later withdraw treatment—when the prognosis is known with a much higher degree of certainty—than it would be never to start treatment on a patient in an acute coma.

It is sometimes easier emotionally for physicians and families to withdraw treatment from a comatose patient than from a patient in a vegetative state—not because one is more conscious than the other, but because it is difficult to consider withdrawing treatment from a patient whose eyes are open and who appears to be awake and "aware." Also, it may be easier for some physicians to withhold or withdraw high-tech treatment (like a respirator) than low-tech treatment (like a feeding tube)—even though, from an ethical standpoint, both treatments and actions are morally equivalent.

SUFFERING

It is now well accepted by neurologists and neurosurgeons that patients in a permanent vegetative state do not experience consciousness and therefore are incapable of suffering. But the eyes-open appearance of these patients and other signs that they may manifest on examination are extremely unsettling to families and healthcare providers, especially to nurses who spend a great deal of time at the bedside caring for these patients. At an emotional level, families have a great deal of difficulty accepting the unconsciousness and lack of suffering of their loved ones when they see signs that clearly indicate to them just the opposite. Families have to intellectually and emotionally accept not only the permanency of the patient's condition, but also the fact that the patient is not suffering and is not aware of his or her condition. These patients gag, cough, suck, and swallow (all on an involuntary basis). They may grimace, smile, and withdraw from painful stimuli. At times, they may even "look" toward sounds or movements, which families may interpret as a sign of apparent awareness. This turning of the head and eyes toward sounds or movements is a manifestation of primitive auditory- or visual-orienting reflexes, reflecting intact brain-stem pathways.

Healthcare providers should refrain as much as possible from giving mixed messages to families concerning the patient's consciousness, awareness, and ability to suffer. They should emphasize to the family that the patient is incapable of experiencing any pain and suffering and does not require analgesic or sedative medication to relieve suffering.

FEEDING TUBES AND STARVATION

Many healthcare providers find it much more troubling, both ethically and psychologically, to withdraw a feeding tube rather than to withdraw a respirator. Although part of this concern is understandable in terms of the symbolic importance of eating and drinking in normal human beings, another part is simply based on a misunderstanding of the facts. The withdrawal of artificial nutrition or hydration in a medical setting does not result in starvation and a prolonged agonizing death over a period of weeks. Unfortunately, even recent federal court decisions on physician-assisted suicide equate withdrawal of feeding tubes with death by starvation. When artificial nutrition and hydration are withdrawn from patients who are permanently unconscious, either in a coma or a permanent vegetative state, the patient cannot experience thirst, hunger, or any other form of suffering. These patients die of acute dehydration, which occurs in 10 to 14 days. They do not experience any signs of starvation and, during the first seven to 10 days, usually manifest no physical signs at all. During the last three to five days there is often dryness of the skin and mucous membranes and then signs of cardiovascular collapse, usually manifested by coolness of the distal extremities. These patients do not manifest any signs of starvation or chronic malnutrition. If there is any question about whether the patient is truly unconscious, then analgesic medications can be given, such as morphine in a concentrated dose through a heparin lock.

COMPUTED-TOMOGRAPHY SCANS

The computed tomography (CT) scan may be very useful in determining prognosis, both in an acute care situation and in a chronic care setting. Severe cerebral edema (diffuse obliteration of the grey-white junction, flattened cortical gyri and small ventricles) usually indicates an exceedingly poor prognosis. Acute brain edema with hypoxic-ischemic encephalopathy is believed to be postinfarction edema—that is, edema that occurs only after extensive destruction of brain tissue, secondary to lack of oxygen or blood. This is not necessarily true, however, with head trauma; patients with head trauma and radiographic features suggesting diffuse brain swelling may do well later, as the swelling and increased intracranial pressure subside. So the cerebral swelling in head trauma may be reversible and treatable with various measures. In patients whose condition evolves into a permanent vegetative state, the CT scan shows signs of progressive cerebral atrophy, starting one to six months after the original injury. This atrophy continues for months, or years, even though the clinical condition of the patient does not change. The importance of this diffuse cerebral atrophy as seen on CT scan is that it indicates irreversible or permanent damage to the brain. The abnormal CT scans may help the family to accept the reality of the hopeless condition—both the devastating nature of the brain damage and its irreversibility. These objective findings of atrophy may help to counter the family's perception of apparent signs of consciousness.

INDIVIDUAL AND FAMILY AUTONOMY

Individual autonomy has been strongly emphasized as an important ethical principle in decision making, but how much attention is devoted to concerns about the family? How relevant is family autonomy when the patient is no longer conscious? In actual practice, the feelings and concerns of the family are often considered in decisions about termination of treatment, but the courts have generally been reluctant to recognize family autonomy as an independent value and principle for ethical decision making.

Is individual autonomy a meaningful concept when someone is permanently unconscious, such as in a vegetative state? This issue has been sidestepped by most courts. This question of family suffering and autonomy seems to be extremely relevant to decisions concerning life support for permanently unconscious patients, or any patients with severe neurologic dysfunction. Families often feel trapped by medical technology and thus lose a great deal of respect and confidence in the medical profession. Aggressive treatment is given in the early stages when the patient is comatose. But later, when the patient evolves into a vegetative state, and the prognosis is equally or even more certain, doctors are reluctant to discontinue treatment once started. Families and healthcare providers sometimes feel strongly about stopping treatment in the early stages, because they fear being trapped later when no one is willing to discontinue treatment. If there is serious doubt about the certainty of the prognosis in a comatose patient, treatment should be initiated and continued for a time-limited period until the prognosis is more definitively determined. Once the prognosis is determined with a high degree of certainty, then it seems morally equivalent to be just as aggressive about stopping treatment as one would have been in the early stages about not starting treatment.

Waiting until the prognosis is more certain, and perhaps for the patient's condition to evolve into a permanent vegetative state, gives the family time to accept the hopeless condition of the patient. Families go through stages of acceptance; they have to live with the guilt of making definitive decisions to withhold or withdraw treatment. Healthcare providers should minimize the family's guilt as much as possible by verifying the prognosis of the neurologic condition and giving the family adequate time to accept the hopeless prognosis. Also, the family should be assured that any treatment started can be stopped later, so that the families don't feel like prisoners of medical technology.

DISCONTINUITY OF CARE

One of the enormous problems in the U.S. healthcare system is the lack of continuity between the critical care unit and the remainder of the healthcare system. A patient may be admitted to an intensive care unit where treatment is aggressive (given the uncertainty of the neurologic prognosis and other important considerations) and then transferred to another unit where other doctors may be reluctant to discontinue treatment for their own ethical reasons. Unless there is some degree of continuity of the care of the patient, and unless the treatment is patient-based rather than institution-based, critical care specialists are faced with a terrible dilemma. They want to give aggressive treatment when the prognosis is uncertain, but they know that other physicians may not be willing later to discontinue treatment once the prognosis is known with a high degree of certainty.

The lack of continuity in healthcare creates an ethical dilemma for critical care specialists caring for patients with neurologic syndromes. By the time a diagnosis of the permanent vegetative state can be made, for example, patients are usually in long-term-care facilities where doctors and nurses may be more reluctant to discontinue treatment, especially artificial nutrition and hydration. The families have nowhere to turn. The promise from the critical care specialist seems hollow.

In addition, physicians may give mixed messages to families. They may tell the family that the prognosis for recovery is exceedingly poor and then, on the other hand, offer coma stimulation or speech and occupational therapy. Or they may mention miracle recoveries. How can a family make a sound ethical decision concerning continued treatment when the physician talks about the poor prognosis and then holds out hope that the patient may recover? When a patient is in a vegetative state and permanently unconscious and the family is caught in limbo, who is really suffering in this situation? The patient or the family? And how much emphasis do we place on suffering in the family?

CONCLUSION

In the future, critical care specialists will face an increasing number of complex ethical dilemmas related to neurologic syndromes resulting from modern medical technology. Managed care will probably put greater pressure on physicians to justify treatment of these neurologic syndromes and show how these patients actually benefit from expensive, high-tech medicine—especially in an acute care setting. Perhaps the most difficult cases in the future will not involve the vegetative state or brain death; instead they will involve patients who are severely cognitively and motor impaired, are not unconscious, and are aware to some extent of their existence and their suffering. When faced with these complex ethical, legal, and social dilemmas, physicians must understand the essential facts and features of these neurologic conditions in order to decide on the most appropriate course of action—for the patient, family, healthcare providers, and society.

NOTES

1. B. Jennett and F. Plum, "Persistent Vegetative State After Brain Damage: A Syndrome in Search of a Name," *Lancet* 1 (1972): 734-47.

2. Multi-Society Task Force on PVS, "Medical Aspects of the Persistent Vegetative State," Parts One and Two, *New England Journal of Medicine* 330 (1994): 1499-1508 and 1572-79.

3. Review by a working group convened by the Royal College of Physicians, "The Permanent Vegetative State," *Journal of the Royal College of Physicians* 30, no. 2 (March/April 1996): 119-21.

4. President's Commission for the Study of Ethical Problems in Medicine and Biomedical and Behavioral Research, "Guidelines for the Determination of Death: Report of the Medical Consultants on the Diagnosis of Death to the President's Commission for the Study of Ethical Problems in Medicine and Biomedical and Behavioral Research," *Journal of the American Medical Association* 246 (1981): 2184-86.

5. See note 2 above.

6. Ibid.

7. See note 1 above.

8. See note 2 above.

9. See note 3 above.

12

Dialysis Dilemmas in the ICU

Jacquelyn P. Slomka
and Emil P. Paganini

INTRODUCTION

More so than other medical technologies, dialysis has brought ethical concerns to the public's attention.[1] The invention and use of the "artificial kidney" not only posed the problem of how to distribute life-prolonging, scarce medical resources equitably, but also led to the question of forgoing life-sustaining technology. The Karen Ann Quinlan case (1976) brought the first question of ventilator withdrawal to the forefront of medical-ethical discussion, but patients' refusals of kidney dialysis were being dealt with long before Quinlan. These cases usually involved competent patients on chronic dialysis who believed they no longer wanted to live by depending on a machine for survival. Nephrologists thus have been facing the ethical issue of forgoing life-sustaining technology longer than most other medical specialists.

Although many ethical issues concerning dialysis are encountered in the outpatient setting, ethical concerns surrounding the use of this technology also arise in the intensive care unit (ICU). Ethical dimensions of decisions about dialysis in the intensive care setting are often related to the use of surrogates for decision making when the patient is mentally incapacitated, the fair distribution of expensive high-technology medical care, and the influence of external factors on clinical decision making. But probably the most frequent ethical concerns revolve around the appropriate use of this technology in dying patients. The decision to provide, withhold, or withdraw dialysis in the intensive care setting can be a critical decision point in the care of the patient for several reasons. First, it may be unclear as to whether the patient's renal failure is an acute or chronic situation, a determination that could affect the physician's and patient's perception of burdens versus benefits of continuing or limiting treatment. Second, dialysis tends to be a popular technology to forgo. According to one study, the withdrawal of dialysis is second to the withdrawal of blood products as a preferred means of forgoing life-supporting therapy in critically ill, dying patients.[2] One reason for this may be that in a critical situation, where the patient is unlikely to survive, the decision to forgo dialysis can be justified by the economic and physical burdens this treatment imposes.

In addition, the withdrawal of dialysis as a means of forgoing life-supporting therapy may be more psychologically comfortable for physicians than withdrawal of other forms of treatment, a factor that may be related to the time lag between withdrawal of therapy and death. The more immediate the death of the patient, the more the physician's action of withdrawal may symbolically resemble active, direct euthanasia. The withdrawal of other kinds of therapies may appear more morally problematic to the physician. For example, the withdrawal of pressors may result in an easy death for the patient, but in too short a time span to avoid the image of the physician's direct responsibility for the patient's death. In ventilator withdrawal, some physicians are reluctant to provide adequate medication when a respirator is withdrawn and may fear causing additional suffering in the patient.[3] The forgoing of artificial

---

Exhibit 12-1

Predicting Outcome of Acute Renal Failure in the ICU: Risk Factors for Mortality

---

1. Male gender
2. Respiratory failure requiring intubation
3. Hematologic dysfunction: platelets <50,000, leukocytes <2,500, or bleeding diathesis
4. Bilirubin >2.0
5. Absence of surgery
6. Serum creatinine at time of first dialysis
7. Increasing number of failed organ systems
8. Increased BUN from time of admission

nutrition and hydration may be uncomfortable for the physician because of the associated images of nurturing and caring for the patient these therapies evoke. On the other hand, death due to the forgoing of dialysis may be viewed by caregivers as a comfortable death because the patient becomes gradually more unaware as toxins build up in the body and he or she slips into unconsciousness and death.[4] Withdrawal of dialysis allows a time lag so that the physician's action is temporally separated from the patient's death. However, one study reports that, in discontinuing life-supporting therapy, physicians prefer to withdraw treatment that results in the patient's death in a shorter, rather than prolonged, time period.[5] These attitudes suggest that physicians may have an ideal concept of a timely death that results from the forgoing of life-sustaining treatment: not too short, yet not too long so as to prolong suffering. More research is needed on the personal values of physicians and how these values influence clinical decision making.

Although many of the ethical dilemmas surrounding dialysis in the intensive care setting revolve around the question of providing dialysis therapy at the end of life, others are more related to the economic, interpersonal, emotional, or political realm. Such dilemmas are rarely purely ethical, but instead involve cultural beliefs and values of patients, families, and professionals, and social and political constraints on medical-ethical decision making. To examine some of the complexities of dialysis dilemmas in the ICU, five cases are presented and analyzed. The final portion of this chapter examines the utility of clinical guidelines for dealing with ethical dilemmas in the ICU.

LIMITING TREATMENT OF A YOUNG, DYING PATIENT

A 19-year-old patient with end-stage non-Hodgkin's lymphoma is admitted to the ICU in respiratory distress. He is intubated and treated with sedation and neuromuscular blocking agents to maintain adequate ventilation. The patient is on an experimental chemotherapy protocol. During the next five days, the patient's liver and kidney function deteriorates, possibly as a result of the chemotherapy. Because the attending physician believes that the decline of all of the physiological parameters is potentially reversible, she consults the renal service to start the patient on hemodialysis. The resident physician and nurse are uncomfortable with the attending physician's decision because they believe this patient is dying and that hemodialysis will only prolong the patient's dying process.

Ethical issues in this situation revolve around the question of how aggressive therapeutic intervention for this patient should be. Should treatment be continued at its present level, or does the patient's situation justify limitation of treatment? The question of forgoing life-supporting therapy is not a new one. In the centuries prior to the discovery of anesthetic agents, surgery was an excruciatingly painful ordeal. The early Church considered whether choosing death over surgical amputation was permissible, given religious prohibitions on suicide and euthanasia.[6] In 1976, the New Jersey Supreme Court decreed in *In re Quinlan* that the withdrawal of a life-supporting ventilator did not constitute homicide.[7] In the 1990 *Cruzan* decision, the U.S. Supreme Court reiterated the right of a competent adult to refuse medical treatment, a value that stems from the common law notion of the right to bodily integrity.[8] Medical-ethical standards support the involvement of appropriate surrogate decision makers in the care of mentally incapacitated patients.[9]

The ethical decision-making process in the forgoing of dialysis parallels the decision-making process in other kinds of therapy withdrawal. Medical prognosis, the burden-benefit ratio, and the patient's wishes are major issues that shape the medical-ethical decision. In an intensive care setting, the patient often does not have decision-making capacity, and the next-of-kin or another appropriate surrogate is asked to reflect the quality-of-life values the patient might express if he or she were able to communicate.[10] If the patient is competent, and significant recovery is possible, the intensive care team and its consultants should evaluate the patient's motivation for refusal of treatment and evaluate and treat any psychiatric conditions. If the patient is able to make a reasoned decision to forgo dialysis, the team should continue to assist the patient and family throughout the discontinuation of dialysis and the dying process.[11]

Although the ethical ideal of decision making involves a physician-patient-family partnership, researchers have reported that physicians often refuse patients' or surrogates' requests to limit treatment if physicians deem the patient's length of life to be more than six months.[12] The same study notes that physicians also make unilateral decisions to forgo treatment if they judge that further treatment would be futile. Nonmedical criteria often influence the ethical decision-making process. As noted earlier, physicians may have biases about which treatments are more acceptable to withdraw when such withdrawal is likely to result in the death of the patient. Anecdotal evidence suggests that physicians may be slower to withdraw therapy when the patient is involved in a research protocol, or when the physician has formed an emotional or psychological attachment to the patient—perhaps as a result of similarity in age, resemblance to a loved one, or an attractive personality.

In a discussion of the initiation and termination of treatment, Kilner suggests that a discrepancy between the patient's and physician's expectations of the caregiver-patient relationship may result in dissatisfaction and even increased suffering for the patient.[13] For example, if the patient desires to be involved in decisions with the physician while the physician prefers a paternalistic role, or vice versa, conflict may result. In making decisions at the end of life, says Kilner, agreement is most likely to be reached when there are shared expectations. In decisions to forgo dialysis in the ICU, the best decisions may be reached when the physician and patient or surrogate understand and accept each other's values through a continuous process of communication.

In the aforementioned case, the patient's prognosis is unclear. Is the patient's need for ICU admission a result of the natural history of his disease, or is it a temporary setback that has the potential for a good outcome? If the patient's worsening condition is due to the former, then his overall condition of multiple organ failure is not likely to benefit from the use of hemodialysis. If his respiratory and liver failure can be reversed, then the patient might benefit from dialysis and return to a reasonable quality of life—whether the dialysis treatment is temporary to reverse acute renal failure, or long-term to treat chronic renal failure. However, the decision-making process in this case may be complicated by other motivations, conscious or unconscious, of the physician. The fact that the patient is on a research protocol may place the physician in conflict between her obligations as a physician and her obligations as a scientist. As a physician, she has a duty to her individual patient. But this duty may conflict with her role as a scientist—to benefit society through research—and her professional goals as a researcher. The physician also may feel a duty to provide the patient with experimental therapy when all other therapies have failed. On the other hand, the physician's decision to provide dialysis may be colored by the possible causal relationship between the chemotherapy and organ toxicity. It has been suggested that physicians who perceive a patient's condition as caused by iatrogenic events are slower to define limits of treatment for a patient.[14]

Another factor that may be motivating the physician is the fact that the patient is relatively young. American culture values youth. A young person's death is seen as tragic because of unfulfilled potential; the death of an elder, although equally tragic, is seen as part of the natural life cycle. The notion that death is unnatural for children and young people is underscored by an apparent lack of interest in palliative care for children in the United States. Aggressive care for a child or young person is considered standard and appropriate. Furthermore, physicians may not always be as objective as they believe they are. Christoffel speaks of the "physician-doctor relationship," a tension between the personal traits of the individual clinician and the role that person plays as a physician.[15] This tension has the potential to affect the medical care of a patient adversely. For example, if this patient reminds the physician of her own teenage son, she may find it difficult to consider limitation of treatment when appropriate for her patient. The intention here is not to overanalyze the mental state of the physician, but to point out some of the potential complexities involved when starting dialysis becomes a critical decision point in the care of a young, seriously ill patient in the ICU.

Finally, communication among team and family members is an issue in this scenario. Disagreeing with the attending physician's prognosis and plan could produce a moral dilemma for the resident physicians and nurses. At least one study has suggested that medical outcomes in the ICU may be improved with collaboration and cooperation among caregivers.[16] If so, one could argue for the inclusion of other team members in the decision-making process, possibly through periodic interdisciplinary patient-care conferences. The family also should be informed of the rationale for starting hemodialysis and the likelihood of the patient benefiting from this treatment. A timed trial of therapy might be negotiated, with discussion of the possibility of limiting therapy if the patient's condition does not improve.

DIALYSIS AND THE ELDERLY PATIENT

An 81-year-old woman has been on chronic dialysis for the past 10 months. She is found lying on the floor of her home and is intubated and admitted to the ICU for possible pneumonia and dehydration. Shortly after admission, her family approaches the attending physician. They state that the patient has a living will and ask that dialysis be discontinued and that she be allowed to die a "dignified death."

The concern of the family that the patient be allowed to die may seem premature from a medical point of view. If this elderly dialysis patient has been able to remain self-sufficient while living alone at home, she may have a good prognosis for returning to her home after discharge.

In some European countries, dialysis would not be offered to an octogenarian, but the question of age *per se* is not considered a relevant medical contraindication for dialysis in the United States. The reason for this attitude is that studies have reported that medical and physiological parameters and comorbidities are more important than chronological age in judging patient outcomes.[17] To refuse a person dialysis solely on the basis of chronological age might be considered "ageism"—discrimination against the elderly.

Ideally, this patient's physician would have discussed with the patient whether therapy should be limited if her prognosis changed. With appropriate treatment, this patient might be able to return to her previous state of health, or to regain the mental capacity to participate in decisions about her treatment. If the patient's prognosis remains poor and the patient remains mentally incapacitated, the physician's decision will be shaped by the patient's goals, as expressed by her family. The weighing of the burdens and benefits of aggressive medical treatment in the context of the patient's perception of quality of life will influence decision making.

The concern of the family is justified in that this elderly patient's condition could deteriorate and result in a prolonged ICU stay with no hope of returning to her previous condition. If, after a timed trial of treatment, the patient does not improve or if she suffers a serious-set back that makes her recovery unlikely, the physician can reevaluate the medical goals of treatment in light of the prognosis and patient's values as expressed by her family. The goals of treatment would then change from aggressive treatment to comfort measures. The patient's execution of a living will does not mean that a trial of therapy would be inappropriate in this case. Patients and family who desire "no heroic measures" may not understand the difference between using "heroic" measures (such as a ventilator) as a temporary measure to treat an acute condition and the use of such measures as chronic life support. A time-limited trial of therapy would permit the continued assessment of the patient's progress toward recovery or provide the necessary prognostic data to justify a shift from aggressive care to comfort care.

DIALYSIS AND THE DIFFICULT OR DISTASTEFUL PATIENT

The patient is a 37-year-old, homeless woman who has been admitted to the ICU for respiratory distress due to sepsis secondary to pelvic inflammatory disease. She is an intravenous-drug user and has tested positive for human immunodeficiency virus (HIV) infection. This is her second ICU admission in a year. Her first admission was also due to sepsis secondary to intravenous-drug use. She undergoes a stormy ICU course, but it appears that she may be able to be weaned from the respirator. However, it also appears that her acute renal failure will now be chronic and she will have to remain on dialysis to survive. The attending physician and head nurse convene a "care conference" because they have noted an undercurrent of resentment toward this patient among the residents and nurses.

A patient who is very different from his or her caregivers may evoke strong emotions of dislike or disapproval, yet professional behavior demands the provision of the highest standards of care without regard to the patient's lifestyle, background, or social situation. An open discussion of the ethics of caring for such patients could be part of a team conference on the best way to care for this particular patient. One way of facilitating such a discussion would be to invite a skilled neutral person—such as a hospital chaplain, liaison psychiatrist, or member of the hospital ethics committee—to lead the discussion.

Some professionals and laypersons alike may hold the attitude that because the patient is a drug addict, she is responsible for her social situation and medical condition and, therefore, not deserving of the same treatment a more responsible patient would get. Such an attitude is what Fitzgerald refers to as the "tyranny of health"—the idea that a failure to take care of oneself is an offense against society because society must pay for the consequences.[18] She cautions against developing a zealotry about healthcare in which we justify the denial of care (or, in this case, the denial of dialysis) to persons of whose lifestyles we disapprove.

Related to the fact of the patient's drug addiction and homelessness is the social context of her illness. It is ironic that we, as a society, are willing to spend thousands of dollars on "rescue" medicine—intensive, expensive, high-technology medical care for an individual—but not on preventive care. Could this woman's medical situation have been prevented through the availability of a drug-treatment program, a needle-sharing program, or the availability of proper housing and rehabilitation? The medical community appears open to consideration of preventive medicine, an openness driven by some of the developments in managed care. Whether this attitude toward preventive medicine can be sustained and operationalized remains to be seen. The current social climate of "blaming the victim" may work against good solutions to social problems that affect the health of individuals and the public.

A secondary issue in this case is the question of whether patients with HIV infection should be dialyzed. With recent advances in treatment, one could argue that HIV infection is no longer a death sentence. The fact that patients with HIV infection can now live many years with a good quality of life would support providing dialysis to this group of patients. An argument against the provision of dialysis would be that healthcare workers would have an added risk of exposure to the HIV virus; however, disagreement exists as to the extent of this risk in the dialysis setting.[19] Because the danger of exposure is constant (even in patients without known HIV infection) and the use of universal precautions is a standard of care, the denial of dialysis on the basis of HIV infection alone cannot be ethically justified in this situation, given the improving condition of this patient.

THE POLITICS OF DIALYSIS: PROFESSIONAL CONFLICT OR COLLABORATION?

A 36-year-old male who has undergone three previous open-heart surgeries due to congenital defects has progressively deteriorated as the result of complications from a fourth surgery. His ICU course has been long and complicated, with several episodes of sepsis and progressive multiple organ failure. The ICU attending physician and the consultants from cardiology and other services all agree that the patient's prognosis is extremely poor because of his irreversible heart and lung failure. The patient's kidneys are failing, and he is in need of dialysis. The ICU staff members agree among themselves that to continue aggressive treatment would be futile and probably result in increased suffering for the patient. They recommend to the surgeon that further discussion with the family include a recommendation for "no CPR," deescalation of aggressive treatment, and a move to provide comfort measures. The surgeon is angered at this recommendation, stating that the patient has always "pulled through" after past surgeries and he is not going to give up on his patient. He insists that the dialysis service begin hemodialysis to treat the patient's kidney failure. This surgeon brings in substantial revenue for the institution and has close friends on the hospital's board of trustees. It is known that colleagues who have disagreed with him in the past have been dismissed from the institution.

In this situation, political rather than medical or ethical indications appear to be the driving force for treatment. The surgeon is able to insist on starting dialysis in the face of his colleagues' assessment of futility because of his powerful position within the institution. But other factors might also be relevant to the surgeon's desire to dialyze the patient. Often physicians believe that they have an ethical and professional obligation to continue to treat in all circumstances.[20] A move to comfort measures may signify, for this surgeon, abandonment of the patient, especially when so much energy, expertise, and resources have already been expended in prolonging this patient's life.[21] Other physicians may simply not accept a concept of medical futility and may wish to continue aggressive treatment even in the face of a dismal prognosis.[22] Cultural beliefs about the unacceptability of death and the power of medical technology also may work against the clinician's acceptance of the reality of the clinical situation.

If the patient has executed a legal advance directive, the document could lend the force of the patient's wishes and the law to the other professionals' unwillingness to pursue aggressive treatment. If the patient has no advance directives, verbal or written, the question is "Why not"? Ideally, the surgeon's discussions with the patient about adverse surgical outcomes would include consideration of end-of-life wishes, given the patient's history of previous heart surgeries. However, physicians and patients may be reluctant to hold such conversations. Researchers have reported that, in spite of knowing patients' advance directives, physicians often make end-of-life decisions unilaterally.[23] A written advance directive can provide a starting point for conversations about decision making at the end of life, but the document should not substitute for such discussions.

When different medical services disagree about the goals of treatment for the patient and one service gives hopeful messages to the family while other services paint a bleaker picture, the family may react with frustration and mistrust. As noted previously, cooperation and collaboration among staff members has been suggested as a significant predictor of improved patient outcome in the ICU. It has been further shown that "closed" ICUs (units in which critical care specialists direct patient care) have better patient outcomes than "open" units (units in which the admitting physician or surgeon directs care of the patient with input from intensive care specialists).[24] In closed units, the intensive care team may be less subject to pressure from a physician or surgeon who is no longer the primary care provider. But if a surgeon admits a patient to a closed unit, he or she may still maintain a relationship with the patient and may wish to participate in decision making. Medical management of the patient should be discussed among the primary physicians or in a patient care conference for caregivers before discussion with the family, so that the team reaches agreement about medical goals and does not give mixed messages to the family. In situations where medical agreement cannot be reached, a mediator (such as the chief-of-staff or an ethics consultant) might be called on to assist. If the surgeon, for reasons of conscience, is unable to forgo aggressive treatment in the face of medical consensus and the patient's or family's wishes, the surgeon is ethically obligated to withdraw from the case by transferring the care of the patient to another physician.

THE POLITICS OF DIALYSIS: WHOSE RESPONSIBILITY?

A 50-year-old, mentally handicapped woman is admitted to the ICU with respiratory distress secondary to sepsis and metastatic breast cancer. She lives with her only relative, an older sister. The patient has become dependent on the respirator and her kidneys are failing. Her sister refuses to discuss any treatment limitations because, she says, the patient is a "fighter" and would want "everything done." As the patient continues to fail, the nurses and physicians become increasingly concerned about continuing burdensome treatment in a situation of apparent medical futility. However, the physicians are reluctant to recommend a move toward "comfort measures only" because they fear the patient's sister may be litigious. They are also concerned that their limitation of treatment might be construed as discrimination against the handicapped. They know that the renal dialysis service has criteria for dialyzing patients and that, in the past, the department has refused to provide dialysis for patients who did not meet certain physiological criteria. They order a dialysis service consultation knowing that this patient may not meet criteria because of hemodynamic instability.

A healthcare team's effectiveness can become seriously undermined in such a situation. The caregivers are unable to act in what they see as the best interest of the patient because they fear legal repercussions from the sister who wants "everything done." They also fear that limiting treatment may be construed as discriminatory; in actuality, the reverse may be true—by continuing treatment instead of providing comfort measures, they could be treating this disabled, dying patient in a manner that is different from their treatment of other dying patients. Why the sister refuses recommendations to limit treatment is an important question. Does she need more time to adjust to her sister's imminent death? As the primary caretaker, will she have difficulty in adjusting to a new role in her life? Does she fear that "stopping treatment" means a kind of abandonment by the healthcare team?

When a family member has fulfilled the role of caregiver for a long time, he or she may have given up outside career opportunities to do so. The care of the patient, in essence, becomes the family member's new career. The threat of losing this role due to the death of the patient may be a frightening prospect for the family member in addition to the experience of personal grief. Furthermore, when forgoing treatment is phrased as "stopping treatment," the images evoked may be those of abandoning the patient. It is more helpful to emphasize what will be done for the patient (for example, the aggressive provision of comfort measures) than what will not be done for the patient (for example, the forgoing of certain treatments). When surrogates demand inappropriate dialysis for a loved one, Keating and colleagues recommend a process based on the patient's best interests. They suggest that a decision to forgo dialysis over a surrogate's objections can be made (1) after a continuing process of communicating with the family; (2) with the agreement of other dialysis team members; (3) with a review by the institutional ethics committee (if available); (4) with detailed documentation of the decision-making process in the patient's medical record; and (5) after providing the family the option of transferring the patient to another facility if possible.[25]

In some large medical centers, the renal dialysis service may occasionally find itself in the position of being asked to decide to forgo dialysis because the primary service is unwilling or unable to consider limitations of treatment in situations of medical futility. (Sometimes other services, such as geriatrics, are also targeted for this role.) Often there are several reasons for this reluctance to forgo life-sustaining treatment. First, the shifting of the responsibility for limiting treatment to the renal service is a measure of the discomfort felt by healthcare professionals when the issue of forgoing life-sustaining treatment arises. Forgoing treatment involves either the withholding or the withdrawing of treatment. The consensus in the medical ethics literature is that while there is no moral difference between withholding and withdrawing a life-sustaining treatment, there is a psychological difference. It is more difficult to withdraw a life-sustaining treatment than it is to withhold it. A reason for this difficulty may be the symbolic meaning these actions have for the physician. When a life-sustaining treatment is withheld from the patient, the moral responsibility for the patient's death is symbolically on the patient, whose body is physiologically unable to sustain life. When life-sustaining treatment is withdrawn from the patient, the moral responsibility for the patient's death is symbolically placed on the physician.[26]

A second reason why the renal dialysis team may be called upon to limit treatment in the ICU is that many physicians, even intensive care physicians, lack skill in making the transition from aggressive care to comfort care. One of the characteristics of U.S. culture is a tendency to deny death; the aggressiveness of our medical care, as compared to European medicine, supports and perpetuates this denial.[27] If physicians are unskilled in the transition from high-technology care to comfort care, patients may exhibit distressing symptoms and caregivers may conclude that stopping treatment leads to increased suffering for the patient.[28] As noted earlier, when discontinuing life-sustaining treatment, physicians view the forgoing of dialysis as preferable to the discontinuation of a respirator. If physicians are not skilled in ventilator withdrawal and fear causing suffering for the patient, then discontinuing dialysis may be considered a more comfortable death for the patient and for the physician. Thus, the reason some dialysis services are being called on to "pull the plug" in the ICU may be rooted in physicians' lack of skill in caring for dying patients. In the wake of research and cost-containment measures, professional organizations are beginning to address the improvement of care for dying patients in the United States.

TOWARD THE DEVELOPMENT OF CLINICAL GUIDELINES FOR DIALYSIS

Limiting the use of life-sustaining interventions at the end of life when the burdens of treatment outweigh the benefits is gradually becoming accepted medical practice in the United States. One of the first limitations of treatment was the forgoing of cardiopulmonary resuscitation (CPR). Originally performed only in select situations of anticipated medical benefit to the patient, CPR eventually was used in virtually every cardiac arrest situation (that is, in every instance of death in the hospital). A growing body of medical data indicated situations in which CPR was virtually futile—the patient with metastatic cancer, the patient who has suffered an unwitnessed arrest, and the patient in multiple organ failure.[29] Individual institutions began to develop guidelines for do-not-resuscitate (DNR) status, which allowed for the withholding of CPR in cases where this treatment would have no benefit for the patient. Eventually, the Joint Commission on Accreditation of Healthcare Organizations mandated the development of DNR policies in all of its accredited institutions.

The call for guidelines for the use of dialysis has not received the same amount of attention as DNR orders. While some of the issues in forgoing dialysis parallel the issues in withholding CPR, the call for "DND" ("do not dialyze") orders has not received widespread attention. One reason for this lack of attention is that the use of dialysis, more so than other medical therapies, has had the official sanction of society for quite a long time. This sanction is in the form of a willingness of the U.S. government to use Medicare and Medicaid money to provide this treatment.

Recently, an interest in maintaining quality care and a concern about rising healthcare costs have fueled current managed care practices and a renewed interest in clinical practice guidelines. Although practice guidelines are intended to promote high standards of care, many are being developed and applied for nonmedical reasons such as cost containment. Such use creates a climate for potentially unethical uses of clinical practice guidelines.[30]

The need for clinical guidelines is suggested by variations in practice patterns in the use of dialysis. In one study, medical directors of dialysis centers displayed variations in attitudes about the appropriateness of withholding or withdrawing dialysis from patients who were demented or in a persistent vegetative state.[31] In the case of chronic dialysis patients, physicians, patients, and families often arrive at decisions to discontinue dialysis only after a series of setbacks such as chronic pain, infection, or ischemic problems.[32] At one institution, a pilot program was initiated to provide patients with a time-limited trial of dialysis before deciding on whether to continue or forgo this treatment.[33] Although patient autonomy is considered a basic principle of medical ethics, physicians often make unilateral decisions about forgoing life-supporting therapy.[34] Another problem is that some patients demand inappropriate therapy. In some circumstances, physicians may be justified in overriding patient autonomy,[35] but physicians often accede to competent patients' requests for treatment. Clinical practice guidelines are viewed as a way of dealing with these variations in practice by encouraging standardization of practice that promotes fairness in addition to quality.

Some measure of the severity of patient illness and projected patient outcomes is extremely important for rational discussions among caregivers. This evidence-based approach to decision making is quite difficult with regard to dialysis. Several severity scores have been used to prognosticate outcomes in the ICU population,[36] but these same systems have been shown to be flawed when applied to patients with acute renal failure undergoing dialysis support.[37] Even disease-specific severity scores may not be valid in hospitals other than their originating institution.[38]

One of the authors of this chapter, with colleagues, has generated a severity scoring system that allows patient outcome identification with a high degree of precision within the ICUs at one hospital.[39] While this system is currently being validated at other institutions,[40] the first institution has begun to use the patient scores as a guide to therapy longevity. Those patients who have a high severity are given full and aggressive therapy, but for a limited period of time (usually seven to 10 days); during this trial period patients are continually reevaluated for improvement, as judged by changing scores. If the score improves, therapy is continued for another defined time period. If, on the other hand, the score worsens, the healthcare team initiates discussion about therapy withdrawal with the patient and/or family.[41]

Acceptance of this approach has been slow, but progressive. Frequently there is a conflict between caregivers who focus on short-term outcomes (for example, discharge from the ICU) and those with concern over the long-term result. A nephrologist who is not the intensive care physician and who is also responsible for the long-term care of the patient on dialysis after discharge from the ICU may take a different approach than a nephrologist who is responsible for only short term or long term. It is precisely for these reasons that practice guidelines must be generated from a multidisciplinary group of caregivers. Also, cost analysis must be used to help determine the financial rationale in supportive care. Supporting everyone with renal failure regardless of their overall status raises questions of appropriate resource utilization.[42]

Arguments have been presented both for and against the use of clinical practice guidelines, and the debate will likely continue for a long time. In regard to the appropriate use of dialysis, various professional groups involved in the treatment of renal disease have developed consensus guidelines for forgoing kidney dialysis. These guidelines recommend not offering dialysis to (1) capacitated patients who refuse it and incapacitated patients who have indicated prior refusal; (2) patients who are unable to relate to others (for example, those in a persistent vegetative state or those with severe, progressive dementia); (3) patients who are terminally ill from a nonrenal disease; and (4) patients who are unable to cooperate in the dialysis process.[43] Whether or not these guidelines become universally accepted in the management of renal disease remains to be seen.

NOTES

1. J. W. Ross, *Handbook for Hospital Ethics Committees* (Chicago: American Hospital Publishing, 1986).

2. N.A. Christakis and D.A. Asch, "Biases in How Physicians Choose to Withdraw Life Support," *Lancet* 342 (1993): 642-46.

3. H. Brody et al., "Withdrawing Intensive Life-Sustaining Treatment: Recommendations for Compassionate Clinical Management," *New England Journal of Medicine* 336, no. 9 (1997): 652-57.

4. N.N. Dubler, "Commentary: Balancing Life and Death: Proceed with Caution," *American Journal of Public Health* 83, no. 1 (1993): 23-25.

5. See note 2 above.

6. R.M. Gula, *What Are They Saying About Euthanasia?* (New York: Paulist Press, 1986), 45-46.

7. *In re Quinlan*, 70 N.J. 10, 355 A.2d 647 (1976).

8. *Cruzan v. Director, Missouri Department of Health*, 497 U.S. 261 (1990).

9. President's Commission for the Study of Ethical Problems in Medicine and Biomedical and Behavioral Research, *Decisions to Forgo Life-Sustaining Treatment* (Washington, D.C.: U.S. Government Printing Office, 1983).

10. J.E. Ruark, T.A. Raffin, and the Stanford University Medical Center Committee on Ethics, "Initiating and Withdrawing Life Support," *New England Journal of Medicine* 318 (1988): 25-30.

11. R. Valdez and A. Rosenblum, "Voluntary Termination of Dialysis: When Your Patient Says, 'Enough!'" *Dialysis and Transplantation* 23, no. 10 (1994): 566-70.

12. D.A. Asch, J. Hansen-Flaschen, and P.N. Lanken, "Decisions to Limit or Continue Life-Sustaining Treatment by Critical Care Physicians in the United States: Conflicts Between Physicians' Practices and Patients' Wishes," *American Journal of Respiratory and Critical Care Medicine* 151 (1995): 288-92.

13. J.F. Kilner, "Ethical Issues in the Initiation and Termination of Treatment," *American Journal of Kidney Diseases* 15, no. 3 (1990): 218-27.

14. See note 2 above.

15. K.K. Christoffel, "The Physician-Doctor Relationship," *Pediatrics* 91, no. 4 (1993): 832-34.

16. W.A. Knaus et al., "An Evaluation of Outcome from Intensive Care in Major Medical Centers," *Annals of Internal Medicine* 104, no. 3 (1986): 410-18.

17. A.H. Moss, "Dialysis Decisions and the Elderly," *Clinics in Geriatric Medicine* 10, no. 3 (1994): 463-73; A.P. Baldyga et al., "Acute Dialytic Support of the Octogenarian: Is It Worth It?" *ASAIO Journal* 39 (1993): M805-08; C. Byrne, P. Vernon, and J.J. Cohen, "Effect of Age and Diagnosis on Survival of Older Patients Beginning Chronic Dialysis," *Journal of the American Medical Association* 271, no. 1 (1994): 34-36; C.R. Blagg and S.S. Fitts, "Dialysis, Old Age, and Rehabilitation," *Journal of the American Medical Association* 271, no. 1 (1994): 67-68.

18. F. Fitzgerald, "The Tyranny of Health," *New England Journal of Medicine* 331, no. 3 (1994): 196-98.

19. P.L. Kimmel et al., "Prevalence of Viremia in Human Immunodeficiency Virus-Infected Patients with Renal Disease," *Archives of Internal Medicine* 155 (1995):1578-84; D.N. Gilbert and W. Bennett, "Patients With Human Immunodeficiency Virus Infection in the Hemodialysis Unit: How Vulnerable Are the Caregivers?" *Archives of Internal Medicine* 155 (1995): 1575-76.

20. N. Wray et al., "Withholding Medical Treatment from the Severely Demented Patient: Decisional Processes and Cost Implications," *Archives of Internal Medicine* 148 (1988): 1980-84.

21. L.J. Schneiderman, K. Faber-Langendoen, and N.S. Jecker, "Beyond Futility to an Ethic of Care," *American Journal of Medicine* 96 (1994): 110-14.

22. J.W. Swanson and S.V. McCrary, "Doing All They Can: Physicians Who Deny Medical Futility," *Journal of Law, Medicine and Ethics* 22, no. 4 (1994): 318-26.

23. The SUPPORT Principal Investigators, "Study to Understand Prognoses and Preferences for Outcomes and Risks of Treatment (SUPPORT): A Controlled Trial to Improve Care for Seriously Ill Hospitalized Patients," *Journal of the American Medical Association* 274 (1995): 1591-98.

24. S.S. Carson et al., "Effects of Organizational Change in the Medical Intensive Care Unit of a Teaching Hospital: A Comparison of 'Open' and 'Closed' Formats," *Journal of the American Medical Association* 276, no. 4 (1996): 322-28.

25. R.F. Keating et al., "Stopping Dialysis of an Incompetent Patient Over the Family's Objection: Is It Ever Ethical and Legal?" *Journal of the American Society of Nephrology* 4, no. 11 (1994): 1879-83.

26. J. Slomka, "The Negotiation of Death: Clinical Decision Making at the End of Life," *Social Science & Medicine* 35, no. 3 (1992): 251-59.

27. M. Osborne and T.W. Evans, "Allocation of Resources in Intensive Care: A Transatlantic Perspective," *Lancet* 434 (1994): 778-80.

28. See note 3 above.

29. American Medical Association, Council on Ethical and Judicial Affairs, "Guidelines for the Appropriate Use of Do-Not-Resuscitate Orders," *Journal of the American Medical Association* 265, no. 14 (1991): 1868-71.

30. J.T. Berger and F. Rosner, "The Ethics of Practice Guidelines," *Archives of Internal Medicine* 156 (1996): 2051-56.

31. A.H. Moss et al., "Variation in the Attitudes of Dialysis Unit Medical Directors Toward Decisions to Withhold and Withdraw Dialysis," *Journal of the American Society of Nephrology* 4, no. 2 (1993): 229-34.

32. K. Bajwa, E. Szabo, and K.M. Kjellstrand, "A Prospective Study of Risk Factors and Decision Making in Discontinuation of Dialysis," *Archives of Internal Medicine* 156 (1996): 2571-77.

33. D. Buonocore and E. Paganini, "Dialysis Trials: Assessing the Value of Renal Therapy in the Compromised Patient," *Nephrology News and Issues* (November 1994): 18-19.

34. M. Danis et al., "A Prospective Study of the Impact of Patient Preferences on Life-Sustaining Treatment and Hospital Cost," *Critical Care Medicine* 24, no. 11 (1996): 1811-17.

35. I. Kerridge, M. Lowe, and K. Mitchell, "Competent Patients, Incompetent Decisions," *Annals of Internal Medicine* 123, no. 11 (1995): 878-81.

36. W.A. Knaus et al., "APACHE II: A Severity of Disease Classification System," *Critical Care Medicine* 13 (1985): 818-29; J.R. LeGall et al., "Simplified Acute Physiology Score for ICU Patients," *Critical Care Medicine* 12 (1984): 975-77; J. Markle et al., "Comparison Between TRISS and ASCOT Methods in Controlling for Injury Severity," *Journal of Trauma* 33 (1992): 326-32.

37. K. MacKay and A. Moss, "To Dialyze or Not to Dialyze: An Ethical and Evidence-Based Approach to the Patient with Acute Renal Failure in the Intensive Care Unit," *Advances in Renal Replacement Therapy* 4, no. 3 (1997): 288-96.

38. W.K. Halstenberg, M. Goormastic, and E.P. Paganini, "Validity of Four Models for Predicting Outcome in Critically Ill Patients with Acute Renal Failure," *Clinical Nephrology* 47, no. 2 (1997): 81-86.

39. E.P. Paganini, W.K. Halstenberg, and M. Goormastic, "Risk Modeling in Acute Renal Failure Requiring Dialysis: The Introduction of a New Model," *Clinical Nephrology* 46, no. 6 (1996): 206-11.

40. G.M. Chertow et al., "Predictors of Mortality and the Provision of Dialysis in Patients with Acute Tubular Necrosis," *Journal of the American Society of Nephrology* 9 (1998): 692-98.

41. E.P. Paganini et al., "Sequential Severity Scoring in ICU Acute Renal Failure Improves Predictive Power and Allows Periodic Objective Patient Reevaluation," (abstract) *Journal of the American Society of Nephrology* 9 (1998): 157A; E.P. Paganini et al., "Physicians' Selective Bias in Choice of Dialysis Support Method as a Predictor of ICU-ARF Patient Outcome"(abstract) *Journal of the American Society of Nephrology* 9 (1998): 157A.

42. M.B. Hamel et al., "Outcomes and Cost-Effectiveness of Initiating Dialysis and Continuing Aggressive Care in Seriously Ill Hospitalized Adults," *Annals of Internal Medicine* 127 (1997): 195-202.

43. A.H. Moss, "To Use Dialysis Appropriately: The Emerging Consensus on Patient Selection Guidelines," *Advances in Renal Replacement Therapy* 2, no. 2 (1995): 175-83.

13

Humanizing Technology: The Future of Critical Care

David H. Beyda

INTRODUCTION

Medicine is addicted to technology. We are infatuated with its remarkable engineering, its prowess, and its mystique. Medicine has become a science of machines with less and less of the human touch that was once the foundation for healing. "High-tech" practices have overshadowed "high-touch" practices. At times technology supersedes caring, leading to a type of pseudo-caring that can leave the patient isolated and empty. Often, as the patient gets sicker, the use of technology increases and the amount of human interaction between clinician and patient decreases. This depersonalization is inconsistent with the purpose of medicine, and the use of unnecessary high-tech interventions can cause human suffering. Although the foundational premise of *primum non nocere* encompasses the basic principle of avoidance of harm, technology has caused iatrogenic events that can harm the patient. This "iatroepidemic" is morally unacceptable.[1]

On the other hand, technology has opened windows into the disease process that has allowed many human lives to be saved. Technology can be a powerful adjunct to the clinician's expertise, and the standard of care in modern medicine expects its use. However, the proper use of technology in a critical care environment should be based on a foundation of humanism, a concept that has lost part of its meaning. Technology is used more often than not as a convenience for the healthcare provider rather than as a necessity for patients and, thus, it takes away from the humanistic approach to the patient. Modern clinicians have become more comfortable treating the disease rather than the patient, and they are more comfortable with curing than with caring. This chapter focuses on two issues: (1) whether there is, or can be, a balance between the use of technology and compassion at the bedside, and (2) how technology can be made to be more humane. This chapter does not address the economic issues of technology but concentrates on what is of primary interest to the patient—the assurance of the patient's comfort and dignity (that is, humanism).

WHAT IS TECHNOLOGY?

The definition of technology is "a general term for the processes by which human beings fashion tools and machines to increase their control and understanding of the material environment."[2] From the scientific standpoint, technology is defined as "systematic application of scientific knowledge and technological skills for the control of matter, energy, etc., for practical purposes."[3]

For the purpose of this discussion, the term *technology* is used in its narrowest sense—that is, a tool or material artifact that assists in a task. By its design and its particular use, technology can be less than neutral in its application. A hammer can be used to build a house or bash in a head. By design, the hammer is supposed to be used as an instrument to pound nails, not heads. Once the artifact is used contrary to its design, it becomes an instrument of questionable purpose. Technology cannot be neutral. It constitutes a way of life and affects human behavior.

Technology changes behavior and culture by virtue of having the ability to change the environment. This change comes as a result of trying to resolve a particular problem but, more often than not, replaces that problem with another. Technology has overpowered patients and healthcare providers alike. Rarely does the patient in the critical care unit give informed consent for the use of technology. The question is not whether technology is good or bad, but whether it is used appropriately and with humane intentions.

Technology threatens to deprive patients of freedom by being restrictive and invasive. On the other hand, its use can also expand freedom by allowing access and mobility (for example, a wheelchair). Finding a balance between these two extremes seems to be difficult.

IS TECHNOLOGY A NECESSITY OR A CONVENIENCE?

Technology has become a convenience for most clinicians rather than a necessity for patients. This should not be misconstrued as an antitechnology statement. Not at all. The advances in medicine have come about as a direct result of this very technology. However, clinicians' technological *knowledge* must become technological *wisdom* in order for technology to be used appropriately.

The controversy over the role and value of technology is nothing new. There is no question that technology is an essential component of modern medicine. Technology has been invaluable in giving clinicians a window into areas of the human body inaccessible by the routine physical examination, and it has given the clinician an early look at the disease process. But the rate of technological change has developed its own momentum; innovations are being implemented at an accelerated rate without respect for the patient's comfort, needs, wants, or dignity. The overwhelming growth of technology has frightened some people, and there is a wealth of literature calling for assessment of technology.[4]

Reiser wrote that diagnostic technology such as the stethoscope has increasingly alienated physicians from patients because it provides "external, objective science [and] the physician no longer relies on his own personal contact with the patient for a diagnosis. The price is impersonal medical care that undermines the physician's belief in his own medical power."[5]

Reiser is correct. By using technology as a substitute for our personal intervention with patients, we force distance between the patients and ourselves. We are who we are as a result of technological changes. We have come to depend on technology and accept it as a way of life. We rely on calculators and computers and other devices to control our environment because they are more convenient. Technology has taken out the human, personal acts of life that once drove our cultures. We picked crops by hand—now by machine; we did math by reason, pencil, and paper—now by computer; and we palpated pulses with fingers—now by doppler technology. Technology is therefore a significant cause of all social change. However, there should be no technological imperative or "one best way." There must be human choices. Some of these choices may be ethical in nature. Who will make them and for whom will they be made? Technology has desensitized physicians to humanism and caring by forcing them to look at what, not who. Technology allows physicians to view the human as machine. Patients become "cases" that are worked up. Technology allows physicians to distance themselves from their patients. If the physician and patient's eyes can't meet, there is a problem. In using technology, physicians mistakenly believe they can reduce uncertainty by changing the patient's problem to one in which there is a technological answer.[6]

At the bedside, some clinicians erroneously believe that technology always gives the right answer. In fact, physicians use technology convinced of its success, fueled by promise of performance rather than performance itself.[7] Technology threatens the patient's freedom of choice and the patient's right to comfort and dignity. The information that technology yields may not necessarily result in better patient care. In fact, some technology contributes nothing of meaning to better the patient. Technological abuse occurs not infrequently in critical care. For instance, tests may be performed when none are warranted. Some causes of technological abuse include physicians' motivation; physicians may perform unwarranted technological procedures motivated by a desire for profit, desire for enhanced prestige in an academic setting, the fascination or pleasure associated with a new procedure, and the simple desire for self-protection against legal action.[8]

An example of technological abuse would be the use of ventilator support for patients with terminal or irreversible illnesses. Ethical issues relate to the appropriate use of such technology. Because of its availability, this technology is used at times with little regard for the patient's comfort. Often high-tech procedures concentrate on the immediate relief of a problem rather than on any future gain. The patient may experience temporary relief but be destined to experience long-term suffering.

When used appropriately, however, technology yields exciting information that can contribute directly to an immediate action by the clinician and to improved patient outcomes. One example is the test for cholesterol. A simple test allows the clinician to use the information to prescribe a therapy that may lower the patient's cholesterol level, thus improving patient outcome. This test can reasonably determine a course of therapy that, in most cases, will benefit the patient. On the other hand, high-tech interventions are unnecessary if they have no benefit to or for the patient.

Technology can prolong the inevitable, such as death. It can be this very use of technology that undermines the essence of medicine by obstructing a process that cannot be changed. On the other hand, technology can push away death and ensure normal survival. The decision regarding when to use technology should be determined by the patient, family, and physician, based on the best guess for outcome. Technology will always be a means for creating new physical and human conditions by interfering in a natural process. Even in everyday life, modern machines are used in contrast to nature: air conditioning for summer heat and artificial heat for winter cold. Some argue that the mere existence of technology dictates that it be used.[9] Technology may have the potential to destroy the essence of humanism.

Although the definition of *humanism* is complex and wide, the term is used here to mean simply an unselfish compassion for another human being that becomes a way of life. Anything more raises expectations that are unreachable. It is unfortunate that humanism has lost part of its meaning. We recognize a deficiency in humanism by simply looking at changes in our culture: pleas for patient care advocates, a patients' bill of rights, and hospices for dying patients; calls for the increased use of alternative forms of medicine; reports of humiliation experienced by clinicians when they themselves have been patients; and the emergence of autonomy rather than beneficence as the dominant principle in medical ethics. In the clinician's defense, humanism may be hard to come by. Patients may impose unrealistic expectations on clinicians and clinicians may be directed by insurance companies that dictate patient care. But simply avoiding self-serving goals may be all that is needed to bring humanism to the bedside.

TECHNOLOGY AND DISEASE

How is the clinician to decide if the use of technology is a convenience or a necessity? A physiologic approach and an understanding of the disease process are invaluable in assessing the need for technology. In the past, human life was a continuum—for the most part uninterrupted. Health lead to disease, which lead to health again or death. Nature directed the course, and humans did not intervene. As medicine became sophisticated, interventional methods (both medicinal and technological) interrupted this continuum. Humans now directed the way and, for the most part, the outcome was in favor of the patient.

From a physiologic standpoint, the sick patient presents in a state of entropy or a state of general disorder, indicating an illness or injury; through a series of interventions, the patient returns to a healthy state or homeostasis. The process can also be reversed, as is seen with iatrogenic complications or physiologic setbacks.

The physiologic state is related to the patient's relative degree of health. Technology plays a more significant role as these physiologic states change. The body in its normal state functions by a series of complex interactions that are self-regulated. As the patient first gets ill, the body enters a predisease state. Organs have a tendency to malfunction that is undetectable in the resting state but may appear when stress is applied. As the degree of malfunctioning increases, the body enters a disease state in which there is an uncoupling among the self-regulated, feedback cascades for metabolic and physiologic functions. The result is a physiologically chaotic state. It is during this disease state that technology becomes a formidable force in patient care.

HISTORICAL OVERVIEW OF THE RISE OF TECHNOLOGY IN MEDICINE

The philosophy of the eighteenth-century philosopher Descartes was influential in establishing the premise that technology is needed to cure. Descartes brought the human body, the earthly machine as he called it, into the sphere of mechanics and physics. He applied the literature and language of physics and mechanics to medicine, leading to the movement of iatromathematics (or iatrophysics) and iatrochemistry. To Descartes, man was simply a machine—except for the pineal gland, where he claimed the rational soul was located.[10]

Following Descartes, La Mettrie published *L'Homme Machine* in 1794, in which he declared that man ought to be considered a machine.[11] This was a classical physiologic doctrine of the mechanist school, one that met with resistance but eventually became a foundation for the science of medicine.

Cartesian dualism, as well, separated the mind from the body and viewed the body as a machine. This philosophy worked well as a foundation for explaining how the body worked. It allowed for the growth of technology to "fix" the broken parts. Today, perhaps, we feel no differently. We tend to view the human as a machine—a soul entrapped, but technology dependent machine.

It is important to understand the difference between *monitoring* and *diagnosis* to understand the difficulty clinicians sometimes have in using technology appropriately. *Monitoring* is defined by *Stedman's Medical Dictionary* as "the watchful observation, usually with the aide of an electronic monitor."[12] Monitoring is simply the continuous observation of physiologic "signs" for the immediate detection of disturbance. It is the "observation of disease." Before the advent of the electronic monitor, nurses played the role of "monitor."

Diagnosis is defined as "the determination of the nature of a disease"; clinical diagnosis is "made from the study of the signs and symptoms of a disease."[13] Diagnosis is simply the "declaration" of disease.

Clinicians for the most part are good diagnosticians, as is technology. Technology is a crutch for the poor clinician and an adjunct for the good one. A diagnostic revolution has taken place over the last century. Technology was recognized as a potential deterrent to patient care back in the late 1800s when S. Meir Mitchell said in a presidential address to the Congress of American Physicians and Surgeons, "You know, alas! that we now use as many instruments as a mechanic."[14]

Since the early 1800s, two revolutions have taken place that have changed the way physicians have evaluated disease: the refinement of the physical diagnosis and the development of technological diagnostic tools.

Before the nineteenth century, physicians practiced primarily at a physical distance from the patient. The practice of "hands-on" examination was done by surgeons who were considered less skilled doctors by virtue of their "mechanical" approach. The better doctors evaluated illnesses by questioning and listening and by a careful visual inspection of the body.

In 1816, the first diagnostic tool was used on a patient. Renee Laennec was making rounds with his entourage when he came upon an obese woman with heart trouble. Unable to use visual inspection or direct auscultation of her heart with his ear on her chest, he fashioned a cone-shaped tube from a rolled sheet of paper, placing the larger end on the patient's chest, and listening through the smaller end. This was the first description of a stethoscope. According to Reiser, the stethoscope increased alienation of physicians from patients.[15]

A threshold for technology is necessary. If a radiograph of the chest for a patient with a cough is too much, would using a stethoscope to listen to the patient's chest be acceptable, or is this practice also too "high tech"? Assessment of healthcare technology should be an interactive process, not a single event.[16]

The second revolution, the development of technological diagnostic tools, came about in the late 1800s. James MacKenzie invented the clinical cardiograph, that depicted heart action on a circular smoke drum attached to electrodes on the patient. For the first time, a device was used to transform data into objective forms of pictorial and graphic data.

The revolution went beyond the evolution of technology. It forced a change in medical culture by labeling physicians, depending on how they practiced medicine. By 1920, Harvard Medical School labeled doctors as either "modern" or "other." Modern doctors relied on laboratory evidence for diagnosis and stood for exactness, precision, and science. Doctors who were not considered modern relied on physical data and stood for diversity, vagueness, and empiricism. These descriptive values may still hold true today in the distinction between specialists and generalists.

THE EFFECTS OF TECHNOLOGY ON PATIENT CARE

This rapid growth of technology has created an environment that is driven by "modern" doctors who choose to use technology to provide patient care. The behavior of physicians is related to the conditions under which they live and practice. It was Descartes who first suggested that the environment plays an active role in the determination of behavior. This observation leads to several questions. Is the technology used today a necessity or simply a convenience? Does the technology used give accurate answers to questions that would otherwise be unobtainable by other means? Does technology contribute directly to patient care or is it used solely as a convenience for clinicians so that they can attend to other things?

Consider, for example, the monitors used in critical care units. Are they used as a means to alert clinicians of a physiologic abnormality, or are they used to allow clinicians to "care" for more patients, go to lunch, or tend to personal needs? The Swan-Ganz catheter made its debut in 1970 and soon became the monitoring and diagnostic norm for all patients admitted to a critical care unit. Today, the Swan-Ganz catheter yields little data of benefit in the majority of critical cases. It is reserved for patients who require a device to monitor direct hemodynamic function.

Asking whether a particular high-tech procedure is a necessity or a convenience will lead to a better relationship between clinician and patient. Unfortunately, the more ill the patient becomes, the more technology is used. There is a gap between high-tech and high-touch care. The patient is often lost in an ocean of machines, medicines, and consultants. The clinician becomes a conductor of a technological orchestra, much of which is out of tune with the patient. Technology has developed its own momentum in medicine without respect for the patient's dignity, comfort, and worth by becoming a convenience for the physician rather than a necessity. Clinical diagnosis has been replaced by technological diagnosis. Technology has perhaps been too successful. Through research and development based on the presumed needs of the patient, new technology is developed. This new technology, in turn, causes an increase in the public's expectation; this leads to an increase in the physician's need to use the high-tech procedure, which then leads to further development of new technologies. Technology has assumed a dominating position in medicine and may lead to its own destruction by becoming so unyielding that it destroys personal choice. Technology has reduced patients to organized systems, and it can become more important than the patient it was designed to serve.[17] Technology should come as a result of a genuine understanding of the disease process, the limitations of the healthcare provider, and the patient's best interest.

When is medical intervention, in particular technology, unnecessary? Friedman argues that inappropriate interventions are dangerous when they interfere with consideration for the patient's welfare.[18]

New technologies should be developed in response to a particular need or as a solution to a particular problem. However, because of marketing pressures, alternative technologies are developed that may or may not lead to the best solution to a problem. Thus, patients experience not necessarily the best care that is available but what is currently available. If research and development centered on finding "optimal" solutions, then better, well-defined technology would be used. Rather than rush to market a device that gives only an alternative solution to a problem, high-tech companies should wait until they have developed the optimal solution. In order to develop the optimal solution, these companies need to use the critical care unit as a "laboratory" for development. Engineers cannot fully understand the patient's needs unless they work in a critical care unit and observe first-hand the patient's dilemma. Clinicians need to encourage and allow these companies to work alongside healthcare providers in a patient-centered environment to encourage the development of technology that is based on patients' needs (patient-centered technology). See Exhibit 13-1 for examples of optimal solutions using patient-centered technology.

Developing technology that is based on optimal solutions starts with ensuring the patients' comfort and dignity. If new technologies are developed only after patients' needs and rights are identified, technology will be more humane.

CURING OR CARING: HUMANIZING TECHNOLOGY

The greatest task physicians face is to decide who they are and what their relationship with their patient is going to be. Physicians' personal "caring principles" will determine their use of technology.

Exhibit 13-1
Optimal Solutions Using Patient-Centered Technology

Patients' Needs	Current Activities/Procedures	Potential Optimal Solutions
Lack of pain	Invasive procedures	Noninvasive measurements
Inability to feel pain	Detection of pain in comatose patients by pin pricking	EEG* monitoring
Awareness	Leads, alarms, EEG* tick, big boxes, brightness of display, frequent visits by clinicians	Volume of EEG* tick, alarms, display brightness, size of equipment, accuracy/amount of remote patient information
Safety and stability	Monitoring trends, predictive alarms, EEG* tick	Elimination of nuisance alarms, better predictors
Lack of fear	Big boxes, alarms, invasive procedures	Equipment ergonomics, minimized testing
Control	Nurse call, self-regulated pain medication, equipment restrictiveness, weaning off technology	Integration of pumps with automatic feedback, telemetry/leadless monitors, pressure/flow loops
To be listened to/attended	Alarms, response time	Volume controls
Calmness	Ergonomics, displays	Psychological healing
Self-esteem	Noisy, exposure, privacy, self-importance	Equipment brought to the patient, remote access to information
Empowerment (choices, control)	Personal preferences	Remote control
Lack of embarrassment	Customizing, naming patient	Identity
Confidence	Monitor is fair game to the public, transportability of technology to patient	..
To be not taken for granted	Reliable products, alarms, soothing without alarms	Humanizing
Dignity	Private use of technology	..

*   Electroencephalogram

Greek physicians were guided by two basic principles: *philotechnia*, the love of the art of healing, and *philanthropia*, the love of man.[19] These principles were called into question years later when it become evident that physicians' care was inconsistent and variable: slaves did not receive the same care as free men, and the poor did not receive the attention given to the rich. This observation may still be true today.

It is important to address *care* as it relates to *cure*. Do patients receive the care they need? Do patients need the care they receive? Today, patients are expected to recover. When they don't, then the assumption is that someone is at fault. This expectation distorts the concept of caring; defensive medicine and "pseudo-caring" (when technology takes precedence over compassion) have become the norm.

Our society may be best described as a pseudo-caring society—one that pretends to care but lacks sincerity. Witness the current trends in business and family life: me first, you second. Today a caring environment is hard to come by. This may be directly related to a change in behavior that has occurred over a long period of time. If the majority holds to a certain behavior, the culture then becomes that behavior.

Technology changes human behavior. Technology is designed to eliminate, fix, or alleviate a particular problem. However, technology often replaces one problem with another.

Technology implies cure and/or life-sustaining treatment. If medicine has progressed to a point of cure first, care if we can, then technology dominates. To counter this problem, we must agree always to care first and cure if we can. This alone puts technology down a step and begins to humanize the relationship. Healthcare providers can then begin to look at themselves as providers of curing and caring.

Curing and *caring*—although different processes—can and should work in harmony. To do otherwise precludes a balanced approach to the patient. A short discussion of these processes follows.

To cure means to make better. Curing can be very objective and without emotion. A patient who was sick has been cured, a relatively easy task to accomplish in most cases. Curing is the process of recovery or relief from a disease by instituting a treatment. Cure is an objective process of correction. Curing promotes wholeness of body, a well-tuned machine. But to cure without caring has drawbacks. Nouwen wrote, "Cure without care is as dehumanizing as a gift given with a cold heart. But cure without care makes us into rulers, controllers, manipulators, and prevents a real community from taking shape. Cure without care can be offending instead of liberating."[20] In summary, curing—which is a task-oriented approach—is associated with "fixing," "getting better," and "getting healthy."

Caring has been described in the literature and by others as painstaking or watchful attention; regard coming from desire or esteem; a person or thing that is an object of attention, anxiety, or solicitude.[21] Caring is a personal matter. The physician or the patient may or may not want to or be able to care. The level of caring can vary, depending on attitude, feeling, or state of mind about a person.[22] To care implies a personal involvement by both the physician and the patient. Pellegrino has eloquently described caring as "[to] have some understanding of what sickness means to another person, together with the readiness to help and to see the situation as the patient does. Compassion demands that the physician be so disposed that his every action and word will be rooted in respect for the person he is serving."[23] Caring is associated with the following qualities: empathy, touching, listening, and attention.

Caring is a process of promoting wholeness of being. It embraces three aspects of humanism that should serve as common denominators for all physicians: preventing and controlling pain, ensuring the patient's comfort, and maintaining the patient's dignity. Curing is certainly our goal, but caring should be our passion.

Just as it is important to understand the difference between curing and caring, it is also important to understand the difference between healthcare and healing. *Healthcare*, which is intuitively objective and scientific, encompasses a process and an institution. Terms associated with healthcare include insurance, hospital, system, process, procedures, and administration. *Healing*, which is more passionate and personal, encompasses the total well-being of the person without boundaries. Terms associated with healing include whole, holistic, involvement, touching, and personal.

CARING AND VALUE PRINCIPLES

Perhaps there is another way of looking at caring. Caring is based on "value principles" individually selected and practiced according to the personality and character of the physician. Physicians cannot be all things to all patients. Physicians must select those "caring principles" that best suit the mutual needs of their patients and themselves with the assumption that a basic foundation of caring principles are held for every patient.

Each value principle produces a different quality. A value principle must be part of an individual's philosophy and is a central component that shapes every plan and decision a physician makes. It therefore defines what physicians do and who they are. Physicians are responsible for all their actions regardless of their intent or lack thereof. Value principles force physicians to make some hard choices about who they are or who they are about to become, and to approach the patient honestly and without pretense.

The four value principles are

1. *Relationship:* What type of relationship will the physician have with the patient—one based on contract or covenant? Will the contract be a commercial or technical one? Will the contract imply success as all contracts do? Or will the covenant imply simply a mutual trust, respect, integrity, and honesty between the patient and the physician?

2. *Priority:* What are the physician's priorities in addressing cure (focusing on the disease) or care (focusing on the patient) or a balancing of both?

3. *Personal commitment:* Does the physician have a commitment to do what he/she should be doing or just what he/she wants to be doing?

4. *Technology use:* Does the physician use technology as a primary resource or as an adjunct?

CATEGORIES OF PHYSICIANS

In trying to solve their patient's medical problems, physicians turn to the things they do best. Physicians make decisions and take actions based in their character and principles. Four types of physicians can be identified, based on value principles (see Exhibit 13-2).

1. *Curing healthcare provider:* This clinician rejects traditional medicine and has a tendency to be concrete, formalistic, and sterile.

Exhibit 13-2
Categories of Physicians Based on Value Principles

Category of Physician	Value Principles			
	Relationship	Commitment	Priority	Technology Use
Curing healthcare provider	Contract	Want	Disease	Primary
Curing healer	Covenant	Should	Patient	Primary
Caring healthcare provider	Contract	Want	Disease	Primary
Caring healer	Covenant	Should	Patient	Adjunct

He or she strives for quantification and promotes wholeness of body through science and technology. The curing healthcare provider is dedicated to the job and committed to making patients better in the name of science. However, this clinician is not willing to take the time necessary to get to know patients other than in the medical sense. This clinician makes no pretense to go beyond the science of curing. A contractual relationship is the norm, a business relationship the format. Thus, the patient who is ill seeks help; the physician offers assistance; a contract regarding the physicians' services is formed; the contract implies a successful outcome and does not allow for the possibility of failure.

2. *Curing healer:* This clinician has an empirical approach, devising new methods and new technologies and seeking new explanations for illness and disease processes. He or she has a concern for theory and, for the most part, is a futurist with a sense of empathy. This clinician is interested in alternative forms of medicine and is curious about their scientific merit.

3. *Caring healthcare provider:* This clinician is contemporary and a professional in the purest sense of the word. He or she has knowledge based on interactions and is driven by such. This clinician is academic and requires scientific evidence of benefit before using a particular therapy. He or she is caring but at times is uncomfortable with it. Science and technology take precedence over caring.

4. *Caring healer:* This clinician ensures patient comfort and dignity by emphasizing quality of life. He or she is a "classical" physician and promotes wholeness of being. The caring healer is much more personal than other physicians in his or her approach to the patient. The physician-patient relationship is not contractual, rather it is based on a patient who seeks help and a physician who is offering it. The relationship is built on trust, integrity, honesty, and respect. No success is guaranteed, although both the patient and the physician do their best in partnership to bring this success about. If the illness persists, there is no blame or fault. The physician and the patient together make an honest assessment of the outcome, and a decision is made.

Thus, value principles can identify the characteristics of the clinician. All four types of physicians may be acceptable, but most patients would prefer the caring healer. The patient must be able to be a partner with the caring healer in order for the relationship to work. Behavior on the part of both the physician and the patient will dictate the type of care given and received. The culture from which the patient and the physician come will also dictate the type of care given.

From the clinical perspective, humanizing technology begins with what type of clinician we are. We agree to do what we ought to do, not just what we can do.

RESPONSIBILITIES OF HIGH-TECH COMPANIES

In the world of medical technology, professional engineers and managers claim to make a contribution to medicine by developing technology that helps physicians and nurses care for patients. Physicians and nurses are the customers of the company. However, the high-tech companies that think this way have the wrong "customer" and, as a whole, contribute little to patient care. In developing technology, they ask physicians and nurses what their needs are. The company should be asking patients what their needs are. The author of a grade school mathematics book writes the textbook with the student in mind, taking into consideration the child's age, level of understanding, language skills, and needs. The author does not write the text for the teacher. The teacher is simply a user of the text. The author writes for the student. However, in medical technology today, the instrument is developed for the physician and the nurse, rather than the patient. Rather than develop technology to fit the patient's needs, the patient is required to fit technology's mold.

The process of humanizing technology should start by recognizing the patient as the person for whom technology is used. If we agree that technology can directly affect a patient's comfort, dignity, and autonomy, we should consider the patient as the center of technology.

In the evolution of critical care, the emphasis has been on technology and practices of care rather than on the patient-physician relationship—that is, cure over care. The use of technology emphasizes cure at the expense of care. There should be a balance between cure and care so that the patient knows that, although technology is helping with more accurate monitoring and diagnosis, the patient can trust and rely on the physician for care. Present assessment of technology focuses primarily on the consequences or effects of human actions rather than on the virtues of moral agents or on actions in accordance with a moral rule.[24] Because clinicians are moral agents of their patients, they are required to approach their patients humanely. Technology has forced depersonalization and has desensitized clinicians to the needs of their patients.

In the past, physicians had few effective means of treatment. The best they could do was to comfort the patient and wait for the disease to run its course. The physician's patience, compassion, and faith in his role served to comfort and heal the sick. In ancient times, the patient was cared for by someone who served. As far as we know, the first physicians may have been priests. As humans acquired knowledge, mystique became fact and physicians were born. But faith in the healer's skills persisted.

Technology has forced the art of healing to become the business of cure. Seneca recognized this phenomenon years ago: "If therefore, a physician does nothing more than feel my pulse . . . instructing me what to do and what to avoid without any feeling, I owe him nothing more than his fee, because he does not see me as his friend, but as a client."[25]

High-tech companies and clinicians alike should consider patient-centered care as a stepping stone to a more sound foundation of human-centered care. By looking at patients as humans, we will be reminded of our intentions—humane caring.

CONCLUSION

Technology affects human values (including respect for the worth of other human beings). It has taken the burden of caring off of clinicians' backs and minds. Clinicians should be bothered by this.

In each complex, critically ill patient, several pathogenic processes may be present—each having its own likelihood of resulting in death and its own probability of reversal with critical care support. Faced with a choice between using technology and using compassion to treat these pathogenic processes, we strive to find a balance between the two. Technology is supposed to minister to human needs. Instead, addictive as it is, it tends to dominate patient care. The patient becomes the object of technology.

In medicine today, we have assumed incorrectly that technology implies better patient outcomes and that healthcare providers and patients need technology. In fact, technology may compromise patient outcomes by prolonging illness and death. In addition, clinicians and patients do not necessarily need technology. Sometimes technology simply allows the clinician and the patient to work more closely together in the healing process. Technology has become a way of life. The critical care unit should not be expected to be a high-tech setting, but rather it should be a haven in which humane care is delivered.

High-tech companies need to accept the responsibility for the appropriate development of technology. They should be looking at "caring principles." Are they doing what they *should* be doing, or are they limiting their efforts by what they *can* do? Are they focusing on the development of optimal solutions or of simply alternative solutions? They need to work with physicians to define optimal clinical outcomes.

There can be intellectual confusion and the misapplication of technology, especially in the transfer of technology to developing countries. These developing countries often find that the use of sophisticated technologies may conflict with the country's cultural and societal values. The level of technology should parallel the level of medical sophistication.

Who is to construct the technological environment and to what end? Who will use a technology and to what end? Individual physicians practice in accordance with a set of caring values that direct their character and practice style. However, technology has had a direct effect on physicians' values by its capacity for creating new opportunities and for making possible what was not possible before. It offers new options to choose from. We must be careful not to allow our principles to be replaced by utility.

It is the responsibility of healthcare providers to ensure the appropriate use of technology by education, by providing appropriate levels of technology to meet the patient's needs, and by understanding that technology reflects human power and also weakness. In trying to solve the technological problems facing us, we should turn to the things we do best. We should play from strength, and our strength is based on our character and principles as physicians. Humanism should be our primary emphasis.

This chapter closes with a list of questions. By addressing these questions, clinicians will force the issue of humanizing technology.

- Just because we are capable of using a high-tech intervention, should we?
- Who should control emerging technology—high-tech companies, clinicians, patients, or society?
- What types of studies are necessary to validate a particular technology's usefulness?

- What type of informed consent is necessary for the use of technology?
- Do clinicians have an obligation to inform their patients about uncertainty of the benefits of a particular technology?

Technology reflects human power and weaknesses, and its use necessitates a relationship of mutual trust and respect between physician and patient.[26] In short, we need to rethink the kind of physician we really want to be. We need to ask ourselves who we are from the patient's point of view. We need to ask who we are in relationship to our patients. We need to identify technological "abuse." We must find a balance between high-tech and high-touch care. We must ensure that patients, and not high-technology companies or clinicians, drive technology. We need to cure; but, foremost, we need to care.

NOTES

1. E.D. Robin, "The Harm That Medicine Does: Iatroepidemics," in *Matters of Life and Death: Risks versus Benefits of Medical Care* (New York: W.H. Freeman, 1984), 65-86.

2. R.H. Merritt, "Technology," in *Microsoft Encarta Interactive Encyclopedia* (Philadelphia: Funk & Wagnall's Corporation, 1993).

3. Committee on the Life Sciences and Social Policy, National Research Council, *Assessing Biomedical Technologies: An Inquiry Into the Nature of the Process* (Washington, D.C.: National Academy of Sciences, 1975).

4. H.V. Fineberg, "Technology Assessment: Motivation, Capability, and Future Directions," *Medical Care*, 23, no. 5 (1985): 663-71; H.D. Banta and S.B. Thacker, "The Case for Reassessment of Health Care Technology," *Journal of the American Medical Association* 264 no. 2 (1990): 235-40; B. Littenberg, "Technology Assessment in Medicine," *Academic Medicine* 67 no. 7 (1992): 424-28; R.N. Battista, "Health Care Technology Assessment: Linking Science and Policy-Making," *Canadian Medical Association Journal* 146 no. 4 (1992): 461-62.

5. S.J. Reiser, *Medicine in the Reign of Technology* (Cambridge, England: Cambridge University Press, 1978), 175.

6. E.J. Cassell, "The Sorcerer's Broom: Medicine's Rampant Technology," *Hastings Center Report* 23, no. 6 (1990): 32-39.

7. G.A. Diamond and T.A. Denton, "Alternative Perspectives on the Biased Foundations of Medical Technology Assessment," *Annals of Internal Medicine* 118, no. 6 (1993): 455-64.

8. F. Vilardell, "Ethical Problems of Medical Technology," *Bulletin of PAHO* 24, no. 4 (1990): 379-85.

9. G.V. Vimpani, "Resource Allocation in Contemporary Paediatrics: The Case Against High Technology," *Journal of Paediatric Child Health* 27 (1991):

354-59.

10. A. Castiglioni, "The Seventeenth Century," in *A History of Medicine,* ed. E.B. Krumbhaar (New York: Alfred A. Knopf, 1958): 504-77.

11. J. La Mettrie, *L'Homme Machine: A Study in the Origins of an Idea* (Princeton, N.J.: Princeton University Press, 1960).

12. *Stedman's Medical Dictionary*, 22nd ed. (Baltimore, Md.: Williams & Wilkins, 1972).

13. Ibid.

14. S.W. Mitchell, "The History of Instrumental Precision in Medicine," *Boston Medical and Surgical Journal* 125, no. 31 (1891): 309-16.

15. See note 5 above.

16. Banta and Thacker, "Case for Reassessment," see note 4 above.

17. D.G. Jones, "Medicine's Future: Technology or a Person-Centered Profession?" *Humane Medicine* 8, no. 1 (1992): 50-55.

18. H.S. Friedman, "Too Much Medicine," *Humane Medicine* 4, no. 2 (1988): 116-17.

19. P. Lain-Entralgo, *Doctor and Patient* (New York: McGraw-Hill Book Company, 1969).

20. H. Nouwen, *Out of Solitude* (Notre Dame, Ind.: Ave Maria Press, 1974).

21. *Webster's Ninth New Collegiate Dictionary* (Springfield, Mass.: Merriam-Webster, 1985), 207.

22. S. Hauerwas, "Virtue and Character," in *Encyclopedia of Bioethics,* ed. W.T. Reich (New York: Macmillan, 1995), 2525-32.

23. E.D. Pellegrino, "Educating the Humanist Physician: An Ancient Ideal Reconsidered," *Journal of the American Medical Association* 227 (1974): 1288-94.

24. L. Walters, "The Concept of Technology Assessment," in *Encyclopedia of Bioethics,* ed. W.T. Reich (New York: Macmillan, 1995), 1650-54.

25. L.A. Seneca, *De Beneficiis* (Cambridge, Mass.: Harvard University Press, 1964).

26. E.D. Pellegrino and J. Carroll, "The Four Principles and the Doctor-Patient Relationship: The Need for a Better Linkage," in *Principles of Health Care Ethics,* ed. R. Gillon (New York: John Wiley & Sons, 1994), 353-65.

14

Emotion and Moral Decision Making in Critical Care Medicine: An E-Mail Correspondence about Hope

Evan G. DeRenzo

Dear Peter,

Thank you for agreeing to think through this case with me. (How did we ever manage before e-mail?) I've been asked to present it for our ethics grand rounds next month—not because it is so unusual, but rather because this is a paradigmatic case.

As I mentioned when I saw you at the New York meeting, this patient was in our ICU for a long time. The facts are as follows. (I'll change the names and enough of the details that you can use the case for your own teaching, if you'd like.)

Mr. Smith was a 61-year-old, white male who came to us, here at ——— University Research Center, in June 1997. Approximately one year earlier, he had undergone abdominoperineal resection and placement of an Infusaid pump for rectal cancer with hepatic metastases. During the procedure, the surgical team noted four lesions, primarily in the right lobe of the liver. He was treated for nine months with chemotherapy and initially responded. His liver disease, however, recurred after six months of therapy. Careful restaging indicated that the patient had no evidence of other sites of metastatic disease. The only evident lesions were the original four tumors in the right lobe of his liver. These had increased in size.

The patient was referred to us for exploratory laparotomy in contemplation of hepatic resection or possible hepatic perfusion based on intraoperative findings. During the procedure, the surgical team found no evidence of extrahepatic disease in any site. There were only four lesions in the right lobe. There was substantial scarring in the porta hepatis from the patient's therapy with the pump, but no evidence of malignant adenopathy. At the completion of the right lobe liver resection, the margin appeared grossly uninvolved with tumor. In sum, his surgeons here considered him to be cancer free.

However, the patient never regained strength or recovered from the surgery. For the first two weeks following the procedure, an occupational therapist was working with him on the ward to help him with ADLs—activities of daily living—particularly mobility, self-care, and endurance. During this period the patient was alert, oriented, and motivated to—as he put it—"exercise my arms and legs so I can go home." But he was never able to maintain even an upright sitting position because of ascites, and his stamina never improved.

During the third week following surgery, the patient's nurse found him comatose, and he was transferred to the ICU. Although his mental status cleared somewhat and he responded to questions in a manner that seemed appropriate, he was not stable enough to leave the unit. Ten days later, he went into respiratory distress and required intubation. By this time he was unresponsive except to grimace in response to needle sticks or when being turned. Although he was severely weakened, his liver and kidneys still functioned. Then, all of a sudden, his kidneys shut down.

On a Friday night, the surgeon told the patient's wife that her husband might not make it through the weekend and that she should call in the rest of the family. In the same breath, he started talking to her about the possible need for dialysis. She declined to discuss much of anything with him until her eldest son arrived the next day.

I'll stop here for now. Is this enough medical information to give you a picture of the patient and his medical status?

Thanks,
Evan

Dear Peter,

Good. Now, to the ethical questions. Because no one from the bio-ethics department participates in surgery department rounds anymore, we did not know that this case was brewing. By the time I was paged, it was late Monday afternoon; the family meeting with the patient's wife, his children (all adult), the surgeon, primary nurse, unit head nurse, and social worker was scheduled for noon the next day.

When the page came in from Mr. Smith's primary nurse, she explained the details and stated that the family was tired and disheartened. She reported that the family did not want to continue aggressive intervention but that the surgeon was presenting dialysis and insertion of a feeding tube as the next appropriate steps. A DNR order had been entered into the patient's chart.

Also, the nurse informed me that the patient's advance directives were noted on his chart and that they were unambiguous. The wife was his durable power of attorney for healthcare, and the patient had indicated in writing that he did not want heroic measures if he were dying. The nurse asked if I would attend the family meeting. After saying that I would, I asked if the surgeon knew that the nurse had called and invited me. She indicated that he did.

The next day, I met with the patient's wife and children before the family meeting. They are lovely people. Mrs. Smith had been here the whole time, and her two sons and three daughters had been driving back and forth regularly. As you know, we are located in the southern tip of the state. The patient's family lives way up north. It's either a long drive or an expensive airplane trip for them, but they came back and forth almost once a week.

These are decent, down-to-earth people. They are deeply religious but not rigid or fanatical. They were appropriately hopeful at the outset but, at the same time, reasonable and realistic. Mr. Smith was a firefighter until he had to retire on disability about a year and a half ago. From what I gather, he has always been a straightforward person, he and his wife have had a loving and uncomplicated relationship, and the siblings are close to one another and to their parents. The nurses told me that this was one of the easiest families with whom they had ever worked. Although medically unsophisticated, each family member is thoughtful and caring. They communicated clearly among themselves and with the staff. Also, they told me in no uncertain terms that, from the time Mr. Smith was diagnosed, he had been very open about anticipating that the cancer would kill him and about not wanting to be sustained on machines beyond the point at which his disease could be reversed or halted.

Are the ethical issues beginning to emerge?

As always,
Evan

Dear Peter,

Yes, you have it. The physician was consciously basing what he thought he ought to do on his understanding of the principle of beneficence, the maxim to err on the side of life and on what he saw as his duties and obligations to act in the best interest of his patient. His recommendations, however, and the developing problems in communication with the family were generated out of a much more complex, subtle, and subconscious process. In short, I think the primary ethical issue was that the physician's emotions, primarily hope that he could save this man's life, clouded his judgment about when it was time to let the patient die. In the language of the Hippocratic corpus, the doctor's emotions had blinded him to the fact that the disease had overmastered the patient.

Because this emotional reaction was invisible (at least initially) to everyone, the surgeon was confident that he had his medical "facts" right and kept insisting that the patient would improve if they just did this or that procedure. The family, however, began questioning his accuracy in assessing what was happening with the patient. The seeds of distrust took root quickly.

Thanks,
Evan

Dear Peter,

You are right. The obvious analysis is the language of futility.[1] I shall take your advice and make some brief remarks in that direction at the beginning of grand rounds. Discussion of emotion in moral decision making is so alien, and perhaps discomforting, to the audience that failing to address futility could give them the opportunity to dismiss all of the talk on the grounds that I missed the point. But the weakness of the futility discussions is that they only address what I call first-line issues. Focusing on the disagreements about what constitutes medical futility allows the underlying emotions that drive these disagreements to go unaddressed.

The heart of the matter is your comment that this experienced surgeon should have known that the patient had entered into what you call "the complication cascade that terminates in death." This surgeon is world renowned for salvaging seemingly unsalvageable cases. To accept the patients he does, he has to have an inordinate degree of confidence in his skills and training. He is not arrogant. He is just very good at what he does and has a career's worth of experience in saving patients in the face of seemingly insurmountable odds. When you bounce that against the backboard of a man whose basic emotional response is one of hopefulness and optimism, you have the recipe for this kind of case.

Yours,
Evan

Dear Peter,

Your example is excellent. Of course the well-established caveat about doctors treating their own family members will be a familiar anchor for the proposition that being emotionally attached to someone can cloud one's judgment. Your comment—that, although the potential for problems in treating family members is well-recognized within the medical profession, physicians have not extended that awareness to emotional attachments to unrelated patients—is intriguing. It is a point that relates directly to the deterioration in communication between the doctor and family in this case. Because the doctor and the family were strangers, the physician did not notice the subtle signs that his views were beginning to be questioned within the family. This lack of awareness relates also to the interplay of the surgeon's emotions with his cognitive processing of the medical data.

Sincerely,
Evan

Dear Peter,

The distrust of the surgeon was never about his surgical skills or his sincerity in caring about the patient, but about the veracity of his assessment of the patient's prognosis. With the exception of one son, the entire family started feeling that the doctor was misreading the medical facts about the patient and was being overly optimistic. Because of their growing lack of confidence in the surgeon's ability to see that Mr. Smith was really dying, they started to think the surgeon was, as the wife said to me in our very first conversation, "doing a fancy sales job" on them.

Yours,
Evan

Dear Peter,

It sounds like you have the picture. Given that this is an oncologic surgeon and this patient was apparently cancer free, it made no medical sense that the patient was declining. Your comments about the specialization of medicine[2] and the discomforts of uncertainty[3] are particularly apt here. Not knowing why a patient is deteriorating when, by all counts, the surgery was successful and the patient seems cancer free, is frustrating. Staying focused on the patient's organs, rather than the patient more broadly, may reduce the surgeon's own emotional discomfort with death.

Nonetheless, the family saw the patient continue to get worse. It did not matter to them that he technically was cancer free. All that mattered to them was that, over a period of many weeks, the patient's body parts were failing, he was no longer able to move or talk, and the physician was not acknowledging the decline. This discrepancy between what the physician said and what the family saw was consistent with a review article about communication between doctor and family in oncology.[4] (This article reported that in the majority of 200 studies reviewed, families' assessments of patients' status were less optimistic than physicians' assessments.)

Because of what the Smith family interpreted as mixed signals, mistrust of the surgeon is growing. The nurses feel trapped (as usual) between the patient's family and the physician. Also, nurses observed the first signs of bickering among the siblings, and between one of the children and their mother, about what should be done.

The youngest son (age 24), the sibling who lived the farthest from his parents and who was the least far along in establishing his own family and career, was the one who seemed to put the most confidence in the surgeon's encouragement. According to the nurses, after the family talked with the surgeon, the family (except for this one son) would say to one another and to the nurses that they could no longer understand the physician. Family members said that what the surgeon was saying to them made sense when he said it; after he was gone, however, they would think about it, look at their husband and father, and realize that what the doctor had just said made no sense at all. Worse still, the youngest son was growing hostile, making comments like, "You all don't know anything. You're not the doctor. It's the doctor who knows and he says if we just give it more time Dad will be okay."

Peter, please let me know what you think so far.

Thanks,
Evan

Dear Peter,

Yes, it does seem that this case represents the long-standing problem created by Western philosophic tradition's insistence on separating reason and emotion in ethical decision making. Although a lengthy discussion of Greek philosophy at grand rounds will put the audience to sleep, a very brief introduction should be acceptable.

It is necessary for physicians to understand that Western philosophy has taught us to be suspicious of our emotions. Classical Western thought is grounded in a rationalist approach to making moral judgments. That is, Western intellectual tradition teaches that persons make moral decisions by dint of reason and that emotion only serves to compromise rationality.

For example, Aristotle taught that, as the acorn's function is to mature into a tree, the proper function of human beings is to exercise their capacity to reason rationally. The view that emotion only mucks up the works has continued to this day. Little more than a decade ago, Feinberg said, "Arguments are one thing, sentiments another, and nothing fogs the mind so thoroughly as emotion."[5]

Recently, however, there has been a growing challenge to this dichotomy. Callahan has proposed a model in which there is a mutual interaction between thinking and feeling in coming to moral judgments.[6] She states: "Certainly, reason should monitor reason as in traditional philosophical critiques, and reason should tutor the emotions as in Feinberg's model. But I would also claim that emotion should tutor reason and that emotions should monitor emotion. The ideal goal is to come to an ethical decision through a personal equilibrium in which emotion and reason are both activated and in accord."[7]

Her proposal makes good sense. But it will be an uphill battle to bring such thinking into mainstream ethics conversation and even harder to integrate such notions into the decision-making practice of scientifi-cally minded physicians. The problem of why feeling has been the lesser half of thinking is made even more difficult when considered in the con-text of deeply held notions of gender distinctions.[8]

Although saying so may cause me to lose my audience to reflexive resistance, the feminist philosophers have made us aware that the human world is divided into two—men who think and women who feel—which is why feeling has been relegated to the back seat. Historically, philoso-phers have subscribed to the position that women could not reason mor-ally because their feelings clouded their ability to think. In his theory of virtue, Aristotle states that virtuous (free) men think and behave in ways required for freedom and political life; however, virtuous women lack the mental machinery, and instead they are submissive and silent.[9] Rousseau, too, clearly differentiated between the genders.[10]

Many other influential Western moral theorists—including Kant, Aquinas, Hegel, Nietzsche, and Sartre—thought women had a signifi-cantly different character from men that caused in their inferiority in moral reasoning. All these philosophers viewed women as too focused on the particular to be able to generalize abstractly.[11]

To focus the thinking-feeling dichotomy only on Western philoso-phers, however, misses the scope of the problem. The scientific study of emotion has lagged far behind other areas of neuroscience. The sorry state of the art was best summed up by LeDoux:

> Despite the obvious importance of emotion to human existence, sci-entists concerned with human nature have not been able to reach a consensus about what emotion is and what place emotion should have in a theory of mind and behavior. Controversy abounds over the definition of emotion, the number of emotions that exist, whether some emotions are more basic than others, the commonality of cer-tain emotional response patterns across cultures and across species, whether different emotions have different physiological signatures, the extent to which emotional responses contribute to emotional experiences, the role of nature and nurture in emotion, the influence of emotion on cognitive processes, the dependence of emotion on cognition, the importance of conscious versus unconscious processes in emotion, and on and on.[12]

Long-winded as he may be, he is correct. There are few data to help us think about how emotion and cognition come together in the domain of moral decision making. The field of psychology, especially, must apply its scientific tools to this task. According to Callahan:

> Psychology and philosophy must complement each other in the study of morality, for it is the whole person who reasons and accepts or rejects moral arguments. When psychology has wrongly ignored the real power of free, rational moral agency and the force of reasoning and philosophical justifications in decision making, it has misread human experience. Similarly, an exclusive focus upon analytic methods of rational moral decision making and the content of arguments wrongly ignores the self who is inevitably informed and shaped by emotions, tacit personal knowledge, intuition, imagery, developmental history, and group experience. Either way, grave distortions appear. Taking account of the full range of human capacities is necessary to adequately understand and map moral functioning.[13]

That is not to say, however, that psychology is the only relevant discipline. With the explosion of work in the neurosciences, one would expect more research investigating interactions between cognitive and emotional functions in the brain.[14]

The recently published book by Antonio Damasio may move the field along.[15] Damasio, who chairs the Department of Neurology at the University of Iowa's Medical School, brings the relevant neuroscience literature together. He states at the outset that his purpose in writing the book is "to propose that reason may not be as pure as most of us think it is or wish it were, that emotions and feelings may not be intruders in the bastion of reason at all: they may be enmeshed in its networks, for worse and for better."[16] His hypothesis is "that certain aspects of the process of emotion and feeling are indispensable for rationality. At their best, feelings point us in the proper direction, take us to the appropriate place in a decision-making space, where we may put the instruments of logic to good use. . . . Emotion and feeling, along with the covert physiological machinery underlying them, assist us with the daunting task of predicting an uncertain future and planning our actions accordingly."[17]

Damasio comes to this postulate by way of his life's work of caring for and studying patients with brain injury. Through the course of this work, some of which he describes vividly in his book, he has come to recognize that brain-damaged patients can have their "cognitive" apparatus intact, but if the parts of their brains that are damaged impair the parts that allow for human emotion, the patient's ability to think (and thereby act) "rationally" will be severely diminished or completely obliterated.

Damasio builds his novel analysis through cases. First is the historical case of Phineas P. Gage. Many at grand rounds will remember this case in which the 25-year-old Gage, a construction foreman, had an iron rod passed through his head during an accidental explosion. The wound healed, but Gage, who seemed rational throughout the event and recovery, changed from a stable, happy man of sound judgment to a cranky, belligerent, emotionally unstable person within weeks after the injury. Damasio reports on a case in which he was involved, which he refers to as a "modern Gage." This is a case of a man named Elliot who, as a result of a benign brain tumor, changed from being a good husband and father with a responsible job to a man who could no longer act responsibly in any venue. Although Elliot presented as coherent and smart and with his memory intact, his judgment and free will were so lacking that he was no longer able to function effectively as a social being.

Damasio supports his novel analysis by marshaling the relevant neuroscience research in a thoroughly coherent and cogent manner. He synthesizes work on brain-body interaction; organism-environment interaction; neural system development and architecture; and forming, storing, and retrieving perceptual images. If he is correct and the neuroscience research progresses sufficiently to support his hypothesis to the satisfaction of scientist and philosopher alike, we may have an important paradigm shift in both philosophy and medicine. We may be approaching that critical mass of new evidence needed to push the ancient paradigm that feeling is the enemy of thinking over the edge.[18]

Do you think this tack will be productive at ethics grand rounds?

Sincerely,
Evan

Dear Peter,

Thanks for being diplomatic. Perhaps it would be interesting to the audience to include a literary illustration of how entrenched the notion is that thinking is good and feeling is bad. Tom Stoppard's play, *Arcadia*, makes just this point. *Arcadia* is about the discomforts people feel when they are forced to admit to the messiness of life. The play pits the symmetries of Newtonian geometry against the asymmetries of chaos theory, played out in the context of the development of English landscape architecture. According to the play, English gardens were neatly laid out in rows prior to the 1750s. But the English garden evolved more naturally, seemingly growing wild. In the play, Hanna, a historian of old English gardens, characterizes this transformation as "the decline from thinking to feeling."

That rather sums up the commonly held view that if we admit that our emotions enter into and contribute to the shaping of our thinking, then somehow the quality of our thoughts and our actions—and, in the case of our ICU patient, the quality of his care—are somehow diminished or threatened. Why can't it be just the reverse? That is, we must learn to become comfortable with our emotions, recognizing that they help us focus on the morally important aspects of patient care.

Sidney Callahan addresses this point explicitly, reminding us that one simply cannot answer the moral questions merely by reference to the scientific data.

> Conscience is integrated, self-committed, conscious activity oriented to moral values and moral standards of the right and the good. Our personal, self-committed acts of conscience are pursuing the right and good thing to do, what we morally ought to do and what morally ought to be. Such acts cannot be equated with knowing or deciding upon the facts of a case, the most efficient or profitable solution to a problem, or even some aesthetic valuation of beauty. We cannot decide how we morally ought to act by appealing to science, economics, biology, aesthetics, etiquette, custom, law, or existing social conventions. Many kinds of active inquiry and pursuits of knowledge and facts may help us to morally decide, but they cannot finally settle a moral question of conscience.[19]

Callahan goes to the core of the case at hand. It was a matter of conscience to Mr. Smith's physician to try every possible technical fix to keep this patient alive, now that he was seemingly cured of his original terminal condition. Although the surgeon thought he was basing his recommendations strictly on the medical facts, his recommendations were coming, instead, from his deeply held (and not necessarily inappropriate) belief that he must do everything in his power to sustain the patient's life. This physician confused having appropriately felt moral distress (a notion that ethicist Christine Grady speaks of regularly) with having a *bona fide* moral dilemma.

There never really was any moral dilemma at all. This family's primary guiding value was to have their husband and father get better, if that was reasonably possible. If not, then they wanted to make certain that he died comfortably and was not sustained by machinery for days and weeks on end. The family was in full agreement on that point, and their intentions were consistent with the patient's wishes as expressed in his advance directive documentation and numerous conversations with family members before he became incapacitated. It was only around the interpretation of how reasonably possible it was going to be for Mr. Smith to get better that there was any disagreement.

Thanks,
Evan

Dear Peter,

You are right, again. I need to explain more about the family dynamics. Although I think that the physician genuinely believed that the patient had a good chance of turning around, the youngest son, it seems to me, was desperate and terrified of losing his father. The physician's authentically felt hopefulness was feeding the son's seemingly unhealthy emotional response to his father's impending death. Here, the son's behavior is a good example of where some kinds and some expressions of emotion are not particularly helpful in the decision-making process.

As I told the patient's wife, I believe that the physician was, unconsciously, ignoring the patient's terminal decline. The youngest son, because he so intensely wanted to believe that the physician's evaluation was right, contributed to the physician's positive interpretation of the medical data by affirming the physician's recommendations for continued aggressive intervention.

Although I accept that it may be necessary for physicians who regularly work with critically ill patients to be particularly hopeful and optimistic persons, we need to learn how to manage that hopefulness better. Just like medication dosages that must often be titrated in highly refined fashion, so too must we learn how to titrate hope and the full range of our emotional responses to pain, suffering, and death.[20]

Roger Bone makes this plea far more eloquently than I ever could.[21] In an article written just before his own death from metastatic renal carcinoma, after an approximately three-year course with the disease, he instructs: "As physicians, we must never give our patients false hopes or unrealistic expectations."[22] Instead he believes we can balance the truth of impending death with appropriately focused hope. "What I have learned, in other words," he says, "is that acceptance and denial can coexist."[23] Although such balancing takes consummate communication skills as well as an awareness of one's own intensely felt emotions in the face of another human's death, we can and must get better at the task.

What do you think? Am I expecting too much?

Thanks,
Evan

Dear Peter,

Yes, even if it is within human capability to have denial and acceptance coexist, it will be difficult to teach physicians how to do it themselves or how to help their patients do it. In 1959 Karl Menninger called on his colleagues to try, and I guess we are not much further along.[24] In giving what was called the "Academic Lecture" at the annual meeting of the American Psychiatric Association, he spoke on the topic of teaching young psychiatrists how to be appropriately hopeful. He told the audience that he had been at first startled to find no entry on *hope* in the *Encyclopaedia Britannica* but that, upon further reflection, he realized that the omission was consistent with his own tendency to avoid consideration of the topic—a resistance he was now reversing. He recounted his change of heart as follows: "Time was when for this occasion I should have chosen as my subject 'Love' or 'Hate' or 'Conflict' or 'Instinct' or 'Sublimation' or 'Symptom Formation' but never such a thing as 'Hope.' It seems almost to be a tabooed topic, a personal matter, scarcely appropriate for public discussion. And yet . . . if we dare to hope, should we not dare to look at ourselves hoping?"[25]

Although psychiatrists may be more introspective than surgeons, most persons can learn to be more attentive to their own emotional reactions. One just needs to accept the need to do so. In medicine, especially with critically ill patients, the need to do so is great if we are to deliver the best that modern medicine has to offer.

If physicians take seriously the age-old medical ethics principle to do no harm, they can learn to think about the application of that principle more broadly. Harm is not only physical, but also psychological and emotional and spiritual. When any psychiatrist, surgeon, or other physician makes recommendations colored by the emotional and moral filters each of us always carries, without being consciously aware that such filters exist, the risk of harm is great. Patients and families, vulnerable from their own hopes and fears, are easily confused—or worse, manipulated—to do things that might not be consistent with their wishes or be in their best interest. If, however, physicians learn how to recognize and modulate their own emotions better—including hope—they will be better at separating their own emotional reactions from those of their patients, thereby reducing or avoiding the occurrence of harm.

The requirement to separate one's own emotional needs from those of one's patients or clients is emphasized in the training of psychiatrists. It needs to become part of the training of all physicians.

As always,
Evan

Dear Peter,

I am going to conclude ethics grand rounds with some practical suggestions. When it comes to recognizing how and when our emotions are involved, I am going to suggest that, for each recommendation, the physician (or nurse or social worker) ask him- or herself: "In addition to the medical data as I interpret them, why do I think this is the best recommendation?" If one then keeps asking "Why?" of every subsequent answer, one ultimately reaches the emotion imbedded in the recommendation.

I am going to suggest following each recommendation to the patient or family with, "My hope in making this recommendation is that it will permit the patient to . . ." and then fill in the blank. By phrasing it just this way, one has forced oneself to shape hopefulness realistically.

This process addresses the concern raised by Kodish and Post that

> Physician reluctance to disclose a grim prognosis may be related to discomfort with putting odds on longevity, recurrence and cure. Treatments may be recommended with few details as to probabilities of success, and definitions of what a "successful" outcome might be are often left vague. While this reluctance to communicate prognosis may be based on the desire to foster hope in the patient, there may be three important additional factors.

First, caution regarding specific prognostic disclosure may be based in the difference between prognosis and prediction. . . . Second, data suggest that oncologists themselves may have inconsistent perceptions of therapeutic benefits, generally overestimating the proven benefits of chemotherapy. . . . Finally, doctors may allow their own hope for a good outcome for the patient to influence the dialogue.[26]

Chronic disinclination to use explicit language allows the physician's (natural) emotional discomfort with death, and hopefulness about holding it at bay, to obscure the reality of the patient's condition. Clearly that is what is going on with Mr. Smith's surgeon.

Yours,
Evan

Dear Peter,

Now to conclude Mr. Smith's case. The family meeting occurred, and went well. The surgeon agreed to wean the patient from the ventilator with the intention of having the patient be able to speak and tell us what his wishes were. Everyone agreed that the weaning process would not start until the patient's other children could return, which they did late that night. The next morning, the patient was successfully weaned.

About 24 hours after the patient was weaned, I was paged by the unit nursing staff. The surgeon had written a reintubation order, if needed, on the chart. I paged the physician. We had a lengthy and reasonably comfortable discussion, during which he told me that of course he would not reintubate within a context of general organ system failure; however, if the patient were up and walking around and developed pneumonia, then under such conditions the surgeon considered it appropriate and morally necessary to reintubate.

It was painfully obvious that this physician was unable to accept that there was no realistic hope that this patient was going to get better. It was unnecessary for me to force the issue, because the patient died within the next 24 hours. But it amazed me that this surgeon could be so unable to verbalize his emotional distress over the patient's impending death and his unwillingness to loosen his grip on the theoretical possibility that a miracle was going to take place.

I am sure you see why this case has been selected for presentation at our ethics grand rounds. Any last thoughts?

As always,
Evan

Dear Peter,

Thank you for all your help on this case. Yes, I think I'm ready for the talk. And I have decided on how I shall close it. I am going to end with a quote from an article by Roger Bone. After being diagnosed with his kidney cancer, he wrote several articles in a series entitled "A Piece of My Mind" in the *Journal of the American Medical Association,* as he experienced his own terminal illness. In his last article he wrote: "Finally, I have come to believe that clinicians must learn to discuss issues of life and death. We are so involved with the scientific that we may unconsciously ignore the dying part of living. Those caring for the dying patient should be less concerned with terminal mechanical ventilation and more concerned with helping him or her find the peace that can come well before the final moments."[27]

Bone gracefully moves his colleagues away from practice that acknowledges only thinking toward practice that incorporates feeling and retains hope for a good end. In so doing, Bone teaches his colleagues that emotion and reason are partners in moral decision making in medicine. He teaches us all that we must end the war between emotion and reason.

Again, many thanks for your time and assistance.

Sincerely,
Evan

ACKNOWLEDGMENT

The author wishes to thank Peter A.F. Morrin, MD, of Kingston, Ontario, Canada, for serving as an imaginary e-mail partner, and for the thoughtful and detailed review of earlier drafts of this chapter provided by Morrin and Christine Grady, PhD, Department of Clinical Ethics, National Institutes of Health.

The ideas and opinions expressed in this chapter are those of the author only and do not represent any position or policy of the National Institutes of Health, any other federal agency, or any other institution or organization with which she is affiliated.

NOTES

1. D.P. Sulmasy, "Futility and the Varieties of Medical Judgment," *Theoretical Medicine* 18, nos. 1-2 (1997): 63-78.

2. M. Foucault, *The Birth of the Clinic: An Archaeology of Medical Perception*, trans. A.M.S. Smith (New York: Random House, 1973).

3. P.L. Bernstein, *Against the Gods: The Remarkable Story of Risk* (New York: John Wiley & Sons, 1996).

4. P.G. Northouse and L.L. Northouse, "Communication and Cancer: Issues Confronting Patients, Health Professionals, and Family Members," *Journal of Psychosocial Oncology* 5, no. 3 (1988): 17-46.

5. J. Feinberg, "Sentiment and Sentimentality in Practical Ethics" (Presidential Address delivered before American Philosophical Association, Sacramento, Calif., 26 March 1982), as cited in S. Callahan, "The Role of Emotion in Ethical Decisionmaking," *Hastings Center Report* (June-July 1988): 9.

6. S. Callahan, *In Good Conscience: Reason and Emotion in Moral Decision Making* (New York: HarperCollins, 1991).

7. Ibid., 9.

8. S.M. Wolf, *Feminism and Bioethics: Beyond Reproduction* (New York: Oxford University Press, 1996); A. Kesselman, L.D. McNair, and N. Schniedewind, *Women: Images and Realities* (Mountain View, Calif.: Mayfield, 1995); E. Fantham, *Women in the Classical World: Image and Text* (New York: Oxford University Press, 1994).

9. E.V. Spelman, *Inessential Woman: Problems of Exclusion in Feminist Thought* (Boston: Beacon Hill, 1988).

10. M. Canovan, "Rousseau's Two Concepts of Citizenship," in *Women in Western Political Thought*, ed. E. Kennedy and S. Mendus (Brighton, England: Wheatsheaf Books, 1987), 86-87.

11. S. Sherwin, *No Longer Patient: Feminist Ethics and Health Care* (Philadelphia: Temple University Press, 1992).

12. J.E. LeDoux, "Emotion: Clues from the Brain," *Annual Review of Psychology* 46 (1995): 209-35, p. 209.

13. See note 5 above, p. 6.

14. J.E. Le Doux and J. Muller, "Emotional Memory and Psychopathology," *Philosophical Transactions of the Royal Society of London. Series B: Biological Sciences* 352, no. 1362 (1997): 1719-26.

15. A.R. Damasio, *Descartes' Error: Emotion, Reason, and the Human Brain* (New York: G.P. Putnam's Sons, 1987).

16. Ibid., xii.

17. Ibid., xiii.

18. J. Polkinghorne, *Beyond Science: The Wider Human Context* (New York: Cambridge University Press, 1996); T.S. Kuhn, *The Structure of Scientific Revolutions* (Chicago: University of Chicago Press, 1970).

19. See note 5 above, p. 17.

20. E. Kodish and S.G. Post, "Oncology and Hope," *Journal of Clinical Oncology* 13, no. 7 (1995): 1817-22.

21. R.C. Bone, "Benediction: A Farewell to My Medical Colleagues," *Journal of Critical Illness* 12, no. 7 (1997): 439-40.

22. Ibid., 439.

23. Ibid.

24. K. Menninger, "Hope," *American Journal of Psychiatry* 116 (1959): 481-91.

25. Ibid., 481.

26. See note 18 above, p. 1819.

27. R.C. Bone, "Lemonade: The Last Refreshing Taste," *Journal of the American Medical Association* 276, no. 15 (1996): 1216.

15

Legal Issues in Critical Care

Paul Greve, Jr.

INTRODUCTION

In the United States, the medical-legal aspects of critical care have been influenced by case law, legislation, regulation, and constitutional law. The courts and the legislatures, including Congress, have sought an appropriate framework of laws and legal principles to govern termination of treatment. Many of these cases and laws have come to fruition since the landmark 1976 New Jersey decision regarding patient Karen Ann Quinlan.[1]

This chapter is not intended to provide clinicians with black-and-white legal solutions to complex situations involving patient care. Instead, it provides a general legal framework for issues in critical care. It is important for clinicians to know all applicable local laws and to seek competent, practical legal advice when needed.

The starting point for clinicians in addressing legal issues in end-of-life decisions is that the patient's wishes regarding treatment should be given the greatest weight. To ignore a patient's wishes as previously expressed or as expressed by loved ones is counter to case law and creates the risk of litigation.[2] However, the number of reported liability cases involving treatment at the end of life is very small.[3] Courts have generally not been willing to impose liability for administering life-sustaining treatment against the patient's wishes.[4]

THE LEGAL FOUNDATIONS OF CRITICAL CARE LAW

CONSTITUTIONAL LAW

Many court decisions involving termination of treatment have been decided on the basis of the right of privacy and the common law right of self-determination,[5] which arises out of the doctrine of informed consent. Case law on termination of treatment has been premised on the common law right of privacy, the constitutional right of privacy, and as a liberty interest under the Fourteenth Amendment.[6] Common law addresses the right to be free from unconsented touching under the doctrine of informed consent.

The New Jersey Supreme Court in the landmark case, *In re Quinlan*, stated: "Although the Constitution does not explicitly mention a right of privacy, Supreme Court decisions have recognized that a right of personal privacy exists and that certain areas of privacy are guaranteed under the Constitution. . . . Presumably this right is broad enough to encompass a patient's decision to decline medical treatment under certain circumstances."[7]

In *Cruzan v. Director* (1990), the first right-to-die case to come before the U.S. Supreme Court, the Court framed its holding under the Fourteenth Amendment as a liberty interest rather than discussing a right of privacy.[8]

In *Cruzan* the court held that there is a constitutional right to refuse treatment premised on the Fourteenth Amendment's liberty guarantee. This is consistent with cases decided by the Supreme Court over the last 100 years: that patients have a constitutionally protected liberty interest in refusing unwanted medical treatment. Physicians are ethically and legally required to honor patient's wishes in this regard.

The court also concluded in the *Cruzan* case that the states have the right to set forth procedural safeguards to protect patients, such as Missouri's requiring clear and convincing evidence of an incompetent patient's wishes. Some state courts have cited both federal constitutional law and state constitutions as the basis for the right to die.[9]

Two United States Supreme Court decisions rendered on physician-assisted suicide in June 1997, *Washington v. Glucksberg*, and *Vacco v. Quill*, reaffirmed the right to refuse life-sustaining treatment.[10] In both cases, the Court upheld the distinction between withdrawing life-sustaining treatment and providing assistance with suicide. In issuing unanimous opinions, the Supreme Court held that there is no right to physician-assisted suicide. Because the Court did not find assisted suicide to be a constitutionally protected right, legislatures must decide its legality.

A discussion of physician-assisted suicide is outside the scope of this text. Of interest to critical care clinicians is the Supreme Court's statements in both cases supporting a patient's right to direct the withdrawal of life-sustaining treatment, although the justices may differ on the sources of law conferring that right. The justices stated that the right to refuse treatment is not absolute.[11]

In *Washington v. Glucksberg* and *Vacco v. Quill,* the Supreme Court decided against the right to assisted suicide but acknowledged the practice of prescribing high levels of sedation for the goal of achieving pain relief, even though the respiration of the patient may be compromised, possibly causing the patient's death.[12] This is known as the principle of double effect. The American Medical Association (AMA) describes this as a physician obligation: "to relieve pain and suffering and to provide effective palliative treatment even though it may foreseeably hasten death."[13]

In both cases, the Supreme Court discusses the state legislatures' clearly distinguishing between withdrawal of life-sustaining treatment and assisting suicide. The Court cites various state legislations that authorize palliative treatment which may hasten death.[14] A majority of the Justices concluded that states shall not enact barriers that prevent the availability of palliative care for terminally ill patients, "including the administration of drugs as need to avoid pain at the end of life."[15]

CASE LAW

Since the 1976 case of Karen Anne Quinlan, the clear trend in case law has been to respect the wishes of patients and their families regarding treatment at the end of life.[16] Furthermore, federal trial courts or state appellate courts in approximately half the states have now recognized the "right to die" premised on common law, state constitutional law, or the U.S. Constitution.[17]

STATE LEGISLATION

The states permit withdrawal of life-sustaining treatment through legislation. Legislation that affects critical care includes living-will statutes, natural death acts, do-not-resuscitate (DNR) statutes, surrogate/family decision-making statutes, and durable power of attorney for healthcare statutes. The overwhelming majority of states have adopted some form of the aforementioned legislation.

All U.S. jurisdictions have enacted some form of legislation regarding advance directives. All jurisdictions have a living-will statute, all but two have a healthcare power-of-attorney statute, and at least half have created a surrogate decision-making statute.[18]

Living will is the term for a written advance directive. It may be a form, often prescribed by statute, or it can conceivably be a handwritten document expressing the patient's wishes in anticipation of future events. Because it is impossible to anticipate all future medical conditions and options for treatment, living wills cannot provide guidance in every situation. Nonetheless, they are a highly desirable form of advance directive.

For the critical care setting, the ideal situation is when the patient has previously executed both a living will and a legal form appointing a healthcare proxy (such as a durable power of attorney for healthcare). By executing both documents, the patient has expressed his or her basic wishes regarding treatment and has legally appointed a spokesperson who can make decisions consistent with the patient's values.

Execution of these documents should take place well before a patient is confined to the critical care unit. However, in some circumstances if the patient is competent and can thus execute the requisite documents, he or she can fulfill the local statutory requirements to create a living will and/or a healthcare proxy appointment form after entering the critical care unit.

For example, a patient confined to a critical care bed who requires open-heart surgery may wish to execute an advance directive prior to being taken to the operating room. The critical care unit may wish to develop a protocol to assist patients at such times. It may include the use of outside legal counsel who can come to the patient's bedside.

Advance directives can be helpful documents, but they are not a panacea. Often they are not specific, because it is impossible for the patient to consider all possible clinical circumstances. Another issue to remember is that patients with decision-making capacity should be consulted or asked to give consent to treatment (rather than next of kin). The advance directive does not take effect while the patient retains the ability to make decisions.

In some states, natural-death acts and living-will acts set forth the legal framework for terminating treatment in situations where the patient has not executed an advance directive. These statutes can give guidance on such issues as seeking consent from the next of kin and identifying which surviving family members are higher in priority. A knowledge of these laws is essential—as is legal counsel—when issues or facts are unclear.

Living-will and natural-death acts vary from state to state on such issues as execution by minors, recognition of documents drafted in other jurisdictions, and the recognition of verbal advance directives.[19]

STATUTES DEFINING DEATH

Critical care clinicians may be confronted with situations in which the statutory definition of death is an issue. Although earlier statutes and the common law consider the definition of death to be the cessation of circulation and respiration (the cardiopulmonary definition of death), the advent of the respirator and other medical technology rendered the definition obsolete. Many states have enacted brain-death statutes to broaden the legal definition of death to include "irreversible cessation of all functions of the entire brain, including the brain stem" (see Chapter 9).[20]

FEDERAL LAW

Congress enacted the Patient Self-Determination Act (PSDA) in November 1990 and the act became effective in 1991. Under the PSDA, all hospitals, hospice programs, nursing homes, skilled nursing facilities, home health agencies, health maintenance organizations, and other Medicaid or Medicare-funded facilities or medical plans are required to have written policies and procedures in place respecting advance directives and to inform patients of their rights (under statute or case law and under the provider's internal policies) to make decisions concerning medical care, including the right to accept or refuse treatment. Written information about advance directives must be provided to hospital patients at the time of admission.[21]

The PSDA requires documentation in the medical record whether or not the patient has executed an advance directive. Providers must educate staff and the community about the PSDA and state laws regarding refusal of treatment. Providers may not discriminate against an individual based on whether the individual has executed an advance directive. The PSDA defines "advance directive" as a "written instruction, such as a living will or durable power of attorney for health care recognized under state law (whether statutory or as recognized by the courts of the state) and relating to the provision of such care when the individual is incapacitated."[22]

From a practical perspective, the critical care unit clinician must know institutional procedure for ascertaining the existence of such key documents through requests of competent patients or families when the patient's condition prevents a response. Even with the most diligent efforts, there will be circumstances where there will be a time lag before such documents can be made a part of the patient's chart. The goal should be to attempt to place advance directives in the patient's chart in as timely a manner as possible.

LIABILITY FOR TERMINATION OF TREATMENT

Clinicians may fear lawsuits from surviving family members who may or may not have been consulted prior to the decision. Many clinicians fear civil liability if life-sustaining treatment is removed. Clinicians are often poorly advised by their personal legal counsel on issues related to termination of treatment. Few lawyers understand the specific laws that affect these difficult decisions; thus, physicians often receive very conservative legal advice, counseling that patients remain on life support well beyond the time when it is clearly beneficial.

Many clinicians believe that, once treatment such as a ventilator or feeding tube has been initiated, it cannot legally be withdrawn. Clinicians who face this issue should focus on the standard of care: if the treatment is not clinically indicated, it is not legally required and no liability can result.

Family dynamics often come into play in cases involving consent to discontinue treatment. Are all family members present for consultation? Is there disagreement amongst the family as to the proper course of action? What opinions do certain family members have and why? Do they have a sufficient understanding of the medical facts? Has there been sufficient time for family members' emotional acceptance of their loved one's condition? Have certain family members been estranged from the patient? Has the patient executed any advance directives? If not, what are the applicable state statutes and/or case law?

These families may have begun the grieving process with the manifestation of anger and denial; such reactions may cause clinicians to be concerned about liability. However, unless an act of negligence precipitated the patient's condition, these situations almost never result in legal action. The passage of time, good communication of clinical information to the family, and counseling (by the attending physician and other resource persons including clergy, chaplains, social workers, and ethics committee members) usually resolve what initially appears to be an intractable problem.

Nonetheless, a few legal cases have imposed civil liability for providing unwanted life-sustaining treatment, including *Leach v. Akron Gen-*

eral Medical Center.[23] Edna Leach suffered from Lou Gehrig's disease (amyotrophic lateral sclerosis). She was admitted to the hospital because she complained of difficulty breathing. After she was hospitalized, she suffered cardiac arrest; she was resuscitated, admitted to the intensive care unit (ICU), and placed on a ventilator despite previous wishes to the contrary expressed by the patient and her husband. When Mr. Leach requested that the respirator be discontinued, the attending physician refused. A court order was obtained from the Summit County (Ohio) Probate Court in a written decision that echoed the *Quinlan* decision's legal reasoning. The patient died, and Mr. Leach subsequently brought suit in civil court on a theory of battery and unconsented touching. The trial court rejected the claim; the appeals court reinstated it, holding that the failure to terminate life-sustaining medical treatment can constitute a battery if legally valid consent to its administration has not been obtained or if consent to its continuation is withdrawn.[24] Upon remand to the trial court, the hospital settled the civil suit with the Leach family.

The author was personally involved in the litigation of a similar case involving a septuagenarian lawyer admitted to a coronary care unit. The patient was competent and requested to the attending physician that he not be resuscitated. The DNR order was not immediately documented in the medical record. The patient was found in a cardiac arrhythmia but not full arrest. He was cardioverted successfully after multiple applications of the paddles. He signed himself out of the hospital and died at home the next day. His widow brought suit, claiming that the patient should not have been cardioverted after his request for no cardiopulmonary resuscitation (CPR). The case went to trial; the attending physician and hospital prevailed, primarily on the argument that the possibility of cardioversion need not be disclosed during the process of consent to the DNR order.[25]

When a patient's condition is thought to be the result of an act of malpractice, there may be a conflict: the ethical interest of the patient may be served by *discontinuing* therapy while the patient's malpractice case is served by *continuing* therapy so that the patient remains alive. These situations must be handled with great care and advice of counsel.

RECURRING LEGAL PROBLEMS IN CRITICAL CARE

INFORMED CONSENT

The doctrine of informed consent had its origins in the principles of common law; many states have enacted statutes regarding informed consent, and other states rely on case law. The basic ethical and legal principle embodied under the law of informed consent is the principle of self-determination. The patient has the right to determine what is to be done with his or her body after having been provided sufficient information by the physician. The right to refuse treatment is thought to be a corollary right.[26]

The ability of a critical care patient to give informed consent is often an issue. The patient's ability to give informed consent is affected by his or her medical condition, drug therapy, underlying disease, and previous and current mental condition (including depression).

Patients who are incompetent cannot provide valid informed consent or informed refusal of treatment. Unfortunately there exists a great deal of confusion regarding the concept of competency and decision-making ability. It is best to avoid the terms *competency* and *incompetency* because the narrower legal definition of those terms seldom applies in an acute care setting. In the critical care setting, one rarely encounters individuals who have been legally adjudicated to be incompetent or competent. A judicial hearing to determine competency focuses on global issues such as the individual's ability to manage personal finances or personal hygiene.

Even for patients who have a court-appointed guardian or ward, it may be proper to involve such patients in limited decision making about their treatment. For example, a patient may be borderline mentally retarded and yet possess the capacity to understand that he will bleed to death without a blood transfusion.

In the critical care setting, clinicians often encounter patients who lack decision-making capacity but who have not been adjudicated to be incompetent. When referring to such patients, it is more precise to use the terms *decision-making capacity* and *incapacity* rather than the legal terms *competency* and *incompetency*.

Adults are presumed to be legally competent unless adjudicated otherwise. The fact that a patient has a history or presentation of mental illness or mental retardation does not necessarily interfere with the capacity to make decisions about life-sustaining treatment.[27] Indeed, patients should be presumed to have decision-making capacity unless demonstrated otherwise. Critical care practitioners commonly err by looking to family members for decisions when the patient is perfectly capable of expressing his or her desires.

When patients do lack decision-making capacity, clinicians should look to family members to make decisions about care.[28] Unless there is a clear and unresolvable conflict among family members or between caregivers and the family, resorting to a court for the determination of incompetency and appointment of a guardian is usually not practical. Court hearings can be expensive, and even an expedited or emergency court hearing may take days. There still may be circumstances where court involvement is necessary to authorize treatment or discontinuation of treatment. A variety of laws can come to bear on these situations (such as probate laws and court procedures for medical treatment, determination of competency, and appointment of a guardian). If life-sustaining treatment is involved, such laws as living-will acts/natural-death acts and surrogate decision-making statutes may all apply.

Competent legal advice is essential, but many seemingly intractable problems may be resolved with good communication with patients and families; counseling from chaplains, clergy, social workers, and others; and, if appropriate, ethics consultations.

DO-NOT-RESUSCITATE ORDERS

There are relatively few court decisions about do-not-resuscitate (DNR) orders because the courts regard these types of decisions as within the purview of the medical profession.[29] Many state statutes have been enacted that address DNR orders and the right of patients or surrogates to direct healthcare providers not to initiate CPR.[30] The DNR statutes can be part of advance directive laws or drafted and enacted as a separate piece of legislation (such as New York's).[31]

In an emergency and when the express wishes of the patient or family are unknown, CPR should be initiated. The law implies consent in an emergency.

Obtaining the patient's or family member's consent to a DNR order is important, as is documenting the consent in the medical record. Miscommunication can be prevented by placing clear written orders or a terminal-care order sheet in the patient's medical record.

In cases involving DNR orders, it is important to ask whether CPR, intubation, and other resuscitative measures are preserving life or merely prolonging the dying process. CPR can inflict trauma on dying patients, and CPR should not be initiated simply because the attending physician avoids a discussion with the patient or family, or because the physician or institution fears liability for "not doing everything" for the patient. If CPR and other measures are not appropriate for a dying patient, the attending physician should obtain informed consent and enter a clear DNR order in the patient's chart.

If a patient has no known family and, thus, clinicians cannot obtain proper consent, an ethics consultation can help to ascertain whether CPR and other measures are clinically indicated and, if not, whether they can be ethically and legally withheld. If all attempts to reach the next of kin are unsuccessful, these attempts should be documented in the medical record. Documenting the ethics consultation and the attempts to reach the next of kin demonstrates that all reasonable efforts were made before deciding to withhold CPR. This documentation would fortify the defense against any potential malpractice case brought by family who later appear.

Sometimes a critical care patient with a DNR order requires surgery. For example, a trauma victim with a poor prognosis might be able to obtain pain relief from a surgical intervention. Such cases raise the question of whether it is appropriate to suspend the DNR order during the intraoperative and recovery period.[32] Many writers urge a reconsideration of the appropriateness of preexisting DNR orders for patients who need surgery.[33] They argue that CPR and other resuscitative measures are less invasive and more quickly administered in the operative and recovery settings and that, in most instances, preexisting DNR orders should not rigidly be applied to critical care patients who undergo surgery. There is no legal prohibition against suspending the DNR order during surgery. If this suspension is clinically indicated, orders can be written in the medical record to that effect. Once the patient has returned to the critical care unit, the DNR order can be reinstituted.

CRIME VICTIMS

When the patient's condition is the result of an alleged criminal act and the family seeks to remove life-sustaining treatment, it may be prudent to advise law enforcement authorities and the local medical examiner or coroner that the patient's life support will be removed. If the consent of a spouse or a parent is needed and that individual is the alleged perpetrator of the crime, legal advice should be sought regarding the need for a court order. In the case of child abuse, officials from child protective services may be authorized to give consent for medical care but may be reluctant to authorize discontinuing life-sustaining treatment. In such cases, a juvenile court order may be necessary. All states have statutes requiring the reporting of criminally inflicted injuries. Even if such statutes do not apply, the institution and attending medical staff may wish to advise the proper legal authorities as a courtesy. Organ donation may be problematic if an autopsy is to be performed. The medical examiner or coroner should be consulted in such cases.

REFUSAL OF TREATMENT BY COMPETENT PATIENTS

The clear trend in the case law over the last 20 years is to recognize the legal right of a competent, adult patient to refuse any treatment including resuscitation, ventilation support, and artificial feeding in almost all circumstances.[34] Courts have agreed with patients that the desire to live without assistance (such as from a ventilator) is not suicide.[35]

This trend in the case law to recognize the right of competent, adult patients to refuse treatment is so strong that it is difficult to envision circumstances under which an institution or physician would be justified in seeking court intervention.[36] The courts balance the patient's legal right to refuse treatment against such state interests as preservation of life, protection of third parties, prevention of suicide, and the maintenance of the integrity of the medical profession.[37]

It is not uncommon for critical care clinicians to encounter cases involving the refusal of a blood transfusion by an adult member of the Jehovah's Witnesses. Although, in the past, case law frequently overrode the patient's wishes, citing such reasoning as the state's interest in the preservation of the family unit and protection of innocent third parties (when the patient was the parent of minor children), recent case law involving Jehovah's Witness patients has held the exact opposite. The courts have found that these patients have a "common law and constitutional privacy right to refuse a blood transfusion."[38] It is doubtful that there is ever justification for transfusing an adult Jehovah's Witness patient in the face of clearly expressed wishes to the contrary. However, when there is doubt about the patient's wishes and the patient cannot communicate during an emergency, consent should be implied, particularly when the treatment seems virtually certain to restore the health of the patient.[39]

It is improper to wait until an emergency develops and/or the patient loses consciousness to then seek the protection of the emergency doctrine in an attempt to override the patient's previously expressed desires not to be treated.[40]

ADULT INCOMPETENT PATIENTS

The number of cases involving termination of treatment that have resulted in court decisions is very small. When patients no longer possess decision-making capacity, the practice in institutions for many years has been for the attending physician to consult the patient's family and to seek their consent to discontinue treatment if clinically indicated. Indeed, these decisions are made daily in critical care units without court intervention or liability suits.

The trend in the case law over the last 20 years is to recognize the rights of incompetent patients to have decisions made on their behalf by next of kin, even in the absence of any form of written advance directives. Meisel states that this represents a "shift toward the absolute end of the spectrum as has been the case with competent patients."[41] Cases involving withdrawal of treatment from incompetent patients most frequently occur when the patient has a terminal illness (such as cancer or AIDS) or when the prognosis is poor (such as patients with stroke or multiple trauma).

Many states have statutes that apply when the patient no longer has decision-making capacity and has not executed an advance directive. To minimize liability risk, clinicians should follow applicable statutes, make a careful determination of the diagnosis and prognosis for the patient, seek a consensus among family members regarding the indicated course of treatment, and then proceed with consent.

PATIENTS IN A PERSISTENT VEGETATIVE STATE

Cases involving patients in a persistent vegetative state (PVS) can be extremely difficult for families, institutions, and healthcare providers. Cases involving patients in this condition have received attention during the past 10 years because several cases have been decided at the appellate court level and one case (*Cruzan*) reached the U.S. Supreme Court.

Situations involving patients in a PVS are fraught with emotion because they usually involve patients who have been in that condition for many months or even years. Their families experience extreme anguish. Terminating treatment means removing a feeding tube, with all the emotional connotations of not providing sustenance to a human being. In examining this issue, the courts have stated that a feeding tube is no different than any other means of mechanical support such as a ventilator.[42]

To minimize the risk of liability in these situations, clinicians must know the state statutes that may apply, especially when there is no advance directive. As in all situations involving termination of treatment, clinicians must also carefully determine diagnosis and prognosis (see chapter 11). Seeking consent from the appropriate next of kin and family consensus also minimizes liability. It may be appropriate to seek court approval for removal of feeding tubes if there is an unresolvable disagreement among family members. Finally, an ethics consultation may help frame all the elements that will lead to a good decision and thus avoid liability.

MINOR PATIENTS

Critical care clinicians are often faced with difficult decisions about the treatment of minors. The most common cases involve parental refusal of life-sustaining treatment; less common are cases involving the withdrawal of life-sustaining treatment.

Clinicians need to know the legal framework that affects minor patients, such as child-abuse and neglect statutes, local court procedures for obtaining emergency treatment orders, case law on parental refusal of treatment, and case law or statute on the mature minor's ability to refuse treatment.

Handicapped newborns are protected by the federal Child Abuse Amendments of 1984 to the Child Abuse Prevention and Treatment and Adoption Reform Act of 1974. These statutes and the resulting regulations define when the treatment of handicapped newborns is medically indicated and when treatment need not be rendered. The statute sets forth five exceptions to the requirement to treat handicapped infants.[43] There is mixed evidence as to whether these federal statutes and regulations have actually changed clinical practice (see Chapter 23 of this text).[44]

When parents are unavailable, the law implies consent for treatment in an emergency; thus, court intervention should not be necessary.[45] When parents are present, they have a legal and ethical duty to act and make decisions that are in the best interest of their child and to provide the necessities of life including medical treatment.[46] Parental autonomy is therefore not absolute; the state may intervene when its interest in preserving the life of the child supersedes parental rights.[47] This is the case when parents refuse treatment that is clearly indicated, such as a blood transfusion or surgery. The ultimate ethical and legal question in these cases involves a determination as to what course of care is in the child's best interest.

Less clear are cases where treatment is not likely to save or preserve the life of the child and, in fact, the treatment poses its own risks. In these instances, it is much less clear as to what course of action truly serves the best interest of the child. Ethics committee consultation can often help parents and healthcare providers work through these decisions. As a last resort, and only if there is disagreement between parents and caregivers, cases can be heard before the juvenile court.

In cases involving mature minors (typically a child age 14 or older), it is important to know if case law or statutes recognize the right of such patients to refuse treatment or to execute advance directives. The statutes setting forth the age of majority and any legislative or judicial recognition of the legal concept of emancipated minors may come to bear in these situations. In recent years, a number of court cases have recognized the ability of mature minors to make their own medical decisions.[48]

CONCLUSION

Many problems in the critical care unit that have legal and ethical dimensions involve withholding and withdrawing life-sustaining treatment. The legal corollary to the ethical tenet that there is no distinction between withholding and withdrawing treatment is that, if treatment is not *clinically* indicated, it is not *legally* indicated.

Critical care clinicians can take the following steps to help avoid legal problems:

- Communicate with patients and families about issues related to treatment.
- Know all the facts before making a decision.
- Try to be certain about diagnosis and prognosis.
- Verify the existence of any advance directives and review them.
- Document family/surrogate consent.
- Get legal advice from a lawyer who is familiar with statutes that apply in critical care and who can balance practicality with legality.

NOTES

1. *In re Quinlan,* 70 N.J. 10, 355 A.2d 647 (1976).

2. M. Crane, "The Latest Malpractice Risk: Saving Your Patient's Life," *Medical Economics* 75, no. 4 (23 February 1998): 226.

3. A. Meisel, *The Right to Die,* 2nd ed. (New York: Wiley Law Publications, 1995), 2: 352.

4. See note 2 above, p. 227.

5. *In re Conroy,* 486 A.2d 1209, 1222 (1985).

6. See note 2 above, p. 1: 54.

7. See note 1 above, p. 663.

8. *Cruzan v. Director, Missouri Department of Health,* 497 U.S. 261 (1990).

9. *Washington v. Glucksberg,* 1997 U.S. LEXIS 4039 at 1; *Vacco v. Quill,* 1997 U.S. LEXIS 1048 at 1.

10. Ibid., 35.

11. *Washington v. Glucksberg,* see note 9 above, p. 131.

12. American Medical Association, *Code of Medical Ethics* (Chicago: AMA, 1997), sec. 2.20.

13. *Washington v. Glucksberg,* see note 9 above, p. 131.

14. R.A. Burt, "The Supreme Court Speaks: Not Assisted Suicide but a Constitutional Right to Palliative Care," *New England Journal of Medicine* 337, no. 17 (October 1997): 1235; *Washington v. Glucksberg,* see note 9 above, p. 150.

15. See note 2 above, 1: xi.

16. Ibid.

17. I.M. Urofsky, *Letting Go: Death Dying and the Law* (Norman, Okla.: University of Oklahoma Press, 1994), 14.

18. F. Rozovsky, *Consent to Treatment: A Practical Guide*, 2nd ed. (Boston: Little, Brown and Company, 1990), 518-19.

19. Uniform Determination of Death Act, 12 U.L.A. 292, 293 (Supp., 1988).

20. 42 U.S.C. 1395, sec. cc (a)(1).

21. Ibid., sec. cc (f)(2).

22. *Leach v. Akron General Medical Center*, 426 N.E. 2d 809 (1980).

23. Ibid.

24. *Galvin v. University Hospital of Cleveland*, No. 115873, (C.P. Cuyahoga City, Ohio, filed 8 September 1996).

25. See note 6 above, p. 271.

26. President's Commission for the Study of Ethical Problems in Medicine and Biomedical and Behavioral Research, *Deciding to Forego Life-Sustaining Treatment* (Washington, D.C.: U.S. Government Printing Office, 1983), 119-26.

27. See note 2 above, 1: 115.

28. Ibid., 1: 138.

29. *In re Dinnerstein*, 380 N.E. 2d 134 (1978).

30. See note 2 above, 2: 555-6.

31. New York Public Health Law, "Orders not to Resuscitate," Article 29-B.

32. R.D. Truog, " 'Do-Not-Resuscitate' Orders during Anesthesia and Surgery," *Anesthesiology* 74, no. 3 (1991): 606-08.

33. S. Youngner et al., "DNR in the Operating Room—Not Really a Paradox," *Journal of the American Medical Association* 266, no. 17 (1991): 2433-34.

34. See note 2 above, 1: xi.

35. *In re Farrell*, 529 A.2d 404, 411 (1987).

36. *In re Jobes*, 529 A.2d 434, 451 (1987); *Browning v. Herbert*, 568 So. 2d 4, 10 (1990).

37. See note 3 above, p. 1225.

38. *Norwood Hospital v. Munoz*, 564 N.E. 2d 1017, 1021 (1991).

39. *University of Cincinnati Hospital v. Edmond*, 506 N.E. 2d 299 (1986).

40. *Holmes v. Silver Cross Hospital*, 340 F. Supp. 125, (1972).

41. See note 2 above, 1: 54.

42. A. Meisel, "Legend Myths about Terminating Life Support," *Archives of Internal Medicine* 151 (1991): 1497.

43. 42 U.S.C.A., sec. 5102 (3)(A) and (3)(B).

44. B.S. Carter, "Neonatologists and Bioethics after Baby Doe," *Journal of Perinatology* 13, no. 2 (1993): 144-50.

45. W.E. Prosser, *Law of Torts*, 4th ed. (St. Paul, Minn.: West Publishing, 1977), 103.

46. N.N. Dubler and P. Nimmons, *Ethics on Call* (New York: Harmony Books, 1992), 272.

47. Ibid.

48. See note 2 above, 2: 276.

16

Language in Critical Care: Humanizing, Depersonalized, or Inhumane

*Dante L. Landucci
and Robert E. Cunnion*

Who, even with words unfettered, could tell in full, though many times narrating, of the blood and of the wounds that I now saw? Every tongue assuredly would come short, by reason of our speech and our memory which have small capacity to comprise so much.
—Dante Alighieri, *The Divine Comedy*

INTRODUCTION

Diagnostic and therapeutic interventions continue to grow in number and complexity. Year by year, discussions about patients among healthcare providers become more technical and include progressively more information. In response to these pressures, the language used by clinicians has become increasingly telegraphic, relying heavily on medical nomenclature, idiomatic expressions, and acronyms. Medical school serves, among other things, as four years of intensive language training, and postdoctoral training is a setting for refining fluency in this dialect. To the layperson, medical conversations have become largely incomprehensible. Even if the words are understood, the concepts may be so foreign as to be impenetrable and the content of medical conversations may even seem repugnant.

A positive aspect of the highly developed jargon of medicine is that its use allows rapid transmission of complicated information and efficient exchange of opinions, helping to facilitate medical decision making. In the intensive care unit (ICU), the time available for these activities may be especially limited, and reliance on such jargon becomes all the more essential. If the result is a temporary detachment from the personhood of the individual patient, no harm is done and much benefit may be derived. On the other hand, talking in such a manner allows clinicians to distance themselves from the focus of their attention so much that their concept of the patient can become not only objectified but downright inhumane.

It is essential to focus on both the origins and the effects of communication from the perspectives of those engaging in and those dependent upon the practice of medicine. Such a focus is the only way to minimize the chasms that so often open when patients, their families, and healthcare workers attempt to engage in dialogue, particularly in the ICU. Ideally, all parties involved should realize that they bring to such conversations not only certain needs but also certain responsibilities. To reconcile individual perceptions, all need to acknowledge that the differing behaviors they encounter represent natural human reactions to many of the same stimuli.

When diseases are life threatening, especially if they develop unexpectedly or rapidly, they evoke profound emotions in everyone they touch. The sense that death may be imminent, together with the accompanying pain and suffering, may be psychically threatening or overpowering for all of us. Distancing allows us to find a suitable perch from which to contemplate these matters fully. Unfortunately, distancing may also unintentionally render us insensitive.

Moreover, in medical discussions, what was understood may not be what was said. Communication relies on the points of view and frames of mind of the participants, which are constantly altered by the surrounding environment. Success in establishing mutual understanding is related to the open-mindedness that each participant brings to the encounter.

In this chapter, the advantages of currently prevailing patterns of conversation among healthcare practitioners are explored in detail. The concepts of objectification and compassion are examined, as well as their proper role in the delivery of holistic care within the critical care setting. In addition, the chapter reviews the pitfalls of speaking, and therefore thinking, in an ly objectified manner and emphasizes the need to dedicate energy and thought to avoiding depersonalized communication when talking with patients or family members. This chapter is written for laypeople as much as for ethicists and healthcare providers, to help them appreciate the reasons for specialized styles of dialogue that might otherwise sound appalling.

DISEASE AND DYSPHORIA

When jazz pianist Billy Strayhorn learned he had leukemia in 1967, there was no hope of a cure. About Strayhorn's compositions, eloquent testaments to the sentiments aroused by affliction with a lethal disease, Robert Palmer wrote the following:

> Not even the final stages of a fatal illness silenced him completely. The titles of his later compositions (*UMMG*, for Upper Manhattan Medical Group, and *Blood Count*) bear grim witness to what his life had become, yet the music itself exudes an indomitable humanity. *Blood Count* in particular has an immediate and devastating impact, speaking simultaneously of fear, longing, resignation, pride, doubt, faith and many more apparently conflicting emotions, all balanced on the knife's edge of a man's life, all vividly brought to life whenever the music is heard.[1]

Few if any of us can hope to express in words what Strayhorn was able to express in music.

At the end of Strayhorn's life, his friend and long-time collaborator, Duke Ellington, summoned together musicians with whom they had both performed. The recording that resulted is . . . *And His Mother Called Him Bill*. Robert Palmer paraphrases their emotions: "This is one of Johnny Hodges' greatest performances. He is still *angry* that Strayhorn has been taken, and for once the familiar adjectives—serene, unruffled—cannot be applied to his playing. He sings, from deep inside, the certain knowledge that any moment can be a man's last moment, and his playing cuts right to the heart."[2]

For most of us, it would be taxing enough simply to have to acknowledge that we may have to give up what we cherish most, life itself. Unfortunately, pain is often an intrinsic aspect of sickness. Intensifying the agony, treatment of life-threatening disease usually requires technology beyond the scope of what patients and their families can readily master. Loss of control starts with an office or hospital visit and often escalates rapidly. For critically ill patients awakening after a lapse in consciousness, there may be no period of adjustment to the mechanical regulation of bodily functions through tubes in every orifice.

Although spared the physical impact of the disease, family members may be sent reeling by its psychological ramifications. While the patient's awareness may be blunted by sedation and analgesia, critical illness takes a relentless toll on those keeping the vigil. As David Todres observed in his pediatric intensive care unit, "The frequent crises the critically ill child experiences, even in the course of 24 hours, produces intense anxiety in the parents; fear overwhelms the parents and the constant uncertainty has the effect of producing irritability or depression."[3]

The fact that diagnostic tests and treatments that may restore health are often administered *to* patients rather than *by* them or their loved ones places the ill into exposed and dependent relationships with strangers. Louise Coulombe proposes, on the basis of her experience with hospice care, that such vulnerability may alter perceptions to such a degree that "what patients fear most is not that they cannot be cured, but that they will be left alone and have no one to turn to."[4] Even medically sophisticated individuals share these perceptions, as attested by a practicing nurse: "During my husband's illness one of the feelings I experienced was powerlessness. . . . On reflection I feel that I was caught up in a power structure where open challenge is difficult because one does not wish to antagonize those on whom one is so dependent in life-and-death situations."[5]

Often, the conditions that bring patients to the ICU are accompanied by loss of higher-order cerebral functions, those which define our very essence. Gradually patients may be stripped of their very identity. Among the worst of these states is so-called ICU psychosis, characterized by delirium, disorientation, paranoia, and disinhibition. Fortunately, the majority of those who recover have little recollection of the experience. What do patients feel during their delirium? Frances Drew, a physician who gradually developed mild dementia and then recovered, offers a clue: "Thinking about dissolution of one's mind, the literal loss of selfness, has no near equal as a source of panic. Pain can be alleviated, death is an ending; but losing one's selfness and still living, losing a self created over a lifetime and cultivated so carefully—that is despair."[6]

Healthcare providers, of course, do not experience despair in the same manner as their patients, but they, just like family members, do experience the vicarious emotional impact. Unlike family members, clinicians must retain the ability to diagnose and treat. They must continue to be as objective as possible, in part because they are professionally bound to preserve an unbiased command of the facts for themselves, their colleagues, and their patients.

However reticent they may be on the subject, those who work at the bedside realize that often, especially in crises, one's feelings must be reined in. This is most important when we are confronted by "senseless" suffering. Paul Peebles, a pediatrician, recalls the impulses he felt while treating a young girl the age of his daughter: "You relate to her as if she was your own. It pushes every rescue fantasy you can imagine. It pushes escape fantasies. You have to be very careful. You have to learn about these emotions and see them for what they are and not let them control you."[7] Clinicians then must walk a fine line. According to Todres, "Marked limitations in closeness result in a cold, aloof, and unsatisfactory relationship. Too much closeness can also be costly—the physician may be incapacitated by the [patient's or family's] anxiety and grief. Supportive discussions may be very time consuming and emotionally draining."[8]

BURNOUT

When the evoked emotions cut very deeply, healthcare workers may simply be striving to preserve their own mental health. A well-adjusted individual may apply "high adaptive level" defense mechanisms such as affiliation, altruism, humor, sublimation, and suppression to this end.[9] Unfortunately, medical education is not focused on helping clinicians develop sophistication in the use of such functions, particularly to "maximize gratification and allow the conscious awareness of feelings, ideas, and their consequences."[10] This may contribute to "the subtle progression by which a young medical student who wants only to care for his sick fellows becomes transmuted unawares into the embodiment of a biomedical problem solver."[11]

In the worst case, clinicians may become dysfunctional when, despite their efforts, the patient is dying or in some other way is prompting them to conclude, often subconsciously, that they have failed. This becomes especially pronounced if a mistake in management of the patient's care is perceived. Under such bitter circumstances, the reaction at the individual or group level may become maladaptive. In technical terms, clinicians may resort to intellectualization, devaluation, denial, rationalization, or passive aggression.[12] Patients and families experience this outcome in the form of comments such as "the gallbladder in bed 6," "gomer," and so forth.

Finally, anguish can arise from the sense of responsibility we have toward others, whether expressed openly or accepted unconsciously. For healthcare workers, the goal of satisfactorily alleviating pain and suffering may provoke irreconcilable stress, as this goal is all too frequently unattainable. Sustained over time, this may result in burnout—the "emotional exhaustion, depersonalization and reduced personal accomplishment that can occur among individuals who do 'people work' of some kind."[13]

At this stage, a clinician may become overwhelmed with pessimism. "No, we don't cure. I never bought that either. I went through the same cynicism—all that training, and then this helplessness."[14] That's the message a dying physician and patient conveyed to Samuel Shem, himself facing a crisis of professional self-doubt during medical internship.

According to Maslach and Schaufeli, "Burnout has been applied to the family sphere, as evidenced by analyses of parental burnout and marriage burnout."[15] Thus, patients' families may succumb to the emotional strain of a loved one's illness. This is probably the "irritability or depression" that David Todres has observed in parents contending with the "roller coaster" pathophysiology of critical illness.[16]

Ironically, it is the patient who has been largely overlooked as a common victim of burnout. "Patients with serious losses that are not life-threatening can have intense emotions, but in time, they come to see beyond the losses to a continuation of life," notes Louise Coulombe. However, for patients with a severe illness that carries a significant risk of death, "the intensity of the problems does not go away; the issues are continually about their life and their death and the meaning each holds for them."[17] In addition, there may be the onerous burden of feeling that one has failed to fulfill personal obligations, especially in the case of parents who are facing the prospect of "abrogating" their most important commitment.

Postulating that stress results in alarm and then in resistance to its cause, Etzion has hypothesized further that what leads to burnout is a varying combination of failure to adapt successfully to the new circumstances and of their persistence for more than a short period. Of great importance is that the ensuing "exhaustion phase is reached before the individual consciously has noticed both preliminary phases [alarm and resistance]."[18] For this reason, burnout often is inapparent to those experiencing it.

Unaware of their own emotional depletion, let alone that which may exist in their caretakers, it is foreseeable that some patients may become completely nonparticipatory recipients of healthcare. As Frances Jarman eventually concluded about her husband's responses to several seemingly unintended conflicts with the medical establishment when he was in the hospital at the end of his life, "He expressed what I believe many other patients feel: that their apparent acquiescence is not necessarily an acceptance."[19]

Depletion and anguish erode the family's and the clinician's ability to contend with what Nuland calls "the reality of what is all too frequently a series of destructive events that involve by their very nature the disintegration of the dying person's humanity."[20] If this erosion is unchecked, it is possible that "most of us will die wondering what we, or our doctors, have done wrong."[21] Even worse, the survivors' memories of the dead may retain a distorted focus on their role as witnesses of a final, personal holocaust rather than on the recapitulation of a memorable life.

DEPERSONALIZATION

There has been extensive research on the aggravation of grief that results from failure to create a suitable environment for the ill. In literally hundreds of articles, authors have attempted to analyze how clinicians routinely fail their patients emotionally while successfully avoiding the more "conventional" types of negligence. Those publications that go beyond anecdote have amassed some dismal statistics:

It is interesting to note that while most interruptions occurred between 5 and 50 seconds of the physician's initial question, most completed statements took less than 1 minute and no patients took more than 3 minutes to complete their statement.[22]

Studies have shown that 50% of psychosocial and psychiatric problems are missed, that physicians interrupt patients an average of 18 seconds into the patient's description of the presenting problem, that 54% of patient problems and 45% of patient concerns are neither elicited by the physician nor disclosed by the patient, that patients and physicians do not agree on the main presenting problem in 50% of visits and that patients are dissatisfied with the information provided to them by physicians.[23]

Although this was the first meeting with a medical oncologist for 79 patients (79%), 82 (82%) made final decisions about treatment by the end of the [on average 50-minute] meeting.[24]

Physicians identify as "most difficult encounters" those in which the patient expresses a strong negative emotion such as anger, sadness, or fear.[25]

In a large number of published analyses, the language used by clinicians is blamed as contributing substantially to the isolation experienced by many patients. Accordingly, analysis of the undesirable, as well as the favorable, aspects of medical communication with patients demands scrutinizing whether there is something inherently inappropriate about the use of medical jargon.

Over the ages, patterns of language development have remained much the same. Cultural evolution necessitates not only the generation of terms, but also the assurance that a "widget" is not confused with a "gizmo." Newly introduced words are comprehensible to those who coin them but recondite to the masses. Eventually, depending on its utility, a word may become a part of the vulgate; jargon becomes language, a process accelerated by modern mass media.

Before finding general acceptance, jargon finds use in the restricted context of conversation among specialists. With jargon, specialists convey complex information, often in vast amounts, with relatively few, seemingly simple words. There can be no more poignant example of the advantages, even the necessity, of jargon than when its use concerns the life or death of the speaker, as in the case of this cockpit voice recording from a jetliner that had inadvertently flown into a volcanic ash cloud:

> *Crew:* Okay we have a light up.
> *Controller:* K L M eight six seven heavy say again.
> *Crew:* K L M eight six seven we have uh complete failure all engines and uh—we are descending now.
> *Controller:* K L M eight six seven heavy Anchorage.
> *Crew:* K L M eight six seven heavy we are descending now we are in a fall. [unintelligible] Anchorage K L M eight six seven heavy we need all the assistance you have give us radar vectors please. [unintelligible] right turning here. K L M eight six seven heavy turning right say again right we are passing two twenty thousand feet we are [unintelligible] in the clear we are turning to the right.[26]

This conversation lasted 76 seconds. During this time, the radio operator had assisted with the ignition of three engines as he simultaneously managed to convey that the aircraft had fallen more than 6,000 feet, that recovery had begun, that they were far off course, and that they had become a collision hazard for other aircraft.

With similarly emotionally barren words, he continued to relay detailed factual information during the ensuing 40 minutes. Despite the fact that almost all instrumentation was disabled, that it was twilight, and that thunderstorms were forming as a consequence of the eruption, the crew successfully landed the plane. This was due in large part to the continuous exchange of voluminous data about the plane's status, location, and direction with air traffic controllers. Yet the radio conversation seems eerily matter of fact.

The image we have of pilots may be enhanced by the facts that their successes are obvious, even when there are casualties, and that their "sins" are mitigated by their own deaths. It is difficult to imagine a cogent argument that the language air crews use during stressful periods is immoral, disrespectful, or inhumane. Because they share the same fate as their passengers, their ability to "remove themselves" from their immediate emotions is readily accepted and even applauded.

Critical circumstances do not permit loquacious conversation, especially not when caring for a severely ill individual. Although healthcare workers have less at stake personally than jet pilots, the result of their actions is nonetheless a matter of life or death. If medical teams are to be effective (whether in the ICU, the operating room, or the emergency department), they must be coordinated, knowing precisely what is happening with each member as well as with the patient. This, too, is dependent on rapid, accurate, and detailed exchange of complex information. Jargon, because it makes this process possible, is of irrefutable merit.

If the language itself is justifiable, then are the implications of its use offensive? Cockpit recordings reveal that, at times of crisis, crews and air traffic controllers instinctively talk about "souls and fuel aboard." It may be startling to hear living beings lumped together with the agent that may imminently incinerate them. But if the crew does not minimize the humanity of those at risk, their emotions—particularly their instinctual fears in the face of such risk—would assuredly paralyze them. Repression of these intense feelings may be the difference between clear thought and panic, successful landing and fatal crash.

Given the obvious magnitude of the potential benefit, we are quick to accept that the passengers on board are objects, to the same extent as the stricken aircraft itself, in the minds of the crew. This is objectification, exemplified in its most extreme form. At such moments, the pilots value even themselves in the same, objectified manner.

Like air crews, healthcare workers are confronted with situations that easily provoke potentially overwhelming reactions, ones that could render them incapable of functioning properly. It is possible to conclude that pilots, who may be seeing the ground rushing at them all too fast, are maximally stressed, thus unimpeachably justified in resorting to psychological defense mechanisms. Still, during most of their working hours, flight crews have time for the usual activities of life: they eat, drink, converse. They also are assured that their passengers are doing much the same with an added emphasis on entertainment and relaxation.

In contrast to pilots, healthcare workers face sustained duress, resulting from nearly continuous exposure to suffering and death. Heightening the contrast further, much of what clinicians do routinely is likely to cause harm to their patients. Patients routinely receive medications with potent side effects or undergo diagnostic or therapeutic procedures that exacerbate their underlying discomfort.

Clinicians must be able to distance themselves from the untoward, but intrinsic, aspects of their work. How else could someone deliberately plunge a needle thicker than a pencil core six inches into the body of another human being? Clinicians must be able to disregard the emotional and physiologic consequences of such an act. Patients, too, must dissociate their intellects and emotions from their bodies in order to consider and consent to necessary maneuvers. Failing this, some become distraught and cannot be "consoled" enough to proceed with tests or treatment.

DYSFUNCTIONAL LANGUAGE

Clearly, depersonalization *per se* is not unnatural or undesirable, but there is a point at which it becomes so. A deed that is inhumane sets itself

---

Exhibit 16-1
Non-Technical Aspects of Care

---

1. Patient's preferences and expressed needs
2. Coordination and integration of care
3. Communication and education
4. Physical comfort
5. Alleviation of fears and anxieties
6. Involvement of family and friends
7. Continuity and transition

---

apart because it is divested of compassion ("sympathetic, kindly concern aroused by the misfortune, affliction, or suffering of another")[27] without the potential of offsetting benefit. It is intended primarily to cause discomfort whether the victim perceives it or not. With respect to language, persisting with depersonalization once the crisis is over renders the objectification cruel and inhumane, even if it had been appropriate initially.

Overhearing healthcare workers speak in depersonalized terms, even when it does not apply to the unintended audience, is likely to arouse anxiety and distaste. For this reason, clinicians must always be circumspect and must always ensure patients' entitlement to confidentiality. This concern serves an additional purpose, for it establishes one of the foundations of sensitivity. As often as possible, we must wonder whether our speech is facilitating our work or whether it has become a means of retaliating against the pain "inflicted by" the patient. In the same vein, we should be attentive to the actions of our colleagues.

In so doing, we safeguard the possibility of constructive conversation with all the people we encounter at the bedside. Patients and their families want and need to trust us so we may collaborate to realize the best possible results. The nature of the interaction may go beyond what is consciously evident. According to Nuland, patients may be "awed by their doctors, create a transference with them in the true psychoanalytic sense, and wish to please them, or at least not to be seen as a source of offense."[28]

Without disciplined introspection, the use of defenses can deteriorate from constructive to destructive. Although the more mature defense mechanisms make it possible for an individual to function optimally in a hostile environment, the less adaptive ones can create problems for the clinician and those around him. Intensive care can devolve into what Sherwin Nuland details with painful clarity:

Despite their best intentions, the staff members have begun to separate themselves from the man whose life they are fighting to save. A process of depersonalization has set in. The patient is every day less a human being and more a complicated challenge in intensive care, testing the genius of some of the most brilliantly aggressive of the hospital's clinical warriors. To most of the nurses and a few of the doctors who knew him before his slide into sepsis, there remains some of the person he was (or may have been), but to the consulting superspecialists who titrate the remaining molecular evidences of his dwindled vitality, he is a case, and a fascinating one at that. Doctors thirty years his junior call him by his first name.[29]

There are other ways in which the characteristics of language can fail the process of communication. The inherent imprecision of language, and how this perennially creates confusion, is epitomized by the existence of contranyms—words whose definitions include meanings that are contrary to each other or whose homonyms are also antonyms. Thus, "he bought a house on the hill, *overlooking* the slums" cannot be properly interpreted unless additional information about the location of the edifice or the frame of mind of the purchaser is provided. When spoken, "the building was *raised*" is not "the building was *razed*."[30]

Similarly, misunderstandings can easily arise when the context of a conversation is insufficient and interpretation becomes a matter of personal bias. The command "dust the room" would cause a detective to go about applying dust in order to detect fingerprints, while the rest of us would attempt to remove dust to improve cleanliness. In everyday use, the term *positive* connotes something good or desirable. In contrast, in medical use a test result said to be "positive" may reveal evidence of malignancy, serious infection, or some other grim diagnosis. Contrary meaning is particularly conspicuous with comparative terms. Higher blood pressure is desirable when the pressure is too low, but undesirable when it is already too high. These examples illustrate that the role of the listener in helping to achieve mutual understanding should not be taken for granted.

Language is more than simply a means for attempting to convey information accurately. Expressions such as "read between the lines" suggest that it concomitantly serves as a conduit, albeit subliminally and far from precisely, of attitudes. It is human nature to narrow one's assumptions about the frame of mind of others by analyzing their modes of conversation.

When specialists and laypeople are talking, they may erroneously conclude that their respective frames of reference are the same. After all, the specialist started out knowing only the vernacular, to which was added technical terminology (that is, the tools of the trade), and this terminology is abandoned when the workday ends and he or she reenters the "real" world. At the same time, the layperson may believe that exposure to technical jargon through the press, television, and movies has engendered an adequate understanding of its meaning.

The number of words an individual learns in mastering medicine may rival the size of that person's entire vocabulary prior to entering the field. These terms include innumerable idiomatic expressions and abbreviations whose proper comprehension is highly dependent upon context. The assimilation of each new stage of words literally creates new perceptions and attentions.[31] Furthermore, at the bedside, each medical term takes on fresh nuances as it is applied in a world unfathomable to the uninitiated. The entire process of medical training can be conceived as one of acculturation; this is not only unavoidable but largely intentional. The students' affinity for their chosen vocation renders them malleable to instructors' purposes.

Even though some jargon may be well understood by laypersons, one should not underestimate the misunderstanding that can result from accumulation of small misconceptions when too many specialized terms are used. Compounding the problem, laypersons do not experience the "rethinking" brought on by intense medical education. What laypersons "hear" and what specialists "say" are reflections of their individual perceptions, which are likely to be as substantively different as their respective belief systems. This chasm between points of reference may be bridged with education.

Unfortunately, in the ICU one often sees patients whose condition does not allow much time. For this reason, the defenses used by healthcare workers for self-preservation are likely to be misperceived. To avoid the sobering impact of the word "moribund," a doctor may casually refer to a patient's status as "circling the drain." Although this does not minimize the seriousness of the circumstances in the mind of the caretaker, the morbid levity may be lost on others.

DISPARATE PERCEPTIONS

European explorers are credited as having successfully navigated the oceans of the world using sextants, compasses, and detailed maps, many of which were fashioned during the trips of discovery. On these parchments are drawn, with as much precision as possible, the detailed outlines of the lands these explorers saw and the waters that they sailed.

Polynesians also explored, then regularly navigated, large expanses of water over the span of centuries during which they settled Oceania and the more remote islands of the Pacific. Their navigators came to ceremonies, usually held the night before departure, armed with their own type of "maps." These seemingly simple fabrications of woven twigs and tied-on baubles (roughly similar to the trivets made by American children with Popsicle sticks) depicted wave patterns regularly encountered at sea. The trinkets were placed at junctures indicating the lands from which they originated. In essence, these pilots used an ancestral, empiric understanding of the pattern of ocean waves resulting from the action of prevailing winds and their diffraction by islands and atolls. This information is analogous to that derived by Western navigators from the terrestrial environment, providing these pelagic people equally reliable data about their course. The Polynesians' understanding of location was based on recognizing how waves converge at different distances from land, coupled with a knowledge of what lies in the vicinity. This method of navigation also afforded them the possibility of locating previously unknown islands. In contrast, Europeans found new places largely by chance, as evidenced by the gyrations they themselves plotted.

Possibly the biggest departure from the Western approach to transoceanic sailing comes from what the Polynesians did with this information. Western cartographers collected ships' charts and attempted to sum their information into ever-more accurate atlases that have been collected in libraries. Our knowledge of the Polynesian equivalent comes from cultural anthropologists because, even today, the "maps" are intentionally destroyed *before* the trip ever begins; it is a part of the ceremony.

The Polynesian process of navigation is so unusual that it is difficult, if not impossible, to comprehend their perception of what appears on our maps as a blue void. But, there can be no denying its merit; in this way, an entire population and its culture were successfully established across the planet's largest body of water. Presented with the task of collectively achieving the same goal, it seems highly improbable that Captain James Cook and his crew would have had much to discuss with their Austronesian counterparts. After all, it has taken us literally centuries to understand that there was substantive meaning to their preparatory ceremony.

Sometimes, it seems that patients and their healthcare providers face similar gaps in perception. While the goals of healthcare workers and their patients are the same, the fundamental approaches by which they seek to achieve them are diametrically opposed. According to Ong and colleagues:

> From a medical point of view, doctors need information to establish the right diagnosis and treatment plan. From the patient's point of

view, two needs have to be met when visiting the doctor: "the need to know and understand" (to know what is the matter, where the pain comes from) and "the need to feel known and understood" (to know the doctor accepts him and takes him seriously). . . . Doctors may define medical information objectively (type of disease, its stage, type of treatment) while patients define it in terms of its personal relevance (will I fully recover? how much pain will I have?).[32]

This is our sense, based on personal experiences and a surprisingly small number of publications, of some of the factors that can disrupt the very intimate conversations between patients and clinicians. These misunderstandings are often misperceived as being engendered by the use of medical jargon; the symptom is viewed as the disease. The deeper reality is that misunderstandings most commonly arise from the different points of reference of the speaker and listener. Although this subliminal contribution to the process is natural, it is undesirable and—more importantly—it can be eliminated. The following section reviews some of the more original and potentially useful suggestions for bridging the gap between speaker and listener.

EMPATHIC COMMUNICATION

A catch phrase used to describe the means of developing common ground among all parties in medical discussions is "empathic communication." Unfortunately, there is little consensus about the definition of *empathy*, let alone *communication*.

Empathy in its broadest sense refers to the responsiveness of an individual to the feelings of another person.[33]

The Golden Rule says to

"Do unto others as you would have others do unto you." While on the surface that could mean to do for them what you would like to have done for you, I think the more essential meaning is to understand them deeply as individuals, the way you would want to be understood, and then to treat them in terms of the understanding.[34]

Grattan and Eslinger define *affectively based empathy* as "an ability to construct for oneself another's emotional experience; a sort of vicarious arousal." They define *cognitively based empathy* as "ability to take another's viewpoint, infer his feelings, and put oneself in his shoes."[35]

Dagenais and Meleis (1982) identify a personality dimension they entitle *empathy,* which has as subdimensions adaptability, sociability, consideration, and sensitivity.[36]

Empathy is conceptualized as a physician's cognitive capacity to understand a patient's needs, an affective sensitivity to a patient's feelings, and a behavioral ability to convey empathy to a patient.[37]

Although intrinsically valid, these definitions can hardly be considered principles readily applicable to the intensive care setting. They are, nonetheless, the necessary substrate for practical guidelines.

The difficulty most people have with empathy is that it involves placing oneself in the position of another, so that one individual can perceive the point of view of another. Traditionally, this has been considered the responsibility of the person attempting to be empathic. As the concept has been explored more extensively, it has become clear that both parties have a role in making this "perceptual shift" a reality.

The responsibility of the healthcare worker is to create an environment that permits the patient and family to fulfill their obligation to present their concerns. The notion of "concerns" should not be narrowly defined. Of course, it is reasonable to anticipate that this includes questions about the nature of the illness, its diagnostic evaluation, and the therapeutic options and their benefits and adverse effects. In addition, it is important to remember that the patient and the family had an elaborate existence prior to the undesired intrusion of disease. As information about this new development begins to sink in, they may begin to remember the dangling threads of the rest of their lives. Most of these aspects of their life remain unaffected, but others take on an entirely new level of complexity amid the changed circumstances.

Exhibit 16-2
Empathic Communication

---

1. Be aware of the affective moment
2. Stop
3. Name the affect
4. Appreciate the affect
5. Affirm the patient's and our own past actions
6. Offer help in the future
7. When in doubt, ask

It is not incumbent on anyone, let alone ICU staff who may have met their patients only recently and who may have other pressing concerns, to be clairvoyant. On the other hand, when clinicians facilitate the expression of personal concerns, the results can be surprising and mutually favorable, as in this example:

> One of our patients . . . was a Lebanese woman, Mrs. A, who had cancer of the endometrium. She was extremely cachectic, was not eating, seemed to be in distress with nausea and pain, but refused to take most of her medications. We all believed that she had very little time to live.
>
> Having talked with her family, we knew that her daughter was to be married in 2 weeks' time, and that this was an extremely important event for her. We talked to Mrs. A, telling her that she was extremely ill and that, if it was important for her to be at her daughter's wedding, perhaps the family should move up the wedding date. We left the decision in her hands to talk over with her family.
>
> Mrs. A clearly understood the seriousness of her illness, but the significance of that news to her was not what we expected. The next day, Mrs. A stated that, if she was that ill, what was most important for her was that she die in Lebanon. Her daughter's wedding was important, but she knew that the wedding would take place and that was enough. She would not wait for the wedding, but would fly back to Lebanon as soon as a flight was available.[38]

The responsibility to help patients express their inner thoughts and feelings is probably intuitively understood and accepted by most healthcare workers. Still, it may not be immediately evident how to do so. There may be some "native empathizers," but most authors concur with Platt and Keller, who regard empathic communication as "a learned intellectual process that requires understanding of feelings. Using and thinking about their own current sensory observations, physicians come to an understanding of the patient's feelings."[39] Platt and Keller emphasize the need to consciously develop this skill as "some physicians may be limited in this area because of a medical training that was itself abusive and unempathic."[40] They believe that healthcare providers may achieve this goal by focusing on the following guidelines:

1. *Be aware of the affective moment.* We begin to dispel our insensitivity to emotions in our patients, or ourselves, by making an effort to be conscious of these emotions when they arise.

2. *Stop.* The pause is essential. It reinforces our awareness of emotion and helps inhibit our well-developed mechanism of repression, our tendency to keep talking until the feeling dissipates.
3. *Name the affect.*
4. *Appreciate the affect.*
5. *Affirm the patient's and our own past actions.* This is done by considering that they may be reactions to the potent emotions we have witnessed.
6. *Offer help in the future.* Patients need reassurance that healthcare workers will not abandon them. In addition, this opens the door to providing constructive guidance on how to respond better in the future.[41]

Thomas Delbanco suggests that eliciting subjective information about the patient's perspective should be an active process incorporated systematically as part of taking the patient's medical history. Specifically, he recommends that inquiries focus on seven nontechnical aspects of care: patients' preferences and expressed needs, coordination and integration of care, communication and education, physical comfort, alleviation of fears and anxieties, involvement of family and friends, and continuity and transition.[42] These lines of questioning cover the majority of issues that may be of concern during the therapeutic process. In addition, this tack reinforces that the clinician is receptive and helps to clear remaining obstacles to the patient's self-expression.

Remedial action naturally follows when this sort of disclosure uncovers a problem. This constitutes the remaining stage of the process of empathic communication, sometimes esoterically termed "empathic mediation." Batson and others have defined the principal steps as "(a) taking the perspective of a person in need which produces an empathic emotional response, with (b) the emotion in turn acting to motivate a helping stance to reduce the need in the other."[43]

This approach induces some additional considerations about empathic communication. Delbanco points out that "it forces us to confront our own attitudes and the range of options we offer or control." He advises that it does not need to be completed during a single encounter. "Moreover, in our clinical teaching, just as we query students and residents routinely about physical signs and symptoms, we can ask them about their patients' values, preferences, knowledge, and support-systems."[44] In this way, the process is perpetuated for future generations of clinicians.

Other authors provide additional suggestions for refining empathic communication:

> Sometimes physicians ask what to do when they are sure that a strong affect is present but are not sure just what it is. We suggest: *when in doubt, be curious.* It is perfectly correct to ask. . . . We also would apply the same rule when we recognize the feeling but not the reasons behind it.[45]

> We can bring ourselves, our honesty, our humility, our compassion, a listening ear, advocacy. Patients can then decide how to use our help. . . . It is patients who choose what help they want, from whom, and the time, the place, and the depth of sharing.[46]

> Listening involves not only hearing what the [patient] says, but also how it is said, i.e. the volume and tone of voice, body posture, eye contact and facial expression.[47]

It is worth emphasizing that empathic communication is a means for exchanging information, a process that "consists of information-giving and information-seeking."[48] Also, it must not be forgotten that clinicians are, in effect, bilingual, while their audiences usually are not. Here, too, healthcare providers are not expected to possess telepathy, but they must actively investigate the level of sophistication of their patients. According to Siminoff and colleagues:

> One simple method is for the physician to mentally outline what would constitute complete information for patients about . . . therapy. The physician can then address each area with the patient beginning with the most general information and gradually progressing to the most detailed. At intervals, the physician can stop to ascertain if the patient understands and if the patient would like more specific information about a given topic. At the end of each topic, the physician can ask patients if they understood what was said and to summarize their understanding of the topic.[49]

With the patient's perspective in mind, the clinician can frame each part of the delivery, "first using terms that the [patient has] offered and then transforming those terms into a more technical vocabulary."[50] The patient's expressed needs also should help to guide the conversation so that each specific concern is addressed. Likewise, there is no need to dwell on issues that are of no importance to the patient.

According to Ong and colleagues, "The ideal medical interview integrates the patient-centered and physician-centered approaches: the patient leads in areas where he is the expert (symptoms, preferences, concerns), the doctor leads in his domain of expertise (details of disease, treatment)."[51] This ensures that patients and families are permitted to participate in the delivery of care to the extent they desire and that is possible.

CONTROL

Some may argue there is no such thing as giving patients too much control over their own healthcare. This point of view ignores several critical facts. In the first place, patients have a legally protected right to opt not to make such decisions. Of greater importance is the likelihood that this is not the sort of advocacy most patients would prefer.

Investigators who have studied cancer patients report that the majority (92 percent) "preferred all possible information to be given (either good or bad) but only 69% preferred to participate in treatment-related decisions. Of those wanting all the information, almost one fourth preferred a more authoritarian relationship with their oncologist."[52] And, in a separate investigation, "many of the interviewed cancer patients actively sought information, however, 63% felt the doctor should take primary responsibility in the decision-making process. Only 10% felt that they themselves should have major involvement."[53] Another review concluded that the "studies taken together debunk the myth that the only alternative to the physician's total control of power in the therapeutic relationship is his or her total abdication of power."[54] This was Frances Drew's conclusion from her experience as physician turned patient. "Twice in the span of three months, I found myself grateful for firm, unambiguous orders, grateful for authority. I wondered whether it is true for most patients? Has our profession, in its headlong pursuit of patient autonomy, ignored the possibility that authority may be therapeutic?"[55]

A group of medical oncologists reported that most of their breast-cancer patients, even after having undergone mastectomy, were not prepared to deal with information pertaining to the next phase of their treatment.[56] As Louise Coulombe concluded, "Even if patients are educated, their emotions are so much at the forefront that their reasoning can be clouded and their understanding diminished."[57] In all these cases, the individuals whose reasoning might have been clouded had been dealing with their diseases for some time and were being interviewed on an elective basis. In contrast, ICU admission rarely follows such a drawn-out course; patients and their families have even less opportunity to assimilate the implications of what healthcare workers need to discuss with them.

Girgis and Sanson-Fisher suggest that the full-disclosure model of providing information to patients may itself be paternalistic, "since it takes no account of the patient's desires about the timing and amount of information disclosed. . . . Denial is used as a coping strategy by some patients. Hence the doctor may be denying patients this way of coping by telling them more than they want to hear."[58] Others have argued that having patients assume too much responsibility for their own care may not be appropriate. If the outcome is undesirable, the patient may feel that they made the "wrong choice."[59] Even worse, this conclusion may be reached by the family, who may carry a burden of irreconcilable remorse long after the death of their loved one.

Healthcare workers are challenged to learn to cede power and control in their interactions with patients and families in a mature and responsible manner. To succeed, they must abandon some other ingrained convictions that are likely to be unnecessary obstacles as providers and patients seek to establish a common ground.

On first experiencing the strong emotional response to a pronouncement of dire facts, a clinician's ability to cope may be temporarily overcome. It is important to learn to anticipate such moments. When they occur, the clinician should pause long enough to differentiate how to talk this through with the patient, rather than talking it away. This is not the time for incomprehensible jargon or technicalities. The clinician may mistakenly conclude that the message was conveyed when, in fact, it was too clouded in euphemisms for the patient to receive and retain it. It may also be improper to attempt to restore hope immediately. Patients may be confused by the implication that the situation is not quite so bad after all, or they may conclude that their perceptions are undervalued or, frankly, misunderstood.

Girgis and Sanson-Fisher provide additional, detailed guidance for conducting difficult discussions.[60] They remind clinicians that it is equally inadvisable to withhold evocative news from patients and families because, in analytic and clinical trials, "the weight of available evidence seems to support a position that disclosure of bad news is not harmful to all patients, with some evidence suggesting that failure to communicate clearly may be."[61] Also, anecdotal experience has shown that "patients don't fall apart; if they do not want to hear bad news, they won't hear it."[62] Nor is it probable that open communication will "put ideas in their heads." In most cases, patients are already subjectively aware; putting a name to their feelings may provide a useful reference point and help dispel phantasms.

CONCLUSION

Once we have mastered these skills, we must concentrate on teaching them to our protégés. Clear comprehension of these relatively subjective issues is a necessity; otherwise, the next generation will be no more successful in integrating these concepts than our generation has been. Individuals conducting research in this area should heed their own advice and avoid another brand of impenetrable jargon, so-called psychobabble. For example, "an interactant may have a characteristic way of communicating yet modifications of this style may be tailored to situational exigencies."[63]

It is not uncommon for the course of a critical illness to become protracted. According to Tzu, "When you do battle, even if you are winning, if you continue for a long time it will dull your forces and blunt your edge; if you besiege a citadel, your strength will be exhausted."[64] Healthcare workers should remain alert to the fact that, under duress, they are far more likely to resort to modes of interaction that limit communication.[65]

To incorporate this mode of interaction into the clinical setting, clinicians must have the necessary skills, the desire to put them to use, and the time. In the ICU, and in an era of managed care, time may be extremely limited. Patients, and those entrusted with making decisions for them, must take this into consideration. The success of the entire communication process also depends on patients' willingness to be open and to accept that they themselves can help minimize miscommunication by volunteering subjective information.

Some researchers report that empathic communication in the healthcare arena has a salutary effect on the outcome of illness. However, even when the patient dies, there is significant benefit from this approach. As Samuel Shem's patient, the dying physician, pointed out, "In spite of all our doubt, we can give something. Not cure, no. What sustains us is when we find a way to be compassionate, to love. And the most loving thing we do is to be with a patient, like you are being with me."[66] We can only achieve this state if we are aware of the patient's feelings and needs and if we can constructively control our own reactions to them.

There is also the surviving family to consider. By learning to be attentive to their needs and wishes, we enhance the likelihood that we will pull them safely through the tempest of the patient's disease. Without understanding, they, like their loved one, will have to endure the battering in isolation as best as they can.

Finally, the experience of those employing empathic styles of communication is inspiring. "Even though we teach empathy as an intellectual activity, we find that an enriched understanding of a patient's feelings leads to something so close to compassion as to be indistinguishable from it," write Platt and Keller.[67] As Ruth MacKay expands on this notion, "The affective quality of the interaction appears to be contagious."[68]

NOTES

1. R. Palmer, recorded on E.K. Ellington, . . . *And His Mother Called Him Bill* (New York: BMG Music, 1967).

2. Ibid.

3. I.D. Todres, "Communication between Physician, Patient, and Family in the Pediatric Intensive Care Unit," *Critical Care Medicine* 21 (1993): S385.

4. L. Coulombe, "Talking with Patients: Is It Different When They Are Dying?" *Canadian Family Physician* 41 (1995): 427.

5. F. Jarman, "Informed Consent. Communication Problems: A Patient's View," *Nursing Times* 91 (1995): 31.

6. F.L. Drew, "Inside Hydrocephalus 1994," *Pittsburgh Medicine* (Fall 1995): 17.

7. A. Trafford, "A Pediatrician's Other Patients," *Washington Post*, 14 November 1995, HM 6.

8. See note 3 above, p. S383.

9. American Psychiatric Association, Task Force on DSM IV, *Diagnostic and Statistical Manual of Mental Disorders*, 4th ed. (Washington, D.C.: American Psychiatric Association, 1994), 752.

10. Ibid.

11. S.B. Nuland, *How We Die* (New York: Random House, 1993), 247.

12. See note 9 above.

13. C. Maslach and W.B. Schaufeli, "Historical and Conceptual Development of Burnout," in *Professional Burnout: Recent Developments in Theory and Research*, ed. W. Schaufeli, C. Maslach, and T. Marek (Washington, D.C.: Tay-

lor & Francis, 1993), 14.

14. S. Shem, *The House of God* (New York: Dell Publishing, 1978), 175.

15. See note 13 above, p. 12.

16. See note 3 above.

17. See note 4 above, p. 423.

18. See note 13 above, p. 10.

19. See note 5 above, p. 31.

20. See note 11 above, p. *xvii.*

21. Ibid., 141.

22. D. Roter and R. Frankel, "Quantitative and Qualitative Approaches to the Evaluation of the Medical Dialogue," *Social Science and Medicine* 34 (1992): 1098.

23. M.A. Stewart, "Effective Physician-Patient Communication and Health Outcomes: A Review," *Journal of the Canadian Medical Association* 152 (1995): 1424.

24. L.A. Siminoff, J.H. Fetting, and M.D. Abeloff, "Doctor-Patient Communication about Breast Cancer Adjuvant Therapy," *Journal of Clinical Oncology* 7 (1989): 1194.

25. F.W. Platt and V.F. Keller, "Empathic Communication: A Teachable and Learnable Skill," *Journal of General Internal Medicine* 9 (1994): 222.

26. R.A. Held, "Transcription Concerning the Accident Involving KLM867 on December 15, 1989, at Approximately 2048 UTC," Federal Aviation Administration, p. 22-23.

27. *American Heritage Electronic Dictionary* (Boston: Houghton Mifflin Company, 1992).

28. See note 11 above, p. 249.

29. Ibid., 149.

30. S.W. Golomb, "Negations and Contranyms," *Johns Hopkins Magazine* (September 1992): 66.

31. J. Jaynes, *The Origin of Consciousness in the Breakdown of the Bicameral Mind* (Boston: Houghton Mifflin Company, 1976).

32. L.M. Ong et al., "Doctor-Patient Communication: A Review of the Literature," *Social Science & Medicine* 40 (1995): 904.

33. R.C. MacKay, "What Is Empathy?" in *Empathy in the Helping Relationship,* ed. R.C. MacKay, J.R. Hughes, and E.J. Carver, (New York: Springer Publishing, 1990), 9.

34. S.R. Covey, *The Seven Habits of Highly Effective People: Restoring the Character Ethic* (New York: Simon and Schuster, 1989), 192.

35. See note 25 above, p. 225.

36. See note 33 above, p. 6.

37. K.M. Feighny, M. Monaco, and L. Arnold, "Empathy Training to Improve Physician-Patient Communication Skills," *Academic Medicine* 70 (1995): 435.

38. See note 4 above, p. 425.

39. See note 25 above, p. 225.

40. Ibid., 226.

41. Ibid., 223-24.

42. T.L. Delbanco, "Enriching the Doctor-Patient Relationship by Inviting the Patient's Perspective," *Annals of Internal Medicine* 116 (1992): 415.

43. See note 33 above, p. 7.

44. See note 42 above, p. 416.

45. See note 25 above, p. 225.

46. See note 4 above, p. 436.

47. B. Lask, "Talking with Children," *British Journal of Hospital Medicine* 47 (1992): 688.

48. See note 32 above, p. 904.

49. See note 24 above, p. 1199.

50. See note 22 above, p. 1102.

51. See note 32 above, p. 904.

52. Ibid., 905

53. Ibid.

54. See note 23 above, p. 1432.

55. See note 6 above, p. 16.

56. See note 24 above.

57. See note 4 above, p. 425.

58. A. Girgis and R.W. Sanson-Fisher, "Breaking Bad News: Consensus Guidelines for Medical Practitioners," *Journal of Clinical Oncology* 13 (1995): 2451.

59. See note 32 above, p. 905.

60. See note 58 above.

61. Ibid., p. 2450.

62. See note 4 above, p. 427.

63. R.L. Street, "Communicative Styles and Adaptations in Physician-Parent Consultations," *Social Science and Medicine* 34 (1992): 1162.

64. S. Tzu, *The Art of War* (Boston: Shambhala, 1991), 11.

65. See note 22 above.

66. See note 14 above, p. 175.

67. See note 25 above, p. 226.

68. See note 33 above, p. 4.

17

Luxury Critical Care, Pluralistic Standards, and Respect for Moral Diversity

H. Tristram Engelhardt, Jr. and Michael A. Rie

DEMANDING BETTER-THAN-USUAL CRITICAL CARE: COMING TO TERMS WITH MULTIPLE STANDARDS OF CRITICAL CARE

Solutions have their own problems. Containing the costs of critical care and establishing criteria for its "more appropriate use" will engender disputes about the nature of appropriate guiding policy. The difficulty is that there are competing accounts of allocatory propriety. The introduction of honest limitations on access to critical care in order (1) to contain critical care costs, (2) to have use conform with established policies of appropriate critical care, and (3) to provide clarity and frankness of policy will disclose controversies about the very core of secular morality and secular moral authority. Even when critical care is excluded on the basis of a thoughtful national policy because it (1) only offers a modest postponement of death, (2) only secures a quality of life that others will judge not worth the resources deployed (such as life in a permanently vegetative state), or (3) only offers a very small chance of full recovery at very high cost, some patients will seek critical care and thus challenge egalitarian aspirations. Individuals and communities who seek better-than-basic critical care will not necessarily be the affluent. They may include individuals and groups with secular or religious moral understandings of how appropriately to postpone death, who will demand more aggressive provision of critical care and be willing to pay for it. This chapter addresses the case of individuals or communities who would demand better-than-basic or "standard" critical care and are willing to pay for it from their own after-tax dollars.

If individuals and communities possess sufficient resources to purchase better-than-basic critical care on the spot or to plan ahead through insurance policies, the notion that there should be a single and universal standard of appropriate critical care will be challenged. This chapter argues in favor of recognizing that morally such challenges should prevail and that, if institutions are willing to offer better-than-basic care for those who can pay, this may not be forbidden with general secular moral authority. The chapter begins by showing why it is morally inappropriate to impose a particular egalitarian morality on a society so as to foreclose the purchase of better-than-basic critical care. This is accomplished by demonstrating that there is no canonical, content-full secular morality, which by its rational force can give a secular state the secular moral authority to forbid such practices. If secular moral authority cannot be drawn from a generally justifiable content-full secular morality, secular moral authority must be acquired from the consent of the participants in a common practice. Because such consent is unavoidably limited, the secular moral authority of common endeavors is unavoidably limited. Limited democracies thus provide the only form of secular polity justifiable in general secular terms. They must, as such, leave space for numerous competing understandings of and standards for appropriate critical care.

If one is to take moral diversity and the limits of reasonable secular morality seriously, one must fundamentally rethink the notions of standards for care, rethink the bearing of tort liability on the obligation to meet such standards, and acquiesce in unequal levels of critical care. Luxury critical care is morally unavoidable.

FASCISM OF FAIRNESS AND THE DRIVE TO UNIVERSAL MEDIOCRITY

Healthcare appears to be a service unlike others: it bears on our very finitude as humans and touches the most intimate passages of life, from copulation and birth to suffering and death. Because of its connections with our finitude, healthcare has notoriously been difficult to limit. Critical care, as the epitome of high-technology medicine, brings with it the hope of dramatically reversing physiological fortunes and allowing those who would otherwise die to survive and return to their normal lives and occupations. Although it is generally successful, critical care in many cases fails to restore health and preserve life. The difficulty in determining when expensive critical care is indicated lies in great measure with the probabilistic character of medical knowledge. It is impossible to know with certainty the outcomes that will be experienced by a particular patient. At best, one can with a very high certainty make predictions of success or failure.

Such predictions take on special moment for critical care, given its costs. Were a treatment likely to save a patient's life in only 0.1 percent of the times it is deployed and to cost only $1, no one would hesitate using it, despite the unlikelihood of success. One would be saving lives at the cost of only $1,000 per life saved. However, if there is a class of patients in critical care units likely to survive only 0.1 percent of the times they are treated with a usual cost of $200,000, one would be saving lives at the cost of $200 million per life saved. The probabilistic character of critical care, combined with the costs involved, impel critical care policy makers to be wise and prudent gamblers with the lives of others. Because the stakes involved are the lives of patients, many find this circumstance discomforting. The disinclination on the part of intensive care practitioners to recognize their role as prudent gamblers is reflected in the tendency for many to characterize care as "futile" and mean only that it is a "bad bet."[1] The moral challenge of deciding between good and bad gambles is further complicated by the circumstance that different individuals assign different values to continuing life. People have different financial and social resources to recruit in their pursuit of better treatment in the attempt to decrease their likelihood of dying prematurely. Generally in our society we accept radical inequalities in access to basic social goods as fortunate or unfortunate, but neither fair nor unfair. It is well known that there are significant differences in life expectancy, depending on the neighborhood in which one lives as well as the level and character of the education one receives, and that those who live in affluent neighborhoods with less crime are at liberty to hire security services to enhance their safety and to decrease the likelihood of having their lives preemptively terminated by intruders. The rich, whose children are already advantaged by more intellectual family circumstances, may further increase that advantage by sending their children to private schools and engaging private tutors. In housing, education, security, diet, and the general circumstances of life, there are radically different levels of access to the resources that contribute to individuals' health and longevity. Although researchers have suggested that access to healthcare in itself comparatively makes only a minor difference in the likelihood of illness and premature death, healthcare has been inordinately the focus of egalitarian passions.[2] Healthcare has become a disproportionate focus of egalitarian concerns to regard fortunate or unfortunate differences as unfair and therefore to employ state coercion in remedy.

In great measure, one may lay blame for the moral distortion of the significance of ensuring equality in healthcare at the feet of the bioethicists who have encouraged an egalitarianism of envy. Here, it is important to distinguish between an egalitarianism of envy, which is concerned with those who have more, and an egalitarianism of altruism, focused on those in need. One can test one's intuitions to determine one's proclivity toward an egalitarianism of envy versus one of altruism by comparing three possible worlds. The first world has 10 individuals, each with equal amounts of that which is good; for the purposes of these considerations, each has six units of goods or benefits. The second world has nine individuals with six units of good and one with 10. The third world has nine individuals with six units of good and one individual with only one. If one regards not only the third world as worse than the first, but the second world as worse than the first, one is an egalitarian of envy. The second world differs from the first only in that one individual is more advantaged and that it has a greater total amount of goods. One individual is fortunate, and none is placed in an unfortunate circumstance other than that of being unequal. If one is disposed to use state force to take from the one who has more, or to forbid anyone from having more, one is a coercive egalitarian of envy. If one celebrates the second world as better than the first and, with respect to the third, asks how one might most cheaply help the individual with less, one is an egalitarian of altruism. This chapter examines luxury care as a case of allowing the second world to come into existence: one in which some have better care than others.[3] An egalitarian of envy would rather have a world in which there is only one basic, albeit mediocre standard of care for all.

In anticipation, it is important to notice the character of the moral issues that support a differential provision of healthcare. We do not share one moral vision of fairness and justice. The thoroughgoing, all-encompassing imposition of a particular view of fairness and justice will likely have severe moral costs. Just as the costs of having an omnipresent police force sufficiently efficient to prevent all crime will likely include imposing a state of fascist proportions in its commitment to law and order, so, too, the all-encompassing imposition of one view of justice or fairness in healthcare can take on the character of a "fairness fascism."

If one forthrightly acknowledges the irreducible pluralism of understandings of justice and fairness, one will be driven to take limited democracy seriously. Taking limited democracy seriously requires allowing willing collaborators peaceably to purchase different standards of healthcare in general and of critical care in particular. One is obliged to acquiesce in the creation and provision of diverse understandings of basic care, as well as of luxury care. This moral circumstance requires us to rethink the very fabric of tort liability obligations. We will need to move from a uniform standard of critical care to diverse standards created through contract.[4]

A diversity of approaches to critical care will be born of (1) different appreciations of adverse outcomes, (2) different levels of willingness to pay for protection against risks, (3) different resources at the disposal of those who would seek health-risk protection, and (4) morally diverse views of the propriety of providing and limiting particular therapeutic interventions (such as Roman Catholic concerns, on the one hand, not to be euthanatized while, on the other hand, not to receive extraordinary care). The moral inevitability of luxury care discloses foundational issues for a critical care ethics. In particular, it leads to the deconstruction of egalitarian aspirations in the provision of critical care.

MORAL PLURALISM AND THE AMBIGUITY OF FAIRNESS: TAKING LIMITED DEMOCRACY SERIOUSLY

There is no single sense of justice. There is no single understanding of fairness waiting to be applied by bioethics to healthcare policy. Instead, one finds repeated in philosophy the babble of the religious sects produced by the Reformation. There are as many accounts of justice and fairness as there are major established religions. The unavoidability of this diversity is easily appreciated if one considers John Rawls's attempt to establish a canonical account of justice.[5] In order for his hypothetical contractors to make the decisions in the original position desired by Rawls so as to endorse that sense of fairness to which Rawls is committed, he must fit them out with a particular understanding (that is, his understanding) of the thin theory of the good, a particular understanding (his) of risk aversiveness, an absence of envy, a view of themselves as heads of families, and so forth. If one provides the hypothetical contractors with a different thin theory of the good, then the expository device of the original position will lay out a different sense of justice. For example, if one gives priority to the notion of being at liberty to act on one's talents as best one can with consenting others, then contractors will approach the fashioning of a constitution quite differently from those in Rawls's portrayal, where they are guided first by a notion of liberty tied to civil rights such as voting, free speech, and so forth, and then by a commitment to equality of opportunity lexically prior to prosperity.

To treat people justly or fairly requires giving to them what they should appropriately receive. As Justinian put it "Justice is the constant and perpetual wish to render everyone his due."[6] The questions are: What is owed and to whom? Does one owe individuals first and foremost an opportunity to prosper? Does one owe individuals an equality of opportunity? Does one owe individuals an equality of outcome? Does one owe individuals the liberty to act on their own visions of the good? Does one owe individuals the liberty to act on a particular content-full vision of the good, such as that endorsed by Rawls?

As recent political discussions regarding the welfare state in America and Europe reveal, there is a considerable lack of consensus regarding the nature of fairness and the substantive character of justice. Postmodernity presents us with a plurality of visions of fairness and justice.[7] As the foregoing arguments show, there is no secular deliverance from this plurality. To recognize one rather than another view of justice as morally binding, one must be guided by an underlying, guiding moral sense. The difficulty is to choose the correct underlying, guiding moral sense. To make that choice, one needs a yet even more foundational moral sense so as to choose the correct underlying, guiding moral sense. Any attempt to supply content recapitulates the challenge of choosing the correct moral guidance at the level of moral foundations. The problem of choosing the appropriate account of justice and fairness, the choice of the appropriate underlying, guiding moral sense, begs the question or involves an infinite regress. For example, one is not able to choose among alternative moral accounts by appealing to the consequences of the choices. In order to make such a choice, one will need to compare the consequences of liberty with the consequences of equality with the consequences of prosperity. But how does one know how to compare such genres of consequences? One cannot simply appeal to consequences. One is thus in the unhappy circumstance of arbitrarily choosing a particular moral perspective or content.[8]

We have approached this problem of plurality in the case of religious visions by refusing to establish any particular religious account. *Mutatis mutandi*, the same should apply for justice and fairness in critical care. Just as it would be inappropriate for a secular polity to establish the Roman Catholic morality of contraception for non-Roman Catholics in the United States, so, too, it is morally arbitrary to establish a particular view of justice and fairness in a thoroughgoing way that would preclude a diversity of options with regard to the provision of healthcare in general and critical care in particular. Moral pluralism, the plurality of visions of justice and fairness, requires making room for people peaceably to collaborate with others and to act upon their particular views of appropriate critical care.

This is the logic of a limited democracy: a polity limited in its claims upon the property of its citizens, as well as with regard to the propriety of establishing a particular moral vision. Insofar as a limited democracy does not involve the exhaustive ownership of the citizens by the citizens—but rather the creation of a structure of limited moral authority to protect the rights of citizens as well as to provide, from common resources, insurance against particular malevents—individuals are at liberty with their after-tax dollars to pursue their particular, diverse visions of the good life. A limited democracy in eschewing the establishment of a particular religion, ideology, or view of fairness must allow individuals, with willing others, peaceably to pursue their own understandings of the good life, proper healthcare, and desirable critical care.

FACING UP TO A PLURALITY OF STANDARDS OF CRITICAL CARE: A CONTRACTUAL APPROACH TO TORT LIABILITY

No one infallibly knows God's wishes for a decent, minimal standard of critical care. Any particular standard involves particular choices regarding the amounts of resources to be expended to avoid particular risks of suffering, disability, and death. There is no canonical secular revelation to guide all to the correct understanding of how critical care should appropriately be provided and with respect to who should be the primary focus of concern. It is very likely that, given different nursing skills, different intensive care units will be more or less advantaged in treating patients afflicted with respiratory versus cardiac versus renal versus hepatic failure. Unless one believes that one can discover from reason the canonically appropriate balance among such alternative policy options, any choice of a standard of care will be an arbitrary contractual creation. It will draw its moral authority from the permission of those who participate. Given the development of new and costly therapeutic opportunities, and given the limits on available resources, standards of care are best approached as the result of contractual agreements.[9]

The implication of this circumstance is that one cannot discover within a general ethos of physicians a particular standard of healthcare in general, or of critical care in particular, that should be provided for all. Given different understandings of morbidity and mortality risks, different available skills, as well as different resources, different standards of care will appear plausible. A single standard of critical care will lead to morally adverse outcomes. Imposing a unitary standard of care by appeal to tort law will foreclose the opportunity to discuss honestly what levels of morbidity and mortality protection should be purchased and at what price. One must not exempt discussions regarding the purchase of healthcare from the kinds of decisions that individuals regularly make in other areas of their lives.

If a family purchases a cheaper home in a less safe part of town, they opt not to invest more in morbidity and mortality protection through housing location. If they purchase a smaller, light-weight car without side-panel air bags, they similarly decide to place themselves and their loved ones at particular risks so as to economize in the area of automobile purchase. Again, since all humans die and no human has infinite resources, all persons must gamble with themselves and those they hold dear. The illusion that there is one appropriate and full standard of healthcare deceives all involved. It suggests that such choices to take prudent risks should not be made with regard to healthcare. In a society of free and responsible individuals, different groups with different values and economic resources would be at liberty to make their own choices regarding the standards of healthcare they wish to purchase. Moved by an egalitarianism of altruism, one might very well act to provide funds to ameliorate the state of the impecunious. Even after that amelioration, both the rich and the poor will still be faced with the choice of how to use their remaining resources and what standards of healthcare they would wish to endorse. The finite character of human life, the limited nature of our resources, the diversity of our moral views, and the limited plausible authority of democratic states should lead to polities abandoning a single standard of healthcare, both in the provision of healthcare and in healthcare tort liability. Instead, standards should be established contractually and enforced by the courts.

In the absence of a single, canonical moral view of an appropriate package of healthcare, and in the face of a diversity of views in this matter, moral authority for standards of care can only be established by agreement. Medical negligence cannot be understood as the failure to provide a standard of care for which one has not contracted. The failure to meet the standard of care can only be a failure to meet a particular standard of care derived from some prior contractual agreement. Moral diversity has significant implications for the character of generally secularly defensible tort law bearing on the provision of critical care. The critical care to which people are entitled is that for which they have contracted.

COMING TO TERMS WITH LUXURY
AND MEDIOCRE CRITICAL CARE

Luxury care is often construed as care (such as cosmetic orthodontics) offering a benefit not necessary for the preservation of life or for the protection of significant bodily integrity or function. In contrast, basic care is used to identify care that meets such needs. In the real world, there are no crisp lines between luxury and basic care. Luxury care cannot be used simply to identify amenities and perquisites such as private or more luxurious rooms. Basic critical care that is in its own way the best of care is expensive care. If it is not to be very expensive care, then it must in some areas be middling in its protection against morbidity and mortality risks. That is, basic critical care cannot include without significant expense all diagnostic and therapeutic interventions that offer a positive balance of morbidity and mortality risks. Once cost becomes a consideration, the matters considered in drawing the line between care to be provided and not to be provided within basic care include financial risks as well as health risks. Basic care becomes mediocre care.

Mediocre care carries an adverse connotation. The word is derived from the Latin *mediocris* ("the middle [mountain] peak") and properly identifies ordinary care, care of moderate excellence. Mediocre care identifies a cluster of possible standards of care that lies in the middle range of morbidity and mortality protection. Such care can be construed as basic care insofar as a commitment to that level of morbidity and mortality relief is endorsed by a society as a floor of treatment for its impecunious.

In any system that does not have sufficient resources to provide the very best of care to everyone, luxury care develops spontaneously in the face of most receiving mediocre care. Luxury critical care identifies intensive care that provides enhanced levels of morbidity and mortality protection. In particular, luxury critical care offers treatment that would only (1) minimally postpone death, (2) secure a quality of life unacceptable for most, and/or (3) involve what most consider a bad gamble in promising only a small chance of success at very high cost.

In the face of human finitude, diverse values regarding risk protection, limited secular moral authority, as well as differences in available resources, all will not contract for luxury care. The result will be that all will not have equal protection through critical care against morbidity and mortality risks. Such circumstances will be of one fabric with the ways in which individuals are currently advantaged or disadvantaged in being male or female, rich or poor, high status or low status (rich, high-status females being most advantaged). Since such differences in human advantage and disadvantage cannot effectively be set aside (1) without invoking a canonical secular moral vision that neither exists nor can be established, and (2) without drawing upon a state authority hostile to the very notion of a nontotalitarian, limited democratic polity, numerous standards of healthcare in general and of critical care in particular are morally unavoidable.

These limitations are moral. In the face of irreconcilable moral diversity, there is no secular moral authority for imposing, in an encompassing fashion, one understanding of distributive justice, fairness, and equality on all. In addition, substantial consequentialist considerations weigh against egalitarian aspirations. The presence of luxury care can allow societies over time to reassess and improve the quality of the basic standard of care guaranteed to all.[10] In the absence of a clear and present illustration of the virtues of luxury care, it will be difficult to understand how, when, and under what circumstances elements of luxury care might be selected to be made available within the basic standard package of critical care. Nor can one easily assess the circumstances under which luxury care will, in the eyes of most, be regarded as not providing a benefit commensurate with its costs. Luxury care can thus function as a basis for correcting and improving mediocre care. It can also show when mediocre care may be judged by most as more than sufficient, since luxury care may frequently entail greater exposure to iatrogenic adverse events. In many circumstances, one will find that less is more.

In American secular culture, a terminal sojourn in critical care prior to death has played a role equivalent to Extreme Unction in a religious community. It has been inconceivable to many that someone in extremis would not be provided with intensive care services, even when there is little or no prospect of survival beyond a few months or when the chances of restoration of physiological function are very limited. This cultural expectation has collided with financial limits. One is constrained to demystify the role of critical care, as societies contemplate fashioning healthcare policy that limits critical care to circumstances in which critical care is likely to offer (1) a more than a minimal prolongation of life, (2) a restoration to conscious life, and/or (3) a considerable chance of having a full restoration of function with less than inordinate costs.[11] If critical care may only be used when there is a reasonable chance of an acceptable quality of life for a significant period of time and without inordinate cost, the moral imperatives surrounding critical care must be transformed. The difficulty is that there are significant disagreements as to what should count as "a reasonable chance," "an acceptable quality of life," "a significant span of life," and "inordinate costs." Many of the disagreements depend on divergent moral, religious, and metaphysical understandings, among which it is not possible to make definitive secular, canonical choices. Any established, general standard of critical care cannot be discovered; it must be created. Given our unavoidable moral diversity and the limits of plausible, secular moral authority, different standards of care are unavoidable.

The consequence of these considerations is that societies will have secular moral authority to establish particular basic standards of critical care, as long as this does not foreclose the possibility of individuals and communities establishing yet other supplementary or luxury standards. The limits of secular morality make plausible the emergence of additional standards of critical care directed to those who wish to subscribe to and pay in advance for health insurance guaranteeing critical care, even when success is likely to be minimal and costs considerable. One can imagine various secular genres of "long-shot care" or "maxicare" being marketed to individuals who wish to protect themselves against being denied treatment under the cost constraints imposed within basic standards of critical care. One can also imagine particular religious groups that would consider it obligatory to maintain life even in a permanently obtunded state. These religions could provide their communities with various genres of "fanaticare." Such insurance associations would then need to approach hospitals with reimbursement schedules in order to reimburse those hospitals for the costs incurred while also providing sufficient excess revenue so that the provision of such care would be economically attractive.

Under such circumstances, the provision of "long-shot care," "maxicare," or "fanaticare" would not deny others access to healthcare. The availability of luxury levels of critical care would bring into the healthcare system after-tax dollars not otherwise available. Those funds would secure not only additional medical resources but also the training of additional medical professionals to meet long-shot, maxicare, or fanaticare commitments. Instead of disposable wealth being invested in video games or luxury cars, the funds would be placed within critical care. This would help to finance the exploration of treatments not clinically assessable with only mediocre critical care.

An approach to critical care that takes moral plurality and the limits of secular moral authority seriously is one that acquiesces in a diversity of approaches to the provision of critical care. Instead of imposing a single, all-encompassing, secular moral view or ideology, one is constrained, on strong secular moral grounds, to tolerate a diversity of moral approaches to the risks of suffering and death. Luxury care is morally unavoidable.

NOTES

1. H.T. Engelhardt Jr. and G. Khushf, "Futile Care for the Critically Ill Patients," *Current Opinion in Critical Care* 1 (1995): 329-33.

2. For data showing the absence of any dramatic increases in life expectancy with significantly increased healthcare investments, see G.J. Schieber, J.P. Poullier, and L.M. Greenwald, "Health System Performance in OECD Countries, 1980-1992," *Health Affairs* 1 (Fall 1994): 100-12. As this article reports, the best predictor of length of life is the sex of the person; women in most OECD countries live five or more years longer than men in their cohort. Also, differences in wealth and status appear to be more reliable predictors of a longer life than the general levels of healthcare investment in a country. See J.K. Iglehart, "Canada's Health Care System Faces Its Problems," *New England Journal of Medicine* 322 (1990): 562-68; M.G. Marmot et al., "Health Inequalities among British Civil Servants: The Whitehall II Study," *Lancet* 337 (1991): 1387-93.

3. These arguments are developed at greater length in H.T. Engelhardt, Jr., *The Foundations of Bioethics* (New York: Oxford University Press, 1996), especially pp. 42, 50, and 375-410.

4. M.A. Rie, "The Oregonian ICU: Multi-Tiered Monitorized Morality in

Health Insurance Law," *Journal of Law, Medicine and Ethics* 23 (1995): 149-66.

5. John Rawls attempts to justify a particular account of justice in terms of how individuals could imagine designing a society such that they would accept any place in it as involving a fair allocation of rights, standing, and resources. In so doing, Rawls develops a hypothetical choice account, or more precisely, a hypothetical contractor account of justice, and as such has to impute to his contractors a particular, thin theory of the good. See *A Theory of Justice* (Cambridge, Mass.: Harvard University Press, 1971).

6. "*Justitia est constans et perpetua voluntas jus sui quique tribuens.*" F.P.S. Justinianus, *The Institutes of Justinian*, trans. T.C. Sandars (1922, reprint ed., Westport, Conn.: Greenwood Press, 1970), 1.1, p. 5.

7. *Postmodernity* identifies our contemporary sociological and epistemological condition regarding our inability to justify a universal content-full account of morality or a universal content-full moral narrative. As a sociological condition, postmodernity marks the de facto recognition that there is no universal dominant account or narrative of justice, fairness, or moral probity, as well as the recognition of our epistemological condition—namely, our inability in principle by rational argument to establish any particular content-full account or narrative of justice, fairness, and morality as canonical. It is postmodern, in contrast with the modern philosophical or Enlightenment aspiration, to establish, by sound rational argument, a canonical, content-full moral vision binding all persons. For a further discussion of these terms and matters, see note 3 above, pp. 20-23.

8. See note 3 above, pp. 32-101.

9. For a discussion of multiple standards of care under fiscal restraint, see H.T. Engelhardt, Jr., and M.A. Rie, "Intensive Care Units, Scarce Resources, and Conflicting Principles of Justice," *Journal of the American Medical Association* 255 (1986): 1159-64; E.H. Morreim, *Balancing Act* (Washington, D.C.: Georgetown University Press, 1995).

10. M.M. Rosenthal, "Beyond Equity: Swedish Health Policy and the Private Sector," *Milbank Quarterly* 64, no. 4 (1986): 592-621.

11. Society of Critical Care Medicine Medical Ethics Committee, "Consensus Statement on the Triage of Critically Ill Patients," *Journal of the American Medical Association* 271 (1994): 1200-03.

18

Advance Directives and Surrogate Decision Making in the ICU

John Schumacher
and John J. Lynch

INTRODUCTION

Surrogate decision making is a fundamental aspect of the intensive care unit (ICU). Illness necessitating ICU admission often interferes with a patient's decision-making capacity, creating the need for some degree of surrogate medical decision making. This chapter explores the connection between surrogate decision making and advance directives (ADs) in the ICU. It begins with an overview of ADs, including their definition and history and comments on the influence of the 1991 Patient Self-Determination Act (PSDA).[1] Second, the chapter explores the utility and role of ADs in the medical decision-making process of the ICU. Third, it discusses elements of an ideal AD in relation to the overall importance of ADs in surrogate decision making. Fourth, the chapter considers some of the challenges posed by ICU patients without ADs and potential reasons for resistance to ADs. The chapter concludes by emphasizing the central role of ADs and surrogate decision making in the ICU and advocating for greater formal integration of ADs into the intensive care setting.

OVERVIEW OF ADVANCE DIRECTIVES
AND SURROGATE DECISION MAKING

DEFINITIONS

The term *advance directives* broadly refers to the conversations and/ or documentation between the physician and the patient that focus on clarifying the patient's wishes and values and projecting the type of medical treatment the patient would want under a variety of circumstances in the event that the patient becomes unable to make decisions. A *surrogate decision maker* is a person who is designated to speak for another person if that person lacks decision-making capacity. A surrogate decision maker may be appointed by means of an AD properly executed according to a state's statutes. In the absence of an AD, some state statutes designate the following default surrogate decision-making order: spouse, adult child, parent, adult sibling, grandparent, friend. However, a surrogate decision maker designated by an AD supersedes the state's default order.

ADs are commonly expressed in three formats: the living will (LW), the durable power of attorney for healthcare (DPA), and a conversation with a physician or others. The LW and DPA are governed by applicable state statute. These state statutes vary in regard to the scope and authority of ADs, witnessing requirements, and other formal provisions.

In general, the LW is the narrowest directive in scope because its provisions are only effective in the event that the patient is certified by two physicians to be (1) unable to make decisions *and* (2) suffering from a terminal condition. Typically, LWs prohibit the use of any life-sustaining or nonbeneficial medical treatment other than comfort measures or palliative care for the terminally ill patient.

In the DPA, the competent person executing a DPA appoints a person as a surrogate decision maker (agent or proxy) for himself/herself. The DPA is significantly different from the LW because the scope and authority for decision making are much broader. The surrogate decision maker can make medical decisions for the incapacitated patient over a range of issues. Importantly, the decision making of a DPA is not limited to the conditions of a terminal illness, as it is for an LW. However, the surrogate decision maker is charged to speak for the patient regarding medical issues and to make decisions based on how the patient would have made particular decisions if the patient were able to speak for himself or herself. The surrogate decision maker does not make decisions based on his or her own values but rather based on the values and prior directions and wishes of the patient. If the patient's preferences are unknown, the surrogate's best estimate concerning how the patient would have made the decision is desired. Generally, the DPA is only effective when two physicians have declared a patient to be incapable of making medical decisions. In addition, state statutes may further specify a surrogate's authority as well as the type of decisions a surrogate may make.

The DPA offers additional flexibility in decision making for patients who lack decision-making capacity. Updated medical information about a patient's status that may significantly influence medical decision making can be presented to the patient's surrogate for consideration. In addition, a patient's surrogate can respond to evolving medical situations that the patient may not have anticipated when completing the AD. Ideally, the DPA can be combined with some form of a LW or other written instructions to provide concrete guidance for the surrogate decision-making process, although this is not necessary.

The third type of legally recognized AD is simply a conversation between the patient and his or her physician that may or may not be documented in the medical record. Because the medical record constitutes a legal document, it is preferable, but not required, that AD conversations are recorded by the physician. As with any form of AD, the validity of the conversation and/or documentation is subject to the provisions of a state's statutes. Regardless of form of AD documentation, it is strongly recommended that a physician be involved at some point in the process of executing an AD. Physicians can provide important technical information that may clarify various medical options. Furthermore, the involvement of a physician early in the process may reduce the potential for conflict and confusion over the implementation of an AD.

HISTORY

Advance directives are not a new concept. An early precursor of ADs, the California Natural Death Act of 1976, states: "Adult persons have the fundamental right to control the decisions relating to the rendering of medical care including decisions to have life-sustaining procedures withheld or withdrawn in instances of a terminal condition."[2] Over the ensuing years, interest in ADs has grown, spurred by two nationally celebrated legal cases. The first case (1976) involved Karen Ann Quinlan, a 28-year-old woman who was in an incapacitated state and dependent on a ventilator. Her family's public agonizing and deliberation over whether to disconnect her ventilator moved the public to consider the situation of incapacity and medical decision making. With the New Jersey Supreme Court's concurrence, the request by Quinlan's parents to remove her from the ventilator was carried out.[3]

The second celebrated legal case, which involved Nancy Cruzan, was ultimately argued at the U.S. Supreme Court. Cruzan was a 25-year-old woman who was left in a persistent vegetative state as the result of an automobile accident. The patient's parents petitioned for the removal of her feeding tube based on the lack of improvement in her medical condition and her prior comments that she would not want to continue living in an incapacitated state. The state of Missouri challenged the parents' petition on the basis of their failure to provide clear and convincing evidence regarding the patient's preference not to be maintained in an incapacitated, debilitated state. Ultimately, the U.S. Supreme Court upheld Missouri's criterion of requiring clear and convincing evidence to limit medical treatment, but the Court articulated a patient's right to limit therapy.[4] Cruzan's parents then gathered additional information regarding her previously stated preferences. This new information was accepted by a Missouri court, and the patient's feeding tube was removed. She died 11 days later.

THE PATIENT SELF-DETERMINATION ACT

In response to the resurgence of interest in biomedical issues as well as the judicial intervention in Nancy Cruzan's case, U.S. Senator John C. Danforth and U.S. Representative Sander Levin introduced the Patient Self-Determination Act. This widely supported legislation, which became law on 1 December 1991, requires hospitals and other healthcare institutions to provide certain information to patients regarding ADs. Specifically, healthcare institutions that receive federal funds must (1) inquire whether a patient has an AD, (2) provide patients written information concerning ADs, (3) accept and properly document a patient's ADs, (4) not condition care on the presence or absence of a patient's AD, and (5) initiate community education projects on ADs. Failure to comply with these provisions could result in the loss of federal Medicaid, Medicare, and other funds.[5]

ADVANCE DIRECTIVES IN THE ICU

ADs are perhaps more important in the critical care environment than in any other hospital setting. Surrogate decision making and AD guidance are often needed for the care of critically ill patients. In general, these patients are in compromised and unstable medical conditions, necessitating continuous care and frequent decision making. Under these conditions an AD can provide important and appropriate guidance that respects the patient's wishes regarding medical decisions. Broadly, ADs in the ICU address one of our society's greatest moral challenges: how to decide for another. The medical community is frequently challenged by situations that involve surrogate decision making for previously competent individuals who develop cognitive impairment (such as patients with Alzheimer's disease and brain-injured and comatose patients).[6] In these morally difficult cases, ADs generated by previously competent patients provide some justifiable, patient-based guidance for decision making.

Because we live in a pluralistic society, ADs are extremely important. There is no clear consensus regarding death and dying among patients, physicians, or society. The type of treatment desired by one person may strike another as pointless, degrading, and horrible.[7] ADs offer a way for individuals to provide guidance about decisions regarding their medical care when they can no longer speak for themselves.

Critical life-and-death decisions are made in the ICU on a regular basis. Without an AD, families and health professionals are often left in the position of guessing what the patient would have wanted under a particular circumstance.[8] Studies report that these surrogate decisions for patients by families are seldom better than mere chance, because these issues were never discussed in the family prior to the patient's admission to the ICU.[9] By default, the absence of patient directives may encourage medical decision making based on the family's or physician's values rather than those of the incapacitated patient. In these situations, a properly executed AD could provide accurate, patient-generated guidance.

Furthermore, there may come a time when aggressive treatment in the ICU has little or nothing to offer the patient except discomfort with-

---

Exhibit 18-1
Requirements of the Patient Self-Determination Act (PSDA)

---

1. Inquire whether patient has an advanced directive (AD)
2. Provide patients with written information on ADs
3. Accept and properly document a patient's AD
4. Do not condition the provision of care based on the presence or absence of an AD
5. Initiate community education projects on ADs

out the likelihood of benefit.[10] In this situation, many patients would choose palliative care rather than continuation of aggressive, nonbeneficial care. In the absence of an AD, it is impossible for an incapacitated patient to suggest such an option. ADs can be designed to articulate a patient's wishes to stop nonbeneficial care in the event that he or she loses the ability to communicate these wishes.

ELEMENTS OF AN IDEAL ADVANCE DIRECTIVE

The ideal situation would be for all ICU patients to have ADs before they are admitted to the ICU. Unfortunately, ICU patients are no more likely to have an AD than any other patient admitted to the hospital.[11] Approximately 85 percent of all patients admitted to a hospital have no formal AD. However, despite the low numbers of patients with ADs prior to admission, a patient's AD wishes may still be documented in the hospital or ICU if the patient retains decision-making capacity. Indeed, admission to the hospital often crystallizes the patient's wishes concerning treatment at the end of life and motivates the patient to document these wishes in an AD. ADs simply document the conversation regarding future medical care between an individual, a designated surrogate, the physician, and the family.

Regardless of whether an AD conversation occurs prior to or during a hospitalization, the patient must be fully oriented and competent in order to execute an AD. Under no circumstances can a valid AD be executed after the patient loses decision-making capacity. Once the patient's decision-making capacity has been verified, several fundamental elements should be considered as part of the AD process. These include

- designation of a surrogate decision maker
- discussion of broad treatment goals and threshold points of treatment
- reflection of the individual's current wishes
- compliance with state laws
- directive's existence known by family and medical team.

DESIGNATION OF A SURROGATE DECISION MAKER

The patient's designation of a surrogate decision maker is desirable in an AD. Ideally, the designated person is intimately familiar with the patient's values and wishes regarding treatment. The surrogate can only make decisions when the patient is no longer able to participate in decision making. An advantage of appointing a surrogate is that this individual can receive up-to-date medical information on the patient's condition by interaction with the medical team. Medical decisions by the surrogate should be based on what the patient would have wanted in light of the evolving medical circumstances. The designation of a surrogate decision maker in an AD can avoid the potential for conflicts among other possible decision makers. Finally, designating an appropriate surrogate decision maker through an AD may facilitate crucial conversations regarding care between the ICU team and the surrogate.

DISCUSSION OF BROAD TREATMENT GOALS AND THRESHOLD POINTS OF TREATMENT

AD conversations in the ICU should focus on articulating broad directions for treatment under a variety of possible medical circumstances. This can be effectively achieved by focusing discussion on overall treatment goals rather than only on a specific list of treatments that the patient may not want. By balancing the broad treatment goals with some reference to specific situations, an AD can more effectively guide the surrogate decision-making process.

In addition, AD conversations are most effective when they include a discussion of threshold points to guide future medical decision making. Emanual and Barry broadly define such threshold points as points "in the spectrum of disability and prognosis, [when] the patient would change from wanting life-sustaining interventions to declining them or asking to have them withdrawn."[12] Discussing threshold points with patients can provide more accurate guidance to decision makers than asking patients simply to list specific procedures or treatments that they would refuse.

It is important to characterize these threshold points for each patient, because different patients have radically different assessments of

---

Exhibit 18-2
Elements of an Ideal Advanced Directive (AD)

---

1. Designation of a surrogate decision maker
2. Discussion of broad treatment goals and threshold points of treatment
3. Reflection of the individual's current wishes
4. AD complies with state statutory requirements
5. Family and medical team are aware that AD exists

---

the points at which the quality of their lives would be so low as to no longer be worth preserving.[13] For example, terminally ill patients develop and express a variety of different ideas about how they want to face the process of dying.

By identifying broad treatment goals and threshold points in an AD, the patient provides guidance for surrogate decision makers, physicians, and nurses.

REFLECTION OF THE INDIVIDUAL'S CURRENT WISHES

The AD and the designation of a surrogate must be relatively current in order to reflect the patient's wishes validly and accurately. Updating ADs on an annual basis (or more frequently if health status changes) is prudently recommended. State statutory guidelines vary with respect to specific timing requirements. In general, ADs lacking review at least annually may be contested because they may poorly reflect the patient's current views. Effective ADs should be updated and relatively current.

Ideally, ADs should be prepared prior to admission to a hospital for an acute illness. As discussed above, ADs ideally reflect and record a conversation regarding a patient's considered values and wishes regarding future medical care. Every effort should be made to begin these conversations prior to the onset of a stressful acute illness and hospitalization. Such preparation allows ADs to evolve as the patient, the physician, and the surrogate develop a history, and the AD has the proper context and authenticity.

At the same time, it should be recognized that a patient's hospitalization may crystallize his or her thinking about healthcare issues. A person may hold strong views concerning future medical decisions but fail to record them in the form of an AD prior to hospitalization. Hospitalization often motivates patients to document their considered wishes in the form of an AD. At least 50 percent of ICU patients are eventually discharged from the hospital, and the consideration of ADs in the hospital or ICU motivates patients to document their wishes in ADs.[14] At minimum, a discussion should occur among the patient, family, and physician regarding the patient's wishes in the future given the same or a similar situation.

COMPLIANCE WITH STATE LAWS

An AD should comply with the specific state laws regarding ADs. The PSDA requires hospitals to provide patients with information regarding state AD statutes, which can vary regarding (1) scope of permissible decision making, (2) necessary forms or documentation, (3) witnessing requirements, and (4) standards of evidence. In order for an AD to be effective, it should meet the minimum state statutory requirements. However, the major purpose of an AD is not to create a legal document, but to communicate a person's values and wishes in the event that the person can no longer speak for him- or herself.

DIRECTIVE'S EXISTENCE KNOWN BY FAMILY AND MEDICAL TEAM

The development of an AD should include plans for distributing the AD to certain individuals. Minimally, the designated surrogate and medical team should receive copies of the document. In addition, the patient's family should be informed of the existence of the AD and discuss its contents with the patient. Ideally, an AD should be placed in the patient's medical record prior to admission to a healthcare facility. In all cases, the existence of an AD should be clearly communicated to the medical team as soon as possible. Unfortunately, ADs are frequently lost as patients and medical records are transported and transferred. It is important for patients and surrogates to keep several copies of the current AD available, and it is their responsibility to see that the treating team receives a copy of the AD.

CHALLENGING ISSUES RELATED TO ADVANCE DIRECTIVES IN THE ICU

Evaluating ADs in the ICU presents many challenging issues. This section addresses three challenges faced by ICU clinicians: (1) ICU patients without ADs, (2) resistance to ADs in the ICU, and (3) physicians' obligation to discuss ADs.

PATIENTS WITHOUT ADVANCE DIRECTIVES

Despite the PSDA, only about 15 percent of patients admitted to hospitals have documented ADs.[15] ICUs need to continue developing procedures to handle patients who do not have documented advance directives. Currently, in many ICUs it is not part of the standard admission protocol to check a patient's record for the presence of an AD.

Admission to the ICU is not necessarily a *carte blanche* approval for aggressive treatment of the patient. Early in a patient's admission to the ICU an appropriate decision maker needs to be identified. However, admission to an ICU does not automatically disqualify a patient from making decisions about his or her care. The patient is the appropriate decision maker unless he or she has lost decision-making capacity. Care that is consistent with the wishes of the patient or the surrogate should be provided.

In extreme cases, failing to address ADs with ICU patients can lead to legal challenges.[16] In such cases, the courts are forced to assume a medical role for which they are poorly suited. In most cases, an institution should seek help from the courts only as a last resort when there are (1) no directions from the patient and/or (2) irreconcilable differences between the family or surrogate decision maker and the healthcare team.

Incapacitated patients without ADs should be assessed for appropriate surrogate decision-making options. Physicians should follow the state's default order of decision making in the absence of an AD. The institutional ethics committee may be an important resource in such cases. The ethics committee or clinical ethics consultant may be able to help clarify ethically permissible options to help determine an appropriate course of action for an incapacitated patient without directives.

RESISTANCE TO ADVANCE DIRECTIVES

Patients, families, and healthcare physicians may resist ADs simply by avoiding the topic. For example, patients may deny critical medical conditions by not asking questions or by waiting for physicians to raise unpleasant topics.[17] In other situations, patients avoid AD discussions by clinging to the idea that their family members will "know" what to do. However, McIntyre reports that, in the absence of AD discussions, family members' preferences for treatment correspond poorly with patients' preferences.[18]

ICU staff can avoid ADs by maintaining that there seems to be "no appropriate time" to discuss ADs with patients. Physicians and staff can perceive patients and families to be too unstable or too upset to engage in discussions about the end of life. Staff may describe discussions of ADs as "premature," "inappropriate," or "cruel." ICU staff who are trained to take action, to intervene, and to prevent death may find their entire value system threatened if a patient states to them, "But I don't want to be treated."[19] To avoid this potentially unpleasant situation, ICU staff can simply fail to make an inquiry about a patient's wishes and ADs. Some physicians feel that, if a patient is salvageable, physicians are duty bound to strive to save the patient's life—regardless of what the patient or surrogate may say or request.

In response to these numerous avoidance strategies, the ICU staff should address ADs before the patient loses decision-making capacity.

Significant "windows of opportunity" regarding ADs exist during the patient's stay in the ICU. Unfortunately, staff may hesitate to initiate an AD discussion at these times because the patient is viewed as too unstable, weak, or upset.

The combination of the patient's avoidance and staff members' hesitation creates a situation of double jeopardy. First, the patient is at risk of losing input into the decision-making process about his or her life. Second, the staff and family lose the guidance of the patient. Once the "window of opportunity" closes, the remaining participants are left with the much more difficult task of making decisions in the absence of the patient's wishes. Unfortunately, some physicians find this more acceptable than dealing directly with a patient.

By addressing ADs early in a patient's admission to an ICU, the patient's wishes can be addressed to the extent that this is possible. Failing to inquire about a patient's wishes and values unjustifiably ignores the patient's intrinsic autonomy.

PHYSICIANS' OBLIGATION TO DISCUSS ADVANCE DIRECTIVES

Several authors suggest physicians have a general obligation to discuss ADs with their patients.[20] This literature documents and laments the fact that conversations about ADs do not occur on a regular basis.[21] Patients and or surrogates have a right to know—and physicians have a duty to state—the diagnosis and prognosis (best medical judgment) and to discuss the various options and likely outcomes open to the patient. A patient cannot provide informed consent unless these discussions take place. A major barrier to open discussion is that patients expect physicians to initiate these conversations.[22] It is not ethical for physicians to maintain that, if patients don't ask, physicians have no obligation to discuss these extremely important issues. In addition, the doctrine of informed consent may support the obligation of physicians to introduce the discussion of ADs before a patient's "window of opportunity" closes.

CONCLUSION

ADs and surrogate decision making occupy a central role in the treatment of ICU patients. The patient-based guidance provided by properly executed ADs and surrogate decision making permits greater justification of the difficult medical decisions that must be made in the ICU.

Unfortunately, the use of ADs in the ICU has been very limited to date. Strategies for increasing the use and improving the content of ADs in the ICU include incorporating ADs into standard ICU protocols, sensitizing ICU staff to AD issues, considering "threshhold points" in treatment for patients and identifying "windows of opportunity" for discussing ADs with the patient. In conclusion, ADs can be an enormous help in making challenging and stressful decisions in the ICU. The use of ADs in the ICU should be supported on every level: the patient, the staff, and the institution. For the sake of patients and the ICU staff, the integration of ADs and surrogate decision making into standard ICU operating procedures should be a strong priority.

NOTES

1. Omnibus Budget Reconciliation Act of 1990, Pub. L. No 101-508.

2. J. Moskop, "Advance Directives in Medicine: Choosing Among the Alternatives," in *Advance Directives in Medicine,* ed. C. Hackler, R. Mosely, and D. Vawter (New York: Praeger, 1989), 9-19.

3. *In re Quinlan,* 70 N.J. 10, 355 A.2d 647 (1976).

4. *Cruzan v. Director, Missouri Department of Health* 100 S.Ct 2841 (1990).

5. See note 1 above.

6. S. Miles, "Conversations in Bioethics," (Paper presented at Case Western Reserve University, Cleveland, Ohio, 12 April 1994).

7. J. Hardwig, "Advance Directives and the Physician: Talking With Healthy Patients About Dying," in *Advance Directives in Medicine,* ed. C. Hackler, R. Mosely, and D. Vawter (New York: Praeger, 1989), 112-19; R. Perlman et al., "Insights Pertaining to Patient Assessments of States Worse Than Death," *The Journal of Clinical Ethics* 4, no. 1 (Spring 1993): 33-41.

8. G. Agich and S. Youngner, "For Experts Only? Access to Hospital Ethics Committees," *Hastings Center Report* 21, no. 5 (September-October 1991): 17-25.

9. L. Schneiderman et al., "Do Physician's Own Preferences for Life-Sustaining Treatment Influence Their Perceptions of Patient's Preferences?" *The Journal of Clinical Ethics* 4, no. 1 (1993): 28-33; K. McIntyre, "Implementation of Advance Directives: For Physicians, a Legal Dilemma Becomes an Ethical Imperative," *Archives of Internal Medicine* 152 (1992): 924-29.

10. See note 2 above.

11. J. LaPuma, D. Orentlicher, and R. Moss, "Advance Directives On Admission: Clinical Implications And Analysis of the Patient Self-Determination Act of 1990," *Journal of the American Medical Association,* 266 (1991): 402-05.

12. L. Emanual and M. Barry, "Advance Directives for Medical Care—A Case For Greater Use," *New England Journal of Medicine* 324 (1991): 889-95.

13. Hardwig, "Advance Directives," see note 7 above.

14. J. Lynn and J. Teno, "After the Patient Self-Determination Act: The

Need for Empirical Research on Formal Advance Directives," *Hastings Center Report* 23, no. 1 (1993): 20-24.

15. G. Sachs, "Empowerment of the Older Patient? A Randomized, Controlled Trial to Increase Discussion and Use of Advance Directives," *Journal of the American Geriatric Society* 40 (1992): 269-73.

16. B. Lo, J. Rouse, and C. Dornbrand, "Family Decision-Making on Trial," *New England Journal of Medicine* 322 (1992): 1228-32.

17. See note 8 above.

18. McIntyre, "Implementation of Advance Directives," see note 9 above.

19. W. White, "Living Will Statutes: Good Public Policy?" in *Advance Directives in Medicine,* ed. C. Hackler, R. Mosely, and D. Vawter (New York: Praeger, 1989), 75-83.

20. See note 11 above.

21. See note 12 above.

22. Ibid.

19

Assessing Competence in Critical Care: Depression, Denial, and the Religious Exception

Philip Candilis

INTRODUCTION

In the crucible of intensive care, patients must make weighty decisions under pressures of time and ill health. The obligation to provide these patients with complete information and the opportunity to reflect is infringed both by disease and by the interventions needed to combat it. These pressures and infringements frequently lead to incomplete knowledge or assessment of the patient's wishes, with resulting uncertainty whether patient's wishes are authentic and volitional or governed by the crisis at hand. The concept that governs such uncertainty is that of competence: are the patient's decisions in the face of life-threatening illness competent, or are they subverted by other influences? This chapter identifies the clinical concepts that guide the determination of competence and the special problems inherent to it.

CONCEPTUAL FOUNDATION

Competence is a legal term whose closest medical approximation is "decision-making capacity." Defined by most contemporary authors as the ability to perform a specific task, competence in the medical setting is applied narrowly to prevent incursion into areas where individuals retain their capacities.[1] Spoken of as "functional" competence, "psychological" competence, or "capacity," to distinguish the informal assessments of the medical setting from those made by a court of law, competence in both arenas relies heavily on the clinical assessment of physicians. In hospital and in court, patients are presumed competent until the burden of proof is met by those wishing to show otherwise. In most jurisdictions, courts apply the "clear and convincing evidence" standard that lies between the civil law's "preponderance of the evidence" and the criminal law's "evidence beyond a reasonable doubt." Modern legal commentary is often traced to the 1914 New York *Schloendorff* case, in which Justice Cardozo pronounced that "every human being of adult years and sound mind has a right to determine what shall be done with his body."[2] A description of state legal interests that may apply in the adjudication of competence is beyond the scope of this chapter, but these interests include (1) the preservation of life, (2) the protection of dependent third parties, (3) the prevention of suicide, and (4) the preservation of the ethical integrity of the medical profession.[3]

In medicine, as in law, competence undergirds the concept of informed consent that governs all patient-physician interactions. Without mental competence, the voluntary action, comprehension of information, and decision making about treatment that comprise informed consent cannot exist.[4] A review of the exceptions to informed consent—incompetence, emergency, waiver, and therapeutic privilege—demonstrates the penetration of considerations of competence. For example, in cases involving incompetent patients, application of alternative decision-making standards (such as substituted judgment or best interest) is important. Emergencies require that physicians know when to operate under the doctrine of presumed, rather than informed, consent. Waiver by patients yielding decision-making authority to their physicians presupposes competence to do so; and therapeutic privilege, by which a physician withholds information for the protection of the patient, presumes incompetence to handle the very currency of informed consent. The latter two exceptions to informed consent are problematic and require careful scrutiny on the part of clinicians. Philosophers since Kant[5] have objected to autonomous agents waiving their autonomy. Pincoffs has written: "How morally can I . . . authorize you to make decisions that I am morally responsible to make? I would be sacrificing my integrity as a moral person by entering into any such agreement."[6] The claim of therapeutic privilege also requires careful attention to the process of competent, informed consent. In *Canterbury v. Spence*, the landmark failure-to-disclose case, the U.S. Court of Appeals observed: "The physician's privilege to withhold information for therapeutic reasons must be carefully circumscribed, for otherwise it might devour the [information] disclosure rule itself."[7]

In bridging the legal and medical paradigms, Appelbaum and Roth have addressed the misperception that competence must fit into a neatly dichotomous all-or-nothing decision. They write that competence is not a fixed attribute of an individual but "a set of deductions from a variety of clinical data that can be as subject to influence and change as the more basic attributes on which it is based."[8] The psychiatrist provides "a factual basis for the legal determination that corresponds to the patient's clinical state." In fact, a psychiatrist may not be required at all. Boisaubin, among others, comments that any physician can assess competence, given a good foundation in mental examination and recognition of disease states affecting mentation.[9] However, psychiatrists are likely best able to identify those patients believed to require a low threshold of suspicion, including: (1) acutely psychotic patients who often suffer a delirium-like clouding of consciousness; (2) chronically institutionalized patients who may have lost the capacity to evaluate critically the proposed interventions; (3) patients with organic brain impairment, often elderly, who may slide slowly into an incompetent state; (4) depressed patients whose hopeless, helpless thinking may handicap reasoning; and (5) mentally retarded patients whose mental status may be confounded by concomitant psychiatric illness.[10] Appelbaum and Gutheil also added a sixth category—patients who face risky procedures with little hope of direct benefit—to alert clinical researchers to a high-risk group that deserves particular attention to their capacity to consent.[11]

When choosing the most useful paradigm for assessing patients who are at risk for decision-making incapacity, the President's Commission for the Study of Ethical Problems in Medicine and Biomedical and Behavioral Research considered three distinct constructs: *function, status,* and *outcome.*[12] The President's Commission found it unacceptable to base competence judgments solely on the decision (or *outcome*) itself, given possible paternalistic influences by medical teams or communities whose choice may simply differ from the patient's. The President's Commission also found it unacceptable to judge capacity by mental or physical attributes such as age or diagnosis (*status*). The literature is replete with findings that even patients with disorders such as depression or schizophrenia may retain decision-making abilities.[13] The President's Commission identified *function* as the most defensible approach for determining competency because of its emphasis on the patient's process, or function, in making the decision at hand.

LEGAL STANDARDS

Legal standards already in use were consistent with the recommendations of the President's Commission. Appelbaum and Grisso's overview of legal standards classified the judiciary's various approaches to assessing decision-making function into four categories: (1) communicating a choice, (2) understanding relevant information, (3) appreciating the current situation and its consequences, and (4) manipulating information rationally. In elaborating these standards, the authors underscored elements of decision making crucial to all clinician-patient interactions.[14]

Communicating a choice, they point out, is not simply the voicing of preference. It also entails the ability to maintain and communicate stable choices. This does not preclude patients from changing their minds but, if the decision-making process is characterized by ambivalence and repeated reversals, the standard may not be met.

Understanding information relevant to the specific decision subsumes the capabilities of retaining and ordering information. In addition, however, this standard requires an understanding of the information applied to possible outcomes and risk-benefit assessments. This goes beyond the simple cognitive elements of the mental status exam.

Appreciating the current situation and its consequences expands the previous standard in that information may be understood but not "appreciated." The meaning of information in the individual patient's valuation of illness, treatment, and its consequences is underscored. As noted previously, it is not the decision reached that is at issue but a realistic evaluation of illness, consequences of treatment or refusal, and the likelihood of consequences. The phenomenon of "denial," which is addressed below, often challenges clinicians to apply this standard.

Manipulating information rationally involves tracing the patient's train of thought. Do the steps incorporating risk and benefit and weighing multiple options evolve logically into a decision that is internally consistent? Do thought processes demonstrate an understanding of the relationship between cause and effect? Appelbaum and Grisso concede, "Although few persons reach decisions by rigorously logical processes, patients should be able to indicate the major factors in their decisions and the importance assigned to them."[15]

TESTS FOR COMPETENCE

In applying the various standards to specific clinical cases, a number of tests for competence have been put forward. Beauchamp has underscored the need to distinguish carefully, however, between the tests and the criteria for competence.[16] He points out that the criteria for competence differ depending upon the question: is one competent to speak French, to recognize a breed of dog, to decide when to seek medical attention? His explication recapitulates the definition of competence as the ability to perform a specific task. However, it also underscores that any test must assess the abilities chosen to meet the criteria of competence in the given clinical situation. Ostensibly, criteria used to assess competence to refuse lifesaving treatment would differ from those used in assessing ability to care for oneself at home. Tests are then the procedures for determining one's abilities; they make the criteria for competence operational.

Roth, Meisel, and Lidz order five classic tests of competence by increasing difficulty: (1) evidencing a choice, (2) "reasonable" outcome of choice, (3) choice based on rational reasons, (4) ability to understand, and (5) actual understanding.[17] Appelbaum and Grisso have noted that these tests have since evolved to match the grouping of legal standards noted earlier.[18] For example, "ability to understand" and "actual understanding" are now subsumed under "understanding relevant information," with actual understanding acting as the test that measures how the standard is met. The test of reasonableness has been discarded for reasons described below, and the appreciation standard, now representing the greatest strictness, has been described more recently by Appelbaum and Roth.[19] All tests are presented here to expand the discussion and include methodologies clinicians are likely to encounter.

The first test, evidencing a choice, is set at a level attainable by most individuals and is most respectful of patient autonomy; it is behavioral, is highly reliable, and can be exercised simply by asking whether the patient wishes to participate. However, it says little regarding the deliberative process.

The second test assesses the "reasonableness" of the patient's decision but threatens to use the medical team's value system rather than the patient's in judging it. As noted earlier, the President's Commission rejected this "outcome" test because it is paternalistic and may, as Roth and his colleagues warn, promote social goals at the expense of patient autonomy.

The test assessing choice based on "rational" reasons is more a test of the quality of the decision-making process and enjoys widespread clinical application. Presentation of vignettes, use of the mental status examination with attention to psychotic symptoms, and even simple conversation have been espoused as clinical applications of this test.[19] The difficulty Roth notes here is with patients whose idiosyncratic or peculiar ideas regarding treatment, disease, or outcome test the bounds of rationality. Clinicians may consequently be unable to trace a decision's derivation to the peculiarity in question.

The test for ability to understand is popular in case law as well as with prominent writers like Stephen Wear, who apply a standard of general competence to medical decisions.[20] In Wear's view, if individuals are generally competent in the ability to understand information, weigh alternatives, and conduct ordinary affairs of living, they are permitted to make unwise or illogical decisions just as they would be in other settings. The way in which specific risks and benefits are assessed, alternatives are weighed, or outcomes are valued is not considered primary. The particular difficulties Roth and his colleagues identify in using this test include the unknowability of what level of understanding establishes competence and the test's dependence on unobservable and inferential mental processes.

The test of actual understanding now provides the measure of ability to understand and asks patients to apply knowledge to the situation at hand.

Appelbaum and Grisso suggest asking patients to paraphrase the information they have been given or even asking explicitly whether patients understand the purpose of the consent process and their role within it.[21]

Appreciation of the situation is now considered the strictest and highest standard. Its test subsumes assessment of the patient's realistic evaluation of the illness, treatment, and risks and benefits. Questions helpful at the bedside to elaborate each test are presented in Exhibit 19-1.

Ultimately it is the type of decision that determines which tests are emphasized and which standard takes precedence. Drane,[22] like Roth, has espoused applying tests on a sliding scale by which patients are held to more rigorous standards and stricter tests as the risk-benefit ratio increases: the more dangerous the consequences or the more unfavorable the ratio, the stricter or higher the standard. Theoretically, this maximizes autonomy at one end of the spectrum, beneficent paternalism at the other. Although criticized for its paternalistic variation of the competence standard, the sliding-scale model still provides the most pragmatic application of standards and takes into account the knowledge and power differential between patient and physician.

Legal jurisdiction also provides an important context. Clinicians are urged to become familiar with the legal standard or standards applicable in their jurisdiction and apply the tests accordingly. This is not to say that courts are the best environment for such decisions. The adversarial nature of courts, with their diminished awareness of clinical variables,

---

Exhibit 19-1
Model Questions to Structure Competence Assessment

Communicating a Choice
1. Have you decided whether to go along with your doctor's suggestions for treatment? Can you tell me what your decision is? (Can be repeated to assess stability.)

Factual Understanding of the Issues
1. Please tell me in your own words what your doctor told you about:
    a. the nature of your condition.
    b. the recommended treatment or test.
    c. the possible benefits or risks/discomforts of the treatment.
    d. any other possible treatments and their risks/benefits.
    e. the possible risks/benefits of no treatment at all.
2. Your doctor may have told you of a (percentage) chance the (named risk) might occur with treatment. In your own words, how likely do you think the occurrence of (named risk) might be?
3. Why is your doctor giving you all this information? What role does he expect you to play in deciding whether you receive treatment? What will happen if you decide not to go along with your doctor's recommendation?

Appreciation of the Situation and Its Consequences
1. Please explain to me what you really believe is wrong with your health now.
2. Do you believe you need some kind of treatment? What is treatment likely to do for you?
3. What do you believe will happen if you are not treated?
4. Why do you think your doctor has recommended (specific treatment) for you?

Rational Manipulation of Information
1. Tell me how you reached the decision to accept/reject the recommended treatment?
2. What were the factors that were important to you in reaching the decision?
3. How did you balance those factors?

Reprinted from P. Appelbaum and T. Gutheil, *Clinical Handbook of Psychiatry and the Law*, 2nd ed. (Baltimore, Md.: Lippincott Williams & Wilkins, 1991), 239-40. © Lippincott Williams & Wilkins, 1991. Used with permission.

questionable timeliness, and occasionally ineffective advocacy combine to make them, according to Presidential Commissioner John Paris, "costly, cumbersome, and traumatic."[23] These weaknesses are compounded by a jurisdictional relativism that forces policy variation by state. The judiciary's emphasis on minimal behavioral standards and its focus on negative rather than positive obligations between citizens further limits its moral authority in discussions of how moral agents ought to behave. Ultimately, it may be medicine with its positive obligations of care and cure that provides the best environment for competence assessment.[24]

PROFESSIONAL STANDARDS

Deliberative bodies within intensive care have also addressed the issue of competence. The Consensus Conference of the American College of Chest Physicians and the Society of Critical Care Medicine adopted the criteria of the President's Commission in writing that patients have decision-making capacity if they have: (1) possession of a set of values and goals, (2) the ability to communicate and to understand information relevant to a decision (including physical condition, the consequences of the treatment being recommended, and the consequences of not receiving treatment), and (3) the ability to reason and deliberate about one's choices.[25]

The Task Force on Ethics of The Society of Critical Care Medicine chose a somewhat expanded set of criteria: (1) the ability to appreciate the significant characteristics of one's condition, (2) the ability to appreciate the impact of the main treatment options, (3) the ability to judge the relationship of options to one's beliefs and values, (4) the ability to reason and to deliberate about one's choices, and (5) the ability to communicate decisions in a meaningful manner.[26] Nonetheless, the standards as grouped by Appelbaum and Grisso are considered benchmark standards in this discussion because of their comprehensiveness and accuracy in describing the ethical and legal landscapes.

CLINICAL EVALUATION

The clinical evaluation for competence generally begins with the question, "competent for what?"[27] This not only keeps to the working definition but enables all parties to discuss criteria by which competence will be assessed. With requests for competence evaluation found to range from ability to care for oneself at home, to ability to properly consent to or refuse treatment, to ability to leave the hospital against medical advice, it is not surprising that individual clinical evaluations might require somewhat different criteria.[28]

When evaluating a patient's competence, it is important to determine what information the patient has received, in what setting, and by whom. Certain authors recommend a reiteration of information by a primary source with the consultant present.[29] Multiple information sources, time pressures, and jargon are common obstacles to retention and comprehension of information. If information for informed consent is conveyed by more than one agent, during a harrowing admission, in a techno-speak that cannot be understood, the patient will certainly be unable to demonstrate competence.

The mental status examination (MSE) is consequently the most useful element of the patient interview. This formal assessment tests attention, concentration, orientation, memory, thought process and content, mood, and affective state. When performed with a neuropsychiatric screen such as the Mini-Mental State Examination (MMSE), the MSE addresses the cognitive element identified by physicians as primary to their competence assessments[30] and the affective component that is often influential in decision-making.

Applying the competence standards and their tests to the patient's clinical predicament completes this stage of the process. Assessing the place and meaning of the hospitalization in the patient's historical narrative or worldview can help discern the patient's cognitive capacity to consider relevant factors. This step also helps establish the presence of interfering pathologic perception or belief (such as delusion), emotional state (such as panic, depression, mania, or lability), or pathologic relationships (such as helpless dependence or coercion).[31]

Diagnostic impression in competence evaluation commonly includes "organic brain" syndrome, substance abuse, depression, or personality disorder.[32] However, functional diagnoses are not valid until confounding factors are eliminated. Metabolic imbalance, hypoxia, hypotension, pain, and isolation influence cognition in clearly recognizable ways that require correction before any final pronouncements can be made.[33] Other interfering factors may include miscommunication or misunderstanding; one study identified this as the primary or secondary reason for treatment refusal in 66 of 114 cases.[34] Appelbaum and Roth, in emphasizing the influence of the setting on decision making, write that personality conflicts or the receipt of "information from a physician the patient

dislikes or in a hospital at which he is furious does not warrant the conclusion that the patient is necessarily unable or unwilling to hear the
information from another person in another place."[35] Morreim describes
cases in which using trusted same-faith or same-race informants may resolve conditions that at first blush appear to confer incapacity. Morreim
is among those who warn physicians from ascribing incapacity without
correcting interfering factors such as "mistrust, miscommunication, poor
education, and emotional exhaustion."[36]

Abandoning patients to their preferences without exploring possible
negative influences is the obverse of this situation and has been called
"pseudoempathy." Without assessing impediments to competence, clinicians may be tempted simply to accept decisions they agree with or ignore conditions that appear appropriate to the setting (such as anxiety,
fear, or depression). For example, the clinical team may believe that an
amputee has good reason to be depressed and accept his or her decisions
without further exploration. The surgical equivalent, one colleague has
wryly observed, would be to allow that a patient has good reason to be
bleeding from a stab wound and not consider treatment.

Documentation of the consultant's findings and formal recommendations constitutes the next important step. Gutheil and Bursztajn suggest articulating the clinical determinants of competence by carefully
detailing the conditions that may be distorting thought processes. They
also suggest, however, that clinicians anticipate future medicolegal even-
tualities; for example, when patients present with a history of incompetent refusal or its imminent possibility, documentation of the patient's
view of illness, medication, and outcome provides valuable clinical data.
Other considerations include the avoidance of extreme or global positions; appropriate concession of islands of competent functioning is more
accurate and more convincing.[37] The patient's responses to the bedside
questions listed in Exhibit 19-1 can also be included in the record.

Restoration of competence by treatment of any or all confounding
factors may consequently require action without informed consent.
Absent a surrogate decision maker or advance directive, intervention to
restore competence without informed consent can be equated ethically
with treatment in an emergency and is equally defensible. This may nonetheless require separate legal recourse. Because competence is not necessarily a fixed state and may be influenced by the variety of factors noted
earlier, observation of the patient on at least two separate occasions on
two separate days has been recommended.[38] Authentication of historical
information during contact with family members or other potential sur-

rogates can occur in the interim. In the event of an intervening clinical emergency, the last known competent wishes and then the emergency exception pertain.

If incapacity persists, consent for nonemergency care remains to be obtained. With passage of the Patient Self-Determination Act in 1990, physicians are required to establish whether patients have enacted advance directives.[39] These directives are, in the usual order of precedence, the living will and the durable power of attorney for healthcare. The former generally elaborates the patient's wishes regarding treatment; the latter names an individual to make all medical decisions in the event that the patient becomes incapacitated. Some states have legislated a hierarchy of individuals who must be consulted should the patient become incapacitated. The hierarchy usually includes guardian, spouse, children, parents, and other relatives in varying order.

DISPUTES AND APPEAL

Resolution of disputes between family members and the medical team or between team members themselves can take a number of different forms. Simply having the disputed elements of the competence evaluation performed with the disputee present may resolve such disagreements.[40] Otherwise, a second opinion and consultation with senior clinicians with forensic training or wider experience in similar cases are universally acceptable. The President's Commission has advised that all institutions establish procedures for such disputes, and many institutions have created ethics committees or similar deliberative bodies to comply.

Absent these resources, or if disputes persist, the courts come into play for appointment of a guardian and determination of treatment. Certain jurisdictions have developed the mechanism of limited or temporary guardianship to address specific lapses of competence and to avoid sweeping findings of general incompetence. Broadly, two standards for surrogate decision making exist. *Substituted judgment* describes the action of a surrogate who knows the prior wishes and values of the patient and decides as the patient would have if competent. *Best interests* describes a decision taken without prior knowledge of the patient's wishes and following more objective determinants. The objectivity of this standard derives from what Beauchamp and Childress describe as "tangible factors—physical and financial risks, harms, and benefits—and makes use of such truisms as 'Health is better than illness,' and 'Life is preferable to death.' "[41]

Creative alternatives to the cumbersome legal apparatus have also been proposed; others are already in place. New York State, for example, has created a Surrogate Decision-Making Committee (SDMC) program that decides on both the need for surrogacy and the need for treatment.[42] Made up of a multidisciplinary task force of trained volunteers, these four-member panels counteract the costly, variable, and unwieldy process of applying for guardianship. Although without jurisdiction in emergency procedures, the SDMC provides a streamlined mechanism for a variety of medical, surgical, and diagnostic interventions.

Other scholars have suggested a legal construct that would permit treatment based on prior consent. Named the "Ulysses" or "voluntary commitment" contract after the Homeric tale in which Ulysses, sailing past the irresistible Sirens, commanded that he be tied to the mast and that his pleas for release be ignored,[43] the contract provides patients with recurrent mental disorders the ability to contract with caregivers to disregard certain instructions (such as treatment refusal) during a relapse. Limited by time and defined by agreed-upon criteria of relapse, the contract includes objective third-party participation and freedom to renegotiate or revoke once the acute episode is resolved. Although criticized as putting another face on involuntary commitment in the patient's best interest, this mechanism may ultimately offer intermittently competent critical care patients a greater voice in decisions concerning their care.

Emanuel—citing the inherent impossibility of formulating objective, societally shared criteria to determine what medical care is appropriate for incompetent patients—proposes a communally federated system by which local communities (including health maintenance organizations, community clinics, and the like) assume the authority to enact their own conceptions of what is acceptable treatment.[44] Consistent with the American Bar Association's move to develop alternative, community-based resources and mechanisms that reduce the need for guardianship,[45] this system would be capable of generating a communally shared vision and allow elements of diversity as well. Whether this relativist model is a significant departure from the current jurisdictional patchwork is open to debate, but the search for objective criteria is already under way in numerous clinical studies.

CLINICAL RESEARCH

The empirical research that informs the discussion of competence comes in two forms: data regarding evaluations and data regarding operational elements of the concept itself. Recent studies have identified the prevalence of competence evaluations as approximately 5 percent of psychiatric consultations.[46] These evaluations fall into four major categories: (1) ability to care for oneself at home, (2) ability to refuse treatment, (3) ability to give informed consent, and (4) ability to leave the hospital against medical advice.[47] Often characterized as urgent or semiurgent,[48] requests are generated most commonly by internal medicine and neurology departments.[49] Patients referred do not appear to fit specific age, sex, or racial demographics but are most commonly diagnosed with an "organic brain" syndrome.[50] Patients found to be incompetent make up half the group referred, with those threatening to leave "against medical advice" and those evaluated for guardianship more likely to be found incompetent.[51]

Katz's study of patients referred for refusing treatment found that incompetent patients tended to be men, to be patients who were the focus of more urgent requests, and to be patients who had refused operations.[52] This group was also found to exhibit more denial of illness, more suicidal ideation, and more delusional ideation regarding their medical situation. Katz categorizes *competent* treatment refusers as "difficult" patients (those with characterologic or substance-abuse disorders) and "patients with difficulty" (those with adjustment disorder or no formal psychiatric diagnosis who are simply struggling to master their predicament). Whether such characterizations can help predict outcome awaits further study, but sensitivity to patient descriptors can increase clinicians' awareness of patients who may be at increased risk for decision-making incapacity.

Farnsworth identified past history of thought disorder and celebrity status as influential in generating competence evaluation.[53] Both characteristics are worthy of comment. As important as psychiatric history is to providing a complete clinical picture, it is not sufficient to generate questions of incompetence. Although psychiatric history is helpful in supporting current clinical data that suggests an incapacitating mental disorder, its use as a trigger for competence evaluation represents use of the "status" standard, which is not an epistemically valid method to screen for decision-making capacity. The celebrity, or "VIP," status of the patient is also not defensible as a vehicle for lowering thresholds for competence evaluation. Consistent clinical use of competence standards and familiarity with the principles espoused here are sufficient for treating similar cases and avoid unnecessary exposure of patients to a potentially dignity-sapping evaluation.

Farnsworth and others emphasize the importance of psychiatric consultation in the management and resolution of brain disorders from delirium and intoxication to psychosis. However, even psychiatrists are not always certain which standards for competence are to be used. Farnsworth's retrospective chart review suggested the use of the Appelbaum-Grisso grouping noted earlier,[54] although this was rarely stated explicitly.

Markson and colleagues' elegant survey of physicians' ability to determine competence examined directly the issues of "status" and "standard."[55] Although psychiatrists were significantly more likely to answer correctly, fewer than half of physicians surveyed were aware that "status" conditions such as dementia, depression, psychosis, and even involuntary commitment do not necessarily render patients incompetent. Most physicians identified their state's legal standard correctly but consequently misapplied it to the case presented. Psychiatrists did not perform better in this area. The authors use the results to emphasize that a legal standard is being applied to resolve a legal question, despite its occurrence in a medical setting. This in no way diminishes physicians' responsibility for diagnosing and treating obstacles to meeting the standard but emphasizes that competence has a clear legal component that governs the clinical findings.

The time pressures of intensive care raise questions concerning the practicality of comprehensive competence evaluations in this setting. However, investigators have reported that reliable information can be generated in a manner that does not interfere with acute care.[56] The appeal to brevity, however, has led to the use of the Mini-Mental State Examination in identifying incapacity.[57] Folstein, the developer of the MMSE, finds that it does not "differentiate competent from incompetent patients with reasonable sensitivity or specificity."[58] He prefers presenting patients with a specific scenario regarding the durable power of attorney and consequently testing their understanding—the Hopkins Competency Assessment Test (HCAT). A unique feature of this test is that the material can be presented at three different reading levels and is also read aloud to ensure comprehension. The HCAT is found to correlate strongly with the findings of a trained forensic psychiatrist.[59] Whether this method will generalize beyond patients' ability to understand advance directives is still a matter of debate; nonetheless, it underscores the need to assess more than simple cognition.

Other writers have suggested elements of psychological or IQ testing to identify incompetent patients, with correlations established in elderly and adolescent populations.[60] Time pressures aside, the statistical frequency model this approach represents has been criticized for ignoring both the affective component of decision making and the hidden values of testing and interpreting population norms.[61] Ultimately, the use of a structured disclosure that incorporates standardized scenarios and reliable scoring may provide the "gold standard" for assessing competence.[62]

The most recent developments in producing such a gold standard arise from the MacArthur Treatment Competence Study—a long-term, multicenter effort.[63] Conceived to answer three major questions—the extent mentally ill patients differ from nonmentally ill and nonill patients in making treatment decisions, the demographic and clinical characteristics of those at risk, and the deficit patterns related to the various legal standards—the study has generated instruments to assess patients' performance of the elements of competence.

For the *understanding* standard, patients were tested on their comprehension of disclosures concerning the nature of their disorder, the nature of recommended treatment, probable risks and benefits, and alternative treatments. *Appreciation* was evaluated as acknowledgment of illness and potential value of treatment, or acknowledgment of these after illogical premises were challenged. For *rational manipulation*, patients demonstrated problem-solving abilities when facing a specific decision. For *communicating a choice*, patients selected a treatment option in a set decision-making task. Separate forms of disclosure were developed for each patient group in order to make content meaningful, and information was disclosed both part-by-part and uninterrupted.

Among the important findings of the MacArthur study is the observation that, although there is considerable heterogeneity within mentally ill groups, patients with mental illness show more frequent deficits than the medically ill or non-ill. However, in another rejection of the "status" standard, the lower mean performance is due to a minority within the group (certain patients with schizophrenia), not identifiable by demographics or diagnosis. Patients also showed significantly improved understanding of treatment following a second part-by-part disclosure, underscoring the need for more information in the clinical setting. Most significantly, the choice of standard for determining competence did not order in lexical fashion the number and type of patients classified as impaired, contradicting the hypothetical hierarchy of increasing strictness. Whether this lack of discrimination by standards of specific competence supports a retreat to a standard of general competence in assessing medical decision making or merely a refinement of existing standards awaits further study.

The clinical application in medical and surgical patients, including intensive care, has taken the form of the MacArthur Competence Assessment Tool-Treatment (MacCAT-T).[64] Preliminary results from the use of this 15-minute instrument support the research finding that demographic variables do not identify poor performance. However, aspects of psychopathology do appear to distinguish poor performers, substantiating the need for trained psychiatric assessment in competence evaluation. Ultimately, it is hoped the MacCAT-T will provide a useful adjunctive tool in assessing even the most seriously ill patients.

SPECIAL PROBLEMS

DEPRESSION

Clinical depression carries with it unique difficulties in the assessment of competence. Underdiagnosed in all medical settings,[65] depression requires clinicians to distinguish neurovegetative symptoms that arise from medical illness or the environment from those that arise from the mental state itself. Disturbances of sleep, energy, concentration, appetite, and mood are all symptoms that may be resolved by modifying an intensive care environment that generally limits visitation, encourages disorientation, and maximizes technological intervention. Including trusted family members in clinical discussions, displaying calendars and time pieces, and providing a constant flow of information can help dissipate symptoms arising from the setting. Consequently, there are a number of approaches to assessing the medical and psychiatric contributions to depression. The *inclusive* approach considers all signs and symptoms without regard for cause; the *exclusive* approach ignores symptoms attributable to medical illness; the *etiologic* approach attempts to distinguish case-by-case whether the depressive symptoms are due to the medical illness; and the *substitutive* approach substitutes certain vegetative symptoms with cognitive symptoms.[66] Sullivan and Youngner's penetrating analysis of depression, competence, and the refusal of lifesaving treatment espouses using the inclusive approach to maximize diagnostic sensitivity, particularly when lifesaving treatment is involved.[67] This is in keeping with the sliding-scale paradigm (greatest caution with greatest risk) and errs initially in favor of preserving life.

Physicians may also experience a bias of training that categorizes suicidal ideation as pathology rather than leaving interpretation of the symptom open to consultation. Although suicidal ideation is among the criteria for depression, this does not establish it as a necessary criterion for incompetence. Although depressive helplessness, guilt, worthlessness, and anhedonia influence patients' appreciation of their situation, a hopeless outlook may nonetheless be accurate. Although treatment of depression and consultation of advance directives is encouraged, clinicians are warned that, once family members verify long-standing patient values and the patient remains consistent, "aggressive psychiatric life-support" itself becomes a burden. Ultimately, some treatment refusals, even in the face of death, may be legitimate.[68]

DENIAL

The importance of denial as a clinical phenomenon is underscored by its proposed, albeit rejected, inclusion as a separate diagnostic category in psychiatry's most recent diagnostic and statistical manual, *Diagnostic and Statistical Manual of Mental Disorders* (4th edition).[69] Cassem and Hackett highlighted its prevalence by identifying eight of 145 critical care unit consultations specifically for "denial of illness."[70] Yet, clarity in its definition, pathology, and relevance has been elusive. Even Anna Freud, who wrote extensively on denial as a psychodynamic defense mechanism, did not specifically define the term.

A number of scholars have attempted to frame the concept of denial. Shelp and Perl identify two discrete meanings within the term that are often conflated by clinicians: (1) the act of disagreeing with another's representation of fact (that is, a conscious disagreement between parties) and (2) a hypothetical unconscious defense mechanism that causes persons to be unaware of certain unpleasant facts.[71] Given the tendency for the second meaning to be used for the first, they suggest substituting the phrase "minimizing illness," both to avoid the pejorative connotation carried by the clinical term and to sidestep reliance on an unconscious thought process as etiology. Laxity in use of the term otherwise diminishes the patient's contribution to medical decision making by characterizing it as out of touch with reality and allows considerations of incompetence to intrude although minimizing illness is neither necessary nor sufficient to a finding of incapacity.

In one of the more widely useful clinical definitions, Moore and Fine subsume both conscious and unconscious elements by defining denial in its most generally recognized sense: "[Denial] repudiates some or all of the meanings of an event . . . avoids awareness of some painful aspect of reality and so diminishes anxiety or other unpleasurable affects."[72] Others emphasize the interpersonal nature of the phenomenon and its purpose in "altering the meaning of events within a social field,"[73] thus expanding the focus on the patient to include the medical team and relevant others. These writers are not alone in pointing out the existence of denial among clinicians who may use it to distance themselves from patients and their serious illnesses. In this context, denial of the patient becomes seeing a "cancer" rather than seeing a person with cancer; more broadly, committing oneself to the cure of cancer or to treatment of terminal patients becomes a mechanism for attempting to deny fear of death or death itself.[74]

Most theoretical constructs of denial have not been tested in the clinical setting. However, Hackett and Cassem used the concept in the critical care unit while developing their 31-item denial scale, the most widely used research instrument of its kind.[75] Using verbal and behavioral cues, the authors recognized typical behaviors and assigned extent of denial to three categories: major, partial, and minimal denial. Major deniers reported feeling no fear during hospitalization or earlier in their lives; partial deniers initially denied fear but eventually admitted some fearfulness; and minimal deniers complained of anxiety or readily admitted fear. Characteristics of major deniers included verbal minimization of fear and symptoms and displacement of symptoms to other organ systems. These patients often reported a history of reckless behavior and regularly downplayed danger. They displaced fear to other areas of their lives such as finances or projected it onto family members ("My wife was scared, but I wasn't."). Their demeanor was found to be cheerful and punctuated with cliches that dismissed the importance of death ("If your number is up, it's up."). The Hackett-Cassem Denial Scale successfully distinguished the three categories of denial and established an important basis for its study. A notable finding in early use of this scale was the identification of denial as a "trait" rather than a "state." Therefore, unlike the frequently state-dependent nature of competence (influenced, for example, by metabolic factors, fluctuating mental state, or environment), denial may be far more difficult to penetrate or reverse. Indeed, as an element of coping, it may serve a useful purpose.

Studies have reported that denial reduces anxiety scores in the critical care unit[76] and correlates with speedier and more likely stabilization of unstable angina.[77] Denial also correlates with improved overall survival[78] and fewer days in the ICU.[79] Therefore, if denial is the patient's predominant coping mechanism during hospitalization for acute care, it may best be left intact. This does not suggest ignoring psychosis or collaborating with a delusional system by abjuring psychiatric treatment, information sessions, or realistic presentations of risk and benefit. Rather, it espouses respect for a fragile but useful defense. At the point where denial interferes with care or results in refusal of treatment or a patient's threats to sign out of the hospital, the mechanisms already discussed for evaluation of competence come into play. The most likely course to be useful, jurisdiction permitting, would be use of the "appreciation" standard, supported by tests of rationality, capacity to understand, and actual understanding.

The differential approach to diagnosis of denial can be helpful in distinguishing stable character traits from organic disorders manifesting as denial.[80] Neurologic, medical, psychiatric, interpersonal, and psychodynamic barriers to sound decision making have all been identified and offer a framework for organizing assessment of such patients.

Neurologically, anosognosia (lack of recognition or acknowledgment of physical defects) can arise from cortical and subcortical brain lesions; it can present as neglect, denial of hemiplegia, and even Anton's syndrome. The latter is a rare neurologic condition resulting from occipital lesions, in which the patient denies visual loss. Psychiatrically, exacerbation of mood disorder and schizophrenia can manifest as disorganization or ambivalence, with psychoses capable of supporting denial of delusional proportions. Obsessive-compulsive disorder may also masquerade as denial because of inordinate procrastination or inability to make a choice. Finally, delirium and dementia, among the most common findings in competence assessments, often result in pathologic minimization or even complete unawareness of illness.

Interpersonal barriers can also contribute to denial. Miscommunication because of language barriers or differing cultural concepts of health and illness is common enough to warrant use of trained interpreters in ambiguous cases. Writing tablets and alphabet boards are oft-neglected tools when lifesaving technologies such as ventilators interfere with verbalization. Concepts from the MacArthur study or clinical questions from Exhibit 19-1 can be used to assess the adequacy of such impaired communication. Otherwise, poor rapport with the medical team may significantly affect the patient's hospital course and have lingering effects on aftercare, as well.

Finally, other characterologic defenses can be considered concomitants of denial, particularly with those patients using such strategies as suppression (conscious submersion of emotions), repression (unconscious banishment of unacceptable emotion or ideas), displacement (attribution to others), or isolation of affect (separation of a situation's emotional meaning from its content). Weddington has even described a medical population with psychiatric history who ascribe physical symptoms to psychological factors, putting a novel spin on the concept of somatization.[81] Familiarity with such coping strategies enables clinicians to use educational and therapeutic interventions most consistent with the patient's style and thereby avoid conflict at times when speed is essential. Questions for assessing denial at the bedside are presented in Exhibit 19-2.

THE RELIGIOUS EXCEPTION

Religion's prominence in the social fabric allows it to lay claim to special consideration in the medical setting. There are, consequently, a wide variety of religious beliefs that influence medical decision making—from the proscription of blood transfusion by Jehovah's Witnesses to the respiratory standard of death used by some Orthodox Jews. The broad concepts of "life" and "death" from which these beliefs are derived are philosophic or spiritual in nature and—although physicians are uniquely placed to assess their medical criteria—are informed by scholarship from fields other than medicine. This discussion does not review the religious exceptions or their theoretical underpinnings but rather examines principles common to religious discussions in the medical setting and what determines their competence.

Exhibit 19-2
Assessing Denial at the Bedside

---

1.   What in reality is denied? Why? To whom?
2.   How is denial evident? In affect, behavior, or cognition?
3.   What are patient's usual coping strategies? General style in approaching threatening information?
4.   What are patient's beliefs regarding physicians/medical care? Prior experiences? Experiences of loved ones?
5.   Is event being denied likely to be repeated?
6.   Has the patient received adequate information?
7.   What is patient's current interpersonal environment? Coercive? Isolated?

Source: B. Cannon, "Pathologic Denial of Medical Illness" (Paper presented at the Psychosomatics Conference at Massachusetts General Hospital, Boston, 9 December 1994).

Religious thought is heavily influenced by casuistry—the study of case examples. In casuistry, moral obligations are derived from specific cases and then expanded or commented upon by developing further cases and analyzing their relevance. This results in practical rather than theoretical advice and is particularly useful in identifying exceptions and excuses to moral rules.[82] Exceptions to well-known sect rules have been granted by community leaders because of the circumstances of a case—such as recent conversion, marriage into the sect, and third-party obligations (for example, to minor children). In these instances, the religious proscriptions were believed to obtain less powerfully than they would otherwise, and competent refusals on religious grounds were withdrawn with the assistance of religious representatives. Awareness of this form of case analysis in religious thought should encourage clinicians to contact religious representatives in emergency-treatment refusals to verify belief systems and investigate salient exceptions. To do otherwise risks the charge of pseudo-empathy and abandonment of patients to their preferences without adequate exploration.

But what is it about a claim of religious exception that makes it competent? This question was underscored some years ago by the case of P.Z., a patient who enucleated his own eye and threatened to amputate a limb because of his unique "covenant with God," who directly ordered his sacrifice and chose him for the purpose.[83] Vanderpool, using his hypothetical Fire Baptized Holiness Christian as a model, suggests that the claim to religious exception should be honored if the patient passes certain mental tests; the patient is not impaired by pain, illness, and so on; and the clinicians discover that (1) a group calling itself by this name exists and is stable, (2) many of its beliefs are relatively consistent with one another, (3) their beliefs can readily support refusal of treatment, and (4) the patient identifies with or is a member of the group. P.Z., by use of this method, belonged to no such group and would fail mental tests for delusion, supporting its usefulness as a construct. Although Vanderpool emphasizes that his model does not address mass delusion, mass hysteria, or established social systems that are internally inconsistent or unstable, he nonetheless offers a useful guide to extending the usual investigations of intensive care.[84]

That a religion or congregation of one could not qualify under Vanderpool's model suggests that there are social or relational factors that also contribute to the religious exception. A psychiatrist might explore such relational factors by applying psychodynamic tests to the evaluation. Competent religious beliefs, rather than being precipitous or newly acquired, are likely to be developmentally related and involve a clearly formed relationship to an important figure or group in the patient's life. This "object relationship," in psychiatric parlance, may describe a tie with an individual or group related to God or with the deity Himself. If the beliefs are not integral to the individual's development or sense of community, psychiatric disorders manifesting as hyperreligiosity may be present. These can include bipolar disorder, obsessive-compulsive disorder, psychotic depression, complex-partial seizures, and delusional disorder. Questions that may augment the mental status exam in these cases are presented in Exhibit 19-3.

Michael Wreen has been particularly thoughtful about the premises that drive society's acceptance of religious belief systems. He identifies religious beliefs as inherently special, representing an attempt to answer ultimate questions—an exercise common to all philosophies—and recognizing the basic limitations of mortality. This recognition subsumes the understanding that the circumstances one is born into, one's genetics, and one's character traits are not of one's own choosing and, thus, that

---

Exhibit 19-3
Assessing Psychodynamics of Religious Decisions

---

1. How did the patient's beliefs develop?
2. Are they related to an important figure or group in the patient's history?
3. If there is a belief in God or other Being, what is the quality of the relationship?
    a. Personal or impersonal?
    b. Familial or alien (e.g., as child to parent or slave to master)?
    c. Caring or uncaring?
    d. One-way or two-way?
    e. Forgiving or punitive?
4. What is required of the individual? Of God? What are the penalties for violation? If the relationship incorporates concepts of good and evil, where does the individual lie on the continuum?
5. How has the patient responded to similar prior challenges? Did religion play the same role?
6. What is God's position in the present clinical situation? Does the patient "deserve" illness as punishment? If the patient suffers or dies because of religious demands, what is God's stand or reaction?
7. In accepting a belief system based on faith rather than demonstration or proof, how does the individual acknowledge and integrate doubt?
8. Is there an external coercive element (e.g., family, congregation, leaders)?

---

external forces influence individual existence. Religious beliefs, therefore, attempt to make sense of the world around us and in so doing appear to follow certain organizing principles.[85] Although assessing these principles may be difficult in the acute care setting, they provide a touchstone for distinguishing the patient who reports, "God told me not to accept transfusion," from the patient who reports, "I am a Witness and transfusion violates my beliefs."

CONCLUSION

The intensive care environment makes serious ethical demands on both the patient and the clinician. Whether in the assessment of the patient's choices, treatment of interfering conditions, or pursuit of appropriate alternatives, considerations of competence are omnipresent. Familiarity with the principles governing current standards and clinical tools will allow more concise and focused attention to proper decision making. Building the framework on which to hang these principles is the essence of the unique collaborative effort of clinician and patient.

ACKNOWLEDGMENT

I am grateful to Ned Cassem, Paul Appelbaum, and Robert Phillips for their suggestions and guidance.

NOTES

1. A.E. Buchanan and D.W. Brock, *Deciding for Others: The Ethics of Surrogate Decision Making* (New York: Cambridge University Press, 1989), 86; T.L. Beauchamp and J.F. Childress, *Principles of Biomedical Ethics*, 3rd ed. (New York: Oxford University Press, 1980), 80.

2. *Schloendorff v. Society Hospitals*, 211 N.Y. 125, 105 N.E. 92 (1914).

3. N.K. Rhoden, "Deciding about Treatment in ICU," in *Medicolegal Aspects of Critical Care*, ed. K. Benesch (Rockville, Md.: Aspen Publishers, Inc., 1986), 31-59.

4. S.J. Youngner, "Patient Autonomy, Informed Consent, and the Reality of Critical Care," *Critical Care Clinics* 2, no. 1 (January 1986): 41-51.

5. I. Kant, *Die Metaphysic der Sitten (The Metaphysics of Morals)* (Frankfurt, Germany: Suhrkamp, 1979), 396-97.

6. E.L. Pincoffs, "Judgments of Incompetence and Their Moral Presuppositions," in *Competency*, ed. M.A. Cutter and E. Shelp (Dordrecht, The Nether-

lands: Kluwer Academic Publishers, 1991), 79-89, 87.

7. *Canterbury v. Spence*, 464 F.2d 772, 789; *cert. denied* 409 U.S. 1064 (1972).

8. P.S. Appelbaum and L.H. Roth, "Clinical Issues in the Assessment of Competency," *American Journal of Psychiatry* 138, no. 11 (November 1981): 1462-67, cited by M. Perl, "Competency Judgments: Case Studies from the Psychiatrist's Perspective," in *Competency*, ed. M.A. Cutter and E. Shelp (Dordrecht, The Netherlands: Kluwer Academic Publishers, 1991), 179-184.

9. E.V. Boisaubin, "Competency Judgments: Case Studies from the Internist's Perspective," in *Competency*, ed. M.A. Cutter and E. Shelp (Dordrecht, The Netherlands: Kluwer Academic Publishers, 1991), 167-77, 179.

10. P.S. Appelbaum and T.G. Gutheil, *Clinical Handbook of Psychiatry and the Law*, 2nd ed. (Baltimore, Md.: Williams & Wilkins, 1991).

11. Ibid.

12. President's Commission for the Study of Ethical Problems in Medicine and Biomedical and Behavioral Research, *Making Health Care Decisions*, vol. 1 (Washington, D.C.: U.S. Government Printing Office, 1982), cited in J.A. Knight, "Judging Competence: When the Psychiatrist Need or Need Not Be Involved," in *Competency*, ed. M.A. Cutter and E. Shelp (Dordrecht, The Netherlands: Kluwer Academic Publishers, 1991), 3-28.

13. D.A. Soskis, "Schizophrenic and Medical Inpatients as Informed Drug Consumers," *Archives of General Psychiatry* 35, no. 5 (1978): 645-47; B. Stanley et al., "Preliminary Findings on Psychiatric Patients as Research Participants: A Population at Risk?" *American Journal of Psychiatry* 138, no. 5 (May 1981): 669-71.

14. P.S. Appelbaum and T. Grisso, "Assessing Patients' Capacities to Consent to Treatment," *New England Journal of Medicine* 319, no. 25 (December 1988): 1635-38.

15. Ibid., 1636.

16. T.L. Beauchamp, "Competence," in *Competency*, ed. M.A. Cutter and E. Shelp (Dordrecht, The Netherlands: Kluwer Academic Publishers, 1991), 49-77.

17. L.H. Roth, A. Meisel, and C.W. Lidz, "Tests of Competency to Consent to Treatment," *American Journal of Psychiatry* 134, no. 3 (March 1977): 285-89.

18. P.S. Appelbaum and T. Grisso, "The MacArthur Treatment-Competence Study. I: Mental Illness and Competence to Consent to Treatment," *Law and Human Behavior* 19, no. 2 (1995): 105-26.

19. P.S. Appelbaum and L.H. Roth, "Competency to Consent to Research: A Psychiatric Overview," *Archives of General Psychiatry* 39, no. 4 (1982): 951-58.

20. S. Wear, "Patient Freedom and Competence in Health Care," in *Competency*, ed. M.A. Cutter and E. Shelp (Dordrecht, The Netherlands: Kluwer Academic Publishers, 1991), 227-36.

21. See note 14 above.

22. J.F. Drane, "Competency to Give an Informed Consent: A Model for

Making Clinical Assessments," *Journal of the American Medical Association* 252, no. 7 (1984): 925-27.

23. J.J. Paris, "Court Intervention and the Diminution of Patients' Rights: The Case of Brother Joseph Fox," *New England Journal of Medicine* 303, no. 15 (1980): 876-78.

24. E.H. Morreim, "Competence: At the Intersection of Law, Medicine, and Philosophy," in *Competency*, ed. M.A. Cutter and E. Shelp (Dordrecht, The Netherlands: Kluwer Academic Publishers, 1991), 93-125.

25. American College of Chest Physicians/Society of Critical Care Medicine, "Ethical and Moral Guidelines for the Initiation, Continuation, and Withdrawal of Intensive Care," *Chest* 97, no. 4 (February 1992): 949-58.

26. Task Force on Ethics of the Society of Critical Care Medicine, "Consensus Report on the Ethics of Forgoing Life-Sustaining Treatments in the Critically Ill," *Critical Care Medicine* 18, no. 12 (December 1990): 1435-39.

27. H.R. Searight, "Assessing Patient Competence for Medical Decision-Making," *American Family Physician* 45, no. 2 (February 1992): 751-59.

28. M.G. Farnsworth, "Competency Evaluations in a General Hospital," *Psychosomatics* 31, no. 1 (Winter 1990): 60-66.

29. P.S. Appelbaum and L.H. Roth, "Clinical Issues in the Assessment of Competency," *American Journal of Psychiatry* 138, no. 11 (November 1981): 1462-67.

30. D.W. Molloy et al., "Factors Affecting Physicians' Decisions on Caring for an Incompetent Elderly Patient: An International Study," *Journal of the Canadian Medical Association* 145, no. 8 (1991): 947-52; see note 28 above.

31. J. Mahler and S. Perry, "Assessing Competency in the Medically Ill: Guidelines for Psychiatric Consultants," *Hospital and Community Psychiatry* 39, no. 8 (1988): 856-61.

32. R.C. Golinge and J.P. Fedoroff, "Characteristics of Patients Referred for Competency Evaluations," *Psychosomatics* 30, no. 3 (Summer 1989): 296-99; A.H. Mebane and H.B. Rauch, "When Do Physicians Request Competency Evaluations?" *Psychosomatics* 31, no. 1 (Winter 1990): 40-46; R. Weinstock, R. Copelan, and A. Bagheri, "Competence to Give Informed Consent for Medical Procedures," *Bulletin of the American Academy of Psychiatry and the Law* 12, no. 2 (1984): 117-25; see note 28 above.

33. S.H. Imbus and B.E. Zawacki, "Encouraging Dialogue and Autonomy in the Burn Intensive Care Unit," *Critical Care Clinics* 2, no. 1 (1986): 53-60.

34. P.S. Appelbaum and L.H. Roth, "Patients Who Refuse Treatment in Medical Hospitals," *Journal of the American Medical Association* 250, no. 10 (September 1983): 1296-301.

35. See note 29 above, at p. 1465.

36. E.H. Morreim, "Impairments and Impediments in Patients' Decision-Making: Reframing the Competence Question," *The Journal of Clinical Ethics* 4, no. 4 (Winter 1993): 294-307, 297.

37. T.G. Gutheil and H. Bursztajn, "Clinician's Guidelines for Assessing

and Presenting Subtle Forms of Patient Incompetence in Legal Settings," *American Journal of Psychiatry* 143, no. 8 (August 1986): 1020-23.

38. See note 29 above.

39. B.A. Venesey, "A Clinician's Guide to Decision Making Capacity and Ethically Sound Medical Decisions," *American Journal of Physical Medicine and Rehabilitation* 73, no. 3 (January 1994): 219-26.

40. L.J. Schneiderman, H. Teetzel, and A.G. Kalmanson, "Who Decides Who Decides?" *Archives of Internal Medicine* 155, no. 8 (April 1995): 793-96.

41. Beauchamp and Childress, *Principles,* see note 1 above, p. 171.

42. S.S. Herr and B.L. Hopkins, "Health Care Decision Making for Persons with Disabilities," *Journal of the American Medical Association* 271, no. 13 (April 1994): 1017-22.

43. R. Dresser, "Bound to Treatment: The Ulysses Contract," *Hastings Center Report* 14, no. 3 (June 1984): 13-16.

44. E.J. Emanuel, "A Communal Vision of Care for Incompetent Patients," *Hastings Center Report* 17, no. 5 (October-November 1987): 15-20.

45. See note 42 above.

46. B. Myers and C. Barrett, "Competency Issues in Referrals to a Consultation-Liaison Service," *Psychosomatics* 27, no. 11 (1986): 782-89; see note 28 above.

47. See notes 28 and 32 above.

48. See note 32 above.

49. Ibid.; see note 28 above.

50. See notes 28 and 32 above.

51. See note 32 above.

52. M. Katz et al., "Psychiatric Consultation for Competency to Refuse Medical Treatment," *Psychosomatics* 36, no. 1 (January-February 1995): 33-41.

53. See note 28 above.

54. See note 14 above.

55. L.J. Markson et al., "Physician Assessment of Patient Competence," *Journal of the American Geriatrics Society* 42, no. 10 (October 1994): 1074-80.

56. L.M. Cohen, J.D. McCue, and G.M Green, "Do Clinical and Formal Assessments of the Capacity of Patients in the Intensive Care Unit to Make Decisions Agree?" *Archives of Internal Medicine* 153, no. 21 (November 1993): 2481-85; J.F. Scott and J. Lynch, "Bedside Assessment of Competency in Palliative Care," *Journal of Palliative Care* 10, no. 3 (1994): 101-15.

57. E. Bruera et al., "Cognitive Failure in Cancer Patients in Clinical Trials," (letter) *Lancet* 341, no. 8839 (1993): 247-48; Ibid.

58. J.S. Janofsky, R.J. McCarthy, and M.F. Folstein, "The Hopkins Assessment Test: A Brief Method for Evaluating Patients' Capacity to Give Informed Consent," *Hospital and Community Psychiatry* 43, no. 2 (February 1992): 132-36.

59. Ibid.

60. H. Thomae, "Components of Competence in the Community Aged,"

Aging 4, no. 4 (1992): 317-25; K.C. Casimir and S.B. Billick, "Competency in Adolescent Inpatients," *Bulletin of the American Academy of Psychiatry and the Law* 22, no. 1 (1994): 19-29.

61. L.M. Kopelman, "On the Evaluative Nature of Competence and Capacity Judgments," *International Journal of Law and Psychiatry* 13, no. 4 (1990): 309-29.

62. See note 18 above.

63. T. Grisso et al., "The MacArthur Treatment Competence Study. II: Measures of Abilities Related to Competence to Consent to Treatment," *Law and Human Behavior* 19, no. 2 (1995): 127-48; T. Grisso and P.S. Appelbaum, "The MacArthur Treatment Competence Study. III: Abilities of Patients to Consent to Psychiatric and Medical Treatments," *Law and Human Behavior* 19, no. 2 (1995): 149-74; T. Grisso and P.S. Appelbaum, "Comparison of Standards for Assessing Patients' Capacities to Make Treatment Decisions," *American Journal of Psychiatry* 152, no. 7 (July 1995): 1033-37; see note 18 above.

64. T. Grisso, P.S. Appelbaum, and C. Hill-Fotouhi, "The Mac CAT-T: A Clinical Tool to Assess Patients' Capacities to Make Treatment Decisions," *Psychiatric Services* 48, no. 11 (1997): 1415-19.

65. K. Wells and A. Stewart, "The Functioning and Well-Being of Depressed Patients: Results from the Medical Outcomes Study," *Journal of the American Medical Association* 262, no. 7 (1989): 914-19; H.G. Koenig et al., "Detection and Treatment of Major Depression in Older Medically Ill Hospitalized Patients," *International Journal of Psychiatry in Medicine* 18, no. 1 (1988): 17-31.

66. M.D. Sullivan and S.J. Youngner, "Depression, Competence, and the Right to Refuse Life-Saving Medical Treatment," *American Journal of Psychiatry* 151, no. 7 (July 1994): 971-78.

67. Ibid.

68. Ibid.

69. American Psychiatric Association, *Diagnostic and Statistical Manual of Mental Disorders*, 4th ed. (Washington, D.C.: American Psychiatric Association, 1994).

70. E.H. Cassem and T.P. Hackett, "Psychiatric Consultation on a Coronary-Care Unit," *Annals of Internal Medicine* 75, no. 1 (1971): 9-14.

71. E. Shelp and M. Perl, "Denial in Clinical Medicine," *Archives of Internal Medicine* 145, no. 4 (1985): 697-99, cited by M. Perl, "Competency Judgments: Case Studies from Psychiatrist's Perspective," in *Competency*, ed. M.A. Cutter and E. Shelp (Dordrecht, The Netherlands: Kluwer Academic Publishers, 1991), 179-84.

72. E.B. Moore and B.D. Fine, *Psychoanalytic Terms and Concepts* (New Haven, Conn: Yale University Press, 1990), p. 50.

73. A.D. Weisman and T.P. Hackett, "Denial as a Social Act," in *Psychodynamic Studies on Aging: Creativity, Reminiscing, and Dying*, ed. S. Levin and R. Kahana (New York: International Universities Press, 1966), 79-110.

74. N. Cousins, "Denial: Are Sharper Definitions Needed?" *Journal of the*

American Medical Association 248, no. 2 (1982): 210-12.

75. T.P. Hackett and E.H. Cassem, "Development of a Quantitative Rating Scale to Assess Denial," *Journal of Psychosomatic Research* 18, no. 2 (1974): 93-100.

76. A. Froese et al., "Trajectories of Anxiety and Depression in Denying and Nondenying Acute Myocardial Infarction Patients During Hospitalization," *Journal of Psychosomatic Research* 18, no. 6 (1974): 413-20.

77. J.L. Levenson et al., "Denial Predicts Favorable Outcome in Unstable Angina Pectoris," *Psychosomatic Medicine* 46, no. 1 (1984): 25-32; J.L. Levenson et al., "Denial and Medical Outcome in Unstable Angina," *Psychosomatic Medicine* 51, no. 1 (1989): 27-35.

78. T.P. Hackett, E.H. Cassem, and H.A. Wishnie, "The Coronary-Care Unit: An Appraisal of Its Psychologic Hazards," *New England Journal of Medicine* 279, no. 25 (1968): 1365-70.

79. J. Levine et al., "The Role of Denial in Recovery from Coronary Heart Disease," *Psychosomatic Medicine* 49, no. 2 (1987): 109-17.

80. J.J. Gonzales, "Denial, Pathologic Denial, and Medical Illness" (Unpublished manuscript); B. Cannon, "Pathologic Denial of Medical Illness" (Paper presented at Psychosomatics Conference, Massachusetts General Hospital, Boston, 9 December 1994).

81. W.W. Weddington, Jr., "Psychogenic Explanation of Symptoms as a Denial of Physical Illness," *Psychosomatics* 21, no. 10 (1980): 805-07, 811-13.

82. M. Eliade, ed., *The Encyclopedia of Religion* (New York: MacMillan Publishing, 1987), 3: 114.

83. See Beauchamp and Childress, note 1 above, p. 412.

84. H.Y. Vanderpool, "The Competency of Definitions of Competency," in *Competency*, ed. M.A. Cutter and E. Shelp, (Dordrecht, The Netherlands: Kluwer Academic Publishers, 1991), 197-210.

85. M.J. Wreen, "Autonomy, Religious Values, and Refusal of Lifesaving Medical Treatment," *Journal of Medical Ethics* 17, no. 3 (1991): 124-30.

20

Conflict Management in the ICU: Intervention and Prevention

Martin L. Smith and Jeffrey Frank

INTRODUCTION

Conflicts in the intensive care unit (ICU) have a variety of manifestations and can have numerous causes. ICU conflicts most often are interpersonal (such as a conflict between physician and family) and interprofessional (such as a conflict between physician and nurse). But conflict can also stem from clinical practice guidelines and protocols, ICU or institutional policies, delivery systems and standards of care, and financial reimbursement mechanisms. Depending on the persons involved and the nature and causes of the conflict, responses to the conflict can run the gamut from quick resolution after a clarifying conversation, to whistle blowing or legal action, to festering for months without resolution.

Although a conflict can be the starting point for positive changes such as increased efforts at communication or quality-improvement initiatives, most serious conflicts produce negative reactions and feelings (such as frustration, anger, anxiety, and fear), and—at least in the short run—have a negative impact on the involved persons' time, energy, resources, commitment, and motivation. When conflicts are resolved satisfactorily, the experience can provide insights for resolving or preventing future conflicts. When conflicts remain unresolved, they can escalate, causing unbearable interpersonal and interdisciplinary pressures that are distressing and destructive for all involved.[1] Further, unresolved conflicts can often have a "rippling effect," becoming a force and factor leading to further conflicts. Rapid resolution of conflicts—or, even better, prevention of conflicts—is usually in the best interest of all those affected or potentially affected by the conflict.

At least three interconnecting factors create a context for clinical conflicts: (1) inequalities of power, (2) differences in knowledge and understanding, and (3) presence of mistrust. The practice of medicine and the delivery of healthcare, by their very nature, contribute to inequalities of power—especially, but not exclusively, between professionals and nonprofessionals. Medicine is a socially constituted practice founded on a body of esoteric knowledge. Simply because medical and clinical personnel know more about illnesses, diseases, and relevant therapies, a structure of inequality is inescapably imposed on interactions between clinical professionals and those who solicit their skills.[2] Further, as Brody has noted, physicians may have greater power (vis-à-vis patients and families), not only because of greater knowledge and skills regarding diagnosis and treatment, but also because of higher socioeconomic and educational status and because of an inherent social or charismatic power.[3] From the patient's side, the situation of illness and the need for professionals' assistance—especially ICU treatment and monitoring—creates an experience of powerlessness, dependence, disorientation, vulnerability, and isolation. This clinically situated imbalance of power can often lead to passivity and acquiescence on the part of patients and families. On the other hand, an unbridled, insensitive, or arrogant use of power by professionals can lead to both overt and covert conflicts if the abuse of power creates reactions of resentment, resistance, or suspicion.

As already noted, inequalities of power partially spring from differences in knowledge and understanding, especially of the human body and of clinical realities. But other differences in knowledge and understanding can create a context for conflicts. For example, although ICU nurses do not have the same training, skill, and clinical expertise as critical care physicians who have ultimate responsibility to make medical judgments about patients' diagnoses and prognoses, ICU nurses often have greater knowledge and understanding about specific patients' family backgrounds, personal values, and reactions and responses to treatment. Similarly, family members ordinarily have more knowledge and understanding of the patient as a person than clinical professionals do.

Finally, professionals and nonprofessionals alike can operate with misinformation or misunderstandings related to the patient's medical condition, psychosocial/spiritual background, or ethically and legally supported options.[4] Because the involved persons may have different knowledge bases, know about different aspects regarding the same patient, evaluate the relevance of their knowledge differently, or simply be mistaken about some aspect of the patient's care, interprofessional and interpersonal conflicts about treatment plans and clinical decisions are not uncommon in the ICU.

A final factor that can create a context for conflict in the ICU is the degree of trust or mistrust that exists among the involved persons. Among the professionals working together in an ICU, mutual respect and trust is either enhanced or diminished on a daily basis; the degree of trust depends on the quality and characteristics of the routine verbal and nonverbal communication that occurs. When joint, patient-centered, interprofessional collaboration is emphasized, with each professional invited to contribute to patients' diagnosis and treatment plans according to professional expertise, the level of trust among the healthcare team will likely be high. If communication is reduced merely to following orders, starting from the top of hierarchically established relationships and moving downward in one direction without mutuality, trust is likely to be replaced by resentment, competitiveness, and mistrust.

Building bridges of trust between patients and families and ICU professionals is especially challenging. Generally the encounters between patients and professionals in the ICU are short-term, with little time to develop trusting relationships. Also, in the complex environment of modern, subspecialty medicine, consultant-physicians and other professionals from outside the ICU are likely to participate in the care of ICU patients. As the number of professionals treating and caring for a specific patient increases, consistency of communication (which helps to build trust) becomes more difficult to accomplish.

This chapter does not address directly every kind of conflict that can arise in the ICU. Rather, it presents and analyzes three illustrative case examples of conflicts that are fairly typical for ICU professionals: (1) an interprofessional (intrateam) conflict between a physician and nurses, (2) a conflict between a healthcare team and a family, and (3) a conflict between a healthcare team and a third-party payer. Each conflict is illustrated by a case example, followed by an analysis of causes and recommended strategies for resolution and intervention. Before presenting these three illustrative conflicts and cases, the chapter summarizes some foundational ideas for conflict prevention and resolution. These foundational ideas are taken from the literature of medical humanities (narrative ethics), law (mediation as a technique for alternate dispute resolution), and anthropology (culture brokering).

FOUNDATIONAL IDEAS FOR CONFLICT PREVENTION AND RESOLUTION

The ultimate goal of ICU admissions, diagnostic testing, treatments, and care plans is the well-being and best interest of patients whose lives are disrupted by critical or acute illness. What is best for patients can range from complete recovery and return to a fully independent life, to a return to a "baseline" of chronic conditions, to a comfortable and peaceful death. The best interest of ICU patients is ordinarily served when conflicts about their treatment are prevented, or when existing conflicts are resolved quickly and to the satisfaction of those involved. Selected ideas, language, and practices from medical humanities (narrative ethics), law (mediation), and anthropology (culture brokering) are helpful for creating a context for thinking about conflict prevention and resolution in the ICU.

NARRATIVE ETHICS

Clinical professionals in the ICU should have an understanding of the fundamental principles of medical ethics including autonomy, beneficence, nonmaleficence, and justice.[5] But beyond this understanding, according to a narrative ethics approach, health professionals must also learn to surmise the texture of a patient's life in all its moral complexity.[6] In other words, a cognitive grasp of the abstract, generalized principles of ethics and morality needs to be particularized and contextualized in the lives of real patients and their experiences of illness.

The methods that are often called *narrative ethics* center the examination of ethical dilemmas and issues squarely in the framework of the patient's culture, biography, and life. When clinicians enter into a patient-centered, narrative approach, they engage and encounter "a powerful, concrete, rich sense of the feelings, values, beliefs, and interpretations that make up the actual experience of the sick person."[7] Within this framework, professionals need to be skilled at evoking and listening to potentially multiple perspectives of the patient's story; examining the contradictions and ambiguities among the story's multiple representations; and discerning the coherence, resonance, and meanings of particular human events.[8] As Charon and colleagues have noted: "Narrative skills can help the clinician to be sensitive to moral questions as they occur, to integrate questions about values and beliefs into the routines of medical care, and to make contact with the conflicts, tragedy, humor, irony, and ambiguity that contribute to each human life."[9] When using a narrative ethics methodology, the clinician can assume the role of articulator—especially of voices either ignored or not usually heard—facilitator and encourager of dialogue; and recaller of contexts, perspectives, and particularities that may be obscured or forgotten.[10] According to Zawacki, this envisioned dialogic approach aims for a "noncoercive 'ethical dialogue' that seeks partnership and collaboration by communicating first to understand and then to be understood; by asking questions, challenging, and seeking to establish a trusting, collaborative, synergistic 'win-win' partnership."[11]

In this narrative approach to patient care, there is also an appropriate role for professionals' self-disclosure of their own personal thoughts, feelings, and vulnerabilities. Drawing upon his own experience as a physician, Zawacki states some benefits to such self-disclosure in situations involving life-and-death decisions:

> When the senior physician, the individual whose role implies the most power, is able to reveal not only information, but also her authentic, individual, and subjective fears, doubts, affections, humor, ignorance, commitments, reluctance, hopes, values, and so on when necessary (and especially if the patient/family in response is able to be similarly vulnerable and authentic), fateful decisions about life and death are regularly made with surprising, at times beautiful, and occasionally even humor-filled serenity and camaraderie.[12]

When such self-disclosure is done carefully, sensitively, and nonmanipulatively, professionals can model for patients, families, and other professionals how to reveal relevant aspects of their own narratives.

An attentive and routine practice of narrative ethics has the potential to prevent the development of many conflicts and ethical dilemmas in the ICU. Professionals who take seriously the tenets of narrative ethics and develop the corresponding skills will frequently counter, in the care of individual patients, the three earlier-stated factors that can create a context for clinical conflict. That is, inequalities of power will be reduced, differences in knowledge and understandings will be diminished, and mutual trust and respect will be enhanced.

MEDIATION

In response to overcrowded U.S. court dockets, disputants are turning to methods other than litigation to resolve conflicts. These methods and mechanisms of alternative dispute resolution come in many forms.[13] Arbitration, on one end of the spectrum, uses an objective third party who, in the context of a formal hearing of arguments from both sides, makes a decision for the disputing parties who have given prior agreement to engage in, and in many instances to be bound by, this method. In arbitration, the parties relinquish their power to resolve their own conflict and place it in the hands of the arbitrator. On the other end of the spectrum is negotiation, in which the disputants try to reach a settlement without the intervention of a third party.

In between arbitration and negotiation falls a variety of facilitation techniques, in which a neutral third person (the mediator or facilitator) helps the disputing parties to reach a resolution, without imposing a decision on them. Mediation, as an example of one of these facilitated processes, is a voluntary, nonadversarial process that allows conflicting parties to establish a workable solution to their problem with the assistance of an impartial mediator.[14] The ultimate authority in mediation rests with the participants, who fashion their own solutions and accept responsibility for the results. Because some of the goals of mediation include preserving relationships, diffusing emotions, promoting communication, and addressing concerns rather than proving persons to be right or wrong, each party is encouraged to tell their story as in a narrative fashion and to present the facts they believe to be relevant.[15]

The role of the mediator is to create an atmosphere of trust in which the parties can express and explore their underlying interests and needs, identify solutions, and work toward consensus. Mediators play a facilitative role; they help the parties to reach an agreement without interjecting their own views into the resolution process.

A recent, innovative application of mediation techniques and skills is in the area of hospital ethics consultation. Mediation (or its close variations) is useful in resolving clinical ethics conflicts because of its ready accessibility (it can be scheduled any time), its informality and flexibility (the parties can agree on any format that seems appropriate), its low cost and minimum preparation, its private and confidential nature (the parties can be open and candid), and its focus on mutual problem solving and mutually acceptable agreements.

Identifying who should fill the role of mediator in the hospital and the ICU is somewhat problematic. Some authors have proposed that ethics committees and bioethics consultants can and should be trained with appropriate skills, techniques, and knowledge about procedural issues and responsibilities to be mediators of conflicts and disputes.[16] Hospital chaplains, social workers, or a designated ICU team member could be added to the list of persons so trained. However, there are problems with this approach. Hospital personnel may lack neutrality.[17] Frequently such persons, especially if they are already involved in the case or have responsibilities in the ICU, may have a personal or professional stance or bias regarding the issues at hand. Further, because mediation focuses on relationships and context and not on principles, ethics consultants and committee members may be unwilling to be neutral about private solutions that violate established ethical principles (such as patient autonomy or justice), institutional ethics policies, or societal standards.

Despite these cautions and criticisms, there is a place for adapting elements of mediation to resolve conflicts in the ICU, even if a complete mediation process is not adopted. Use of mediation skills, techniques, and procedures can enhance the autonomy and self-determination of the parties; create a greater balance of power; emphasize context and circumstances in the application of ethical principles; and promote communication, mutual respect, and trust.

CULTURE BROKERING

Culture, in its broadest definition, can be understood as the conceptual framework of shared values, beliefs, and behaviors by which people understand themselves, their environment, and their experiences. Culture is not equivalent to race, nationality, or ethnic group; however, these categories frequently are contributors to culture, as it is understood more narrowly. In the broadest sense, medical and healthcare systems (including the ICU) can be viewed as cultural systems.[18] For example, many patients enter the hospital and its ICUs much like immigrants entering a foreign country. The ICU or the hospital can have all the characteristics of a cultural system—its own values, beliefs, customs, behaviors, symbols, and language. When patients and their families enter this unfamiliar world, they often experience "culture shock."

Culture brokering, which has been practiced for many years by anthropologists, is defined as the act of bridging, linking, or mediating between groups or persons of differing cultural backgrounds for the purpose of reducing conflict or producing change.[19] The functions of culture brokering include interpreting, educating, advocating, clarifying, empowering, implementing, facilitating, and resolving. Attributes of the culture broker include the ability to function where unequal relationships exist. According to LaFargue, the culture broker has the respect of both parties, is knowledgeable about both systems, and can introduce and translate ideas into a language understood by both systems.[20]

Although the framework of culture brokering in healthcare has been most often applied to nursing,[21] it has utility for all health professionals who strive to prevent and resolve conflicts in the ICU. For example, when a conflict arises because of differences in knowledge and understanding, what may be needed is education, interpretation, and "information brokering" to help the patient and family understand ICU technology and its meaning for the specific patient. In a situation involving conflict among family members, what may be needed is facilitation of discussion and mediation that helps family members understand one another's thoughts, feelings, and perspectives, as well as those of the patient and the professionals. If a patient's lack of economic power or the constraints of a third-party insurance program are preventing the patient from receiving reasonable medical care, what may be needed is a network of relationships (formal or informal) that uses the power of the broker to give the patient access to needed healthcare.[22]

Recognition and anticipation of the need for culture brokering are first steps that can prevent conflicts in the ICU. When conflicts do arise, interventions such as those mentioned above, performed by professionals willing to act as culture brokers, can help to resolve conflicts in a timely manner.

THREE TYPES OF CONFLICT

Three commonly encountered types of conflict in the ICU are (1) interprofessional, (2) team-family, and (3) team-payer conflicts. This section presents cases that illustrate each of these types of conflict, with a subsequent analysis of the basis for the conflicts and recommendations for prevention and intervention. Many of the recommendations are transferable to other types of conflict not illustrated here.

CASE 1: INTERPROFESSIONAL (INTRATEAM) CONFLICT
Patient information. A 46-year-old man had a six-year history of amyotrophic lateral sclerosis (ALS), a degenerative disease of motor neurons. He gradually adapted to his progressive disability characterized by

quadriplegia and the inability to speak. Difficulty swallowing led to progressive malnutrition which, coupled with loss of respiratory muscle strength, led to acute respiratory failure after an episode of aspiration.

The patient was transferred to the ICU after he had been resuscitated with intubation and mechanical ventilation at a local emergency department. Upon ICU admission, he was hemodynamically stable on mechanical ventilation with adequate oxygenation, despite mild bilateral basilar aspiration pneumonitis. Although he was quadriplegic, some limited leg adduction allowed him to communicate with a laser-triggered computer. Also, he was able to indicate "yes" and "no" with eyebrow elevation and weak head shaking.

The patient wanted all stabilizing and life-sustaining treatment to be instituted. His supportive wife and three young children allowed him to see purpose and quality in life, even with his severe, dependent disability. In the month before his hospitalization, he had continued working in his managerial position for a large corporation. The slow pace of his progressive disease created the opportunity for him to redefine his life around his disability. The patient and his wife were well-educated professionals, and they had insight into the implications of decisions about life and death for their family and lifestyle.

Acute medical treatments. The first several weeks of hospitalization included full treatment for the pneumonitis. Artificial nutritional support was instituted and well tolerated. A systematic weaning program tailored to the patient's ALS defined the permanent need for mechanical ventilatory support with tracheostomy to increase the patient's chances of stability and survival following discharge. Swallowing evaluation revealed severe aspiration. Permanent tracheostomy and percutaneous endoscopically guided gastrostomy were performed. In addition, laryngectomy was performed to allow continued eating without risk of aspiration.

The restrictions stipulated by the patient's health insurance plan made it difficult to arrange home care with mechanical ventilation. The patient's insurance plan provided payment for treatment at an extended-care facility but did not cover the home care services necessary for his medical profile and needs. Difficulties with the insurance company resulted in a significant delay in discharge from the hospital.

Setting the stage for the conflict. The patient was a very positive and optimistic individual, but the prolonged hospitalization in the ICU with seemingly endless obstacles to discharge home led to his increasing disappointment and depression. His lengthy hospital stay, coupled with his prolonged recovery from the recent surgical procedures and the associated discomfort, led to a loss of optimism and a loss of perspective.

The ICU nurses were encouraging and supportive of the patient; however, several nurses were troubled by the degenerative nature of his disease, appreciating that his future held only continued neurological decline with further disability and morbidity. Several nurses viewed life-long dependence on mechanical ventilation as inappropriate for patients with severe degenerative disease. Early in the patient's hospitalization, the ICU physician and nurses held frequent discussions that took into consideration the patient's prehospitalization perspective and quality of life. These discussions contributed to the nurses' understanding of the goals of the critical care plan and its congruity with the patient's wishes for his projected quality of life following discharge.

The ICU physician, because of his patient-centered, narrative approach to the case, understood well the patient's prehospitalization quality of life and his desire to remain alive with the assistance of mechanical ventilation. The physician viewed continued life-sustaining treatment as appropriate for this patient. The patient's wife shared this view. However, as the physician's focus shifted toward improving the patient's disposition, he neglected to communicate with the nurses about the patient.

The conflict. As the patient began to feel more hopeless about his situation and home discharge, he communicated his general discontentment to his nurses and the ICU physician. The ICU physician perceived the growing discontentment as a sign of the patient's narrowing perspective due to the prolonged ICU stay, insufficient contact with his children, and the possibility of discharge to an extended-care facility rather than home. In contrast, several nurses interpreted the patient's change in outlook to be a result of his gradual realization that his situation was indeed hopeless. These nurses, seeing themselves as "patient advocates," became increasingly uncomfortable with the aggressive treatment plan; and they also disagreed with the persistent attempts by the physician and the patient's wife to help the patient develop renewed perspective. The conflict festered, increased in intensity, and undermined patient care. A summary of the conflicting viewpoints and the corresponding desired actions can be found in Exhibit 20-1.

The basis for the conflict. Because nurses usually spend more time with patients and their families than physicians do, nurses are often more aware of acute psychosocial issues. This critical role appropriately serves as the

Exhibit 20-1
Case 1: Conflicting Viewpoints and Corresponding Actions

Player	Viewpoint	Necessary Action
ICU physician and patient's wife	The patient has lost perspective of the projected quality in his discharge disposition (home) due to his situation and delays in discharge.	Accelerate discharge by challenging insurance company more aggressively. Renew the patient's optimism by conducting bedside discussions, taking the patient on wheelchair expeditions through the hospital, providing psychosocial support from social workers and pastoral counselors, and arranging for regular family visits with all of the patient's children.
Nurses	The patient finally realizes his dismal situation. The ICU physician and the patient's wife have an unrealistic outlook, not victimizing the patient.	Advocate the patient's new perspective. Redefine the level of care to reflect the patient's new perspective.

foundation for nurses' power and perspective as strong patient advocates. However, several factors can limit a nurse's perspective, including limited scope of nurses' encounters with patients and families due to changing work shifts and limited understanding of disease processes and their natural history.

Physicians, on the other hand, often focus on long-term goals and overlook strategies to enhance patients' short-term coping. Because physicians do not spend as much time at the bedside as ICU nurses do, physicians generally have a limited awareness of acute psychosocial issues. Physicians' insufficient respect for and recognition of nurses' vital role in providing continuity of care and communicating with families frequently detracts from the potentially powerful partnership that can exist between ICU physicians and nurses and can affect patient care.[23]

Good communication, coordination, mutual assistance, and competence can bridge the "perspective gap" between physicians and nurses to achieve a more consistent, holistic, dynamic plan for treatment.[24] However, the intensity of this communication can be highly variable, particularly with respect to long-term ICU patients. In the case above, the lack of ongoing communication between the physician and the nurses resulted in unnecessary conflict.

Recommendations to prevent and resolve intrateam conflict. ICU professionals can prevent and resolve many intrateam conflicts by incorporating the following action steps into their clinical practice.

1. Strive for patient-centered analysis of decisions regarding treatment, with a full understanding of the particular patient, the disease, and its natural history. Avoid generalized preconceptions for what is "appropriate" or "inappropriate" treatment.

2. Bridge the "perspective gap" by frequent, planned, and comprehensive communication among professionals. This requires an appreciation of the special role of each team member in patient care.

3. Avoid biased "editorializing" during reporting procedures. This can hurt patient care and result in issue-focused conflict that may not apply to the individual patient's situation from which it was derived.

4. When conflicts arise, institute early intervention through candid communication, ICU team meetings, and mediation if appropriate.

5. Initiate a primary nursing model for long-term ICU patients to enhance continuity of care and consistent family interactions. Physicians should also consider a primary ICU physician model for long-term ICU patients if the care is not already organized in that manner. Both of these "primary professional" models refer to the identification of a single health professional championing uniformity of care for complex patients.

Case resolution. The ICU physician arranged a two-day period for the patient's wife and children to visit the patient in the ICU. The patient was dressed each day in his own clothes, and the projected vision of his day-to-day life at home was simulated in the hospital. To prepare for this intervention, ICU staff held a meeting to discuss the patient's life and the vision for his long-term disposition. A letter summarizing the details of the meeting was sent to all ICU nurses and respiratory therapists (with the family's permission). Meeting participants also identified a core group of primary nurses who were comfortable with the treatment plan.

The patient was eventually discharged to his home, and four years later he was doing well. Although he continued to be severely disabled and required around-the-clock assistance (including mechanical ventilation), hospital readmission was never necessary. He remained well-nourished and without the breathlessness that characterized his condition before he entered the ICU. He communicated through a computerized word processor, and he attended all of his son's high school basketball games.

The patient summarized his retrospective view of his hospitalization and coping when he thanked the ICU team for their care and support:

There were two great adventures I never got to do but still I dream about them. One was to climb a significant mountain (I was diagnosed with ALS the summer that I went to mountaineering school). The other was to sail the Strait of Magellan. However, life's great adventures sometimes occur in places that one never dreamt about. The last month of my hospitalization has been the greatest adventure of my life; a life filled with considerable adventure including flying off aircraft carriers. The adventure has had high drama. It has been a life-or-death struggle that has tested the limits of my endurance and spirit. Through it all I have had in you the best partner who was there with solutions each time I felt I couldn't go on. I know you have saved many lives, but I doubt you have saved the same life as many times as you have saved mine. I will never be able to adequately thank you for all you have done.

CASE 2: TEAM-FAMILY CONFLICT

Patient information. A 32-year-old man had a three-year history of a brain-stem tumor, inoperable due to location and extent of invasion. He received maximum exposure to radiation therapy and participated in an experimental chemotherapeutic protocol. Although these treatments slowed the tumor's growth, the tumor ultimately progressed with subsequent neurological deterioration.

During the month prior to ICU admission, the patient became bedridden with quadriplegia and an inability to articulate, swallow, and move his eyes. His level of consciousness declined to a stuporous state most of the time, and he was unable to interact meaningfully with his environment. As a result of this gradual decline and tachypnea (increased rate of respiration), the patient was hospitalized.

The patient had been unwilling to confront his own mortality with his wife. His parents knew through many of his comments (made before his neurological deterioration) that he was preparing emotionally for the inevitability of his death. However, he and his wife coped primarily through denial, never acknowledging the evolving medical problems and the progression of his disease.

Acute medical treatments. The patient was admitted to the hospital with severe dehydration, malnutrition, and anemia. His most acute problem was respiratory insufficiency requiring intubation and mechanical ventilation to achieve short-term survival. The respiratory insufficiency was caused by the tumor's invasion of essential respiratory control centers. There were no remaining therapeutic options to enhance the patient's neurological function.

Setting the stage for the conflict. The patient's wife, who failed to appreciate that her husband had a terminal condition, was unprepared for his inevitable decline. Profound denial allowed her to view his deterioration as an event that would resolve with medical intervention. She came from a Fundamentalist Christian background and believed that "only God can make decisions that will result in death." She believed that the use of all available medical technology to achieve survival was a moral obligation, and she frequently reported that she was praying for and expecting a miracle.

The conflict. The patient's admitting physician believed that the directives of the patient's wife dictated the plan for medical treatment. His perspective reinforced the wife's belief that ventilatory support was an acceptable and reasonable medical option. The ICU physician reviewed the patient's medical history and acute condition and held detailed discussions with a neuro-oncologist and the patient's wife and parents. The ICU physician concluded that mechanical ventilatory support would be futile, inhumane, and should not be offered.

The patient's wife resisted any process of discussion or education and was unwilling to acknowledge the reality of her husband's terminal condition. She became angry because of the ICU physician's refusal to allow intubation and mechanical ventilation. The admitting physician was alarmed about the potential legal ramifications of challenging a family's directives. The wife's demand for a "second ICU opinion" was honored. The second physician concurred that resuscitative intervention was not an acceptable medical option.

A summary of the conflicting viewpoints and the corresponding desired actions appears in Exhibit 20-2.

The basis for the conflict. The patient and his wife did not adequately understand the natural history of progressive brain-stem tumors, despite regular contact with physicians. The patient's tendency to avoid confronting his own mortality prevented him from communicating his advance directives for medical treatment. His grief-stricken wife was poorly informed about the disease process and the inherent limitations of medical alternatives in halting tumor progression. In addition, she sustained an image of divine intervention that focused on a narrow perspective regarding miracles and death.[25] Her displaced anger over her loss was directed at the medical system.

The ICU physician believed that medical interventions should only be instituted when defined goals and outcomes are achievable. In his view, burdensome, nonbeneficial treatments should not be offered to patients and families.

Recommendations to prevent and resolve team-family conflict. ICU professionals can prevent and resolve many team-family conflicts by incorporating the following action steps into their clinical practice:

1. Educate patients and families about the natural history of disease processes or potential complications of interventions. Clinicians should especially focus on possible situations that could require decisions about life and death. An ICU professional, functioning as an "culture broker," may be necessary.

Exhibit 20-2
Case 2: Conflicting Viewpoints and Corresponding Actions

Player	Viewpoint	Necessary Action
Patient's wife	Death is an unacceptable outcome. Medical technology must be used to achieve survival. Only God can choose when and how a person dies, and miracles can occur.	Demand that all life-sustaining treatments be provided.
Admitting physician	Ventilator support is futile. The patient's wife is appropriate surrogate for decision making. Family can dictate medical treatments. Legal reprise is a potential concern.	Institute ventilator support despite its futility.
ICU physician	Ventilator support is futile. Medical technology should be used only to achieve beneficial outcome. Offering futile medical options is irresponsible and fosters dysfunctional family coping. The patient's wife is unprepared for the situation; needs education/guidance The patient's wife is not a rational surrogate.	Educate family by reviewing disease progression and inevitability of death. Refuse ventilatory support. Consult hospital legal counsel to address concerns of admitting physician. Support family via pastoral care, social work, and nursing. Communicate to family palliative care plan and nonabandonment of patient.

2. Interpret the patient's unwillingness to discuss issues of mortality as a medical problem requiring multidisciplinary interventions.

3. Identify significant persons, supportive of patient and family (such as family clergy, hospital chaplains, social workers, or bioethicists), who should be included in important meetings dealing with sensitive issues.

4. Clarify the differences in perception that are causing conflict to determine the necessary interventions to resolve the conflict (for example, review imaging scans with family members, address prior concerns about treatment).

5. Remain patient-centered when dealing with a team-family conflict. Remember that the medical team's primary goal is to promote the patient's best interest (which may be a comfortable death).

6. Sensitively and patiently interpret family reactions and emotions in the clinical context as a manifestation of their current coping mechanisms (for example, avoid reflexive responses of anger to a family member's anger).

Case resolution. The patient's wife returned to her husband's bedside two hours after angrily leaving the hospital, and the ICU physician requested the services of the hospital chaplain and a social worker. The ICU physician had obtained advice from a bioethics consultant and the hospital legal counsel that validated the appropriateness of the medical team's position. In the presence of the hospital chaplain and the patient's parents, the ICU physician reviewed the medical issues and affirmed the prior conclusion that respiratory resuscitation was not a medical option. He also reaffirmed that the patient would continue to receive comfort-enhancing medical and nursing care. The medical team's consistency and patient-centered reasoning helped the patient's wife appreciate the unequivocally terminal nature of her husband's condition. The chaplain counseled her regarding her apparent religious conflict about the role of medical technology with respect to "God's ways and plan."

The patient died six hours later. His wife wrote a letter to the ICU physician one month later indicating the importance of his unwavering resistance to respiratory resuscitation. The physician's stance helped her confront the reality that her husband's situation was unambiguous. She agreed that offering futile medical options would have perpetuated her misconceptions and made her husband's death much more difficult to endure.

CASE 3: TEAM-PAYER CONFLICT

Patient information. A 42-year-old male dancer suffered an acute sub-arachnoid hemorrhage from a ruptured basilar artery aneurysm. The initial hemorrhage did not cause disability, but the aneurysm clipping and subsequent vasospasm (contraction of the blood vessel) led to a large brain-stem infarction. This caused the patient to develop "locked-in syndrome," a condition characterized by normal cognitive function with severe motor limitation. The patient could not readily interact with his environment, and his only means of communicating was through eyelid blinking (he blinked once for "yes" and twice for "no").

Despite his new disabilities, the patient had a strong will to live, which he continued to communicate through eyelid blinking. He underwent tracheostomy and gastrostomy, and he was successfully weaned from the ventilator. As he achieved medical stability, discharge arrangements were made.

Setting the stage for the conflict. Significant improvement in function was possible for this patient, but he would require a highly specialized, neurologically focused, multidisciplinary rehabilitation program with experience in caring for patients with this type of severe disability. The closest rehabilitation program adequate to meet this patient's needs was 300 miles from the acute care facility. The patient's insurance plan did not cover care at the distant institution and would only provide care at an "in-plan" regional facility.

The conflict. The ICU team knew that the regional rehabilitation alternatives could not provide the specialized program needed to ensure the best possible neurological and functional outcomes for this patient. The insurance company personnel insisted that the patient's entitlements allowed for care at regional facilities only, and that several regional facilities were "approved" to provide care for neurologically disabled patients who had tracheostomy and mechanical ventilation. The team feared that transfer to one of these facilities would lead to possible death or life-threatening complications and poor long-term neurological outcomes.

The conflict delayed the patient's discharge and required time-consuming interactions among the ICU team, the hospital discharge coordinators, and the payer's case-management representative. The hospital discharge coordinators were unable to persuade the payer's representatives that the patient was an exception to the payer's practice guidelines. A "discharge deadlock" resulted.

A summary of the conflicting viewpoints and the corresponding desired actions is presented in Exhibit 20-3.

Exhibit 20-3
Case 3: Conflicting Viewpoints and Corresponding Actions

Player	Viewpoint	Necessary Action
Payer	The patient's neurological disability limits his qualifications for acute rehabilitation. His nursing and medical needs can be provided locally. We have a responsibility to all policyholders to ensure responsible resource utilization.	Uphold the policy entitlement restrictions for this patient.
ICU team	The patient has a special neurological disability. The patient requires a highly specialized and focused program. The facilities proposed by the payer are inadequate and seriously jeopardize the patient's survival and long-term neurological improvement.	Advocate for the patient. Insist on appropriate discharge arrangements. Challenge the payer to consider this patient's special circumstances.

The basis for the conflict. Payers of healthcare have a responsibility to ensure that policyholders receive program benefits according to contractual agreements. This responsibility requires planned allocation and utilization of limited resources. Frivolous expenditures on one patient without clear benefit can potentially jeopardize the availability of resources for other policyholders. Payers must provide for individuals without losing sight of all the other "covered lives."

The payers' front-line personnel (usually clinical professionals who review patient situations on a case-by-case basis) must interpret policies and practice guidelines, usually without authority to individualize entitlements in special circumstances. Because many patients believe that their circumstances are an "exception to the rule," front-line personnel may be instructed that individualization is not even a possibility.

Physicians, for their part, are often intimidated by the presumed impenetrability of payers' systems and processes that are perceived to result in unwavering adherence to restrictions on patient entitlements. Challenging such restrictions is time-consuming. Many hospitals have personnel assigned to work with payers, but these individuals' skills and commitment to advocating for patients may vary. In addition, because they are not caregivers themselves, the medical information they provide to the payer's representative is second-hand.

These different perspectives among payers, hospital personnel, and physicians can create barriers to the kind of collaboration necessary to achieve the best possible patient disposition in complex cases. As a result, patients can be victimized by "the system."

Recommendations to prevent and resolve team-payer conflict. Clinical ICU professionals can prevent and resolve many team-payer conflicts by incorporating the following action steps into their clinical practice:

1. Acknowledge payers' important responsibility to ensure the availability of benefits to all policyholders and payers' usual good intentions to provide the best possible patient outcomes in individual cases.

2. Approach payers collaboratively, assuming their mutual interest in the patient's well-being. This can set the stage for proactive planning, with both the medical team and payers acting as partner-advocates for the patient.

3. Proactively initiate communication with key individuals in the payer's organization regarding complex cases that may require individualization of entitlements to achieve the best possible patient outcomes. Comprehensive letters communicating a particu-

lar patient's special circumstances can help to crystallize issues and clarify why policy restrictions might not be in the best interest of the payer and patient.

4. Organize, educate, and train hospital support staff who are involved with patient care and disposition to be "power brokers"—that is, to work with payers to achieve individualization of entitlements when appropriate.

Case resolution. An individual within the payer's organization was identified who had the authority to consider special circumstances that would require "out-of-policy" coverage. The ICU physician telephoned that person and explained in detail the patient's situation, disease, prognosis, and necessary rehabilitation. The physician then wrote a letter that identified the patient's special circumstances and explained that appropriate disposition arrangements would benefit both patient and payer.

Discussions of mutual concern for the patient's best interest led to the payer's approval of the patient's transfer to the appropriate rehabilitation program, including air transportation. Two years after discharge, the patient was doing well with some residual disability. He had achieved almost total independence in his activities of daily living and had started a new business as a dessert caterer.

CONCLUSION

The intensity of the critical care environment is often overwhelming. That same intensity and the many diverse relationships and interactions in the ICU breed unlimited potential for distracting conflicts. This chapter reviews strategies for conflict prevention that should be used by all ICU personnel.

However, even with the best preventive measures, conflicts will occur in the ICU. When conflicts occur, early and aggressive intervention is necessary to prevent conflicts from escalating to the degree that patient care is affected and the effectiveness of the ICU is hindered.

Professionals must strive to be effective communicators, as well as assertive, respectful, and compassionate. These essential qualities enable ICU professionals to engage patients and families in the narration of their stories; to facilitate impartially the exchange of understandings, opinions, and ideas when conflicts do arise; and to bridge the "culture gap" that exists between the ICU and the everyday world of ordinary people faced with a medical crisis. A deeper understanding of the basis for conflict, and the personal character traits and behaviors that prevent or minimize conflict, will empower ICU personnel to function as a unified team and to avoid unnecessary distractions and detractions from patient care.

NOTES

1. Y.J. Craig, "Patient Decision-Making: Medical Ethics and Mediation," *Journal of Medical Ethics* 22, no. 3 (1996): 164-67.

2. B.J. Crigger, "Negotiating the Moral Order: Paradoxes of Ethics Consultation," *Kennedy Institute of Ethics Journal* 5, no. 2 (1995): 89-112.

3. H. Brody, *The Healer's Power* (New Haven, Conn.: Yale University Press, 1992).

4. A. Meisel, "Legal Myths about Terminating Life Support," *Archives of Internal Medicine* 151 (1991): 1497-502.

5. T.L. Beauchamp and J.F. Childress, *Principles of Biomedical Ethics*, 4th ed. (New York: Oxford University Press, 1994).

6. R. Charon et al., "Literature and Medicine: Contributions to Clinical Practice," *Annals of Internal Medicine* 122, no. 8 (1995): 599-606.

7. Ibid., 602.

8. R. Charon, "Narrative Contributions to Medical Ethics: Recognition, Formulation, Interpretation, and Validation in the Practice of the Ethicist," in *A Matter of Principles? Ferment in U.S. Bioethics*, ed. E.R. Dubose, R.P. Hamel, and L.J. O'Connell (Valley Forge, Penn.: Trinity Press International, 1994), 260-83.

9. See note 6 above, p. 602.

10. D. Leder, "Toward a Hermeneutical Bioethics," in *A Matter of Principles? Ferment in U.S. Bioethics*, ed. E.R. Dubose, R.P. Hamel and L.J. O'Connell (Valley Forge, Penn.: Trinity Press International, 1994), 240-59.

11. B.E. Zawacki, "The 'Futility Debate' and the Management of Gordian Knots," *The Journal of Clinical Ethics* 6, no. 2 (Summer 1995): 112-27, at p. 119.

12. Ibid., 122.

13. M.B. West and J.M. Gibson, "Facilitating Medical Ethics Case Review: What Ethics Committees Can Learn from Mediation and Facilitation Techniques," *Cambridge Quarterly of Healthcare Ethics* 1 (1992): 63-74.

14. F.C. Daskal, "Mediation for Health Care Providers: An Exciting Alternative for Dispute Resolution," *Journal of Health and Hospital Law* 22, no. 11 (1989): 338-42.

15. Ibid., 340.

16. See note 13 above; "Introducing Mediation to Hospital Ethics," *California Lawyer* 12, no. 12 (1992): 69-70, 72.

17. D.E. Hoffman, "Mediating Life and Death Decisions," *Arizona Law Review* 36, no. 4 (1994): 821-77.

18. A. Kleinman, "Concepts and a Model for the Comparison of Medical Systems as Cultural Systems," *Social Science & Medicine* 12 (1978): 85-93.

19. M.A. Jezewski, "Culture Brokering as a Model for Advocacy," *Nursing*

and Health Care 14, no. 2 (1993): 78-85.

20. J. LaFargue, "Mediating between Two Views of Illness," *Transcultural Nursing* 7 (1985): 70-77.

21. Ibid.; T. Tripp-Reimer and P. Brink, "Culture Brokerage," in *Nursing Interventions*, ed. G.M. Bulechek and J.C. McCloskey (New York: W.B. Saunders, 1984).

22. See note 19 above.

23. W.A. Knaus et al., "An Evaluation of Outcome from Intensive Care in Major Medical Centers," *Annals of Internal Medicine* 104 (1986): 410-18.

24. P.A. Prescott and S.A. Bowen, "Physician-Nurse Relationships," *Annals of Internal Medicine* 103 (1985): 127-33.

25. R.B. Connors and M.L. Smith, "Religious Insistence on Medical Treatment, Christian Theology and Re-Imagination," *Hastings Center Report* 26, no. 4 (1996): 23-30.

21

Ethical Issues in Critical Care Obstetrics

Phillip J. Goldstein

INTRODUCTION

Critical care decisions in obstetrics are often complicated by complex ethical issues. The physician managing the critically ill, pregnant mother must consider the effects of maternal therapy on the fetus. Conversely, decisions made on behalf of the fetus have obvious health implications for the mother. Even a simple amniocentesis to assess pulmonary maturity at term confers the risk of sepsis on the mother.

The American College of Obstetricians and Gynecologists (ACOG) has issued several guidelines to help care providers make decisions in obstetrics and gynecology (OB/GYN).[1] Based on the fundamental principles of medical ethics, the guidelines are useful for managing the ill, pregnant woman. Essentially, the mother's autonomy outweighs the autonomy of the unborn child. Autonomy is best expressed by informed consent. When the patient cannot give informed consent, the legally designated next of kin may become involved. The difficulty with this hierarchical arrangement is nowhere more obvious than in cases involving a dying, pregnant woman.

But even with informed consent, limits may be established as to ethical boundaries. A critically ill patient may undergo a procedure or receive a drug based on her family's "substituted judgment"—a judgment about what the patient would have wanted if competent.[2] Similar therapy may be given under the ethical principle of beneficence, using the values of the provider as the cornerstone of an action.

It is reasonable to assume that, under ordinary circumstances, a pregnant woman who is beyond 24 weeks of gestation expects to have a healthy outcome to pregnancy. Such expectations are socially and medically appropriate. That is to say, motherhood is a good, desired expectation for a pregnant woman beyond 24 weeks' gestation. Prior to this gestational age, when extrauterine viability is unlikely, one can separate pregnancy and motherhood into two distinct entities; thereafter, the distinction blurs, and the fetus has rights independent of the mother.

According to the President's Commission for the Study of Ethical Problems in Medicine and Biomedical and Behavioral Research, "Health care professionals serve patients best by maintaining an assumption in favor of life."[3] What remain unresolved and therefore controversial in decision making about critical care in obstetrics are issues related to the unborn baby and the responsibility of the father, the family, and society in such matters. Although there are many thorny ethical issues in gynecology (such as assisted reproductive technology and abortion), the great majority are not of a critical care nature. This chapter focuses on the issues related to critical care in obstetrics—especially the controversial issues related to the fetus.

CONGENITAL MALFORMATIONS

Occasionally, physicians are confronted with critical care issues in obstetrics where an unknown neonatal outcome makes medical decision making difficult. The following is an example of such a case:

A 27-year-old woman, pregnant with twins, was told by her physician following an ultrasound at 25 weeks' gestation that one of the twins had marked hydrocephalus [excess cerebrospinal fluid within the cranial cavity] and ventriculomegaly [enlarged-ventricles]. An extensive evaluation of the mother and the fetuses revealed that the hydrocephalus was probably an isolated birth defect and probably the result of an aqueductal stenosis [a narrowing of the cerebral aqueduct]. Recent studies had reported success with ventriculo amniotic shunts in reducing hydrocephalus *in utero*,[4] allowing fetal growth and maturation to proceed. The results on "all comers" (taking all fetuses for surgery without regard to the cause of the problem) was not good, however, usually because of other congenital malformations.[5] In addition, no such procedure in twins had ever been reported. The parents were informed of the options and agreed to the experimental procedure.

The hospital's institutional review board (IRB) met with the physicians associated with the case and discussed the risks, benefits, and consequences of the surgery. Some IRB members, as required by law, were from nonmedical, nonscientific backgrounds. The IRB considered several options. Because the hydrocephalic twin had no noted associated anomalies and exhibited sonographic functional cortical tissue, immediate delivery was considered; however, because this plan posed a risk to the affected twin from prematurity as well as surgery, and because the unaffected twin would also be born prematurely and therefore at risk, this plan was rejected. It was unlikely that early delivery would result in survival with good quality of life. On the other hand, delay in delivery increased the likelihood of at least one healthy neonate. After considerable deliberation, the IRB approved the *in utero* procedure.

Three weeks after the procedure the twins were delivered. Eight years later, they are doing well and attending school at the appropriate level.

INFORMED CONSENT

In the case presented above, the mother granted permission for an experimental procedure on her body. She knew that the procedure would threaten not only her life and health but the health and lives of the twins.

The informed-consent discussion and the mother's understanding were critical. She was consenting to an experimental procedure for both twins. The discussion of several options for treatment, ranging from early delivery to no intervention, was part of the informed-consent process. The physicians' well-meaning but perhaps coercive support for the procedure required balance by the IRB.

If the mother had not consented, could the providers have obtained a court order? Probably not in this case, because of the experimental nature of the procedure.[6] Although court orders for treatment of a newborn are not uncommon, court orders for treatment of a fetus are far more problematic. In fact, the ACOG considers such practices to be relatively unacceptable because they interfere with maternal autonomy.[7]

When the IRB met to consider the case presented above, a group of national experts had just recommended a moratorium on such *in utero* shunts; this panel's report suggested that unnecessary surgery was being done because several infants with multiple lethal malformations had been operated on.[8] However, critical evaluation of the same data considered by the national panel suggested that *in utero* surgery on selected cases of hydrocephalus was indeed effective. Aware of the recommended moratorium, the IRB believed that in this particular case, *not* granting approval was unethical. The mother's informed consent required her understanding of the moratorium and the reasons for it.

A national debate on the *a priori* ethical basis for surgically intervening in children with lethal anomalies remains to be held. Intrauterine surgery continues to be performed without much apparent public condemnation.[9]

FETAL AUTONOMY

In the case presented above, the risks of fetal surgery included the initiation of premature labor or an intrauterine infection, which could have been disastrous to both twins. The purpose of the shunt was to reduce the expanding head size, damage to the brain, and the likelihood of preterm labor. Although one could argue that the rights of the unaffected fetus were clearly being compromised in an effort to operate on the affected twin, the procedure to reduce the size of the affected twin's head and to reduce the likelihood of preterm labor was also on behalf of the unaffected twin. On the other hand, one could argue that surgery compromised the rights of the affected twin (an uninformed subject) by exposing it to unnecessary risks in order to reduce the likelihood of preterm labor for the unaffected twin.

Selective termination of fetuses is an option in the late twentieth century.[10] A severely anomalous twin may be sacrificed to reduce the likelihood of preterm birth for the "normal" sibling. In *in vitro* fertilization, where three or more embryos may develop, selective termination down to one or two embryos significantly improves the chances for a healthy birth.[11] The psychosocial and societal effects on the individuals born under such circumstances are not yet known. Should they be told of the manipulations that allowed them to be born? By whom? Will these individuals in late adolescence and adulthood understand the complex circumstances surrounding their birth?

DECISION-MAKING CAPACITY

A 16-year-old honor student learned that she was eight weeks pregnant and notified her boyfriend of the pregnancy and her intention to terminate it. She met him near her home, where he—disagreeing with her decision to abort—shot her in the head. The bullet entered the left frontal area of the skull, traversed the cerebral cortex, and fragmented against the occipitoparietal skull table.

She underwent a craniotomy, debridement of the bullet track, decompression shunting for raised intracranial pressure, and partial amputation of her index finger (which, presumably, had been hit as she raised her hand to protect herself). She had a remarkable recovery in the intensive care unit (ICU). Yet, because of her severe injury and critical condition, her caregivers questioned her competence to provide informed consent to terminate the pregnancy.

Her parents were solidly in favor of her decision to terminate the pregnancy. However, because one of the physicians was concerned about the patient's capacity to understand the circumstances, the hospital sought legal counsel. Although the legal counsel was content that the patient was competent, a psychiatrist's lingering concern about the patient's understanding pushed him to suggest a court order. The patient recovered rapidly (less than three weeks from the injury) and was eventually judged competent to make her decision, which was to terminate the pregnancy. Consequently, no court order was required. After her informed consent, she underwent an uneventful abortion and was discharged.

In this case, who has the responsibility to make the decision whether to terminate the pregnancy? Who should give consent for this pregnant adolescent who was shot because she wanted to terminate the pregnancy?

In this case, the father—the attempted murderer—was clearly not an option. But what are the rights of the father of an unborn child? Review of the most recent world literature reveals that the issue of a father's rights has not been well examined. Fathers have been excused from responsibility by legal decisions during the past several decades, and they have been seen as, somehow, not responsible. The concern about "deadbeat dads" is overshadowed by larger questions surrounding abortion. Although it seems reasonable that the contribution of one-half of the genetic material should confer one-half of the responsibility for the pregnancy and related decisions, that is not the case.

In 1992, the Supreme Court struck down a husband-notification clause in the Pennsylvania abortion statute.[12] In an opinion written by Justice Sandra Day O'Connor, the Court found that the husband (father) need not be notified in pregnancy terminations, reasoning that laws regarding pregnancy "inescapably" affect the mother's physical integrity far more than the father's. This recent legal decision, along with the clinician's ethical duty to protect the rights of the mother (that is, not to cause harm to the mother in order to further the interests of the fetus), mitigates against the father's role in decision making.

In the case above, the parents of the pregnant adolescent approved of the abortion. However, their daughter—who was the "apple of their eye" and for whom they had high expectations—was in critical condition. One must wonder whether, even if the girl had been considering continuing the pregnancy, the parents would have opted for termination. The psychiatrist who examined the patient believed her to be possibly not competent to sign informed consent. So a legal consultation was called. The lawyers were concerned that the parents might be making a decision based *not* in their daughter's best interest but in their own. If their daughter had not terminated the pregnancy and had remained incapacitated, the parents would have felt responsible for the newborn. Additionally, the parents' dreams were shattered when their daughter was shot, and the pregnancy was the reason for the shooting. The parents' emotional need to "strike back" at the pregnancy might have been the motivation for termination, rather than the best interest of the patient.

Kanoti describes moral dilemmas that represent putative alternative choices regarding treatment.[13] All rational physicians encounter conflicts between what they believe is right and what the patient or the surrogate believes is right. In the case above, the question is: the "right" for whom? The parents? The daughter? The fetus? This case demonstrates the need to individualize ethical standards. Ethical standards are clearly dynamic and vary among individuals and groups.[14]

ANGELA CARDER REVISITED

The 1990 Angela Carder case (*In re A.C.*), which has far-reaching implications, illustrates the blurring of what is "right," and for whom. Carder was a young, married, pregnant woman with metastatic and incurable cancer, who experienced an inexorable decline toward death. Because of her condition, she was intubated and given drugs for pain and to reduce respiratory distress.[15]

Because the mother was incapacitated, her physicians depended on guidance from the husband concerning their 26-week fetus. He essentially abrogated his responsibility in determining the baby's future. The pregnant woman's mother was very clear, however, about not wanting the baby delivered. With the baby's father apparently out of the picture, it was likely that the mother of the patient felt overwhelmed by the prospect of raising a grandchild.

To confound the situation, there was conflicting medical opinion about the fetus's viability and quality of life.[16] The hospital's general counsel requested a judicial proceeding to help sort out the moral and ethical dilemmas presented by this case. Clearly the mother had no prospectus of survival, and the fetus's chances of survival were uncertain. The court approved a cesarean section. The newborn baby died within hours of the delivery, and the mother died a few days later. The medical community was devastated—not only by the tragic result but by the continuing ignorance about what was "right" for everybody in the case.

FETAL RIGHTS

The Carder case recognized the rights of the fetus as a person, but this issue continues to be a focus of contention. Some have argued that conception or implantation signals the beginning of life. Others have argued that life begins only when the child has achieved the ability to exist outside the uterus. Others may argue that, because a newborn still requires warmth, sustenance, and nurturing to survive, the question of "rights" should not be considered until adolescence.

The different schools of thought regarding the ontogeny of fetal "humanness" or when the fetus becomes a "person" are beyond the scope of this chapter, but the considerable consternation about when human life (and hence human rights) begins concerns the concept of *life potential* in any pregnancy as well as in biological life.

Even in the adult ICU, the most troubling questions arise about life potential. The most comatose, elderly patient—if revived or even if left in a fragile state—may have a value to family or friends. Moreover, in the neonatal intensive care unit (NICU), one generally expects survival with unlimited potential. Thus, it is not surprising that the rights of the unborn fetus is such a sensitive issue. Hence, the agony of the Carder case. Was the therapy an unethical decision? A bad medical decision? These questions are unresolved.

POSTMORTEM CESAREAN SECTION

A 33-year-old woman who was 27 weeks pregnant and diagnosed with acquired immunodeficiency syndrome (AIDS) developed unrelenting *Pneumocystis carinii* pneumonia. During her treatment, as her condition worsened, she and her family were asked to consider the unborn child's future. Options ranged from doing nothing to delivering the child for adoption by family members. The woman developed candida septicemia, and her condition became grave. The patient care advisory committee was informed of her status, and they explained the options to the patient and her family. The woman and the family felt that the child should be allowed to survive if at all possible. They also agreed that the family would care for the child, regardless of the child's human immunodeficiency virus (HIV) status.

On the 20th hospital day, the patient, who was now intubated, developed marked hypotension, and the electrocardiogram revealed acute myocardial infarction. The ICU staff, who had been informed of the family conferences, immediately called the obstetric team. When the patient developed asystole, clinicians initiated cardiac resuscitation, which was unsuccessful. A cesarean section was performed in the ICU, in accordance with the patient's and family's wishes. A preterm (30-week), male infant was born. He had Apgar scores of 2 and 6, who required ventilator support in the NICU. Although the baby was born with hepatosplenomegaly [enlarged liver and spleen], all cultures were negative.

Katz reports essentially unanimous opinion concerning postmortem cesarean section. Neonatal survival and quality of life are major considerations in postmortem cesarean sections. In cases such as the one described above, there is a risk of neonatal complications due to a combination of prematurity and asphyxia. Conventional wisdom suggests that multiorgan failure due to asphyxia begins after about four minutes of maternal demise. Obviously, the disease causing the mother's demise is a consideration. For example, if the mother has a prolonged course toward death, the infant is more likely to have complications.[17]

In *Roe v. Wade*, the U.S. Supreme Court indicated that viability is the earliest point at which the state has an interest in fetal life. The decision implied that the state has the right to intervene in the third trimester on behalf of the fetus. Experience suggests that obstetricians have little ethical controversy in delivering a child in an emergency situation such as acute maternal cardiopulmonary collapse. If the life of the mother is over, conventional medical protocol indicates saving the fetus. Perhaps this convention would apply in the Carder case.

THE BRAIN-DEAD, PREGNANT WOMAN

As technology has created options for preserving life in critical care situations, ethical issues have arisen. The pregnant woman who is declared brain dead certainly pushes the envelope of ethical considerations. In a highly reasoned and balanced article, Kantor and Hoskins discuss the ethical ramifications of a pregnant woman who has been declared brain dead.[18] First, they lucidly discuss pathophysiologic changes in such patients that adversely affect the fetus. A fetus of 24 weeks, which weighs about 500 grams, or 1 pound, has a likely survival of less than 30 percent and very significant risk of major morbidity.[19] So the question of preserving life in a woman who is 24 weeks pregnant and declared brain dead to improve the outcome of the fetus is probably not medically justifiable. It is when the woman is 27 or more weeks pregnant that terrible conflicts arise. Clearly, the fetus under such circumstances has rights that override theoretical considerations of the dead mother's rights. Part of the justification to prolong the mother's life in such a situation is based on the presumption that she would have expected a healthy infant. Wear and colleagues suggest that, where no clear wish of the mother is known, one seldom-discussed maternal interest is the birth of the fetus. The long investment in gestation is an interest comparable to inheritance and disposition of remains. They argue that "implied consent may be assumed" but that a "legitimately functioning surrogate could decide otherwise."[20]

THREE MODELS OF CONSIDERATION

Kantor and Hoskins cite three models for considering brain death in pregnant women: (1) the mother as a competent, living person; (2) the mother as incubator; and (3) the mother as organ donor.[21]

THE MOTHER AS A COMPETENT, LIVING PERSON

In the first model, the mother is treated as a competent, living person. Significant diversity of moral and religious opinion exists about the definition of death. For the competent, *healthy* pregnant woman, issues of informed consent for the fetus are straightforward. The *minimum* legal duties of the pregnant woman remain to be defined. For example, is a woman legally allowed to take drugs that may do harm to the fetus?

Kantor and Hoskins conclude that the physician "may not override the wishes and interests of the mother in order to use her to further the interests of the fetal patient."[22] They argue that a pregnant woman who is brain dead may have only wanted the pregnancy to continue if "she would be present to raise a normal child."[23] In an era where surrogate parenting is becoming ever more frequent, such a statement loses some validity. The husband or father may be involved in decision making about the fetus carried by the brain-dead woman. However, as in the *Carder* case, there are no fetal interests being served when the protective parent or grandparent simply does not want the baby. The parent or grandparent, then, may decide against maintaining the pregnancy, for their own interests. Such actions seem unethical.

INCUBATOR MODEL

In the incubator model, the woman is treated as a useful object. According to Kantor and Hoskins, this approach is objectionable at several levels—most importantly, our societal obligations toward the dead. As a result of their efforts to connect the "normal" model and the "incubator" model, Kantor and Hoskins propose the third model—the organ-donation model.

ORGAN-DONATION MODEL

Kantor and Hoskins argue that the organ-donation model is legitimate "if there is no evidence that the brain-dead individual would have objected."[24] They argue that this model should take into account the mother's values while alive and that the mother's wishes cannot be ignored simply to use her body.

In a provocative response to Kantor and Hoskins, Frader says that he is appalled by the consideration of fetal preservation because (1) the circumstance is rare and (2) preservation of dead mothers to allow fetal growth will bring "yet another motherless child into the world."[25] However, Frader does not seem to consider the likely possibility that "life" for a newborn is of potential value, even if the child is "motherless."

Glover, also responding to Kantor and Hoskins, suggests a family-centered model.[26] She argues convincingly that the concept of a "dead" mother reverberates through a society, with the family being the first concentric ripple affected. She states that maternal autonomy ceases with death and reports that, as of 1992, 35 states *prevent* women from refusing life-sustaining treatment if they are pregnant. She suggests that the confusion about fetal rights is in part a reflection of the deep division over the question of abortion in the United States "tending to support the woman's right of autonomy ('right to choose') and simultaneously not supporting abortion as an entity in itself."[27]

CONCLUSION

The maternal-fetal relationship is associated with complex ethical questions. This complexity is compounded in critical care situations. The lack of consensus about when fetal rights begin contributes to the over-all confusion. A clear definition of when fetal rights begin would help clinicians treat patients, because concepts of fetal rights affect ethical considerations about managing a critically ill mother.

If the mother is dying and the fetus is not salvageable, the decision about medical care is clear, even if painful. If a pregnancy is killing the mother, as in decompensating heart disease or eclampsia, delivery may save the life of the mother; once again the decision is painful but clear—save the mother at the expense of the fetus.

Postmortem cesarean section near term is based on the belief that the baby has the "right" to be well born. Yet, when the mother is dying, with no hope of survival, the fetus is also essentially dispensable. In addition, the father's wishes may be helpful but are not completely binding in such cases. Even ACOG, in trying to establish clear guidance regarding fetal rights, waffles more than a little.

In today's world, where fetal surgery is performed without randomized, controlled clinical trials, multifetal reductions are commonplace, and mothers abuse their fetuses by using alcohol and tobacco, it is only ethical to assume that the fetus has rights.

NOTES

1. American College of Obstetricians and Gynecologists, *Ethical Decision Making in Obstetrics and Gynecology*, Technical Bulletin 136 (Washington, D.C.: American College of Obstetricians and Gynecologists, 1989); American College of Obstetricians and Gynecologists, *Patient Choice: Maternal-Fetal Conflict*, Committee Opinion 55 (Washington, D.C.: American College of Obstetricians and Gynecologists, 1987); American College of Obstetricians and Gynecologists, *Ethical Dimensions of Informed Consent*, Committee Opinion 108 (Washington, D.C.: American College of Obstetricians and Gynecologists, 1992); American College of Obstetricians and Gynecologists, *End of Life Decision Making: Understanding the Goals of Care*, (Washington, D.C.: American College of Obstetri-

cians and Gynecologists, 1995).

2. J.J. Glover, "Incubators and Organ Donors," *The Journal of Clinical Ethics* 4, no. 4 (Winter 1993): 342.

3. President's Commission for the Study of Ethical Problems in Medicine and Biomedical and Behavioral Research, *Final Report on Studies of the Ethical and Legal Problems in Medicine and Biomedical and Behavioral Research* (Washington, D.C.: U.S. Government Printing Office, 1983).

4. F.A. Manning et al., "Catheter Shunts for Fetal Hydronephrosis and Hydrocephalus: Report of the International Fetal Surgery Registry," *New England Journal of Medicine* 315 (1986): 336.

5. P. Goldstein et al., "Ventriculo-Amniotic Shunt for Treatment of Hydrocephalus in One of Twins: Medical, Ethical and Legal Considerations," *Fetal Diagnosis Therapy* 5 (1990): 84.

6. American College of Obstetricians and Gynecologists, *Ethical Dimensions*, see note 1 above.

7. American College of Obstetricians and Gynecologists, *Patient Choice*, see note 1 above.

8. See note 4 above.

9. M.T. Longaker et al., "Maternal Outcome after Open Fetal Surgery: A Review of the First 17 Human Cases," *Journal of the American Medical Association* 265, no. 6 (1991): 737.

10. U. Chitkara et al., "Selective Second Trimester Termination of the Anomalous Fetus in Twin Pregnancies," *Obstetrics and Gynecology* 7, no. 30 (1989): 690.

11. P. Schreiner-Engel et al., "First Trimester Multifetal Pregnancy Reduction: Acute and Persistent Psychologic Reactions," *American Journal of Obstetrics and Gynecology* 172 (1995): 541.

12. *Planned Parenthood Association of Southeastern Pennsylvania v. Casey*, 112 S.Ct. 2791 (1992).

13. G.A. Kanoti, "Ethics and Medical-Ethical Decisions," *Critical Care Clinics* 2, no. 1 (1986): 3.

14. D.R. Field et al., "Maternal Brain Death During Pregnancy," *Journal of the American Medical Association* 260, no. 6 (1988): 816.

15. *In re A.C.*, 497 U.S. 261 (1990).

16. M. Hack et al., "Very Low Birth Weight Outcomes of the National Institutes of Child Health and Human Development Network," *Pediatrics* 87 (1991): 587.

17. B.L. Katz, D.J. Dotter, and W. Droegmuller, "Perimortem Cesarean Delivery," *Obstetrics and Gynecology* 68 (1986): 571.

18. J.E. Kantor and I.A. Hoskins, "Brain Death in Pregnant Women," *The Journal of Clinical Ethics* 4, no. 4 (1993): 308; D. Callahan, "The Abortion Debate: Can This Chronic Public Illness Be Cured," *Clinical Obstetrics and Gyncology* 35, no. 4 (1992): 783.

19. See note 16 above.

20. S. Wear, W.P. Dillon, and R.V. Lee, "Maternal Brain Death During Pregnancy," *Journal of the American Medical Association* 261, no. 12 (1989): 1728.

21. See note 18 above.

22. Ibid., 310.

23. Ibid., 310.

24. Ibid., 312.

25. J.E. Frader, "Have We Lost Our Senses? Problems with Maintaining Brain-Dead Bodies Carrying Fetuses," *The Journal of Clinical Ethics* 4, no. 4 (Winter 1993): 347.

26. See note 2 above.

27. Ibid., 343.

22

Ethical Issues in Pediatric Intensive Care

James P. Orlowski

INTRODUCTION

Many of the ethical issues discussed in this book apply equally to adults and children, but others change dramatically when the patient is a child or a minor. This chapter focuses on ethical issues that are unique to pediatrics or that are drastically different when the affected individual is an infant, child, or adolescent. The ethical issues involved with the critical care of neonates and premature infants are covered in chapter 23.

PAIN AND ITS TREATMENT IN CHILDREN

Major advances in the knowledge about pain in children and its treatment have occurred in the past decade, commensurate with increased recognition of the importance of pain and the adequacy of its therapy in the overall humanistic care of patients. Some of these advancements have revolutionized the care of pediatric patients.

Until recently, clinicians assumed that babies do not feel or recognize pain; this assumption was based on the belief that the neurologic system of babies is still immature.[1] This premise was supported by evidence that a neonate or infant could be calmed and would stop crying after a painful procedure if given a pacifier soaked in sugar water or a bottle to drink.[2]

This barbaric belief was perpetuated by an anesthetic technique called the "Liverpool technique," which was widely used for major surgical procedures in newborns and infants. The Liverpool technique consisted of completely paralyzing the infant with neuromuscular blocking agents and then operating on the infant without analgesics or with very small, clearly subtherapeutic doses of analgesics. The proponents of this technique believed that they were protecting the infants from the adverse hemodynamic effects of opiate analgesics. The Liverpool technique was widely employed for open-heart and abdominal surgery on infants. Many children's hospitals in this country as well as abroad used the Liverpool technique for all surgeries on neonates, infants, and young children.

We now know conclusively that newborns and infants feel pain and that, although their expression of pain is different from that of older children or adults, their perception of pain is not. We now know that the fetus can feel pain as early as 20 weeks of gestation, and perhaps earlier. For example, pain receptors are present in the human fetus's perioral area at seven weeks of gestation and encompass the entire face, palms of the hands, and soles of the feet by 11 weeks. The trunk, arms, and legs develop pain receptors by 15 weeks of gestation. These findings have obvious ramifications for abortion.[3]

Lack of myelination has been invoked to support the argument that neonates are not capable of pain perception. However, even in adults, nociceptive impulses are carried by unmyelinated or poorly myelinated fibers. All that incomplete myelination implies is a slower conduction of pain impulses in the neonate, which is usually offset by the shorter distances traveled by the impulses. Investigators recently reported that the pain pathways to the brain stem and thalamus are completely myelinated by 30 weeks of gestation.

Another example of the belief that babies do not feel pain is the practice of performing circumcision on male neonates without anesthesia or analgesia. Only in the recent past have penile nerve blocks come into vogue for circumcisions, and a study showing the effectiveness of a topical local anesthetic for circumcision was only published in 1997.[4]

Much work still needs to be done to determine the most effective analgesics and their doses in pediatric patients. Unfortunately, much work also needs to be done to educate healthcare providers that babies and children feel pain, are adversely affected by pain, and deserve to be pain free.

It is only within the last few years that studies have demonstrated a significantly increased mortality when infants and neonates undergo cardiac surgery without complete and deep anesthesia.[5] The natural stress response to surgery in conscious or only partially anesthetized patients adversely affects surgical outcome.[6] Anesthesia should be used for all surgical and painful procedures on infants and children, as well as for other stressful therapies such as mechanical ventilation, burn care, and intensive care.[7]

A NEW UNDERSTANDING OF CONSENT IN PEDIATRIC PRACTICE

The standard of practice in pediatrics is to obtain consent from parents for any procedure or research involving a child. In the past, it was assumed that adolescents and children were incapable of decision making until they reached the legal age of majority, typically 18 years of age in most states. Recently the courts have allowed children and adolescents to participate in medical decision making to a degree that is commensurate with their maturity and understanding. This trend has culminated in the new standard of care of seeking the assent of minors for procedures and research.

A recent example in Florida involved a 15-year-old boy who had undergone two liver transplants at the University of Pittsburgh and was now in the process of rejecting his second transplant. He decided that he could no longer take the side effects of his antirejection medications and was adamant that he did not want to undergo another liver transplant. With the support of his parents, he stopped taking his immunosuppressive medications. When the transplant team at the University of Pittsburgh became aware of what he was doing, they had the Florida protective services officers take the boy into custody, hospitalize him against his will, and force him to take his medications. The case came before a judge, who ruled in favor of the boy and his decision, stating that this young man probably understood better than even his transplant physicians the adverse effects of the medicines he had to take and the consequences of his decision.[8]

At about the same time, a young man in New York, only days short of his 18th birthday, wished to stop taking chemotherapy drugs for cancer because he found the side effects intolerable. A judge in New York ruled in favor of the physicians; the young man was forced to be hospitalized and received chemotherapy drugs against his will.

The current approach in pediatrics is to seek assent from children to undergo procedures and participate in research studies once they are able to comprehend information and participate in decision making (generally around seven years of age). Adolescent patients should participate fully in the consent process, and their consent to procedures or research should be sought. If either the parents or the adolescent dissent or refuse to consent, then healthcare providers should not proceed.

Children or adolescents may refuse a procedure or therapy for reasons that adults might consider inconsequential, immature, lacking in perspective, or short-sighted. Such reasons might include fear of needles, fear of pain and suffering, loss of bodily integrity, or an unwillingness to be perceived as different from their peers. Rather than seeking a court order, healthcare providers and parents should work with the pediatric patient to gain the patient's confidence and cooperation.

When parents refuse clearly beneficial or lifesaving therapies for their child, healthcare providers should attempt to reason with and convince the parents of the importance of the therapy. If reason fails, the healthcare team should seek legal guidance and a court order.

RESEARCH INVOLVING CHILDREN

Research involving children is becoming increasingly common. At one time, children were specifically excluded from research studies, and most new drug development and testing excluded pregnant women and children. This trend has been corrected in the recent past. Children are how being entered into research studies, especially in oncology; pharmaceutical companies are being pressured by the Food and Drug Administration (FDA) to include children in drug trials; and pediatric research studies are becoming more commonplace.

In the past, children were excluded from research studies because they were recognized as a vulnerable population that needed protection, and because they were unable to consent directly to participate in research studies. The fear that children might be exploited was not totally unfounded. Some of the most egregious examples of unethical research studies were conducted on children in the not-too-distant past, such as the infamous Willowbrook School hepatitis studies.[9]

The Willowbrook School was a residential school for retarded children in New York State. Hepatitis was endemic at Willowbrook, as it was in many other state institutions, and all children admitted to the school developed clinical hepatitis within a year. Saul Krugman, the medical director of the institution, desired to understand the epidemiology and pathophysiology of this infectious disease, including its transmission, latency, contagiousness, and course. Krugman devised a series of studies that included feeding filtered stool samples from infected residents to new inmates, following the course of the disease, and testing the ability of gamma globulin to ameliorate the disease. Although Krugman claims to have obtained consent for the research studies from parents, in fact the parents were coerced. The Willowbrook School, like most other state institutions, was overcrowded; the school had few openings, and only children whose parents agreed to allow their children to participate in the research study were admitted to the institution. Although much knowledge of infectious hepatitis was gained from these studies, some children died of viral hepatitis. The ends do not justify the means. Ironically, Krugman was recently honored by the American Academy of Pediatrics for his pioneering research into viral hepatitis, with no mention of the ethics of the research.[10] If a study is unethical, it is not justifiable simply because it produces useful results.

In a famous 1966 study of the ethics of human experimentation, Henry Beecher examined 22 studies that he identified as unethical and which were published in prestigious medical journals.[11] Two of these studies involved research on fetuses. In the first study, researchers from Case Western Reserve University and the University of Helsinki decapitated eight fetuses of 12 to 20 weeks' gestation, to examine whether the fetal brain could metabolize ketones. The severed heads continued to function metabolically for hours. In the second study, U.S. scientists immersed 15 fetuses in salt solutions to determine whether they could absorb oxygen through their skin. One fetus survived for 23 hours.

Cancer patients, one of the most heavily represented groups in clinical research studies, are also especially vulnerable as research subjects. Many cancer patients are willing to participate in research studies because they want to try all of their options, and many are trying to hold on in the hope that a cure will be found. A few patients participate for altruistic reasons of helping others and furthering scientific knowledge. Some patients participate to reduce the cost of their medical care, and still others become research subjects for the social interaction or because they fear abandonment.

Harth and colleagues examined the psychological profile of parents who volunteered their children for clinical research studies and compared their results with the profile of parents who had refused to allow their children to be research subjects.[12] Volunteering parents tended to place more value on beneficence, whereas nonvolunteering parents were more concerned with power and prestige. The self-esteem of volunteering parents was much lower than that of nonvolunteering parents. Volunteering parents were more introverted and exhibited greater anxiety and low superego; nonvolunteering parents appeared to have greater social confidence and emotional stability.

Another area of recent concern in research ethics has been the use of placebo controls. The 1964 *Declaration of Helsinki* states: "In any medical study, every patient—including those of a control group—should be assured of the best proven diagnosis and therapeutics method."[13] Unfortunately, the FDA considers placebo-controlled studies to be the "gold standard" of research studies to evaluate new drugs or therapies. The FDA requires placebo-controlled studies as part of the process of approval for an investigational new drug. As long as the control group of patients is receiving standard therapy for their disease plus a placebo, this is not a problem. But if the control group is deprived of standard therapy and receives only a placebo, then the research study violates the *Declaration of Helsinki*. This distinction is especially important in research studies involving critically ill patients or children, or involving diseases where placebo therapy would cause unacceptable progression of disease or harm to patients.

The important rule of thumb in research ethics is that if a conflict between a research protocol and a patient's care develops, the ethical obligation is to protect the patient.

FUTILITY

A number of authors have suggested that *futility* is too vague and undefinable a concept to be of value in medicine, or that futility is a medical attempt to counteract patient autonomy.[14] These authors claim that the concept of futility should be abandoned and not employed as a reason for withholding medical therapy. However, anyone who has practiced clinical medicine realizes that clear-cut examples of futility are encountered routinely in critical care medicine and clinical practice. A treatment is futile when it will offer no physiologic benefit to the patient.

Examples of clinical futility in pediatrics include the use of cardiopulmonary resuscitation (CPR) in patients with brain death. CPR is also futile in the instance of an ongoing chemical code—the situation in which a patient is on the highest concentrations of vasopressors (agents to increase or maintain blood pressure) and/or inotropes (agents to increase or maintain heart muscle contractions) and yet remains hypotensive and does not respond to therapy.[15] CPR and the use of advanced life-support drugs will not work if the patient is already receiving suprapharmacologic doses of these drugs. This situation is also referred to as refractory shock.

Another example of clinical futility would be the patient with refractory hypoxemia and respiratory failure. If the patient cannot be oxygenated and ventilated and he or she progresses to cardiac arrest, CPR is not going to work. CPR is also futile in patients in a persistent or permanent vegetative state. A treatment is futile when it cannot—within reasonable medical probability—cure, ameliorate, improve, or restore a quality of life that would be satisfactory to or for the patient.

Other examples of situations in which the use of CPR is futile include the failure to respond to CPR and pediatric advance life support in 30 minutes, decapitation, and putrefaction (criteria commonly employed by emergency medical services). Many emergency medical services also use charred or burned beyond recognition as futility criteria for not employing CPR.

A number of other examples of futility in pediatrics exist. Most intensive care clinicians consider mechanical ventilation and CPR to be inappropriate and futile in anencephalics. For patients in a persistent vegetative state, mechanical ventilation, ICU admission, and CPR are all considered inappropriate and futile. Other examples of futile therapy in pediatrics include the use of antibiotics for viral illnesses and use of antipyretics for febrile seizures.

One of the reasons that the concept of medical futility has fostered so much debate is that futility means different things to different people. To some, continued existence—no matter how poor the quality of that existence—means that the therapy is not futile. To others, therapy is futile if a sentient, functional existence cannot be achieved. To some, any therapy is worth a try; to others a therapy must offer a reasonable chance of success. Because the principle of autonomy has gained such preeminence in Western ethics, many ethicists believe that any patient's request that stands even a remote chance of working, must be honored. Autonomy is not a trump card and does not overrule all other principles and factors.

Conflicts over the issue of medical futility often signal a breakdown in communication. In cases where the family makes inappropriate demands and the healthcare team insists that continued treatment is futile, the two sides are often not communicating effectively. Two factors will usually resolve such conflicts. First, it is necessary to reestablish good communication, using clear and understandable language to help the family fully appreciate the situation. At times, the use of a neutral third party or family advocate can facilitate the reestablishment of effective communication. A great deal of empathy is necessary to understand the family's reluctance to see their hopes and dreams for their child dashed. Likewise, the heroic efforts of the healthcare team have been unsuccessful, engendering a feeling of failure and remorse. The second factor is time. Families may need hours or even days to come to grips with the reality of the situation, and patience and understanding on the part of the healthcare team can do a lot to resolve conflict.

Another factor that fuels the futility debate is that medicine is not an exact science. What has worked or not worked in previous patients may have a completely different effect on the patient at hand. As the public becomes more sophisticated and knowledgeable, families may realize these subtleties. Medical predictions of outcome may be based more on assumptions or hunches than facts. A solid statistical basis for prediction is usually lacking because the appropriate studies have never been performed. An individual physician is unlikely to have seen a large enough number of similar patients to form a statistically relevant basis for predictions. Each patient is sufficiently unique as an individual, that even large data bases cannot be used to predict accurately the outcome in individual cases. That is, even an experienced physician backed by statistically relevant studies cannot predict outcome with a high degree of accuracy. A physician can state that a therapy is highly unlikely to work, but he or she can never state conclusively that it will not work.

Physicians can and should refuse to provide a therapy that violates professional, ethical, or moral tenets. A unilateral decision to stop medical treatment based on futility arguments may require ethics committee and perhaps judicial backing. The best approach is to work with the family and gain their concurrence.

The following recent cases may elucidate some of the issues surrounding medical futility:

Theresa Hamilton was a 14-year-old diabetic who presented to a hospital in Sarasota, Florida, in severe diabetic coma; her condition rapidly progressed to brain death. The parents, partly out of guilt over having waited too long to seek medical attention, refused to accept the diagnosis of brain death. Numerous consultants and experts were brought in, all of whom confirmed the diagnosis of brain death and recommended discontinuing ventilatory support. The parents continued to refuse; the case was brought to the ethics committee, which also recommended disconnecting the ventilator. The parents sought support from the news media, and a number of well-meaning but misinformed people came forward with stories that they or a loved one had been pronounced brain dead by the medical profession and were now living a normal life. Meanwhile, the hospital sought legal guidance from the state attorney general's office, who opined that there was no issue and that, because the patient was brain dead, artificial support could be withdrawn. At the same time, the hospital's own legal counsel waffled and recommended that the hospital do whatever the family demanded. The hospital acquiesced and arranged for the patient to be sent home on mechanical ventilation. This corpse was ventilated at home for five months before cardiac arrest ensued.[16]

Baby K was an anencephalic infant born at Fairfax Hospital in Virginia. The mother insisted that everything—including CPR and mechanical ventilation—be performed, believing that only God could take a life. At first, the hospital complied with the mother's wishes. After a few months, the baby was transferred to a chronic care facility. Hospital physicians and nurses began to question repeatedly admitting and ventilating the baby whenever respiratory problems or apneas developed. The hospital sought judicial guidance on the claim that continually resuscitating and ventilating this anencephalic infant was futile, based on the prognosis. The mother countered that she believed that physicians have an obligation to do whatever possible to maintain biologic life. Her lawyers cited the Emergency Medical Treatment and Active Labor Act (EMTALA) to support their case. The case was heard at the federal level and appealed to the Federal Appeals Court. The judges ruled in favor of the mother, citing EMTALA and Consolidated Omnibus Budget Reconciliation Act (COBRA) regulations. However, the judge stated that he did not believe that this was what Congress had in mind when they wrote EMTALA. He stated that his job was only to interpret the law, and that it was up to Congress to right the wrongs they had created in the way they wrote the law.[17]

Increasingly, our society has come to believe that the maintenance of nonsentient, noninteractive biologic life with artificial, mechanical means represents a technologic intrusion and indignity, and that such individuals should be permitted to die without such an assault and insult.

There is also increasing societal sentiment that the consumption of scarce resources for the maintenance of these lives could be better used for other purposes.

REFUSAL OF TREATMENT
BASED ON RELIGIOUS BELIEFS

It is an accepted medical ethics principle, supported by numerous court decisions over the past century, that a mature adult of sound mind can refuse any medical therapy, even if the therapy is potentially lifesaving. On the other hand, courts have consistently ruled, and medical ethics dictates, that parents cannot deprive their children of medical treatment or lifesaving therapy, no matter what their beliefs. Adults can refuse medical therapy or lifesaving therapy based on religious beliefs, idiosyncratic beliefs, or no beliefs at all, but they are not free to impose their beliefs on their children. The theory is that children should be allowed to grow and develop and then make their own decisions about what they believe.

Classic examples of religion-based refusal of treatment have included Jehovah's Witnesses' refusal of blood and blood products and Christian Scientists' refusal of medical and surgical treatment. The American Academy of Pediatrics has campaigned in recent years to reverse state and federal laws that exempt parents who refuse treatment on religious grounds from prosecution under child abuse and neglect laws.[18]

On occasion, a child or adolescent strongly professes religious beliefs or opinions that may or may not coincide with the parents' beliefs and may affect the child's willingness to accept recommended medical therapy. Intelligence, experience, and the relationship between the child and parents can all influence the maturity and decision-making capability of the child. The little empirical information that exists regarding the development of mature medical decision-making capacity in children generally suggests that the decision-making ability of minors by the age of 14 years cannot be distinguished from that of adults.[19]

Although courts routinely grant court orders to treat infants or children when parents refuse treatment on religious or other grounds, courts should assess, and are assessing, the maturity and decision-making capacity of adolescents before ruling on treatment. Obviously, if the adolescent is critically ill, his or her participation may not be possible. Another factor that has entered into the equation when deciding on a petition for court-ordered medical treatment is the prognosis. In one recent Delaware case involving a child with non-Hodgkin's lymphoma—a cancer with an exceptionally poor prognosis—the court sided with the Christian Scientist parents who refused treatment. This decision was based on the difficult course of treatment being recommended, the less than 40 percent probability of one-year survival, and the considerably smaller likelihood of long-term survival.[20]

Most pediatricians and ethicists now agree that children who can experience and enjoy life, including the vast majority of patient's with Down's syndrome, have legitimate, independent moral and legal claims to lifesaving therapy—including intensive care—even if the parents prefer the child to die. Inherent in this moral consensus is the notion that the quality of the lives of these patients is sufficiently high to justify complex, difficult, or expensive treatments, despite the views of the parents who would be the ordinary decision makers. Most of the time, communication and counseling with parents leads to parental understanding and acceptance of the proposed treatment. When these measures fail, foster-care arrangements may be necessary.

More problematic are the situations where physicians are uncertain about survival, neurologic outcome, or other major medical prognoses, and where the proposed treatment may have a profound impact on the family. Such situations might require the parents to give up employment to care for the child (for example, in cases where continued dependence on technology will demand 24-hour vigilance) or require parental attention that significantly detracts from the time and care available for other siblings or dependents. Fortunately, with the growth of home care, respite and assistance for parents is often available, but we should not lose sight of the tremendous demand and drain that a medically needy and technology-dependent child can place on a family.

FORGOING LIFE-SUSTAINING THERAPY

Although forgoing life support is a major source of angst for any intensive care physician, this anguish is magnified many-fold when the patient is a child.

See chapter 5 for a discussion of the medical and ethical aspects of withholding or withdrawing treatment. Several points are important for a discussion of forgoing life support in pediatric patients. The first concern is that many physicians, including pediatric intensivists and pediatric neurologists, are reluctant to make predictions about outcomes, especially in children with neurologic trauma or anoxic-ischemic injuries.

Part of this reluctance may stem from remarkable recoveries that have occurred in children after traumatic injuries or anoxic injuries associated with hypothermia. Despite the occasional amazing recovery, the likelihood of good neurologic outcome following global hypoxic-ischemic brain injury in children remains low, especially if no recovery has occurred following a suitable period of observation. It is important for clinicians to address the likelihood of a poor outcome and to allow families to prepare for the worst, because the result is often a neurologically devastated child in a permanent vegetative state (PVS). For most of us, PVS is a fate worse than death.

Clinicians often use the lack of statistical or clinical certainty as an excuse to avoid discussing probable poor outcomes. Clinical uncertainty should not be used as a means of forestalling disclosure of reasonably available alternative courses, including withholding further treatment or withdrawing therapies already in use.

Clinical uncertainty also should not preclude decisions to forgo life support. Except in unusual circumstances, the patient's or family's values should largely dictate the direction for medical care. Healthcare professionals should not impose their personal beliefs concerning life with mental or physical handicaps or life dependent on medical technology on others.

A second point about forgoing life support concerns guilt or duress on families. Many physicians feel that parents are unable to handle the emotional distress and guilt attendant with making the decision to allow a child to die. However, one study reported that families that had endured such a painful experience later expressed appreciation for their involvement. These families had no demonstrable adverse psychologic sequelae compared with families who did not participate in the decision to limit respiratory support for their child.[21] Families who do not wish to carry this responsibility usually find ways of making their views known, and families with strong feelings or beliefs favoring continued treatment usually make their desires clear.

The art of pediatric intensive care usually requires as much time and effort devoted to communication and interpersonal interaction with families as to the scientific knowledge and necessary skills.

NOTES

1. K.J.S. Anand and P.R. Hickey, "Pain and Its Effects in the Human Neonate and Fetus," *New England Journal of Medicine* 317 (1987): 1321-29.

2. E.M. Blass and L.B. Hoffmeyer, "Sucrose as an Analgesic for Newborn Infants," *Pediatrics* 87 (1991): 215-18.

3. See note 1 above.

4. A. Taddio et al., "Efficacy and Safety of Lidocaine-Prilocaine Cream for Pain During Circumcision," *New England Journal of Medicine* 336 (1997): 1197-201.

5. K.J.S. Anand and P.R. Hickey, "Halothane-Morphine Compared with High-Dose Sufentanil for Anesthesia and Postoperative Analgesia in Neonatal Cardiac Surgery," *New England Journal of Medicine* 326 (1992): 1-9.

6. F.A. Burrows and C.B. Berde, "Optimal Pain Relief in Infants and Children," *British Medical Journal* 307 (1993): 815-16.

7. J. Bauchner, A. May, and E. Coates, "Use of Analgesic Agents for Invasive Medical Procedures in Pediatric and Neonatal Intensive Care Units," *Journal of Pediatrics* 121 (1992): 647-49.

8. I. Traugott and A. Alpers, "In Their Own Hands: Adolescents' Refusals of Medical Treatment," *Archives of Pediatric and Adolescent Medicine* 151 (1997): 922-27.

9. S. Krugman, "The Willowbrook Hepatitis Studies Revisited: Ethical Aspects," *Reviews of Infectious Diseases* 8 (1986): 157-62.

10. W.P. Parks and J. Dancis, ed., "Saul Krugman Festschrift," *Pediatrics* 90 (1992): 133-77.

11. H.K. Beecher, "Ethics and Clinical Research," *New England Journal of Medicine* 274 (1966): 1354-60.

12. S.C. Harth, R.R. Johnstone, and Y.H. Thong, "The Psychological Profile of Parents Who Volunteer Their Children for Clinical Research: A Controlled Study," *Journal of Medical Ethics* 18 (1992): 86-93.

13. B. Freedman and C. Weijer, "Placebo Orthodoxy in Clinical Research: I. Empirical and Methodological Myths and II. Ethical, Legal, and Regulatory Myths," *Journal of Law, Medicine, and Ethics* 24 (1996): 243-59.

14. S.J. Youngner, "Who Defines Futility?" *Journal of the American Medical Association* 260 (1988): 2094-95; D.B. Waisel and R.D. Truog, "The Cardiopulmonary Resuscitation-Not-Indicated Order: Futility Revisited," *Annals of Internal Medicine* 122 (1995): 304-08.

15. S.G. Stern and J.P. Orlowski, "DNR or CPR: The Choice Is Ours," *Critical Care Medicine* 20: (1992): 1263-72.

16. "Lack of Futile Care Policy Compromises Hospital's Authority," *Medical Ethics Advisor* 10 (1994): 51-53.

17. G.J. Annas, "Asking the Courts to Set the Standard of Emergency Care—The Case of Baby K," *New England Journal of Medicine* 330 (1994): 1542-45.

18. American Academy of Pediatrics, Committee on Bioethics, "Religious Exemptions from Child Abuse Statutes," *Pediatrics* 81 (1988): 169-71.

19. L.A. Whitehorn and S.B. Campbell, "The Competency of Children and Adolescents to Make Informed Treatment Decisions," *Childhood Development* 53 (1982): 1589-98.

20. *Newmark v. Williams*, 588 A.2d 1108 (Del., 1991).

21. D.G. Benfield, S.A. Leib, and J.H. Vollman, "Grief Response of Parents to Neonatal Death and Parent Participation in Deciding Care," *Pediatrics* 62 (1978): 171-77.

23

Ethical Issues in Neonatology

Kathleen E. Powderly

INTRODUCTION

Newborn intensive care is a highly successful service, by many parameters. Technological innovation has allowed many very-low-birth-weight (VLBW) infants and others with catastrophic illnesses to survive, often with an excellent quality of life. Virtually all infants born at 28 weeks gestation (12 weeks early), weighing approximately 2 pounds, will survive if born in a hospital with a neonatal intensive care unit (NICU). Indeed, the vast majority of such infants are healthy and developmentally appropriate on long-term follow-up. On the other hand, some survivors of NICUs would not have survived in the days before such units and, some would argue, should not have survived. Such survivors may have profound multiple handicaps and experience great suffering and a poor quality of life. Still other NICU patients do not survive but suffer in a prolonged dying process.

There is a great deal of uncertainty about prognosis in the NICU. In addition, the patients, by definition, cannot speak for themselves. Although parents are most often looked to for decisions about their infants, there are problems in some cases. The questions of who makes decisions and what criteria are used to make decisions in NICU are explored in this chapter. Technology has evolved and societal attitudes have changed since the early days of neonatal intensive care. What has not changed is the presence of difficult ethical dilemmas and the need to explore mechanisms for dealing with them. This chapter discusses the history of neonatology and ethical issues within neonatology. In addition, it identifies some strategies for coping with ethical dilemmas in the NICU.

HISTORICAL PERSPECTIVES

Modern technology has allowed some VLBW babies and babies with congenital anomalies to survive. Although many of these babies would not have survived in the past without technological support, some clearly did survive before modern neonatal intensive care and aggressive interventions. How such infants were treated varied by culture and over time. In some cultures, mothers may have abandoned their less-than-perfect offspring who were deemed not fit to survive. Thus, there are stories of mothers abandoning infants on the mountainside and of selective infanticide. Demographic statistics from the Middle Ages suggest that selective infanticide, particularly of female infants, was practiced. On the other hand, one must be careful not to generalize too much from such statistics. It is also clear that some blind, lame, hunchbacked, and mentally disabled individuals did survive and were embraced by their cultures.

Even in the nineteenth century, physicians and midwives did not focus much attention on which babies should live and which should not. Their foremost concern was to get the mother safely through childbirth. The survival of the infant was desired, but certainly secondary. At that time, there were few available interventions for infants and children, much less for fetuses and neonates. Modern neonatal intensive care and technology contributed to a very different approach to newborns' survival. As technology evolved in the first half of the twentieth century, maternal mortality and morbidity dramatically decreased, and clinicians focused more attention on the fetus and neonate. In addition, technology specific to the neonate was developed. L. Stanley James, a pioneering neonatologist at Columbia-Presbyterian Medical Center, has identified the development of plexiglass as a critical parameter for the development of neonatal intensive care.[1] For the first time, the baby could be undressed and observed inside the incubator. Thus, color changes and other subtle signs of illness could be observed. There was, of course, a good deal of trial and error in the early days of neonatology. For example, clinicians knew that the administration of oxygen to a cyanotic baby sometimes improved its color; they hypothesized that, if a little oxygen was good, more must be better. As we know now, too much oxygen caused a dramatic increase in blindness in premature infants. Other experiments, such as those with antibiotics, caused side effects such as deafness.

The history of technological innovation in neonatal intensive care is essentially one of "miniaturization." As technology was developed and proved successful in adult intensive care, it was made smaller and tried on infants.[2] Catheters, ventilators, and other technological innovations have made a contribution to the survival of many infants who would have died only a decade ago. A good case to illustrate the accomplishments of technology in neonatal intensive care is that of Patrick Bouvier Kennedy. The only infant born to an incumbent President of the United States, Patrick arguably had all the technology in the world available to him when he was born in 1963. Born by Cesarean section five and one-half weeks before his due date, he weighed 2,100 grams (four and one-half pounds). He died on the second day of life, succumbing to respiratory distress syndrome.[3] Only a few years later, with the perfection of techniques to ventilate neonates artificially, Patrick would have been much more likely to survive.

Technological innovation continues in neonatal intensive care, as it does in all areas of critical care medicine. Extracorporeal membrane oxygenation (ECMO) and sophisticated surgical interventions are examples of such innovations today. With the successes that result from such innovations come the ethical issues that parents and clinicians must face daily in the NICU. Although most of the survivors of NICUs are "successes," there are also clearly "failures" along the way—that is, infants who experience prolonged suffering before they died, or who survive with catastrophic disabilities.

WHO MAKES DECISIONS FOR NEONATES?

Once childbirth moved into the hospital, decisions about what to do with and for anomalous and sick newborns became medical decisions. Most of the time, the physician paternalistically suggested what ought to be done and the parents were given little choice. Such decisions, which were made in every nursery, were not very public and there were no clear guidelines. These decisions became much more open and public as a result of the regionalization of perinatal care. As more and more new technologies became available, special nurseries were set up to provide increasingly specialized care. Because it was too expensive and inefficient for every hospital to have such a nursery, regional special-care nurseries were set up to provide specialized care for infants who were transported from local hospitals. Thus, instead of occasional problem babies for whom decisions were made privately between parents and the physician, these central nurseries had many such babies. By necessity, the process of decision making became more public and visible. This was probably not a bad thing, but it raised a new set of questions.

Questions about the application of neonatal technology—such as who should get it and who should decide—had been raised even before the establishment of the first special-care nurseries.[4] The landmark article on decision making in neonatology was published in 1973 in the *New England Journal of Medicine* by Raymond Duff and A.G.M. Campbell.[5] Duff and Campbell described the decision-making process that was used in the special-care nursery at Yale-New Haven Hospital, the regional center for Connecticut. They also described the group of infants who had died in the nursery because of decisions to withhold treatment. Based on a review of the records of infants who had died in the special-care nursery between 1 January 1970 and 30 June 1972, they reported that 43 of the 299 deaths (14 percent) were related to withholding treatment. These included infants with multiple anomalies, trisomies, cardiopulmonary disease, meningomyelocele, other central nervous system disorders, and short-bowel syndrome. Duff and Campbell believed that parents should be actively involved in decision making for their catastrophically ill newborns. They advocated and practiced a consensus model of decision making, in which all individuals involved with an infant's care—including the parents—would review the options for treatment. If the group decided that the prognosis for meaningful life was extremely poor or hopeless, treatment was withheld. The advantage of this process was that the parents had an active voice in the decision-making process and were supported by others who were involved with their infant who could provide knowledge and expertise. On the other hand, parents did not have to feel that the entire burden of such a decision was on their shoulders. In addition, in this type of "public" decision making, decisions were open to more scrutiny than those made in private encounters between parents and one physician. Recognizing that the law was unclear in this area, the authors ended their article with the following statement: "What are the legal implications of actions like those described in this paper? Some persons may argue that the law has been broken, and others would contend otherwise. Perhaps more than anything else, the public and professional silence on a major social taboo and some common practices has been broken further. That seems appropriate, for out of the ensuing dialogue perhaps better choices for patients and families can be made. If working out these dilemmas in ways such as those we suggest is in violation of the law, we believe the law should be changed."[6]

Duff was criticized by some of his colleagues, and he and the special-care nursery were subject to intense scrutiny. However, he and Campbell had broken the silence about decisions in the NICU. The media and lay literature began to cover such issues. In addition, the professional literature carried more discussions and opinions. Most notably, pediatrician Norman Fost and attorney John Robertson warned about the possible legal ramifications for parents and clinicians if treatment was withdrawn or withheld.[7] They also questioned whether parents were always in a position to make the best possible decision for their infant. Even the best-intentioned parent was generally anguished, grief stricken, and overwhelmed in such cases. Although increased public discussion promoted more thoughtful inquiry into decision making in the NICU with its emerging technologies, it was clear that these decisions would remain difficult.

THE BEST-INTEREST STANDARD

We have reached a consensus in our society, albeit an uneasy one at times, that an adult with decision-making capacity has the right to make his or her own decisions regarding healthcare. Respect for autonomy is at the core of American bioethics. Thus, in the life-threatening situations that arise in the adult intensive care unit (ICU), patients with capacity make their own decisions about treatment. On the other hand, the reality in the ICU is that patients have often lost capacity, either temporarily or permanently. In such cases, there is an attempt to make a substituted judgment for such patients. Respect for autonomy dictates that decisions be made, as much as possible, based on what was important to the individual patient. A substituted judgment is one that reflects what the individual would have chosen in a particular situation, based on what was important to him or her. Advance directives and surrogates are often used to try to guide decision making in such cases.

In the NICU the substituted-judgment standard cannot be achieved. Neonates have not yet developed a value system and are unable to communicate. The problem is not only who will speak for them, but also what ethical standard will be used to guide decision making. The standard most often referred to for infants and children is the best-interest standard, which is more subjective than objective. A decision guided by the best-interest standard reflects what a "reasonable" person would decide is the best balance of benefits over burdens.[8] Of course, because any group of individuals trying to determine what is in an infant's best interest is composed of individuals with their own set of values, it is difficult to achieve a completely objective decision. The ambiguity in prognosis that often exists in the NICU only compounds this problem. What is important, however, is that decision makers attempt to avoid making quality-of-life judgments for infants who are vulnerable and cannot speak for themselves.

Parents are generally the best spokespersons and advocates for their infant. They also have a vested interest in seeing that their baby survives with maximum potential. On the other hand, they need information and guidance from the experts assessing and caring for their baby in order to make the "best" decisions. In some cases, however, parents may be unwilling to accept the limitations that a catastrophically ill infant may present. It is very important that the institution has safeguards in the system and advocates for the infant so that a best-interest standard, rather than a quality-of-life judgment, truly guides decision making.

THE "BABY DOE" REGULATIONS

Concern about nonaggressive treatment of catastrophically ill newborns contributed to several legal challenges to parental authority in the 1970s and early 1980s. Consider, for example, the case of conjoined twins in Danville, Illinois, who had a single trunk below the waist and shared three legs and internal organs.[9] The parents and their obstetrician decided against resuscitation, but the babies breathed spontaneously. When an order was written not to feed the babies in accord with the parents' wishes, an anonymous caller reported the case to the Illinois Department of Children and Family Services. The parents and the attending physician were charged with conspiracy to commit murder, and temporary custody of the twins was granted to family services. As no witnesses came forward to link the parents and the physician directly with the decision not to feed the babies, the charges were dismissed. The parents regained custody of the twins and took them home. Although the twins were not expected to live long, they were successfully separated. One twin survived for four years and the other continues to survive.

Such challenges to parental authority during the 1970s were not common. In fact, a film made at Johns Hopkins in the early 1970s portrayed doctors' decision to respect parental refusal of surgery for an infant born with Down's syndrome (trisomy 21) and a surgically correctable, life-threatening anomaly.[10] Although the film was distributed nationally and widely viewed, it produced no public outcry.

Public discourse and concern about appropriate treatment for catastrophically ill newborns reached a critical level in 1983 when the federal government issued the "Baby Doe" directives. Baby Doe, an infant with Down's syndrome and a commonly associated, surgically correctable, life-threatening, gastrointestinal anomaly, was born in Bloomington, Indiana, in 1982. After much anguishing discussion with their physicians, which yielded conflicting opinions, the parents decided not to consent to surgery to correct the gastrointestinal anomaly. Their decision was contested in the Indiana courts, with the Supreme Court of Indiana upholding the right of the parents to refuse consent for surgery.[11] The baby died at six days of age.

Although Baby Doe died, his case came to the attention of the federal government and then Surgeon General C. Everett Koop and resulted in regulations and legislation meant to promote treatment of catastrophically ill and handicapped newborns and infants. In 1983, the U.S. Department of Health and Human Services published new regulations in the *Federal Register*.[12] These regulations set up a "Baby Doe Hotline" to receive calls reporting discriminatory treatment (or, rather, lack of treatment) of infants in hospitals. The regulations also required hospitals to display signs prominently in obstetrical units, pediatric units, and nurseries, warning that it was a violation of the Federal Rehabilitation Act of 1973 to deny food or medically beneficial treatment to infants solely because of their handicaps.

The Baby Doe regulations were quickly overturned by a federal court on procedural, rather than substantive, grounds. They were reissued following appropriate administrative procedures but were essentially unchanged. The rules were in effect for only a short time before they were overturned by the Second Circuit Court in a New York State case involving a baby known as Jane Doe.[13] Baby Jane Doe had hydrocephaly, microcephaly, and a meningomyelocele. Her parents did not want her aggressively treated (and surgically repaired), because they believed she would live a life of intractable pain and suffering and they did not want to prolong her suffering. The appeals court invalidated the Baby Doe regulations, finding that the Federal Rehabilitation Act was never intended to apply to medical decisions about catastrophically ill newborns. During the time that the Baby Doe regulations were in effect, approximately 50 cases were reviewed. In no case was there a finding of medical neglect.

At the same time that the Baby Doe regulations were being proposed and subjected to legal scrutiny, Congress was working on legislation to recognize the withholding of "medically indicated" treatment from an infant as a form of child abuse and neglect, rather than discrimination. Compromise legislation amending the Child Abuse and Neglect Prevention and Treatment Act was passed in 1984.[14] This legislation required each state to establish a procedure to investigate potential cases of medical neglect or denial of medically indicated treatment for infants. Medically indicated treatment is defined in the legislation as: "treatment (including appropriate nutrition and hydration and medication) which, in the treating physician's . . . reasonable medical judgment, will be most likely to be effective in ameliorating or correcting all such [life-threatening] conditions."[15] Exceptions to this requirement for medically indicated treatment were as follows: infants who are irreversibly comatose; infants for whom such treatment would merely prolong dying, not correct all of the life-threatening conditions, or be useless in ensuring survival; or infants for whom such treatment would be "virtually futile" and its provision would be inhumane. This legislation left most decisions up to "reasonable medical judgment." The exceptions were also difficult to interpret and open to clinical judgment. In addition, failure to comply would result in loss of a state's federal child-abuse funding, rather than intervention in any individual patient's case. In summary, the "Baby Doe directives" may have cast a shadow over clinical decision making in the NICU, but they are often not helpful and have little effect on day-to-day decisions in the NICU.

IS THE PROBLEM UNDERTREATMENT OR OVERTREATMENT?

The Baby Doe regulations and the public discourse surrounding them focused on the rights of neonates to receive indicated medical treatment. However, overtreatment of neonates is as much of a problem as undertreatment. Many of the day-to-day decisions regarding treatment of catastrophically ill newborns are much more subtle than the decision about whether to perform surgery on an infant like Baby Doe. The care of a typical low-birth-weight infant involves decisions about ventilation, feeding, transfusions, antibiotics, and so on. Sometimes it is only after many aggressive interventions that parents and clinicians realize that further treatment is futile.[16] It is often far harder to withdraw treatment after many months than it is to withhold it initially. Parents may be unable to accept the ultimate futility of further treatment and demand that it be continued. In addition, nurses and physicians may have bonded with the infant and be unwilling to accept the futility of the situation. In some cases, clinicians may believe that there are legal prohibitions regarding withholding of treatment. Although the law does not require the continuation of futile treatment, the debate about the definition of futility in any individual case often contributes to continued treatment, and suffering, for infants with little or no hope of survival.

A good illustration of problematic overtreatment is the case of Baby K. Baby K was an anencephalic infant born in 1992, in a Virginia hospital. Her mother refused a do-not-resuscitate order and demanded aggressive treatment for her baby. There is probably no clearer and better example of futility in neonatology than the anencephalic infant. The standard of care is to provide comfort for these infants, who lack an upper brain, and to support them in their dying while promoting bonding with the parents if they so desire. Virtually everyone believes that anencephalics have no ability to interact and no potential for meaningful existence. They generally die within hours or, at the most, days after birth. Baby K, with aggressive treatment, survived for more than two years. She was transferred from the acute care hospital to a nursing home, but was repeatedly readmitted on an emergency basis for respiratory crises. Attempts to challenge the mother's request for aggressive treatment in the courts failed. Legal decisions were based on the Americans with Disabilities Act and later, in the Circuit Court in Virginia, on the Emergency Medical Treatment and Active Labor Act (EMTALA).[17]

The case of Baby K is a troublesome example of futile overtreatment. The infant's treatment was expensive and emotionally burdensome to many of those providing it, although possibly not burdensome to her, as she lacked the ability to feel suffering. In addition, there was no hope of fixing her underlying problems in order for her to have a meaningful life. The support of the courts for the mother's demands, however, indicates a lack of consensus in this regard. Although other cases may be more subtle, it is clear that overtreatment is an issue and a concern to many neonatologists.

THE ROLE OF THE ETHICS COMMITTEE

Ethics committees have taken on an increasingly prominent role in day-to-day decision making in hospitals, particularly in difficult end-of-life decisions in the ICU. The ethics committee's role in neonatal intensive care is similar to its role in an adult ICU. It includes providing education on ethical issues, helping to develop hospital and unit policies related to ethical issues, and facilitating communication and providing recommendations in difficult cases. Ethics committees generally serve in an advisory capacity to clinicians, patient, and families. Most committees allow an issue or case to be brought by a patient, family, or staff member. Committees are interdisciplinary in composition and generally include community representation.

Although ethics committees in NICUs generally function in a similar fashion to other ethics committees, there are some important differences. As indicated above, there are unique ethical issues in newborn intensive care. In addition, patients are never involved in discussions and are always represented by surrogates (generally the parents). Because of these unique characteristics, some institutions establish separate ethics committees for their NICUs. In fact, some jurisdictions, such as New York State, require a specific review mechanism in institutions with NICUs.

NICU ethics committees usually fall into two categories: infant ethics committees (IECs) and infant care review committees (ICRCs). IECs generally follow a model recommended by the President's Commission for the Study of Ethical Problems in Medicine and Biomedical and Behavioral Research and the American Academy of Pediatrics.[18] These committees are multidisciplinary and include physicians, nurses, social workers, chaplains and/or ethicists, and community representatives. Persons familiar with an infant's care who can enhance the discussion are included on an ad hoc basis. IECs generally seek to enhance communication, clarify misunderstandings in basic knowledge, mediate disputes, and assist in identifying the course of treatment likely to be in the infant's best interest. In cases where there is agreement that a specific course of treatment is in the infant's best interest or where it becomes clear that treatment is futile, the IEC's recommendations in that regard are generally followed. However, in cases where parents continue to demand treatment that is viewed by the IEC and clinicians as futile or where the parents refuse what is viewed as appropriate treatment, the IEC may involve the hospital administration and the case may go to court for resolution. Medical decisions are best made in the clinical setting, so it is best to avoid the courts. On the other hand, the courts are a last resort in cases in which parents are viewed as making decisions that are not in their child's best interest.

ICRCs were recommended, although not required, in the later versions of the Baby Doe regulations and in the Child Abuse Amendments. They are also likely to be multidisciplinary and may be involved in education and policy development, but they may have a very different mission from that of IECs and general hospital ethics committees. ICRCs are more likely to be involved in reviewing diagnosis, prognosis, and treatment in a given case to determine if medically indicated treatment is being provided as required by the Child Abuse Amendments. Parents may not be involved in such discussions that focus on regulatory requirements rather than ethical decision making.[19]

Ethics committees, in and out of the nursery, are not without their problems. Although most are interdisciplinary, at least on paper, some may not include all desired constituencies. Group dynamics may be a problem. Institutional politics may interfere with the dynamics of the committee and preclude successful functioning. Many committees consist of high-level administrators who may not be well suited to deal with clinical issues and may create an environment that is viewed as unfriendly by staff members, patients, and families. On the other hand, many committees are working hard and struggling to gain expertise in dealing with ethical issues and providing support to patients, families, and staff. They are probably the best mechanism currently available to deal with complex ethical issues in the NICU and deserve support in the institutions that they serve. The legal system should only be used as a last resort when infants need to be protected from decisions that are clearly not in their best interest.

CONCLUSION

Clinicians who provide neonatal care have made a great deal of progress in the care of catastrophically ill newborns. In addition, ethicists and institutions have improved their strategies for dealing with ethical issues in the NICU. Such strategies are vitally important, because the providers of care in NICUs are constantly bombarded with ethical stress and quickly burn out if they are not supported in dealing with this stress. There is a reasonable consensus that parents are best suited to make decisions for their children, but they also need support in dealing with the ethical issues and their own grieving for their very sick babies. Together, parents and care providers struggle to identify what is in the best interest of patients in the NICU. Ethics committees should support them in this struggle, because parents and care providers are best suited to identify appropriate treatment. The courts should be used only as a last resort.

As difficult and ambiguous as decision making is in the NICU, there is even more controversy surrounding decisions regarding fetuses. Although a discussion of maternal-fetal conflict is beyond the scope of this chapter (see chapter 21), it is important to recognize that aggressive treatment of newborns and increased success in the technology of neonatal intensive care has contributed to a concern about appropriate treatment for fetuses—especially in the third trimester. In such cases, not only can the patient not participate in decision making, but it is inside the body of the mother and subject to her decisions for herself. Just as most parents struggle to make the best possible decision for their newborn, most mothers strive to provide the most healthy environment for the fetus. There are exceptions in both cases, however. It is those exceptions that will continue to present ethical dilemmas and challenges in the future.

ACKNOWLEDGMENTS

The author greatly appreciates the knowledge gained from her colleagues during her participation in the Hastings Center's Research Project on the Care of Imperiled Newborns from 1984 to 1987. To review the work of that project, see "Imperiled Newborns," *Hastings Center Report* 17, no. 6 (December 1987): 5-32. In addition, the research assistance of Ms. Dillan Siegler is greatly appreciated.

NOTES

1. Dr. L. Stanley James, Department of Pediatrics at Columbian Presbyterian Medical Center, New York. Personal communication with the author.

2. W.A. Silverman, *Human Experimentation: A Guided Step into the Unknown* (New York: Oxford University Press, 1985).

3. The Hastings Center Project on Imperiled Newborns, "Imperiled Newborns," *Hastings Center Report* 17, no. 6 (December 1987): 8.

4. J.M. Gustafson, "Mongolism, Parental Desires, and the Right to Life," *Perspectives in Biology and Medicine* 16, no. 4 (1973): 529-57; J. Lorber, "Results of Treatment of Myelomeningocele: An Analysis of 524 Unselected Cases, with Special Reference to Possible Selection for Treatment," *Developmental Medicine and Child Neurology* 13, no. 3 (1971): 279-303.

5. R.S. Duff and A.G.M. Campbell, "Moral and Ethical Dilemmas in the Special-Care Nursery," *New England Journal of Medicine* 289, no. 17 (1973): 890-94.

6. Ibid., 894.

7. J.C. Ahronheim, J. Moreno, and C. Zuckerman, *Ethics in Clinical Practice* (New York: Little, Brown and Company, 1994), 18.

8. Ibid.

9. See note 3 above; J.A. Robertson, "Dilemma in Danville," *Hastings Center Report* 11 (October 1981): 5-6.

10. A. Hellegers, "Problems in Bioethics: The Johns Hopkins Case," *Obstetrical and Gynecological News* 8, no. 40 (15 June 1974).

11. *In re Infant Doe*, No. GU8204-00 (Cir. Ct. Monroe County, Ind., 12 April 1982).

12. *Federal Register*, 15 April 1985; 45 *CFR* 1340, DHHS Part IV.

13. *Weber v. Stony Brook Hosp.*, 60 N.Y.2d 208, 456 N.E.2d 1186, 469 N.Y.S.2d 63, cert. denied, 464 U.S. 1026 (1983); *United States v. University Hosp.*, 575 F. Supp. 607 (E.D.N.Y. 1983), aff'd, 729 F.2d 144 (2d Cir. 1984).

14. Child Abuse and Neglect Prevention and Treatment Program: Final Rule.

15. Ibid.

16. R. Stinson and P. Stinson, *The Long Dying of Baby Andrew* (Boston: Little, Brown and Company, 1983).

17. *In re Baby K*, 832 F.Supp. 1022 (E.D. Va. 1993); *In re Baby K*, 16 F.3d 590 (4th Cir. 1994).

18. President's Commission for the Study of Ethical Problems in Medicine and Biomedical and Behavioral Research, *Deciding to Forego Life-Sustaining Treatment* (Washington, D.C.: U.S. Government Printing Office, 1983); American Academy of Pediatrics Bioethics Task Force and Consultants, "Guidelines for Infant Bioethics Committees," *Pediatrics* 74, no. 2 (August 1984): 306-10.

19. See note 3 above, pp. 20-21.

24

Enhancing Trust and Subjective Individual Dialogue in the Burn Center

*Bruce E. Zawacki
and Sharon Imbus*

*If someone were to ask me with regard to a particular person the
location of the soul, I would examine that person for a wound
because the soul would most likely be there.*
—Richard Selzer, Interview in *Cambridge Quarterly of
Healthcare Ethics*

Whatever *matters to human beings, trust is the atmosphere in which
it thrives.*
—Sissela Bok, *Lying: Moral Choice in Public and Private Life*

BACKGROUND

In scholarly reviews about decision-making discussions with patients
(or their appropriate surrogates), the *professional community standard* of
disclosure is sometimes referred to as the "reasonable doctor standard."[1]
It is the oldest of the three commonly cited standards and legally requires
revelation of only that which is customarily disclosed by an appropriately trained and experienced physician in a given locality. It is a "fun-
nel" model of educational discourse, that is, the careprovider simply
"pours" information into the patient and requires in return only com-

munication of compliance in order to proceed.[2] It is commonly used in situations of extreme emergency, as at the time of admission for a grave injury, if only because there is little or no time available for discussion in greater detail. The second and more recent *reasonable person standard* legally requires disclosure of what a hypothetically typical and "reasonable patient" in the patient's condition would want to know and seeks from the patient (or if necessary, from an appropriate surrogate) not just an expression of compliance, but of consent. This *legal* standard of "informed consent" is currently recommended for use by surgeons in achieving *morally* adequate decisions in relatively stable and nonemergent clinical circumstances.[3] By this standard, once the appropriate information about the diagnosis, recommended and alternative courses of action, and so forth are provided, comprehended, and deliberated upon, the patient's competence verified, and the patient's voluntary consent communicated, a professionally competent surgeon meeting the "standard of care in the community" may morally and legally carry out the course of action agreed to by the patient. When seeking informed consent about medically and morally routine matters associated with good prognoses from those who appear to be "competent" patients (or patient-surrogates) with mild to moderate burdens of bio-psycho-social trauma, one or the other of the two standards described above may well be morally as well as legally adequate. But these are neither the circumstances, nor the kinds of decision-making discussions, that most trouble the persons providing and receiving care in the Burn Center and the Burn Intensive Care Unit (BICU). The bio-psycho-social wounds sustained by extensively burned persons and their families are probably the most severe that are regularly seen in clinical practice. Burned persons are abruptly stripped not only of the buffers and defenses provided by social roles, clothing, and bodily privacy, but also of their skin and often (because of facial burns) their customary sense of identity. Severe burn wounds typically require many operations, prolonged rehabilitation, and a *very* long time to heal fully and finally. On average, those providing care for a woman or man surviving an acute 80 percent body-surface-area burn can expect to be in virtually daily contact with that person and that person's family during 80 days (about 50 to 60 days for a child) of hospitalization for acute care.[4] This is often followed by at least as long a cumulative duration of in-hospital care for rehabilitation and surgical reconstruction, and many years of follow-up outside the hospital.

If they choose to appreciate their opportunity and Selzer's insight, those who care for seriously burned persons and their families will discover themselves to be in prolonged and intimate contact with unusually vulnerable and "transparent"[5] persons, whose spiritual and moral center or "soul" (to use Selzer's language) may be exposed and "visible," extraordinarily close to the surface. In such circumstances, we have found relatively superficial bedside discussions between personas acting out the roles of "reasonable doctor" and/or "reasonable patient" to be unsatisfactory. In a carefully constructed "atmosphere of trust" such as that detailed below, we have found that no less than moral dialogue between named, particular, and substantially authentic persons is adequate to appreciate and honor that moral transparency, and, to approximate on at least some occasions, the "finely aware and richly responsible"[6] relationship it allows.

It is axiomatic that the more severe and complex the malady, the more medical careproviders should seek to heal the bio-psycho-social wounds of their patients, seeing them one at a time as subjective-individual persons, and not merely as an instance of a general type or category. By analogy, we believe individually tailored and person-centered disclosure to be most appropriate for complex and momentous moral decision making at the bedside of persons with severe burns. Under these conditions especially, we, like McCullough et al., try to "switch gears" from the "reasonable doctor" or "reasonable patient" disclosure standard to a variation of the third standard commonly cited, that is, the *subjective individual standard.*[7] As usually understood, this standard requires the physician to disclose all that this particular patient, here and now, needs to know in order to discuss and decide "what should be done" in a comprehending, adequately appreciated, substantially autonomous and noncontrolled, deliberate, and voluntary way. For severely burned persons and their significant others, however, disclosure is not enough. In addition to information and "talking-to," they need, among other things, "listening-to," self-reflection, respect, safety, patience, compassion, support, and empowerment. The greater the bio-psycho-social injuries affecting burned persons and their significant others, the more care and effort is required to empower them to make substantially autonomous decisions. The greater their vulnerability, the more trustworthy we must be, and the more compelling it is to avoid coercion, manipulation, undue control, or even the appearance of disrespect, discourtesy, or conspiracy.

Our approach is probably best described as a "subjective-individual dialogue-partner standard," seeking to achieve, not just informed consent to treat "a patient," but mutually empowered collaboration to dis-

cover through dialogue how we should or should not care for a particular person with severe burns. Moral dialogue was for Socrates, and (in
our experience) remains today, a major tool for examining and living the
moral life we share with others, including our patients.[8] Unlike Socratic
dialogue, however, moral dialogue with patients and/or their surrogates
in the BICU (or its adjacent conference and patient-care rooms) should
almost never be abrasive or confrontational. At its best, it engages the
careproviding person/s and a burned person (and/or the person/s) acting as his or her supporter or surrogate) in a caring, self-reflective, and
open-minded willingness not only to convince, but to be convinced; not
only to educate, but to be educated; not to prevail-over, but to work-
with and thereby approximate a relationship of mutual commitment and
responsibility.[9] It seeks to accomplish this by: (1) removing barriers to
mutual proactive collaboration by careproviders and burned persons (or
their surrogates), (2) increasing trust, thereby making the Burn Center
and its ICU a "safe place" for searching moral dialogue, and (3) listening
to, questioning, and supporting dialogue partners as subjective and particular individuals having unique life stories, world views, moral commitments, and character traits. We present below a description of those
attitudes, structures, and processes in a large Burn Center that we have
found to be of help and daily practicability in working to achieve these
goals.

SOME MORAL AND ORGANIZATIONAL ASSUMPTIONS

Let us begin with a few of our most important assumptions. *First,*
careproviders' continual self-improvement of their professional competence and technical expertise is a *sine qua non*; without this medical practice is, or rapidly becomes, unsound ethically as well as pathophysi-
ologically.[10] *Second,* we maintain a strong presumption in favor of sustaining life and keeping options open at least until the relevant facts are
in and the relevant stakeholders' assumptions, opinions, values, and arguments are aired, analyzed, and balanced critically. At its best, "ethics
doesn't answer in a day."[11] Therefore, we stipulate that for our patients

> maximal therapy should be given: at and during delivery from the
> site of the [injury]; at and during transfer to the Burn Center, while
> expert evaluation of the [burned person] is being completed; until or

unless there is . . . [valid] rejection of maximal therapy by the [burned person]; or, if the [burned person] is [without decision-making capacity], by persons having the right and responsibility to make decisions for the [burned person] regarding . . . medical care.[12]

We may at some point recommend a do-not-resuscitate (DNR) order and/or a comfort-measures-only (CMO) order, but will not carry out such an order unless the patient or his or her appropriate surrogate(s) agree. *Third*, absent violation of valid law, prior contract, or the like, a mutually collaborative "win-win seeking" covenant between a careproviding person and a burned person requires that one not coerce, manipulate, conspire against, or otherwise improperly seek (or appear to seek) to control the other by methods designed to abridge or violate his or her moral integrity. If differences develop that are irreconcilable (by counseling, mediation, ethics consultant or committee, and so on) any party to the relationship may withdraw or elect to seek judicial relief.

Fourth, we believe that, at their ethical best, "patient-centered conferences"[13] about end-of-life and similar moral issues should not treat burned patients (and/or their surrogates) as people we careproviders are concerned about but nevertheless exclude from the conference room while we, the "real burn team," deliberate privately to achieve "consensus" before emerging to request "compliance with" or "informed consent" to "our team's decision." Rather, we believe such conferences should, *prima facie* and as much as reasonably possible, accept burned persons and their supporters and surrogates as genuine and fully ratified members of the burn team and whose moral life stories, life plans, world views and opinions are of at least equal value to those of other members. No less than careprovider-members of the team, their views and opinions should be considered at the same time, in the same room, and as part of the same deliberating or negotiating process culminating (hopefully) in a "team consensus collaborated in" and not merely "consented to." Similar in many ways to Nuland's experience during meetings of this kind, we have never found "that the intimacy of a long, caring conversation . . . [at] the side of a [burned person's] bed has interfered with the detachment so necessary to the subsequent skillful accomplishment of a surgical procedure in the operating room. . . ."[14] or with the benevolent deliberation and commitment appropriate for momentous decision making with or on behalf of a seriously burned person.

> If anything, it ["sharing the pains and pleasures of our species" in such conversations] will help us make those crucial . . . decisions. . . . If we do not know the people who put their lives, literally, into our hands—if we have not listened to them tell the narratives of their lives . . . and allowed the element of choice—we are depriving ourselves of a crucial factor in that decision-making. . . . Why not see and feel . . . who our patients really are, and feel like what it is to be in their place? We are not the single-minded craftsmen of the past.[15]

And if "subjective individual disclosure" of some portion of our personal life stories can help friends and colleagues reflect on morally relevant portions of theirs, we believe it can be wise, unselfish, and professional, on an appropriate occasion, to do something similar with burned persons or their surrogates.[16]

Our *fifth* assumption follows from our fourth, and is perhaps organizationally the most important. In our BICU, burned persons and their families are *prima facie*, and from the moment the patient is admitted, assumed, and to be and treated as valuable, competent, and responsible members of the burn-care team, able to teach and be taught. Attractive posters and personal orientations expressing this assumption are provided on admission and when questions are answered. In most hospitals and burn centers, head administrators, doctors, and nurses are placed at the top of the "table of organization," and patients (if they appear at all) are placed at the bottom. We believe this contradicts mission statements that "put the patient first." The prominently posted "table of organization" of the LAC+USC Burn Center inverts the organizational pyramid, placing "patients and their significant others" at the top, those supporting and working most closely with the patients (attendants, aides, technicians, interns, and others) next lower, and finally, at the bottom, are those "bearing the burden of supporting, encouraging, and empowering all those above": the head administrator, doctor, and nurse. Burned persons are often very sensitive to touch and are, therefore, touched and submitted to painful procedures only with permission. Decision-making rounds with the responsible attending physician ("attending," for short) are virtually never made away from the bedside or without addressing the patient, who is assumed always to be aware and competent, even when he or she may appear otherwise. Families or significant others, or at least their representatives, are *aggressively* solicited to attend any and all non-emergency bedside discussions and rounds (especially afternoon teaching rounds with the attending) which typically form a single-tiered circle that includes the patient, a non-family translator (if necessary), family representatives (in the ICU, no more than two), a pharmacist, a physical therapist (PT), an occupational therapist (OT), nurse, social worker, and so on. After presentation by the resident, each person in the circle is invited to ask his or her questions and/or provide input. The discussion finishes with a lay-language summary by the attending and response to questions and comments, first from the family and finally from the patient (all through an interpreter, if necessary). Physician-friends, pastors, professional providers of second opinions, and others are genuinely welcomed. Instead of constantly searching for information and finding only distorted or incomplete versions from different sources, severely burned persons and their families are submerged in the details of the "one-most-current-and-most-accurate story we know"; and, *mirable dictu,* they rapidly learn how to surface, swim, and occasionally even teach us new strokes with surprising comfort and sophistication.

APPROACHES

During admission of a critically burned patient, our usual approach is to focus attention predominantly on pathophysiological matters. The history and physical examination are completed to establish a diagnosis. Initial burn care—fluid replacement, respiratory and metabolic stabilization, and pain control—are instituted and monitored to maximize survival. The most experienced physician establishes the prognosis, aided by standard references, recent burn literature, and the cumulative experiences of other careproviders, all of whom (except two out of three rotating surgical residents) are permanent or relatively stable (rotating every six or 12 months). The staff also shares any available social and family history.

Very often, usually a matter of hours after relative hemodynamic and respiratory stability has been achieved, the burned person's consciousness clears to a point that suggests that meaningful communication is possible.

A. The careprovider present (usually a nurse or resident), by him- or herself or through an interpreter—and if necessary reading head-nods and hand-signals from the intubated patient—determines if the patient is adequately oriented: does she know who she is and the roles of the people around her, where she is, why she is there, the date, and so on? If so, the attending is summoned, because the dialogue that is to follow is so crucial and demanding that it *must be* postponed, for a short time at the most, until the attending can be present to preside, in order to avoid misunderstandings that may be irreparable.

B. The attending introduces himself or herself, confirms the patient's orientation and decision-making capacity (often asking "silly" questions, answerable by "yes" or "no," such as, "Are you at the beach?" "Am I a postman?") and then summons other available careproviders to assist with, witness, and participate in the conversation and commit to the often quite solemn covenant that is being fashioned.

C. The attending introduces herself (or himself) and colleagues, says that they have come to explain and discuss the burned person's injuries, to outline present and planned management, and to obtain the patient's permission for and collaboration in future management.

D. If the burned person appears to understand and is able to express herself, she is encouraged to express her thoughts and ask questions, using a writing tablet if necessary and if possible. Always, but especially if the patient belongs to a cultural group that is unfamiliar to the attending, it is important to ask what her understanding of her injury is, why it happened, and so on;[17] and how, in her ethnic group, and, sometimes more importantly, in her own judgment, significant medical decisions are to be made in her case.[18]

E. To make autonomous decisions, a competent patient must, as much as possible, comprehend and appreciate the facts of the case, the nature of the "usually indicated" and other plausible options, and, for each option, the expected risks, benefits, discomforts, outcomes, and effects on values that the patient, as a subjective individual with a particular life story, holds to be important. Because important points are regularly misunderstood (and at times grossly misunderstood), the patient should be asked to paraphrase what she has heard, if possible. To accomplish all this, and to make or hear important points gently and sensitively, several trips to the bedside may be necessary. A nod from an intubated patient doesn't always mean agreement; an abrupt change of subject may indicate a need to pause or temporary unwillingness to deliberate on an important decision. An explicit demand "not to be told and let my family decide" should ordinarily be respected.

The five-step procedure shown in Exhibit 24-1 provides a framework to recall major areas for collaborative decision making with the patient in the BICU and serves as a teaching model for surgical house officers. In practice these guidelines function not as a rigid *"Miranda"* rule proforma, but rather as a flexible foundation upon which to build an ongoing discussion and alliance. The guidelines address five problems:

1. Permission to treat present illness
2. Release of information about present illness
3. Decision making about changes in present illness
4. Decision making should patient become incompetent
5. Decision making should patient's condition be or become one in which, based on past experience, survival has been rare or unprecedented.

The first three problem areas apply to all patients with life-threatening injuries, admitted with burn injuries, even if they don't require intensive care. All competent patients are asked for permission to treat their injuries after they have been told their diagnoses. As described above, the usual treatment course and plausible alternatives are explained, along with the risks and benefits of each. Questions regarding facts and values are answered or explored, and the surgeon's and other careprovider team members' recommendations are stated. Questions are answered and patients are informed of their right to consent, decline, or obtain a second opinion.

Patients are told that their diagnoses and the details of their condition are confidential and will be revealed to people other than the usual hospital, insurance, public health personnel and the like only with the patient's permission and only to those people specified by the patient. Since the careproviders in the team rarely know patients before their first admission, this provision offers patients privacy and control over an important segment of their stay. Most burned persons place no restrictions on the flow of information. Other patients, especially those whose burns were intentionally inflicted by others, welcome such restrictions.

During the various phases of burn care, there are invariably changes in the patient's diagnoses and treatment. Most of these changes are expected as part of the natural history of burn-wound care and healing; some are not. Patients are assured that careproviders are available to them every day to answer their questions. They are warned that the careproviders will not lie to them nor withhold information from them; neither will they force on them painful truths if they do not wish to hear them.

The fourth problem, decision making should the patient become incompetent, is addressed specifically to the burned person in the BICU. The patient is told that, at some point during the hospital stay, it is quite possible (for example, because of infection or high fever) that she might lose decision-making capacity. Should this occur, the careproviders still would need consent for surgery or other major treatment changes. The burned person is asked: "Who do you want to speak for you should you

Exhibit 24-1
Guide to Autonomous Decision Making by Patients When They Are Competent

Patients	Problem	"These are the facts"[1]	"It is your right . . ."	"Please may we . . ."
			Approach	
All	1. Permission to treat present illness.	Diagnosis: Treatment: usual; recommended. We advise; patient decides.	. . . to consent, to decline, to get a second opinion.	. . . have permission to treat your present illness as recommended?
	2. Release of information about present illness.	Your diagnosis and treatment are privileged information and can be revealed only with your permission.	. . . to decide who is told what.	. . . have your instructions about telling what to whom?
	3. Decision making about changes in present illness.	Changes may occur in your condition. A change in treatment may be appropriate.	. . . to be told of changes; to decline, consent, or get a second opinion about recommended changes in treatment.	. . . approach you about future changes as we are now about your present illness?
Critically ill	4. Decision making should patient become incompetent.	During some period of your illness, you may become so ill with fever, etc., that you cannot speak for yourself.	. . . to choose who should speak for you should you become unable to speak for yourself.	. . . have the name of your designee and ask if he or she will accept this role?

5. Decision making should patient's condition change to one in which the chances of survival are rare or unprecedented.[2]

Your diagnosis is serious; the death rate in the past has been _____.[3] We are committed to prolonging life and to rapid, efficient, pro-life action as long as it is in your best interest as you see it, regardless of the cost. This is true now and will remain so even if you take a turn for the worse and your condition becomes one in which, to our knowledge, survival has been rare or even without precedent. We will continue maximal treatment unless you or your chosen spokesperson tells us to stop.

. . . to receive maximal therapy no matter what, even should your condition change to one in which survival has been, to our knowledge, rare or even unprecedented. However, you may wish to decline treatment at a certain point.

. . . have your instructions about continuing or stopping maximal treatment with respirators, feeding tube, and dialysis machines, etc., should your condition change to one in which survival has been, to our knowledge, rare or unprecedented?

NOTES

1. To make proper decisions, competent patients must be told the facts. They may, however, be disenfranchised by their own denial should any but the gentlest and most sensitive exposition of facts be made. It will take time and repetition to make a point gently, but the truth must be available if the patient wants it. A patient's desire not to be told must also be respected.

2. The patient-designated spokesperson should join the discussion at this point.

3. Before continuing, questions such as "Would you like to discuss this further?" and "Would you like me to be more specific?" help gauge the patient's willingness to discuss these matters.

An earlier version of this exhibit appeared in S.H. Imbus and B.E. Zawacki, "Encouraging Dialogue and Autonomy in the Burn Intensive Care Unit," *Critical Care Clinics* 2, no. 1 (1986): 53-60. © 1986, W.B. Saunders Company. Used with permission.

become unable to speak for yourself? May we speak with the person you name and ask if he or she will accept this responsibility?" To facilitate an uninhibited answer, these questions are put to the patient only when no friends or family members are present.

The fifth problem area is explored with all patients who have a 50 percent or more expected mortality rate and any others who express a desire for such a discussion. It is the most difficult to discuss and is often omitted during the first round of dialogue so that the spokesperson designated by the patient can, if willing, be called to be present to hear the patient state his or her choices. Asking burned persons if they want to discuss the seriousness of their illness requires tact by the caregivers and courage on the part of the burned person. Some of the language used includes: "Would you like to know how serious your burn is?" "Would you like to know the expected survival rate?" "Are you sure you'd like to know? We can give you a rough estimate of the percent expected survival rate if you'd like to hear it . . . or would you rather discuss this at another time?" The vast majority of patients insist then and there on hearing a percentage and often require clarification of what it means. The patient's instructions about continuing or stopping treatment if her condition is, or changes to, one in which the chances for survival are either rare or unprecedented demand undistracted attention. We believe at this juncture that our patients must understand and be assured that their caregivers are committed to providing the best possible therapy without regard to cost or difficulty for the caregivers. The policy in our BICU is to continue all efforts at prolonging life—even if, for example, the patient's condition worsens beyond a point beyond known precedent of survival—until or unless the patient or his or her spokesperson tell us to stop, or survival is, to our knowledge, physically impossible (examples might be the burned person with a 100 percent full-thickness skin loss, or the patient consistently unresponsive to unabridged and well-managed CPR). This is done for two reasons: (1) A large majority of our patients are uninsured, have at most a marginal income, and know that transfer to another burn center is virtually impossible financially. Many enter the hospital fearing they will "not receive all the care they would get is well insured." From the beginning, therefore, we wish to disarm the patient's fear of loss of control in deciding what she needs and the treatment she wishes to receive or not to receive. (2) "Survival without precedent" is not synonymous with "survival cannot happen." In the past, we have, on rare occasions, "made history" by discharging alive and well (on one occasion directly to home) patients who were, for our

BICU, (and apparently for at least one other)[19] "without precedent for survival,"—for example, a 72-year-old man with an unequivocal 72 percent body-surface-area burn. Nevertheless, we as careproviders need to know, and need the surrogate(s) to know, by hearing for themselves in the burned person's own words (if possible), if there is a point at which the patient would no longer wish to receive mechanical ventilation, dialysis, or other invasive life-support measures. So we ask the patient for his instructions and respect them. Occasionally we have, in the same way, asked patients for instructions regarding a condition or change in condition to one which, in the patient's judgment, would entail disproportionate burdens in relation to the benefits experienced or anticipated (for example, amputation of four limbs or persistent vegetative state). Patients are then told that we plan to continue discussion of their condition and these matters in their presence on daily rounds, and that they have the right to change their minds. If the patient wants more time to reflect before deciding, that is also her right.

After discussing these issues with the patient, the attending (or more usually, the responsible resident assigned to the patient) documents the following on the medical record: the patient's mental status, language (if other than English), diagnosis, prognosis, and the treatment proposed; the patient's acceptance or rejection of treatment, instructions about release of information, and any other relevant details about the dialogue; the name and phone number of the person designated to speak for the patient, special instructions given by the patient if his or her condition worsens to a state associated in the past with rare or unprecedented survival (or, if discussed, other state beyond which, for the patient, the benefits are outweighed by the burdens of continued life support); the name of the caregivers present, and any general impressions or areas of ambivalence. If, after reading this note, any of the careproviders on any other work shift disapprove of the agreement arrived at in step 5 of Exhibit 24-1, they are invited to state and discuss their objections for consideration by the whole team, which of course includes the patient.

THE PATIENT WITHOUT DECISION-MAKING CAPACITY

Sometimes after emergency care, a burned person is found to be without decision-making capacity due to potentially reversible conditions (such as head trauma, hypoxia, substance abuse, or metabolic imbalances) or irreversible conditions (such as mental retardation or Alzheimer's disease). On other occasions, a patient with decision-making capacity initially, becomes, with the passage of time and progressive illness, unable to make decisions. If there is no legally appointed guardian or health-care decision-making agent named in a durable power of attorney for healthcare, all available family members or significant others can be asked to pick a spokesperson from among themselves to substitute for the patient in decision making and convey the decision they believe the patient would make if able. Whenever possible, however, we have found it more effective for the attending, responsible resident, nurse, and social worker to hold a "family meeting" for this purpose. Occasionally 25 or more family members and friends attend; none are turned away. In our experience, it has been at these meetings especially—where patient representatives and loved ones are strained but physically healthy and present in large numbers—that lengthy dialogue occurs that is often open, searching, and rich in detail and revelation of the values held by the patient and her representatives.

We have found it especially valuable to start such a meeting (with a hospital-employee interpreter if necessary) by sitting all attendees in a circle and asking each (including the nurse, resident, attending, and social worker) to take as much time as they would like telling the group who he or she is, why they are there, and what each would like to accomplish by the meeting. This can, and probably should, take a long time, but this trust-building exercise is time very well spent. No matter how large and varied the group, and no matter how much dissent or misplaced affect might be expressed throughout this initial sharing process, and no matter how often family members choose to leave the room to control their emotions, we have never found a group that could not unanimously agree to begin deliberations with a single goal when it was expressed as, "I think we are here to discover together how we can best love and honor Mrs. X," or words to that effect. Family members (and careproviders) have to work through their own values, especially if they conflict in some way with the goal expressed as above. They do this best by teaching us about themselves and their values. The first portion of the meeting is, therefore, not a good time to "shut up" family or careproviders by saying things like, "Your values aren't relevant; what were Mrs. X's values?" Sooner or later, the goal of "best loving Mrs. X" usually leads someone, often the family member who emerges as a leader, to suggest, in effect, that "Perhaps the way to best love Mrs. X is to honor what her wishes and values were; and she always said '. . . .'." If asked their opinion about "how best to love Mrs. X," careproviders should express their authentic opinions only. As suggested by Socrates, in places made safe for moral dialogue, authenticity counts, and the "flattery of rhetoricians" and the suggestions of devil's advocates do not.[20]

Some patients have no relatives but have a friend who consistently exhibits care and concern. A staff member, usually the social worker, interviews this friend to gain insight about the patient and his or her value system. If this individual appears to have no significant conflict of interest (for example, because of anticipated secondary gain), gives evidence of knowing the values of the patient and of caring for the patient by frequent visits, and so on, they are treated as the patient's surrogate and given the level of support usually given to surrogate decision-making family.

Occasionally, a patient admitted to the BICU is found, after diligent search, to be without a legal guardian, advanced directive, family or friends; often they haven't even a name we can discover. This burned person may be the most vulnerable of all: she typically comes without a life story, medical history, or community, and the chart lists her as "a transient." In these cases, the social worker contacts the police for relevant "missing persons" information, and the nurses keep close watch on the patient's level of consciousness to piece together any clues about her, her name, her wishes, and so on. Sincere and sustained efforts are made to reverse possible causes of the patient's clouded sensorium, in part because, if such efforts fail, we come to experience (still another time!) how relatively colorless and cold, how relatively blind and empty bedside decision making can become when bereft of the subjective-individual story and values of a particular flesh-and-blood patient. In this circumstance we are forced into discerning for ourselves what an abstract "reasonable person" would see as her "best interests" and act accordingly. Not much substantive and positive information is available in this effort, but a few helpful but largely cautionary signposts, extrapolated from the *Guidelines for Foregoing Life-Sustaining Treatment for Adult Patients at LAC+USC Medical Center,* are available to us when we are backed into this arid and largely statistical-data-free wasteland of guessing what a "reasonable person in this patient's circumstances" might decide; readers should consult analogous guidelines from their own particular institutions:

Decisions should be made [by the healthcare team] based on medical judgment and in what is believed to be the best interest of the patient. . . . Two mechanisms of resolving conflict are consultation with the [ethics committee] and solicitation of opinions from profes-

sionals who are not primarily involved in the care of the patient. . . .
[Moral propriety requires] when contemplating forgoing life-sustaining measures [or making other major treatment decisions] in a patient in this category: 1) a diligent search has been made and no surrogate is available; 2) all persons involved in the patient's treatment have disclosed any real or apparent conflicts of interest; 3) all relevant medical information has been obtained and reviewed; 4) one or more physicians in addition to the attending physician have examined the patient and concur in the prognosis; 5) opinions of the entire health care team [except of course the unavailable patient/surrogate members thereof] have been reviewed; 6) the burden and benefit from the [hypothetically reasonable] patient's view have been examined; 7) consideration of economic impact on health care providers and the hospital have been excluded; and 8) steps have been taken to ensure that the "benefit of continued life to a disabled patient is not devalued or underestimated.[21]

With or without family or friends, when or if the burned person regains decision-making capacity, she resumes responsibility for collaboration in her healthcare decisions.

FOLLOW-UP REPORT

Changed only slightly since it was first reported in 1986, the five-step procedure described in Exhibit 24-1 has been used with over 200 patients.[22] Discussion of the first four questions in Exhibit 24-1 has always been unproblematic. Patients have occasionally surprised us by naming an unexpected person as surrogate, but only once did a homeless man designate (apparently by default) a physician-careprovider to that role. At times it was difficult to understand intubated patients' answers to question 5, or they declined to answer it at all. In that circumstance the answer to question 4 served to save many hours of anguish and distress for all involved. At times, especially early in their hospitalization, very severely burned patients or their surrogates said, and persisted in saying, that they wanted "everything done" in answering question 5, despite careproviders' recommendations to the contrary. Often, however, with progressive appreciation of their predicament and routine review of "moral issues" as part of the "problem list" discussed with them openly at bedside rounds, they gradually changed their minds and accepted a recommendation that a DNR and/or CMO order be written.

Occasionally (usually associated with the arrival of a new physician on the team), the five questions were not explored at a time of mental clarity for the burned person, or there was no opportunity to do so (for example, when anoxic brain damage prevented such a period of clarity from occurring). In such circumstances, especially if there were no friends or family available, the considerable turmoil expressed at regular teaching rounds forced us into the painful position of trying to guess what the patient's wishes might be. No patient and no surrogate has expressed disapproval at our temerity in asking these questions. Inappropriate (in our judgment) demands for CPR still occur occasionally (for example, when many organ systems have failed and a recommendation to forego life support is not trumped by what we judge to be valid psychosocial or conscientious moral, cultural, or religious objections).[23] This usually occurs when we have not gained the trust of patient or surrogate. In such cases, the temptation to perform a deceptive "slow code," in violation of our word and our own integrity, has, to our knowledge, been yielded to only once (when a new and uninitiated resident and attending were in charge.) Rather than reflecting virtue, this record of resistance to temptation may reflect lack of opportunity because of the typically short lifespan of severely burned patients with multiple organ-system failure (often only a few days), no matter what is done.

When the University of Southern California (USC) chose its current president several years ago, he articulated a new mission statement, which read in part: "The mission of USC is the building up of the individual and society by the cultivation and enrichment of the human mind and spirit." This became a major stimulus for reaching toward a goal of "cultivating and enriching" the moral dimension of "mind and spirit" we shared with burned persons, their families, and the health professionals we are responsible for teaching at our Burn Center. At that time we formally undertook and increased our efforts to make the changes needed to realize the inversion of the Burn Center organizational pyramid described above. We believe that this organizational and attitudinal change, added to the interviewing approach[24] and autonomy-encouraging guide[25] previously published, improved trust and the quality of moral dialogue at our Burn Center, but we cannot prove it. At that time there was available no approach to measure the moral adequacy of clinical decision-making that enjoyed widespread approval by a consensus of authoritative experts. Even now, despite recent impressive scholarship in this area, we are aware of no tested, validated, and widely accepted instruments measuring moral values such as stakeholder education and empowerment, or ethicality of the process and outcome of moral dialogue in clinical decision making.[26] At this time, therefore, we are able to offer not "results," but only "follow-up" impressionistic statements about the changes associated with this overall approach.

We have, on virtually all Burn Center inpatients, and without fail except on holidays and weekends, made "large-group-circled-around-the-bed" rounds at least daily as a complete team, with family members invited. Family members were almost always present at the bedside during rounds on burned infants and young children, less often when patients were older children or adults. When the anticipated mortality rate of a patient in the BICU was approximately 50 percent or greater on admission, we, by protocol, made a concerted effort to have two members of the family of each seriously burned patient make rounds with staff at least during our afternoon teaching rounds in the BICU. Patients were addressed directly during teaching rounds, using as little editing of discussion as possible. Teaching of residents was not interfered with by this process, and, after a few days, family members regularly asked excellent questions about, for example, a BUN (blood urea nitrogen) level falling after discontinuing a nephrotoxic antibiotic, or made remarks such as, "Doesn't that x-ray of the chest appear to show some improvement today?" Families often expressed admiration of and appreciation for the clinicians' skill demonstrated in managing multidimensional problems and were pleased and even flattered to hear "the inside story everyday." In general, the frequency of miscommunications attributable to families "ambushing" caregivers one-by-one in the hall outside the BICU was greatly reduced. Recognizing the patient and family as full team members, and avoiding any appearance or suspicion of a "conspiracy behind closed doors," the attending, when appropriate and with prior permission from patient and/or family but without prior private "caucusing" and/or "consensus building" among careproviders, encouraged explicit dialogical discussion at bedside in the BICU by the entire team about problems, such as the appropriateness of CPR. Usually this occurred with explicitly stated balancing of bio-psycho-social and moral pros and cons in the presence of, and with participation by, the family and (if well enough) the patient. In the private "family meeting" described above, family story telling and active participation was usually much more extensive and often more open but required patience. For example, in dealing with a patient and his family belonging to a particular religious sect, it was not until the last 10 minutes of an hour-long family meeting that we learned their ultimate criterion for moral decision making. It was not the answer to our question, "How best can we together love Mr. X?" but "How quickly can we get the Chief Priest here to decide this matter?" Jehovah's Witnesses and Orthodox Jews and their families agonized in such sessions, changing their minds often as we listened more than persuaded them. In discussions with patients, we learned, for example, that drug addicts, alleged arsonists, alleged arson victims, very "take-charge-and-never-give-up" business executives, and homeless vagrants might or might not adhere to stereotypical expectations in making decisions and might or might not change their minds with time. One nearly lifelong narcotic addict, after seeing how damaged he was, swore he would shake his habit, and several years later he returned, clean and sober with a book he had published recounting his conversion experience and new life as a drug counselor. Only after hours of discussion during three hospitalizations did one patient (a woman who was sometimes psychotic, who had immolated herself three times in two years in attempted suicide, despite maximum available psychiatric intervention and medication) confide to us that she repeatedly burned herself in order to return to the one place she felt loved—our Burn Center—and that she knew she would continue to burn herself if she survived. At bedside and separate family meetings, in short, we learned, in greater detail than we ever thought available, how courageous, sophisticated, discerning, maddening, weak, tough, intelligent, sympathetic, and loving patients and exhausted family members can sometimes be when faced with moral and other problems after abrupt disaster and prolonged stress. To rationalize these matters, deal with the details, and to better plan financial, social, and other supportive measures for burned persons and their families, a separate weekly multidisciplinary conference became mandatory. When we learned what a patient in the BICU who was facing a difficult moral problem consistently wanted or probably would want, moral controversy usually disappeared, or at least greatly diminished. Lawsuits were extremely rare, and mortality rate by age and size of burn changed little: but no formal "before-and-after" measures of trust or the adequacy of moral decision making were made. We are grateful for the lessons we have learned, the virtue we have seen, and the friends we have earned. Mutually supportive and sympathetic conversations, and even hugging between nurses or therapists and families, have become more common. We know them so well that meeting former patients in clinic at an outside rehabilitation facility or at our annual Christmas party is regularly like a family reunion. We believe the "minds and spirits" of all involved have been "cultivated and enriched," but, of course, until compared to an alternative approach in an appropriately controlled prospective study, we cannot prove it scientifically.

To remain authentic in dialogue and to "love the patient" as best we could, careproviders on our burn team have often recommended that DNR and CMO orders be written. Such orders, however, have never been written or acted upon without due moral process, that is, without prior and valid explicit consent from a competent patient, substituted consent from an appropriate surrogate, or consent reasonably deducted or assumed when neither a competent patient nor an appropriate surrogate was available. We continue to reject "futility policies" from HECs or professional societies which, although written without propositional and valid community representation, nevertheless recommend unilateral action and/or decision making by careproviders without these or other forms of prior and morally valid dialogue resulting in patient and/or surrogate consent. Although we are unaware of existing examples, the "other forms" referred to might include a prior and validly entered upon health insurance contract, or valid law enacted by elected and appropriate representatives of the entire community. Our's often appears to be a minority position. We take it because we believe that with the death of dialogue, civility and due process die; and with their death, respect for persons and perhaps even democracy itself is endangered. Even on rare occasions when we have been forced to "triage" patients out of the BICU temporarily to make room for patients who needs intensive care more, or who could use it with greater prospects of success, we have fully informed the involved families (and patients, if competent) of our rationale before the move was carried out. No lawsuits or noticeable damage to health or trust occurred on these occasions.

DISCUSSION

Socrates saw his greatest task to be not the resolution of moral dilemmas, nor the discernment of propositional truth, but to answer the question: "How ought one to live?"[27] Moral dialogue was his major tool for examining not only how his interlocutors did live, but how they and he himself should live.[28] After years of training first in a distinguished academic environment in which the sickest patients, without prior discussion with patient or family, were repetitively given CPR virtually "until they were cold," the senior author (BEZ) moved to another, similarly distinguished academic burn-care environment in another country.

There, many elderly burn patients with severe burns were given only morphine, dextrose, and water intravenously and allowed to die, again with no prior discussion with patient or family. Neither approach was satisfactory. Now, after over 30 years devoted almost exclusively to burn care, the senior author is still looking for some "golden mean" between these extremes, some "finely aware and richly responsible" environment that might "cultivate and enrich" the moral lives of those who deliberate, work, live, and sometimes die in the Burn Center and its BICU.

Like Socrates, as reflected in his early dialogues, we have come to believe the most valid response to such problems probably doesn't lie in some "one size fits all" slogan, nor in an un-Socratic quest to develop some unanswerable rhetorical position or public policy with or without the sanction of law. Rather we believe it more likely to lie in: (1) continuous reflection upon and improvement of one's skill and ability to learn from repetitively performing the one-on-one and one-person-at-a-time verbal dance called moral dialogue between a careprovider and a seriously burned person and/or her family; and (2) seeking "how we ought to live" collaboratively with patients in a relationship committed to moral as well as bio-psycho-social health. Careproviders who arrange never to talk seriously to burned persons or their surrogates obviously cannot "learn to dance" in moral dialogue with them. Careproviders who, ahead of time, together and away from burned persons and their families, plan for themselves a rigid series of agreed-to and locked-in steps before stepping on the moral dance floor, will be in danger of learning little from, and, at the very least, of stepping on the moral toes of their partners. As unlikely as it sounds, before stepping on the moral dance floor some careproviders develop a written plan for how to escape and how to arrange that other careproviders in the hospital, who might be available and willing to dance in their place, will not be allowed to do so should the interchange not "go their way." They appear to see moral dialogue as a kind of verbal contest or even verbal warfare. Dance instructors know they probably won't accomplish much when called to the scene of a "dance gone bad" in which partners have been hurt or are trying to overpower one another. As experienced dancers, they realize it would be better to teach preventative approaches and to coach participants in how to collaborate in a more balanced, more sensitive and aware dance. *Mutatis mutandis* for moral dialogue, dance lessons are needed, teaching how to listen better, provide a better environment, ask and respond to questions without overpowering partners, and so on. The dance of moral dialogue is a metaphor we hope careproviders and burned persons and their surrogates will find helpful in visualizing their partnership, and this chapter is meant to be a contribution to that effort.

A few final comments are appropriate about what burned persons and their families may have in mind when, during end-of-life discussions, they ask for "everything!" As indicated above, personal life stories can sometimes help those who hear them to examine morally relevant portions of their own lives. The senior author (BEZ) is more than a little shaken to admit that he has, for a long time, failed to reflect on what might be meant by words such as "everything," "never," or "nothing" when used in important relationships in his life. For example, as a surgical resident and fellow, he (like every physician) worked *very* long hours. His children often said, "Dad, you *never* come home! You're *always* at that hospital, and you *never* play ball with us!" In response, he often said, "Well, I came home and played ball with you just a few weeks ago . . . and I'm home now . . . so don't be silly and say I 'never' come home. Now off to bed with you."

After about 10 years of marriage, his wife said: "You really are *always* at that hospital. *Everything* important to you seems to be at that hospital, and I'm not one of them. And when you do come home, you *never* talk to me!" And he would say: "I came home at 6 p.m. last Saturday, and we're talking right now, so don't be silly . . . and by the way, what's for supper?"

How obtuse! His family members used words like "always," "everything," and "never," but were actually saying, "We need you . . . desperately. We need your caring, presence, and attention. We need your time and our relationship." Instead of taking them *seriously*, he took them *literally*, and even used their own words against them.

Could it be that patients and families who ask for "everything" are really asking careproviders for the same things the senior author's family wanted and had a right to? If so, we will never hear them, when, instead of taking them *seriously*, we take them *literally*. Gail Gazelle suggests that when a request for "everything" is mistakenly "taken at face value," caregivers may be led to perform a "slow code" as an appearance-saving way out of what they see as a threat to their moral integrity.[29] Could much of the heat, resentment, and confusion about demands for "futile interventions" originate in a similar failure to "listen with the third ear" for what our patients and/or their families really want when they ask for "everything" to be done? A successful effort to enhance trust and subjective individual dialogue in the Burn Center and its ICU just might provide the answer.

NOTES

The quotation at the beginning of this chapter by Richard Selzer is from an article by T. Kushner, "CQ Interview: Richard Selzer on Death, Resurrection, and Compassion," *Cambridge Quarterly of Healthcare Ethics* 4 (1995): 494-98.

The quotation from Sissela Bok is from her book, *Lying: Moral Choice in Public and Private Life* (New York: Vintage Books, 1978), 33.

1. R.R. Faden and T.L. Beauchamp, *A History and Theory of Informed Consent* (New York: Oxford University Press, 1986), 23-89.

2. M. Buber, *Between Man and Man* (London: Collins, 1961), 109-31.

3. L.B. McCullough, J.W. Jones, and B.A. Brody, "Informed Consent: Autonomous Decision Making of the Surgical Patient," in *Surgical Ethics*, ed. L.B. McCullough, J.W. Jones, and B.A. Brody (New York: Oxford University Press, 1998), 15-37.

4. B.E. Zawacki, *Annual Report of the LAC+USC Burn Center, 1994* (Los Angeles, Calif.: LAC+USC Burn Center, 1994); B.E. Zawacki, *Annual Report of the LAC+USC Burn Center, 1995* (Los Angeles, Calif.: LAC+USC Burn Center, 1995).

5. T.C. Brickhouse and N.D. Smith, *Plato's Socrates* (New York: Oxford University Press, 1994), 85; B. Zawacki, "The 'Futility Debate' and the Management of Gordian Knots," *The Journal of Clinical Ethics* 6, no. 2 (Summer 1995), 112-27.

6. M. Nussbaum, *Love's Knowledge: Essays on Philosophy and Literature* (New York: Oxford University Press, 1990), 84.

7. L.B. McCullough, "Informed Consent and Refusal," in *Critical Care, 3rd Edition*, ed. J.M. Civetta, R.W. Taylor, and R. Kirby (Philadelphia, Pa.: Lippincott, 1997), 81-87.

8. Zawacki, "The 'Futility Debate' and the Management of Gordian Knots," see note 5 above.

9. S.K. White, *The Recent Work of Jurgen Habermas* (Cambridge, Mass.: Cambridge University Press, 1988), 56 and 73; Zawacki, "The 'Futility Debate' and the Management of Gordian Knots," see note 5 above.

10. E.D. Pellegrino and D.C. Thomasma, *A Philosophical Basis of Medical Practice* (New York: Oxford University Press, 1981).

11. W.F. May, personal communication.

12. B.E. Zawacki, "The Doctor-Patient Covenant," *Journal of Trauma* 19, no. 11 Supplement (1979): 871-73.

13. R.B. Fratianne et al., "When is Enough Enough? Ethical Dilemmas on the Burn Unit," *Journal of Burn Care and Rehabilitation* 13, no. 5 (1992): 600-04.

14. S.B. Nuland, "The Past Is Prologue: Surgeons Then and Now," *Journal of the American College of Surgeons* 186, no. 4 (1998): 457-65.

15. Ibid.

16. Zawacki, "The 'Futility Debate' and the Management of Gordian Knots," see note 5 above.

17. A. Fadiman, *The Spirit Catches You and You Fall Down* (New York: Farrar, Straus and Giroux, 1997), 260-61. Quoting the work of A. Kleinman, this book is an unforgettable illustration of the importance of such questions.

18. L.J. Blackhall et al., "Ethnicity and Attitudes Toward Patient Autonomy," *Journal of the American Medical Association* 274, no. 10 (1995): 820-25.

19. R.B. Fratianne and C.P. Brandt, "Determining When Care for Burns Is Futile," *Journal of Burn Care and Rehabilitation* 18, no. 3 (1997): 262-67.

20. T.C. Brickhouse and N.D. Smith, *Plato's Socrates,* see note 5 above, p. 7.

21. Ethics Resource and ICU Committees of LAC+USC Medical Center, *Guidelines for Forgoing Life-Sustaining Treatment for Adult Patients at LAC+USC Medical Center* (Los Angeles, Calif.: LAC+USC Medical Center, 5 May 1993).

22. S.H. Imbus and B.E. Zawacki, "Encouraging Dialogue and Autonomy in the Burn Intensive Care Unit," *Critical Care Clinics* 2, no. 1 (1986): 53-60.

23. Zawacki, "The 'Futility Debate' and the Management of Gordian Knots," see note 5 above.

24. S.H. Imbus and B.E. Zawacki, "Autonomy for Burn Patients When Survival Is Unprecedented," *New England Journal of Medicine* 297 (1977): 307-11.

25. Imbus and Zawacki, "Encouraging Dialogue and Autonomy in the Burn Intensive Care Unit," see note 22 above.

26. E. Fox and R.M. Arnold, "Evaluating Outcomes in Ethics Consultation Research," *The Journal of Clinical Ethics* 7, no. 2 (Summer 1996): 127-38; J. Andre, "Goals of Ethics Consultation: Toward Clarity, Utility, and Fidelity," *The Journal of Clinical Ethics* 8, no. 2 (Summer 1997): 193-98.

27. Plato, *Gorgias* 487e7-488a2, in *Plato: The Collected Dialogues including Letters,* ed. E. Hamilton and H. Cairns (Princeton: Princeton University Press, 1989), 270.

28. T.C. Brickhouse and N.D. Smith, *Plato's Socrates,* see note 5 above, p. 14.

29. G. Gazelle, "The Slow Code: Should Anyone Rush to Its Defense?" *New England Journal of Medicine* 338, no. 7 (1998): 467-69.

25

Critical Care Nurses: Moral Agents in the ICU

Ginger Schafer Wlody

INTRODUCTION

Developments in society and within the nursing profession in the past 20 years have created heightened awareness of ethical struggles and ethical behavior. This has resulted in moral discourse observed in the media as well as within the healthcare professions.[1] Feather notes that, due to the pressures of rapid medical and social development in healthcare and the professional status nurses have acquired, moral dilemmas have emerged as urgent topics of discussion.[2] In a study of staff nurses, Wilkinson found that, in the course of their duties, nurses frequently experienced strong negative feelings of moral distress resulting from being unable to implement a moral decision because of contextual constraints.[3]

This chapter discusses the underlying threads in the role of critical care nurses as moral agents: protecting the autonomy and rights of patients as decision makers, assessing each situation clearly, promoting advocacy, opening interdisciplinary lines of communication, and creating an ethical environment in which critical care nurses can advocate for patients and their families. The current healthcare and ethical environment is described, the historical background and causes of ethical conflict in critical care are presented, and the role of the nurse as a moral agent in critical care nursing is defined. Components of an ethical environment are described, and concepts related to individual, professional, and institutional values are put forth. Finally, specific ethical conflicts facing critical care nurses are identified, and a nursing model to address ethical issues is presented. A case study illustrates use of the model. As we move forward into an age of ever-increasing technology and managed care, the importance of the ethical role of critical care nurses must not be underestimated.

THE CURRENT ENVIRONMENT IN CRITICAL CARE

The ethical environment is profoundly affected by the economic environment. In the current unstable healthcare environment where leaders are challenged daily by economic, administrative, and ethical issues, it is essential to create and sustain an environment that is ethical and provides excellence in management of the critically ill patient. It is the patient-centered, "customer-oriented," healing environment, created by the multidisciplinary team that seeks to provide excellence in patient care—excellence that is based on recognized standards, shared processes, and measurable outcomes. As we move into the twenty-first century, nurses are in a unique position to create ethical environments where patients' needs can be met.

HEALTHCARE TRENDS AFFECTING THE ETHICAL ENVIRONMENT

Review of current healthcare trends provides a perspective of factors affecting the ethical environment and demonstrates that consideration of ethical issues will play an increasingly important role in healthcare. Current healthcare trends in the United States include those related to the changing, unstable financial climate; variations in types of healthcare services; streamlining of healthcare management; and a growing emphasis on legal issues. Triaging, resource allocation, and rationing are occurring in various forms. Another important trend that will raise ethical issues and affect the delivery of critical care services more directly in the future is the aging of the U.S. population. According to Rowe and colleagues, "[e]stimates of the number of older Americans who will need specialized care by the year 2000 and the number of physicians who will be trained to provide that care foretell a serious disparity."[4] It is estimated that the number of people over 85 years old—now 2.1 million—will double by the end of the century. Critical care nurses need to be prepared to care for and create an ethical environment for these patients, because the needs of this aging population differ substantially from those of younger patients.[5]

Another trend that affects the ethical environment is the tremendous increase in the number of hospital beds devoted to care of the critically ill. This trend will probably continue. As more healthcare services to the chronically ill are delivered in the home, there will be an increase in the acuity of patients admitted, and hospitals will have a greater percentage of critically ill patients. With the new drugs available for patients infected with the human immunodeficiency virus (HIV) there may be increased use of critical care services. Use of improved techniques and continued progress related to organ transplantation have been tremendous during the last decade, and these patients will continue to require critical care services as well. Healthcare costs continue to grow and, according to the U.S. Commerce Department, a decade of cost containment has done little to slow spiraling healthcare costs. In 1990, U.S. spending on healthcare reached $661.3 billion.[6] Problems related to widespread lack of insurance, an aging population, and immigration waves of low-income minorities are factors that provide the impetus to restructure the U.S. healthcare system.

Critical care services continue to expand to care for patients in the home. Patients are being discharged connected to ventilators, taking vasoactive drugs, and dependent on other high-technology patient-care equipment. With the advent of new technology, it is believed that there will be fewer invasive procedures performed on critically ill patients and an increased use of assistive devices such as pulmonary or cardiac-assist devices. Increased telemetry and intermediate care (step-down units) to care for the increasing number of high-acuity patients must be made available. Critical care physicians may increasingly choose to work for hospitals or large practice groups.

CHANGING SOCIAL ENVIRONMENT

Although technological advances have occurred with great rapidity during the past 25 years, societal and cultural belief systems have not kept pace. During this time span, societal changes have occurred in attitudes and beliefs regarding access to care, the infallibility of the physician, death and dying, informed consent, and people with disabilities.

Universal access to care was a major issue in the early 1960s, when the concepts of Medicare and the Great Society deemed that everyone was entitled to equal access to care. Today, our society has returned to the concept of limited access to care, with patients having personal responsibility to provide for their own care. Current reimbursement policies are creating changes in the way healthcare is delivered. Capitation is popular, and use of the managed care model escalates annually. Reimbursement for outpatient ambulatory services has increased, whereas reimbursement for inpatient hospital care has declined. Hospital beds in the United States will be closed or eliminated.[7] The need for further efficiency has led to new initiatives and programs such as managed care or case management. Already there is greater delegation of nonnursing activities to nonlicensed personnel such as patient technicians.

CRITICAL CARE NURSING, MORALITY, AND ETHICS

HISTORICAL BACKGROUND AND CAUSES OF CONFLICT

Concern for moral decision making and moral behavior has been a topic in nursing education and nursing literature for decades; literally no decade has passed since 1900 without publication of at least one basic text in nursing ethics.[8] Ethics was so important at the turn of the century that the *American Journal of Nursing* published an article on ethics in its very first volume in 1901, and during the 1920s and 1930s the journal carried a regular column of ethics cases.[9] Lagerlof supports the importance of ethics in nursing and believes that nurses are the healthcare providers most interested in the ethical aspects of their work.[10] Nursing has a strong tradition of ethics teaching, and nursing curricula frequently included ethics courses until they were pushed aside after World War II by burgeoning courses in science and healthcare technology.[11] The American Nurses Association (ANA) published the code of ethics for nurses in 1926[12] and, as ethical interest grew, nursing schools again began to offer the study of ethics as an integral part of the baccalaureate program.[13]

Although in the past nurses frequently studied and discussed ethical issues, their stances were frequently based on acceptable behaviors for women in those times. Nursing carries a tradition of deference, obedience, and loyalty to physicians, nursing supervisors, and hospital administrators.[14] In the 1970s the emerging concepts of feminism and assertiveness modified that tradition. Nursing has evolved to have a more autonomous role and a much stronger patient advocate role.[15] This leads one to conclude that the ethical role of the nurse is also changing. Inherent situations exist today that compound ethical dilemmas for nurses and complicate their ability to deliver the best possible nursing care.

CONCEPT OF THE NURSE AS A MORAL AGENT

Nurses are involved with ethical and moral decision making throughout their nursing careers. Some experts believe that advocacy is the basis of patient care. Jecker asserts, "It is often assumed that the chief responsibility medical professionals bear is patient care and advocacy."[16] She sees a tension existing between different kinds of moral principles.

Concepts identified by Curtin,[17] Ketefian,[18] and Daley[19] shape our view of the nurse as a moral agent. Leah Curtin believes, "The end or purpose of nursing is the welfare of other human beings. This end is not a scientific end, but rather a moral end."[20] She goes on to say that nursing involves the seeking of good and relationships with other human beings and that the science that nurses learn and the technological skills that they develop are shaped and designed by that moral end. These beliefs lead Curtin to the following conclusion: "The wise and human application of our knowledge and skill is the moral art of nursing."[21]

Ketefian holds that, as healthcare professionals, nurses often find themselves in the position of client guardian and caretaker and, as such, nurses must make decisions and act on those decisions. She believes that it is also critical that nurses' ethical practice be based on thought and reflection (higher levels of moral reasoning), rather than the lower-level processes of intuition, self-interest, or pragmatic considerations.[22]

MORAL DEVELOPMENT

Moral ideals are those beliefs, values, and attitudes considered so important to an individual or group that they serve as general guidelines for conduct.[23] Quinn postulates that the moral ideals of nursing are fundamental beliefs and values and include advocacy, respect for autonomy, and concern for the patient's well-being. Kohlberg developed a major theory of cognitive-moral development.[24] His explanation of moral development is aligned with cognitive development and emphasizes the child's ability to reason (about moral problems) and to choose values. Kohlberg's research identified three levels of moral judgment reasoning and six stages into which these levels are divided; the stages are categories that represent successively more adequate ways of handling moral/value reasoning. Kohlberg claims that all persons move through these stages in an invariant sequence, and that a person's reasoning is predominantly from one stage.[25]

On the other hand, Feather questions the development of social wisdom, stating: "In time a new graduate with proper instruction has sufficient intelligence to operate sophisticated critical care life support systems; yet, will that person also develop the moral wisdom to decide in what context it should or should not be used?"[26]

ADVOCACY

The concept of advocacy has been an integral component of nursing since the founding of the profession.[27] Advocacy means active support of an important cause, frequently used in a legal context to refer to the defense of basic human rights on behalf of those who cannot speak for themselves.[28] Advocacy in nursing practice involves an implied contract in which each party fulfills a specialized role and incurs corresponding duties and obligations to be discharged. For example, in 1985 the California Board of Registered Nursing adopted regulations defining competency to include the following: "[The nurse] acts as the client's *advocate,* as circumstances require, initiating action to improve healthcare, to change decisions or activities which are against the interests or wishes of the client, giving the client the opportunity to make informed decisions about healthcare before it is provided."[29]

Advocacy in the nursing literature. Thomas notes that the climate for patient advocacy has never been more favorable in terms of external pressures from the public and internal concessions from institutions. He says that patient advocacy is an idea whose time has come and is a role that can be effectively and sensitively played by nurses who have a distinct contribution to make to patient care.[30]

The goal of advocacy is to promote the autonomy, self-actualization, and individual uniqueness of the patient.[31] According to Fry, the role of the advocate is to assert the patient's choices or desires on his or her behalf, similarly to the way an attorney pleads a case for his client or defends the client's right in the case.[32]

Advocacy requires the development of moral reasoning and maturity of the nurse as an individual and as a skilled practitioner. The processes of moral reasoning must be developed, the concept of the therapeutic environment must be understood, and nurses must acquire skills as moral agents. A process of addressing ethical issues is developed and involves looking at the ethical principles and facts in each situation. The

ANA code of ethics requires nurses to protect the client from "incompetent, unethical, or illegal practice of any person," and the ensuing interpretive statements describe the advocacy role.[33]

Vulnerable persons require even more protection by nurses. The concept of vulnerable persons includes children, retarded persons, the aged, the critically ill, mentally ill or incompetent, and others. For example, researchers report that the risk of suffering an injury in a hospital increases with a patient's age. In the injuries cited, age was clearly a risk factor. Patients over 65 years of age who often suffer from complex medical problems were judged to have twice the chance injury as patients between 16 and 44 years of age.[34]

Conceptual models of advocacy. Winslow, who is not a nurse, wrote extensively about advocacy in nursing and described it as a changing metaphor. He believes that, during the past decade, nursing has gone from a framework of loyalty (to superiors, physicians, and so forth) to one of advocacy. Winslow views changes in nursing ethics through two metaphors and the norms and virtues consonant with them. In the past, nursing could be viewed as a military effort in the battle against disease. This metaphor permeated many of the early discussions of nursing ethics and is associated with virtues such as loyalty and norms such as obedience to those of higher rank. Currently, nurses can be viewed as advocates. The concept of nurses as advocates is a "legal" metaphor that has been espoused by nursing leaders and represents a change in nursing's self-image.[35]

Advocacy behaviors and skills. Nurses in the advocacy role must understand the concept and develop skills as moral agents. In becoming moral agents they must have opportunities to observe role models. In addition, they must pursue ethical inquiry, use ethical reasoning, analyze ethical dilemmas, use moral intuition, and learn to use a framework for addressing ethical issues. They must learn to work through the steps in a reasoned process, using certain facts and principles as tools of ethical inquiry. Ethical questions must be addressed in a reasonable, logical manner. Facts and information must be shared, and the information must come from multiple perspectives. Ethical dilemmas are profoundly affected by details of care, and the nurse needs to ensure that patients' wants and needs are met.

Nurses involved in ethical decision making must be able to use ethical theories and principles and understand conflicts such as those between utilitarianism and deontology, paternalism and autonomy, and beneficence and nonmaleficence. In their development as moral agents, nurses must learn to assess how choices reflect these basic ethical principles, using consistency and coherence.[36] During the past 30 years, the model of ethical instruction for nursing students has changed from a focus on rule ethics to a focus on situational ethics.[37] Then, beginning in 1975, the focus moved from professional codes of behavior to specific moral dilemmas, and the role of the nurse changed to that of a moral agent and patient advocate.[38]

Gadow[39] and Curtin,[40] both nurses, view advocacy as the philosophical foundation of nursing. Corcoran believes that, if advocacy is indeed the philosophical foundation of nursing, then appropriate methods for implementing it need to be developed and tested.[41] Advocacy can be viewed several ways, but the view most commonly taken by critical care nurses appears to be the "values-based decision model."[42] This view of advocacy portrays the nurse as helping patients to discuss their needs and interests in addition to helping them to make choices congruent with their values. Kohnke views the true advocate as one who informs the patient and supports the patient in his or her decision.[43] Nurses are expected to prevent others from limiting freedom of patients, thus allowing patients to make decisions.

AACN position statement: the nurse as a patient advocate. The American Association of Critical Care Nurses (AACN) believes that patient advocacy is an integral component of critical care nursing practice. To articulate this concept, the organization developed a position statement related to advocacy that presents definitions of advocacy and defines the essential behaviors that typify advocacy. This position statement was developed by ethical experts and reviewed by peers. This view of critical care nurses as active patient advocates may involve personal and professional risks for nurses. The AACN document also extends the continuum of advocacy from the individual (patient) to societal concerns.[44]

The AACN defines advocacy as respecting and supporting the basic values, rights, and beliefs of the critically ill patient. The AACN states that, as a patient advocate, the critical care nurse shall do a number of specific behaviors (see Exhibit 25-1). These are very specific behaviors not previously pulled together as strongly in the general or the critical care literature. In its position statement, the AACN also recognizes that healthcare institutions are instrumental in providing an environment in which patient advocacy is expected and supported.[45]

Risks and benefits of advocacy. Advocacy has risks as well as benefits, and a number of problems related to the advocacy role have been identified.[46] Levine notes that the functions of the advocate can, at times, be at odds with the institution's cultural norms. Nurses may find themselves blocked and or admonished for taking on the role of the advocate.[47] Nelson observes that the traditional perception by the public of the physician as the authority and decision maker is an obstacle to nursing advocacy.[48] Leddy and Pepper point out that physicians tend to view patients as their exclusive domain and may view nurse advocates as troublemakers.[49] Corcoran states that implementing an advocacy role is difficult and sometimes threatening because it promotes patient self-determination and because a professional's moral rights and obligations may not be compatible with institutional policies or legal regulations. She believes that although patient advocacy has become a slogan for nursing, it has not been thoroughly carried out.[50]

A second problem related to advocacy is that components of advocacy have not been described clearly. Curtin described confusion about the scope and nature of the nurse's relationship with the patient or client.[51] This confusion may be related to the fact that the role of the nurse as a moral agent has not been well developed. Pursuit of ethical inquiry, analysis of ethical dilemmas, use of ethical reasoning, and development of an ethical environment are behaviors and skills that need to be advanced before one can act as a true advocate.

A third problem related to the advocacy role is the lack of a preferred model for advocacy. The literature describes models of advocacy

---

Exhibit 25-1
Behaviors of the Critical Care Nurse as a Patient Advocate

- Respect and support the right of the patient or the patient's designated surrogate to autonomous informed decision making.
- Intervene when the best interest of the patient is in question.
- Help the patient obtain the necessary care.
- Respect the values, beliefs, and rights of the patient.
- Provide education and support to help the patient or the patient's designated surrogate make decisions.
- Support the decisions of the patient or the patient's designated surrogate or transfer care to an equally qualified critical care nurse.
- Intercede for patients who cannot speak for themselves in situations that require immediate action.
- Monitor and safeguard the quality of care the patient receives.
- Act as liaison between the patient, the patient's family, and healthcare professionals.

---

wherein the nurse behaves in various modalities (on behalf of another versus loyal and obedient, as a mediator, as a protector of patient self-determination, or as a patient's rights advocate). It is not known which model is preferred. In a study of models of patient advocacy as perceived by critical care and noncritical care nurses, the author found that the "advocate" model reflected the behaviors most frequently selected (as opposed to the nurse acting as a mediator or protector) in a case scenario.[52]

Winslow described five problems related to the advocacy role: (1) the meaning of advocacy needs clarification; (2) the states' practice acts need revision; (3) patients (or their families) are often unprepared to accept nurses as advocates; (4) advocacy is frequently associated with controversy; and (5) as advocate, the nurse is bound to be torn at times by conflicting interests and loyalties.[53] The concept of advocacy in nursing is valued despite these and related problems, including personal and professional risks, lack of clarity of components or dimensions of the role, exclusion of ethical content from nursing curricula, and a number of models of advocacy with no one model clearly preferred.

VALUES

The identification and adaptation of some mutual values is important in a critical care unit where nurses are empowered to act as moral agents. The nurse manager sets the stage for the development of unit values. Values education and clarification is important to a nurse's development as a moral agent or mastery in addressing ethical issues. According to Raths and colleagues, any belief, attitude, or other value indicator that is chosen freely and thoughtfully, prized, and acted upon consistently is defined as a value.[54] Omery asserts that there are many views of values, but "the common pattern that emerges is of a subjective, strongly motivational preference or disposition toward a person, object or idea that is more likely to be manifest in an affective situation."[55] Additionally, these preferences are organized in the individual and are more likely to be mobilized by the individual in a hierarchical order. Values then direct choices of the individual. Discomfort occurs when decisions conflict with individual values.

Uustal believes that, before nurses can minister in a significant way to any patient, they must first critically examine their own personal and professional values and identify those clinical situations that might pose value conflicts, causing the nurse to interfere with another's autonomous decision making.[56] Values influence decision making in several ways; perception of a problem, of one's responsibilities, and of one's beliefs is influenced by values. For example, as Taylor says, "Only when I value life, do I begin to raise questions about death."[57] Values are influenced by cultural variations, as shown by different beliefs about the importance of health and healthcare and views related to death and dying. Personal values are developed from childhood and reflect cultural heritage and environment.

Importance of values. Values are central to decision making, but they can only be used when identified and given priority. Humanitarianism and the concept of service remain as prominent values in healthcare today, as they did when Florence Nightingale exemplified these values in the nursing profession.[58] Without values, there are no standards and hence no moral code; there is no identification of right or wrong and, ultimately, there is chaos.[59] Uustal asserts that nursing is a behavioral manifestation of the nurse's value system, rather than merely a career.[60] Value systems are thought to guide behavior. Some authors pose the questions about changing ethical values. Braun and colleagues postulate that, although humanism remains a vital link in the evolution of this society, more recently it has become overshadowed by the quest for technological advancement.[61] Uustal holds that the literature amply documents that the value of caring has been sharply eroded by the development of the team approach, specialization, and the increasing use of technology.[62]

Professional values. Nurses' professional values develop during their formal education and training and serve as standards for their conduct as nurses. These values are based on the American Nurses' Association (ANA) *Code for Nurses,*[63] which has provided guidance for the profession for many years, as well as the beliefs and values of historical figures in nursing such as Florence Nightingale and Lavinia Dock.

The American Association of Colleges of Nursing's Essentials Document also outlines values essential to professional nursing and gives examples of personal qualities and behaviors that reflect a commitment to those values.[64] The seven values to which the professional nurse should be committed are altruism, equality, aesthetics, freedom, human dignity, justice, and truth. Students are exposed to these values early and learn the professional ethics of nursing through many mechanisms, only one of which is the use of formal documents. Styles noted that the development of the individual as a professional is a very personal process; it represents a continuous journey into the self, seeking to know and strengthen the I-Nursing relationship.[65]

It is vitally important that nurses understand the theoretical framework of values—identifying these values and recognizing their influence on decision making and behavior as a nurse. Values shape the individual's nursing philosophy and are the basis of the individual's actions. The result of unexamined values is often confusion, indecision, and inconsistency.[66] The quality of decisions made in difficult situations is a direct reflection of the clarity one has of one's values; additionally, once values are clarified, it is easier to face an ethical dilemma or conflict.

Institutional values. Institutional values affect the practice of nursing and nurses as individuals because of the strong cultural norms in the workplace. Institutional values may be reflected in policy, workplace behaviors, and rewards and punishments. Acceptance of a position within an institution involves making a commitment to the value system of that institution.[67] Frequently anger, frustration, and dissatisfaction occur when there are conflicts between institutional and personal value systems.

TECHNOLOGY, ETHICS, AND CRITICAL CARE

Tremendous technological and scientific advances in healthcare have propelled complex ethical issues to the forefront of concern.[68] Ethical conflicts, such as those related to transplantation, feeding, and withholding and withdrawal of care, have made frequent newspaper headlines during the past few years.[69] Nurses become involved with these conflicts because they are closest to the patients. Nurses must face the patient and family 24 hours a day, 365 days per year. They are not able to delegate their responsibilities to anyone. Technological advances have occurred in every aspect of healthcare, and as medicine's ability to sustain life increases, healthcare professionals encounter more and more ethical dilemmas. Each new technology—such as replacing body parts, predicting genetic defects, treating the fetus in utero, and using embryonic tissue to combat specific illnesses—engenders a multitude of conflicts, legal questions, and ethical dilemmas.[70] Some believe that technology comes at the expense of the individual patient's rights. Others suggest that improved technology enhances the patient's rights by providing more options.

Thus, one of the greatest challenges to our society today is to address the ethical issues that arise from the use of technology. As technology has become more complex and more intertwined with human life and more choices are available for the healthcare team, ethical conflicts emerge.[71] Use of technology actually creates situations never before encountered. Technology provides us with procedures to save and prolong life but also presents dilemmas about the quality of those lives and the responsibility of having power over what was previously beyond the influence of human hands.[72] Decisions involving care of the hopelessly ill, transplantation, appropriate withholding or withdrawal of life-support systems, and a patient's right to refuse treatment arise and require recognition, discussion, and action. The 1991 passage of the Patient Self-Determination Act demonstrates the national concern related to these ethical issues. This act mandates that hospitals receiving Medicare funds provide a variety of treatment options to patients upon admission. These options are related to the patient's wishes about care in the event that the patient becomes unable to make decisions. In a study of members of the general public and patients at three major hospitals, Boston researchers found that more than 70 percent of people who were questioned claimed that they would refuse life-sustaining treatment in cases of coma and terminal illness. In addition, nine out of 10 patients said that they wanted to make preferences for treatment known through living wills or advance directives.[73]

These technology-induced dilemmas affect nurses, particularly nurses caring for more vulnerable patients (such as neonatal, gerontological, and critically ill patients). Nurses in acute and long-term care are faced with issues such as withdrawal of artificial feeding in the hopelessly ill; critical care nurses face these and other ethical dilemmas daily. Critical care units were developed with the intent to save lives. Frequently, the critical care nurse may be bound to provide life-sustaining care hour after hour, day after day, to a patient who does not respond and has no hope of ever doing so. Additionally, the same nurse must cope with a confusing and highly charged emotional situation in which she or he constantly gives to, yet receives no psychological support or fulfillment for, a patient who does not know the nurse is there and who most likely will not recover.[74]

It may be that nurses in the intensive care unit (ICU) experience more moral distress and concern over ethical issues than nurses in other settings because of the numerous conflicts related to life and death. They are faced with the problems more frequently, and rapid decision making is required. However, nurses working in other settings are also faced with various kinds of problems creating ethical conflicts. For example, long-term care patients frequently pose "right-to-die" questions;[75] obstetrics patients might want to refuse a needed cesarean section; and HIV-positive patients may want to refuse AZT (zidovudine), a drug that has been proven to prolong the life of patients with acquired immunodeficiency syndrome (AIDS).

Lagerlof believes that, in a world of modern medicine that is ever-more technology driven, the basic human element of caring for the sick has been left more and more to nurses and that, subsequently, nurses have the closest personal contact with sick and dying patients.[76] Nurses must be skilled at moral reasoning and ethical decision making to meet the demands of these responsibilities.

IDENTIFICATION OF ETHICAL CONFLICTS

Ethical dilemmas occur when a solution to a conflict encroaches upon the interests and welfare of another. Usually conflicts occur when two "good things" conflict with each other, or when there is a choice between two competing desired values. For example, prolonging life may conflict with the patient's autonomy to make decisions about his or her care. Our society strongly values prolongation of life, but it also places great importance on patients' rights to decide about their own care. Ethical decision making in nursing practice engenders tremendous cognitive dissonance in the decision maker.[77] Jameton identified three types of moral conflict in nursing: (1) the inability of the nurse to recognize the nature of the ethical problem (*moral uncertainty*), (2) a conflict between two or more ethical principles with no obvious solution (*moral dilemma*), and (3) conflict between the nurse's knowledge of the ethically appropriate action and institutional constraints that prevent or make that action difficult (*moral distress*).[78] Nurses can experience any of these types of moral conflict in the daily patient care environment.

The American Association of Critical Care Nurses administered an opinion survey to more than 1,100 critical care nurses attending their annual educational conference in 1991. Several of the questions dealt with ethical issues. The survey inquired about areas where respondents could foresee maximum opportunities for critical care nurses to assert new professional skills. Respondents indicated that critical care nurses see an expanded role in the area of ethical or advocacy behaviors (see Exhibit 25-2).[79]

An array of dilemmas occur in caring for acute and critically ill patients. Although many conflicts have ethical and administrative components, nurses need to discriminate and separate ethical from administrative conflicts. However, from analysis of the literature, it seems that dilemmas in patient care most frequently center around three ethical conflicts: autonomy versus paternalism, justice versus utilitarianism, and veracity versus fidelity. Various ethical dilemmas and case types reflect these three conflicts (see Exhibit 25-3).

AUTONOMY VERSUS PATERNALISM

Individual freedoms are highly valued in the United States and are supported by the U.S. Constitution and societal norms. On the other hand, American medicine has a strong history and tradition of paternalism.[80] This causes conflicts when individuals are pressured by physicians to use a specific technology or undergo a specific therapy. These conflicts occur more frequently with patients in ICUs because of the high-technology environment.

Autonomy refers to the right of the patient to self-determination and freedom of choice. Husted and Husted believe that contemporary bioethical standards are all derived directly or indirectly from the standard of autonomy.[81] The principle of autonomy asserts that human be-

Exhibit 25-2
Results of AACN Critical Care Choices

% Respondents Who Indicated Maximum Opportunity (n = 1,100)*	Behavior
91	Helping a family make decisions that relieve and satisfy the grieving process.
88	Playing a critical role as patient advocate, acting as champion of their concerns with physicians and family members.
87	Participate in caring for patients who receive new therapies and for whom technology is employed.
86	Illuminate and help choose decisions on organ donation and procurement.
84	Given proximity to patient and family members, advising physicians in thinking through decisions to use life-support systems.
80	Acting as mediator for decision making, explaining a variety of procedural options to patients when they encounter negative side effects, identifying choices and "stop gaps" for patient and family consideration.
72	Monitoring premature and endangered babies at home to nuture their support network.
68	Running businesses as AIDS home caretakers, focusing on needs of AIDS patients as physicians relinquish attention.

* Percentage who indicated 4 or 5 on a five-point scale, in which 1 = minimum opportunity and 5 = maximum opportunity.

ings have incalculable worth, deserve respect, and have the right to self-determination.[82] If a competent patient makes a clear statement about his or her wishes, then these wishes should be respected. Freedom of choice requires that full information be given to the patient; thus, informed consent is defined as the right of competent adults to accept or refuse medical treatment on the basis of full information.[83] The right of competent adult patients with incurable, but not immediately terminal illnesses, to refuse treatment—even over the objection of physicians and hospitals—was affirmed by the California Court of Appeals in 1984[84] and by the U.S. Supreme Court in the *Cruzan* decision in 1990. Ensuring informed consent is the first step in ensuring that patients are able to make autonomous decisions.

Paternalism, on the other hand, claims that beneficence (doing good for others, being helpful) should take precedence over autonomy. Beneficence also involves balancing the benefit of some therapy with the burden of it. For example, in the paternalistic approach, a healthcare worker makes a decision for the patient, saying, "It's in the patient's best interest." This type of conflict (autonomy versus paternalism) occurs frequently with decisions about treatment—particularly high-technology treatments. If a patient needs a technological therapy that the physicians view as lifesaving, but the patient views the technology as unnatural and unbearable, he may make an informed decision that the benefit does not

---

Exhibit 25-3
Critical Care Patient Care Dilemmas

Dilemma	Case Type
Withholding medications	Patient with quadriplegia with other medical problems
Code versus no-code	Cardiac patient who needs ventilator, patient with severe chronic obstructive pulmonary disease
Right to die at home	Transplantation patient
Technology versus cost	DDD pacemaker vs. VVI
Nutritional dilemmas	Withdrawal of food and fluids vs. tube feeding
Who gets the bed?	Resource allocation
Triage decisions	Patient with DNR order
Technology versus quality-of-life decisions	Patient with left ventricular assist device
Informed consent	Patient scheduled for bilateral above-knee amputations versus death

---

outweigh the psychological and physical costs. The patient may then refuse the therapy. Case law in most states supports the right of competent patients to make these decisions for themselves. The federal Patient Self-Determination Act seeks to ensure this right.[85]

JUSTICE VERSUS UTILITARIANISM

Justice is an ancient concept that has accumulated a variety of meanings over the centuries.[86] Justice refers to what is just or what is right. One deserves to be treated fairly and should not be discriminated against on the basis of social contribution or mental capability. To some, justice is based on responding to people with what they deserve—whether this is rewards, burden, or punishments. Jameton maintains that others associate justice with harmony and balance, and he includes the concept of overall harmony and fundamental equality of human beings. He cites three types of justice: distributive, retributive, and procedural.[87] Distributive justice, which focuses on allocation of goods and services, has the greatest application to healthcare. Justice demands that individuals have an opportunity to obtain the healthcare they need on an equitable basis.

Utilitarianism is an ethical theory whose principal architects were Jeremy Bentham and John Stuart Mill. The name is derived from "utility" (usefulness). Utilitarians believe that an act is right if it brings about a desirable outcome. Utilitarianism, as Mill developed it, is understood as seeking the "greatest possible balance of value or disvalue for all persons who would be affected.[88]

Utilitarianism is one of the most basic teleological or consequentialist theories of ethics. According to Mill, agreement on moral beliefs is the most important single factor making for cohesion in society.[89] Two main elements of utilitarianism as proposed by Mill are concern for general happiness and balancing benefits and losses. These principles are found today in welfare economics, risk-benefit analysis, and to some extent in healthcare economics.

Utilitarianism states that the morally right thing to do is that act which produces the greatest good (for the greatest number of people, or society). The current state of expensive or limited resources has forced healthcare leaders to review outcomes of care. Critically ill patients consume vast resources such as personnel, time, space, highly sophisticated equipment, and pharmacological products. Patients are discharged prematurely from hospitals to decrease resource utilization. One of the earliest studies reported that maximum therapeutic support of patients in one ICU resulted in a one-year survival rate of 27 percent.[90] Other studies report that most resources are used within the last few days of life.

Provision of intensive care to critically ill patients ultimately has effects on other patients (the moderately ill), from whom resources may be diverted. Therefore, clear benefit should be gained by the critically ill patient in order to justify the vast expenditures of resources.

Conflicts over decisions about treatment occur because some physicians and nurses want to provide every available therapy for their patients, even though the psychological and financial costs may outweigh the benefits or eventual outcome. Currently there is an overriding concern for the costs of healthcare in the United States and for the lack of uniform availability of basic healthcare. Can funds more justifiably be spent on the needs of many, rather than on the needs of the few?

VERACITY VERSUS FIDELITY

The concept of veracity refers to truth telling, honesty, or integrity. Veracity is vital to meaningful communication, which is an absolute necessity in any moral system or relationship between two or more human beings. Nurses, as professionals, have an obligation to tell the truth and strongly support practices related to informed consent. Nurses frequently find themselves caught in the middle when someone else has not told a patient the truth about his or her condition. Aroskar holds that nurses do not have a clear legal right or obligation to disclose information in most states, but nurses do have a moral right and, in some instances, a moral obligation to do so.[91]

Fidelity is related to trust, or keeping the promises we make. Professional nurses promise to care for patients to the best of their ability. Fidelity is integral to the nurse-patient relationship; in nursing, fidelity may be interpreted to mean faithfulness and loyalty to patients as a primary foundational aspect of the professional relationship.[92] Husted and Husted maintain that many of a nurse's ethical dilemmas concern disagreement or confusion over the details of various promises.[93] Thus, fidelity is related to implicit trust and an implicit agreement to meet the expectations conveyed by the healthcare system. Without fidelity to commitments, a moral community cannot exist.[94]

The ANA Code of Ethics puts forth the ethical standards for professional nurses and sets the standards for a trust relationship between nurses and their patients (see Exhibit 25-4).[95] Critical care nurses care for some of the most vulnerable patients in the hospital. Because the patients are so vulnerable and dependent upon the nurse, the trust relationship established is strong. As the nurse carries out this trust relationship and strives to deliver safe, quality care to the patient, conflicts may arise with the nurses's other responsibilities (such as to perform a painful or potentially dangerous procedure). Veracity conflicts with fidelity in these situations. Telling the patient truthful information (veracity) that could cause the patient distress may conflict with protection of that patient (fidelity).

OTHER CONFLICTS

Conflicts between professional integrity and remaining true to one's own ethical and moral beliefs occur in various situations because personal values influence professional behavior. For example, nurses may participate in abortions even when this practice conflicts with their own religious or philosophical beliefs. Such conflicts cause great personal and psychological distress and must be dealt with so that the nurse can continue to function, yet maintain integrity. Many nurses have removed

---

Exhibit 25-4
American Nurses Association *Code for Nurses* (1986)

- The nurse provides service with respect for human dignity and the uniqueness of the client, unrestricted by considerations of social or economic status, personal attributes, or the nature of health problems.
- The nurse safeguards the client's right to privacy by judiciously protecting information of a confidential nature.
- The nurse acts to safeguard the client and the public when healthcare and safety are affected by the incompetent, unethical, or illegal practice of any person.
- The nurse assumes responsibility and accountability for individual nursing judgments and actions.
- The nurse maintains competence in nursing.
- The nurse exercises informed judgment and uses individual competence and qualifications as criteria in seeking consultation, accepting responsibilities, and delegating nursing activities to others.
- The nurse participates in activities that contribute to the ongoing development of the profession's body of knowledge.
- The nurse participates in the profession's efforts to implement and improve standards of nursing.
- The nurse participates in the profession's efforts to establish and maintain conditions of employment conducive to high-quality nursing care.
- The nurse participates in the profession's effort to protect the public from misinformation and misrepresentation and to maintain the integrity of nursing.
- The nurse collaborates with members of the health professions and other citizens in promoting community and national efforts to meet the health needs of the public.

themselves from specific job situations in order to spare themselves daily conflict.

CREATING THE ETHICAL ENVIRONMENT

To create an ethical environment, the critical care nurse must understand concepts related to creating a framework for the healing environment or therapeutic milieu. The environment must be caring and therapeutic, focus on the patient, and utilize team decisions. The critical care nurse as a moral agent promotes patient autonomy, creates an ethical environment, communicates and clarifies information, and uses patient advocacy concepts and behaviors. Collaborative practice is an essential component of the healing environment, and the dynamic interaction of nurses with other caregivers must be supported by promotion of the interdisciplinary process. By promoting and supporting the interdisciplinary practice environment, nurses enhance patient care. Intangible components of the therapeutic environment (such as ethical issues) and tangible components (such as problems related to informed consent, safety, risk management, and infection) are important considerations in the healing environment. The concept of the nurse as a moral agent is not new. The ethics of care, the role of the nurse as a key player in addressing ethical issues, and strategies for patient advocacy are introduced. Nurses are expected to be able to use an ethical model to address ethical issues at the bedside.

Essential elements of an ethical environment further include an ongoing assessment of the patient's ability to make healthcare decisions, a determination of the patient's preferences, and an early initiation of the decision-making process. All patients in the ICU are not "healed," but the concept of the healing or therapeutic environment brings to mind a place where therapeutic goals are on a continuum and change in relation to patient responses and goals. The highly technological environment requires nurses to model a humanistic philosophy and create an ethical environment where nurses are able to act as patient advocates.

ETHICAL DECISION MAKING AT THE BEDSIDE

MECHANISMS FOR ETHICAL DECISION MAKING: A MODEL

With the expanded use of technology and the need for moral decision making in healthcare, there is growing pressure on nurses to be proficient in ethical decision making. In fact, current nursing practice requires that nurses become involved in ethical decision making.[96] Roles of professional nurses (prepared at the baccalaureate level or higher) include patient advocate, change agent, risk taker, and consumer activist. All of these roles require a clear conceptual framework through which to understand and make decisions regarding ethical issues and skill in using this framework.

There is no recipe for solving ethical dilemmas or for ethical decision making. However, Fry believes that ethicists recognize that there are many components or variables in ethical decision making and puts forth four fundamental questions of ethics that must be considered in an orderly fashion when addressing ethical dilemmas: (1) What makes acts right? (2) What types of acts are right? (3) How do rules apply to specific situations? (4) What ought to be done in this specific situation?[97]

Part of the difficulty in caring for hopelessly ill patients is that critical care nurses are unsure of their roles in addressing ethical issues. At the end of the shift they leave their patients, and they are burdened with dilemmas, unanswered questions, and frustration. As coordinators of patient care, critical care nurses are in a unique position to work with physicians and other members of the healthcare team in addressing these issues and to provide a climate in which patients' rights are protected and ethical issues are addressed.

THE CRITICAL CARE NURSE: CENTRAL PERSON TO IDENTIFY ETHICAL CONFLICTS

Because critical care nurses treat some of the most vulnerable patients in the hospital, this vulnerability engenders a unique relationship between the nurse and the patient. It is this implicit relationship that creates ethical dilemmas for nurses. Haddad states that ethical dilemmas involve conflicts between rights and responsibilities and require a choice between two or more alternatives.[98] The nurse's primary responsibility is to ensure delivery of safe, quality care to the patient. When this responsibility conflicts with other responsibilities, nurses must choose which obligation to honor.

Another area of conflict occurs as an internal struggle in which critical care nurses are torn between feeling that they must meet multiple needs (the needs of the patient, family, and physician—all of whom may have differing ethical beliefs and practices) and following institutional policies. This might involve a conflict between duty and veracity (for example, the duty to perform a specific treatment versus the duty to be truthful and tell a family that a patient's outcome is hopeless).

It is the critical care nurse who often must administer or withhold therapy in these days of cardiopulmonary resuscitation and advanced cardiac life support. It is the critical care nurse who cares for the hopelessly ill patient 24 hours a day, and it is the nurse who is pressured by the family for information. As critical care nurses encounter these issues in daily practice, they will be called upon to play a more active role in assisting patients and families caught in ethical dilemmas. As a moral agent, the critical care nurse is involved with identifying the conflict, protecting the patient from harm, assisting with clarification of issues, providing support for the patient and family, and initiating discussions with physicians and other members of the healthcare team. A nursing model helps nurses to deal with ethical dilemmas.

USING A MODEL

Critical care nurses have emerged as the caring link to the patient in today's technological environment. The individual nurse has taken on a broader role as patient advocate. By use of a model, nurses may incorporate this role into practice by methodically examining and addressing ethical issues as they arise in the clinical setting. Models provide nurses with consistent methods of addressing issues. The model should be used in a multidisciplinary context, ensuring team participation.

A practical model that critical care nurses may adopt consists of three components: assessment, advocacy, and action ("the three *A*s"). These components are related to the patient, not the physician or the hospital. As nurses use problem-solving techniques within this framework, they develop an increased awareness of their values and ability to address various ethical situations (see Exhibit 25-5).

Assessment. The assessment phase occurs first. Nurses need to assess the variety of factors that affect ethical issues—assessing the patient's response to illness; looking at quality of life from the patient's perspective, and identifying what quality is likely, should therapy change. In addition to assessing the patient's response to his illness, the patient's ability for decision making is considered. Is the patient informed about his or her illness and options for treatment? Is the patient competent? What is the patient's or surrogate's understanding of the diagnosis, prognosis, alternatives to treatment, consequences of therapy, and availability of resources? Are principles from the ANA's code of ethics, which focus on the role and responsibilities of the professional nurse, being used?[99]

After assessing the patient's response to illness and decision-making capacity, the nurse must consider a number of other factors in the assess-

Exhibit 25-5
Wlody Model for Addressing Ethical Issues

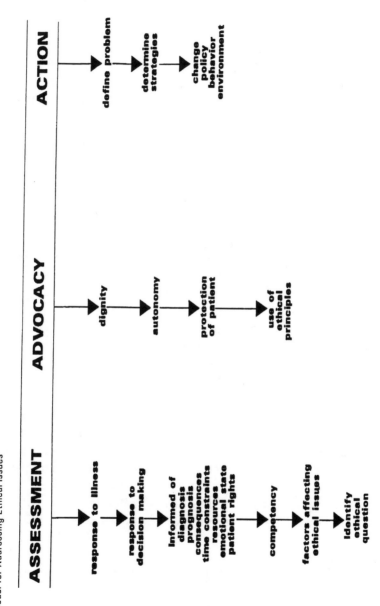

ment phase of the model. These include the patient's needs, the disease process, the patient's rights, the patient's feelings and wishes, the family's wishes, the goals of the treatment team, and societal factors (see Exhibit 25-6).

- *Patient needs.* Are the patient's physiological needs being met, even though the patient has a terminal disease? The airway should be kept clear, generally food and fluids are given, and the patient should receive pain medication and basic nursing care (comfort measures and cleanliness). Does the ICU "dump" (transfer) the patient from the unit as soon as he or she is made a "no code" or "DNR"?

- *Disease process.* Which disease processes are affecting the patient? Is the disease process reversible, terminal? Is it superimposed on a chronic, irreversible process? For example, does the patient have multiple sclerosis and pneumonia?

- *Treatment team.* The goals of the treatment team need to be articulated. Do they fit in with the overall picture? The attitude of the members, composition of the team, and the specific specialties involved all influence the decision-making process.

- *Patient rights.* These rights revolve around the ethical principle of autonomy. Patients should be consulted and participate in decisions that affect their care. If the patient is not competent, does the next-of-kin or guardian have the opportunity to participate in the decision-making process? The patient also has the right to privacy, competent care, and informed consent regarding special procedures and various aspects of therapy. The *Patient Bill of Rights,* published by the American Hospital Association, outlines what patients can expect and includes the right to respectful care, informed consent, refusal of treatment, privacy, confidentiality, and other components of care.[100] The patient's feelings and wishes must be considered and followed. For example, if the patient wishes to have a living will or to have a DNR order (if he or she is hopelessly ill), these wishes should be honored.

- *Family wishes.* A major focus in recent years has been the promotion of greater patient and family participation in decision making. In the case of Karen Quinlan, the family decided, with the advice and consent of the medically responsible individual, to disconnect the patient from the respirator.

Advocacy. Advocacy is based on the value of human dignity and, hence, autonomy. This implies the right to privacy and the right to self-determination of one's best interest. The patient (or family) must be protected from inadequate information, a single viewpoint, undue haste (or delay), coercion, lack of support, unjustified intrusion, and clear violation of their best interest. Nurses learn to become skilled patient advocates once they realize that advocacy is an essential component of contemporary nursing practice.

Advocacy can be viewed several ways, but the view most commonly taken by critical care nurses appears to be the "values-based decision model." This view of advocacy portrays the nurse as helping the patient to discuss his or her needs and interests in addition to helping the patient to make choices congruent with the patient's values. Kohnke views the true advocate as one who informs the patient and supports him or her in the decision made.[101] Nurses are expected to prevent others from limiting the freedom of the patient, thus allowing patients to make their own decisions. The ANA code of ethics requires nurses to protect the client from "incompetent, unethical, or illegal practice of any person," and the interpretive statements describe the advocacy role.[102] Although advocacy is a primary component of this phase of the *Wlody Model for Addressing*

Exhibit 25-6
Factors Affecting Ethical Issues and Ethical Decision Making

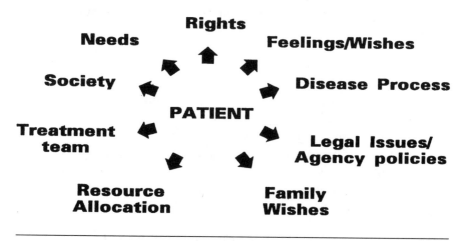

Copyright 1986 by Ginger Shafer Wlody. Used with permission.

Ethical Issues, nurses need to identify, consider, and apply all the ethical principles that come into play in the specific dilemma. For example, a conflict may entail autonomy versus paternalism (for example, the concepts of patient self-determination versus paternalism, which claims that beneficence—doing good for others or being helpful—should take precedence over autonomy). In the paternalistic approach a healthcare worker makes a decision for the patient, saying "It's in her best interest." This type of conflict occurs frequently in regard to decisions about treatment.[103]

Action. Action is the third step in the framework for addressing ethical issues and occurs after the conflict has been defined or located. The depth of the problem is assessed, and then strategies are determined. The strategies and activities occur in the multidisciplinary context. The nurse considers who should initiate action, who can contribute expertise, who can contribute legitimacy, who needs to be involved, and who may be resistant to the action. For example, in protecting a patient's right, nurses may need to work to change a policy. They may need to change the behavior of the family (for example, assist them in interacting with the physician) or change the behavior of some of the other nursing staff. Nursing administrators have special obligations because of their unique professional role in the health organization. Administrators need to be more involved with ethical issues, more supportive of staff in protecting patients' rights, and more involved in development of policies related to ethics (such as DNR or withdrawal-of-treatment policies). Other options for action include changing the environment (such as actual physical alteration or perhaps moving the patient to another, more suitable environment).

APPLYING THE MODEL

An array of ethical dilemmas confronts the nurse caring for the critically ill. However, dilemmas in the critical care environment most frequently center around the four ethical conflicts previously described: autonomy versus paternalism, duty versus outcome, justice versus utilitarianism, and veracity versus fidelity. In this section, a case study is presented, the ethical conflict is identified, and then the model is used to help the nurse identify and address the ethical conflicts involved.

CASE STUDY: A PATIENT'S REQUEST FOR NO FURTHER TREATMENT

A 75-year-old female, Ms. Beethoven,[104] has been a patient in your ICU several times before. She has had multiple operations for carcinoma of the liver, and each time she has come through the procedure without complications. The surgery has extended her life.

Ms. Beethoven is a retired nurse and has always had a positive attitude toward her illness. The more recent palliative procedure did not go well. In addition to a severe postoperative wound infection, she sustained an iatrogenic pneumothorax. Now that these complications are resolving, the medical team is planning to initiate a chemotherapy regimen. You are changing the patient's dressing as the resident physician begins a discussion with Ms. Beethoven. Information is given to the patient describing her diagnosis, the course of chemotherapy, prognosis, risks, benefits, and so forth. She listens, asks pertinent but superficial questions, and seems to accept what the physician has told her.

During the next few hours, the patient becomes increasingly withdrawn and tearful. She tells you that she has changed her mind and that she wants no further surgery, no chemotherapy, no antibiotics, no total parenteral nutrition (TPN), no food, and no resuscitation. She states that she has "lived a wonderful and happy life." She ends the conversation by saying, "You're such a good nurse, I know you'll understand and tell the doctors for me." Ms. Beethoven seems be saying, "I know that you'll help me."

You discuss the case with the chief resident, who feels that Ms. Beethoven should receive full therapy, including chemotherapy, TPN, antibiotics, and any extraordinary measures necessary. You, the nurse, disagree with his "all-out" approach. What is your next step?

CASE ANALYSIS

Assessment. What are the medical/surgical facts of the case, diagnosis, prognosis, and the treatment plan? How is the patient responding to her illness? Has the recent pneumothorax caused a temporary depression? What does Ms. Beethoven really want? A discussion with the patient can elicit more information about her frame of reference.

What type of family support does Ms. Beethoven have? Do they visit frequently or live 3,000 miles away? Or are they estranged and have no contact? Are there significant others? Does she live alone? Are finances a problem? The critical care nurse gathers information, consulting with the patient, physicians, and other healthcare professionals during this assessment phase of the model.

Advocacy. What can the nurse do to act in the patient's behalf? What are the ethical principles or conflicts here? Why is the nurse concerned? Is the patient enduring pain and suffering? The conflict appears to be one of autonomy versus paternalism.

Autonomy. This refers to the rights of the patient to self-determination and freedom of choice. Autonomy asserts that human beings have valuable worth, deserve respect, and have the right to self-determination.[105] If a competent patient makes a clear statement about his or her wishes, then those wishes should be respected. Paternalism, on the other hand, claims that beneficence (doing good for others) should take precedence over autonomy. For example, in the paternalistic approach, a healthcare worker makes a decision for the patient, saying, "It's in her best interest." This type of conflict (autonomy versus paternalism) occurs frequently in regard to decisions about treatment of critical care patients. Critical care nurses find themselves in the midst of the conflict because of their identified role as patient advocate.

In the case of Ms. Beethoven, the nurse is obligated to ensure that the patient has all the information needed for decision making. It is this analysis by critical care nurses that must precede the *action* phase of the model. Without analysis of the ethical conflicts, the critical care nurse may become involved in actions that do not aid in resolving the conflict.

Action. The third phase of the model is characterized by strategic activities aimed at clarifying or perhaps resolving the conflict. Rather than provoke the physicians (some nurses might say to the physician, "Ms. Beethoven doesn't want chemotherapy. You'd *better* talk to her!"), the nurse might begin by documenting the patient's feelings in the record, using direct quotes. The critical care nurse uses the information gained in the first two phases to plan strategic activities. For example, the nurse might plan a family or team conference that involves all disciplines. Or the action might be as simple as asking the decision maker on the medical/surgical team to talk with the patient regarding treatment plans and options. The nurse should be there to help clarify issues and assist the patient to express herself.

CONCLUSION

Today's critical care nurses play an important moral and ethical role in patient care. To help nurses deal with the ethical conflicts that they encounter on a daily basis, this chapter presents a model for ethical decision making. The model incorporates use of ethical principles; is readily adapted to the nursing process; and consists of the concepts and activities of assessment, advocacy, and action. Critical care nurses and their leaders, as the caring link to patients in a highly technological environment, are in a unique position to provide a climate in which patients' rights are protected and ethical issues addressed.

NOTES

1. A. Omery, "Values, Moral Reasoning and Ethics," *Nursing Clinics of North America* 24, no. 2 (1989): 499-508.

2. R. Feather, "Hypothetical Dilemmas: A Teaching Strategy for Moral Development," *Journal of Nursing Education* 24, no. 7 (1985): 298-301.

3. J.M. Wilkinson, "Moral Distress in Nursing Practice: Experience and Effect," *Nursing Forum* 23 (1987-1988): 16-29.

4. J.W. Rowe, E. Grossman, and E. Bond, "Academic Geriatrics for the Year 2000: An IOM Report," *New England Journal of Medicine* 316, no. 22 (1992): 1425-28.

5. E.L. Schneider and T.F. Williams, "Geriatrics and Gerontology: Imperatives in Education and Training," *Annals of Internal Medicine* 104 (1986): 432-35.

6. A. Rehm, "Legislative Update" (Organizational letter to members of American Association of Critical Care Nurses, Newport Beach, Calif., January 1990).

7. "Health Care Costs Keep Skyrocketing," (editorial), *USA Today*, 6 April 1993, 11A.

8. A. Jameton, "Basic Moral Concepts and Theories," in *Nursing Practice: The Ethical Issues* (Englewood Cliffs, N.J.: Prentice Hall, 1984), 124-51.

9. Ibid.

10. J.M. Lagerlof, "Nurses and Ethics," *California Nursing Review* (September-October 1987): 12-18.

11. See note 8 above.

12. American Nurses Association, "A Suggested Code," *American Journal of Nursing* 26 (1926): 599-601.

13. T. Stanley, "Nursing," in *Encyclopedia of Bioethics*, 1st ed., ed. W.T. Reich (New York: Free Press, 1978), 1138-46.

14. B. Kalisch and P. Kalisch, "An Analysis of the Source of Physician-Nurse Conflict," in *Socialization, Sexism, and Stereotyping: Women's Issues in Nursing*, ed. J. Muff (New York: C.V. Mosby, 1982), 25-35.

15. Nelson, "Advocacy in Nursing," *Nursing Outlook* 36, no. 3 (1988): 136-41; C. Murphy, "The Changing Role of Nurses in Making Ethical Decisions," *Law, Medicine & Health Care* (September 1984): 173-75; see note 10 above.

16. N.S. Jecker, "Integrating Medical Ethics with Normative Theory: Patient Advocacy and Social Responsibility," *Theoretical Medicine* 11, no. 2 (1990): 125-39, at 125.

17. L. Curtin, "The Nurse as Advocate: A Philosophical Foundation for Nursing," *Advances in Nursing Science* 1, no. 3 (1979): 1-11.

18. S. Ketefian, "Moral Reasoning and Ethical Practice in Nursing: Measurement Issues," *Nursing Clinics of North America* 24, no. 2 (1989): 509-21.

19. B. Daley, "Ethical Issues in Critical Care," in *Critical Care Nursing*, ed. J. Clochesy (St. Louis, Mo.: C.V. Mosby, 1992).

20. See note 17 above, p. 9.

21. Ibid.

22. See note 18 above.

23. C. Quinn, "A Conceptual Approach to the Identification of Essential Ethics Content for the Undergraduate Nursing Curriculum," *Journal of Advanced Nursing* 15 (1990): 726-31.

24. L. Kohlberg, "The Development of Children's Orientation Toward a Moral Order: Sequence in the Development of Moral Thought," *Vita Humana* 1, no. 6 (1963): 11-33.

25. Ibid.

26. See note 2 above, p. 300.

27. See note 15 above.

28. S.T. Fry, "Ethics: Issues in Nursing," *Nursing Clinics of North America* 24, no. 2 (1989): 461-62.

29. *California Administrative Code*, sec. 1443, 5.

30. J.E. Thomas, "Patient Advocacy: A New Role for Nurses" *Registered Nurse* (1988): 32-33.

31. See note 15 above.

32. S. Fry, "Autonomy, Advocacy, and Accountability," in *Ethics at the Bedside: A Sourcebook for Critical Care Nurses,* ed. M.D.M. Fowler and J. Levine-Ariff (Philadelphia: J.B. Lippincott, 1987), 39-49.

33. American Nurses Association, *Code for Nurses with Interpretive Statements* (Kansas City, Mo.: American Nurses Association, 1985).

34. J. Goldman, "Four Percent Got Disabling Injury in N.Y. Hospital Study Finds," *Los Angeles Times,* 1 March 1990, p. A17.

35. G.R. Winslow, "From Loyalty to Advocacy: A New Metaphor for Nursing," *Hastings Center Report* 14 (1984): 32-40.

36. See note 19 above.

37. S.J. Smith and A.J. Davis, "Ethical Dilemmas: Conflicts among Rights, Duties, and Obligations," *American Journal of Nursing* 80 (1980): 1463-66.

38. Ibid.

39. S. Gadow, "Existential Advocacy: Philosophical Foundations of Nursing," in *Nursing: Images and Ideals,* ed. S. Spickes and S. Gadow (New York: Springer-Verlag, 1979), 99-101.

40. See note 17 above.

41. S. Corcoran, "Toward Operationalizing an Advocacy Role," *Journal of Professional Nursing* 4, no. 1 (July-August 1988): 242-48.

42. G.S. Wlody, "Addressing Ethical Issues in Critical Care: A Nursing Model," *Dimensions of Critical Care Nursing* 9, no. 4 (1990): 224-30.

43. M.E. Kohnke, "The Nurse as Advocate," *American Journal of Nursing* 80 (1980): 2038-40.

44. American Association of Critical Care Nurses, *Role of the Critical Care Nurse as Patient Advocate, AACN Position Statement* (Newport Beach, Calif.: American Association of Critical Care Nurses, 1989).

45. Ibid.

46. J. Levine and D. Groh, *Creating an Ethical Environment* (Baltimore, Md.: Williams & Wilkins, 1990); S. Leddy and J.M. Pepper, *Conceptual Bases of Professional Nursing* (Philadelphia: J.B. Lippincott, 1984); see notes 15 and 41 above.

47. Levine, see note 46 above.

48. See note 15 above.

49. Leddy and Pepper, see note 46 above.

50. See note 41 above.

51. L. Curtin, "Ethics in Nursing Practice" (editorial), *Nursing Management* 5 (1988): 8-9.

52. G.S. Wlody, "Models of Patient Advocacy as Perceived by Critical Care and Non-Critical Care Nurses," *Critical Care Medicine* 22, no. 1 (1994): S72.

53. See note 35 above.

54. L. Raths, M. Harmin, and S. Simon, *Values and Teaching*, 2nd ed. (Columbus, Ohio: Charles E. Merrill, 1978).

55. See note 1 above, p. 500.

56. D.B. Uustal, "Values: The Cornerstone of Nursing's Moral Art," in *Ethics at the Bedside: A Sourcebook for the Critical Care Nurse*, ed. M. Fowler and J. Levine-Ariff (Philadelphia: J.B. Lippincott, 1987), 136-53.

57. S. Taylor, "The Effect of Quality of Life and Sanctity of Life on Clinical Decision Making," *AORN Journal* 41, no. 5 (1985): 928.

58. T.L. Braun et al., "The Future of Nursing: Combining Humanistic and Technological Values," *Health Values: Achieving High Level Wellness* 8 (1984): 12-15.

59. See note 56 above.

60. Ibid.

61. See note 58 above.

62. See note 56 above.

63. See note 33 above.

64. American Association of Critical Care Nurses (AACN), *AACN Essentials Document* (Aliso Viejo, Calif.: AACN, 1986)

65. M.M. Styles, *Nursing: Toward a New Endowment* (St. Louis, Mo.: C.V. Mosby, 1982).

66. See note 56 above.

67. See note 1 above.

68. See note 18 above.

69. See note 1 above.

70. G.S. Wlody, "Technology, Ethics, and Critical Care," in *Advanced Technology in Critical Care Nursing*, ed. J. Clochesy (Rockville, Md.: Aspen Publishers, Inc., 1989), 169-96; see notes 10 and 15 above.

71. See notes 10 and 15 above.

72. See note 10 above, p. 12.

73. L. Emanuel et al., "Advance Directives for Medical Care: A Case for

Greater Use," *New England Journal of Medicine* 324, no. 13 (1991): 889-95.

74. M. Cameron, "Moral and Ethical Components of Nurse Burnout: Ethical Anguish," *Nursing Management* 17 (1986): 4B, D, E; G.S. Wlody and S. Smith, "Ethical Dilemmas in Critical Care: A Proposal for Hospital Ethics Advisory Committees," *Focus on Critical Care* 12, no. 5 (1985): 41-46.

75. See note 10 above.

76. Ibid.

77. A.L. Gaul, "Ethics Content in Baccalaureate Degree Curricula: Clarifying the Issues," *Nursing Clinics of North America* 24, no. 2 (1989): 475-88.

78. See note 8 above.

79. American Association of Critical Care Nurses, *Critical Choices Survey* (Aliso Viejo, Calif.: American Association of Critical Care Nurses, 1991).

80. W.R. Harlan et al., "Ethics of Biomedical Technology Transfer: Committee Report on Ethics," *Circulation* 67, no. 4 (1983): 942A-946A.

81. G.L. Husted and J.H. Husted, *Ethical Decision Making in Nursing* (St. Louis, Mo.: Mosby Year Book, 1991).

82. A. Haddad, "Ethics: Using Principles of Beneficence, Autonomy to Resolve Ethical Dilemmas in Perioperative Nursing," *AORN Journal* 46, no. 1 (1987): 120-24.

83. *Cobbs v. Grant,* 8 Cal. 3d 229 (1972).

84. *Bartling v. Superior Court,* 163 Cal. App. 3d 186, 195 (1984).

85. S. Hassmiller, "Bringing the Patient Self-Determination Act into Practice," *Nursing Management* 22 (1991): 12, 29-32.

86. See note 8 above.

87. Ibid.

88. M.D.M. Fowler and L. Levine, ed., *Ethics at the Bedside: A Sourcebook for Critical Care Nurses* (Philadelphia: J.B. Lippincott, 1987).

89. J.S. Mill, "Utilitarianism," in *Moral Problems in Medicine,* ed. E. Gorovitz (Englewood Cliffs, N.J.: Prentice Hall, 1963).

90. D.C. Cullen et al., "Survival, Hospitalization, Charges and Followup Results in Critically Ill Patients," *New England Journal of Medicine* 294 (1976): 982-87.

91. M. Aroskar, "Fidelity and Veracity: Questions of Promise Keeping, Truth Telling, and Loyalty," in *Ethics at the Bedside: A Sourcebook for Critical Care Nurses,* ed. M. Fowler and J. Levine-Ariff (Philadelphia: J.B. Lippincott, 1987).

92. Ibid.

93. See note 81 above.

94. See note 91 above.

95. See note 33 above.

96. See note 18 above.

97. See note 28 above.

98. See note 82 above.

99. See note 33 above.

100. American Hospital Association (AHA), *Patient Bill of Rights* (Chicago: AHA, 1978).

101. See note 43 above.

102. See note 42 above.

103. See note 35 above.

104. The name and nonessential characteristics of the case have been changed for confidentiality. Any similarity to any actual person is coincidental.

105. See note 82 above.

26

Barriers to Effective Critical Care Bioethics Consultation: A Social Work Perspective

Ed Silverman

INTRODUCTION

As acute care hospitals continue to anticipate and adapt to the revolutionary changes in healthcare delivery, social work and other healthcare professions have been forced to search for fertile ground on which to develop expanded clinical roles. Often eclipsed by the ongoing reform-focused policy debate and subsequent administrative reengineering is another major change in the healthcare landscape—efforts to empower the healthcare consumer. Patient's rights, advance directives, and formal ethics committees are now an important part of the healthcare environment.[1] The Patient Self-Determination Act (PSDA), passed by the U.S. Congress in 1990, mandates hospitals to inform and ensure patients of their right to control the care they receive. Patients also have the option of appointing a proxy to act as their healthcare decision maker should they become incapacitated.[2]

As a result of the educational efforts required by the PSDA, patients have become more educated and assertive healthcare consumers. The fact that an empowered healthcare consumer and an increasingly restrictive managed-care-driven healthcare system have arrived simultaneously has created a variety of challenges for healthcare professionals and medical ethicists. For example, a healthcare team can encounter the case of an 88-year-old, terminally ill, ventilator-dependent patient whose husband of 50 years insists on continued futile treatment that insurance will not cover. Another scenario may involve the treatment of a vegetative, head-injured patient whose advance directive requests withdrawal of food and water but whose family adamantly resists withdrawal and demands full-code status.

As clinical and ethical concerns tend to arise together, the opportunity exists for the medical social worker to assume an expanded, consultative role in critical care bioethics. The social work profession's historical concern for justice and autonomy, coupled with its knowledge of psychosocial issues, allows for a natural partnership between social workers and hospital-based bioethics programs.

Following a brief contextual overview of medical social work, this chapter discusses the social worker's potential role and contribution to critical care bioethics. The chapter focuses on the assessment and subsequent resolution of barriers that impede constructive bioethics consultation and concludes with a brief discussion of ethical issues and training for medical social workers.

HISTORICAL PERSPECTIVES

THE PROFESSION: SOCIAL WORK

In 1958, a commission of the National Association of Social Workers defined social work practice as a constellation of value, purpose, sanction, knowledge, and methods.[3] This widely accepted definition identified three purposes of social work practice:

1. To assist individuals and groups to identify and resolve problems arising out of disequilibrium between themselves and the environment.
2. To identify and prevent areas of disequilibrium between individuals, groups, and the environment.
3. To identify and strengthen the maximum potential of individuals, groups, and the community.[4]

Certain philosophical values and an identifiable knowledge base are basic to social work. The concern of society for the individual, the interdependence between individuals in the society, and the need to overcome disequilibrium between individuals and their environment are fundamental to basic social work. In addition, social work, like all professions, derives knowledge from a variety of sources. Typically, social work practice is guided by psychology, sociology, group process, communication theory, organizational theory, and human development. This theoretical and value foundation has guided medical social work practice and is consistent and identifiable with ethical principles.[5]

Social workers have been engaged in hospital-based practice since Richard Cabot, the Chief of Medicine, established the first department of social work at Massachusetts General Hospital early this century.[6] Cabot believed that the function of social work was to supplement the physician's treatment of patients by alleviating, to the extent possible, the patient's social problems that interfere with the plan for medical care.[7] Thus, traditional medical social work has emphasized enhanced social functioning, focusing on special concerns about the consequences of illness and disability on the social role of individuals and families.[8] These concerns are integrated with a knowledge of life-stage development, allowing the social worker to evaluate effectively the individual's potential ability to function under the stress of trauma, illness, or physical disability.[9]

The task of defining hospital social work is difficult. The medical social worker responds simultaneously to the needs and demands of patients and their families, hospital administrators, and colleagues from a variety of disciplines. Donnelly writes that hospital-based social work, with its emphasis on discharge planning, is often perceived by other social work professionals as something less "clinical" and, therefore, less desirable than mental health practice.[10] Social work educators, too, have underestimated the clinical complexity of medical social work, and often curricula fail to prepare students to enter a medical setting.[11]

Still, the role of the medical social worker is described consistently in the literature. Blazk and Canavan report that the role of the medical social worker is to assist the patient and family to adapt to illness and injury and to help with the transition from the acute stage of illness to discharge from the hospital.[12] The specific contributions of medical so-

---

Exhibit 26-1
Services of the Medical Social Worker

---

1. Counseling
2. Emotional support
3. Provision of resources
4. Consultation

---

cial work include assessing the patient's environmental and psychological strengths and weaknesses; understanding the illness and its relationship to the patient, family, and friends; and assisting the patient to adjust to the illness to allow the best possible physical and psychosocial functioning.[13]

Estes writes that the medical social worker typically provides the following services: counseling and support, resource provision, and consultation.[14] Counseling helps the client to address the pain, fear, isolation, and grief associated with illness. In addition, the social worker can provide the emotional support that helps the client's "system"—which typically includes the patient, family, and significant others—to manage the confusing environment of an acute care hospital.[15] These psychosocial skills are useful in assessing and diffusing the underlying barriers to successful ethical resolutions.

THE ENVIRONMENT: INTENSIVE CARE UNIT

Although the generic roles and functions of medical social work that are described above are consistent with the practice of critical care social work, the intensive care environment creates unique challenges. A hospital can be a cold and confusing system for patients and family members. Often, the intensive care unit (ICU) can become an emotional hazard for patients and their families.[16]

Patients and their families are often overwhelmed by the ICU's intricate machinery—its lights, buzzers, respirators, and suctioning devices. Faced with the potential or impending loss of a loved one, the family's equilibrium is further shaken in the ICU. The family must confront and adapt to a host of healthcare providers who are rapidly responding to technically complex, life-and-death situations. Families find themselves in a tense, enclosed environment, surrounded by professionals who perform tasks that family members do not understand.[17]

It is on this crisis-loaded terrain that multidimensional, often delicate, bioethical dilemmas arise. Similarly, it is within this context that barriers to resolution must be accurately assessed, identified, and ameliorated. It is here, at the bedside, that the medical social worker can make his or her most significant contributions to the ethics process.

THE SOCIAL WORKER AS
CLINICAL ETHICS CONSULTANT

Much of the bioethics literature lists social work as an appropriate discipline represented on the large, hospital-based bioethics committee.[18]

However, the potential for expanded social work activities in a fully integrated ethics program has not been explored.

An exception can be found at the Washington Hospital Center, in Washington, D.C., where social workers routinely serve on bioethics consultation teams. These multidisciplinary teams are physician-led, with a nurse and social worker as team members. Additionally, each team has access to a pastoral counselor, a psychiatrist, and an attorney. Team members rotate on-call responsibilities. This ensures that a team will be available 24 hours a day, seven days a week.

ASSESSMENT ISSUES

It is important that the members of the multidisciplinary consultation team, including social workers, avoid role confusion between their identified profession and their consultation responsibilities. However, it must be noted that each discipline brings a unique theoretical perspective and training experience to the consultation process. For example, the ability of a social worker to assess complex, psycho-social systems is a valuable component of consultation practice. The components of the bedside ethical workup are well documented in the literature.[19] Often these include establishing the facts, determining the decision maker, identifying treatment options, determining the relevant ethical principles, and recommending sound resolutions. In contrast, the elements and conflicts that can affect consultation have not been extensively outlined. Still, it is necessary to identify and remove these barriers to productive bioethics consultation. This is especially true in the high-stress, disorienting critical care environment.

Several sources of potential conflict between the patient/family and healthcare team have been identified:

- cultural diversity issues
- lack of trust with the healthcare system
- psychological issues
- communication issues.

These potential sources of conflict may not always be easy to identify. What often presents as denial regarding a grim prognosis, may actually be an underlying communication issue. Furthermore, observed dysfunctional family behavior may not be historical in nature. Rather, the behavior may be the result of acute crisis reaction or general distrust of the healthcare system.

Often the consultation team fails to assess for and integrate the likelihood of potential conflict into their ethics workup, which increases the possibility of their being blindsided by angry, confrontational family members. This adversarial beginning makes subsequent constructive working relationships unlikely.

The practice of social work is often directed at identifying and resolving problems that arise from the disequilibrium between individuals and the environment. The social worker can contribute to the consultation process by identifying trust, communication, and psychological issues masking as ethical concerns. Additionally, when true ethical issues are present, the social worker can intervene to diffuse conflict, an intervention that is essential to subsequent resolution of ethical issues.

CULTURAL DIVERSITY

Lack of respect for or, more often, inadvertent insensitivity to cultural differences are often the underlying reason for conflict between the healthcare team and the patient system. Not all cultures are driven by similar value systems. For example, although autonomy is highly valued in most cultures, some cultures do not value self-determination. A practitioner's lack of knowledge of cultural differences may impinge upon good medical and ethical decision making. It is unreasonable to expect patients and families to surrender historical belief systems at a time of serious or terminal illness. Sometimes informed consent and patient autonomy must be superseded by cultural norms. For example, some cultures may deny patients access to their own medical information. Others may refuse standard and routine medical procedures and blood products. Although dramatic examples of cultural differences are well documented,[20] the healthcare team must also be sensitive to subtle differences in beliefs about health, disease, and treatment among and within various ethnic groups.[21]

Even patients who have lived in the United States for generations may have traditional ties to their own specific cultures.[22] This is especially so for the poor and disadvantaged. Congress and Lyon write that, although people may assimilate some healthcare beliefs, it is inaccurate to assume that a "melting pot" theory is consistent with providing healthcare to culturally diverse patients.[23]

Sometimes the consultation team and healthcare staff are confronted with scenarios that conflict with their own knowledge base and value systems, such as minority patients and families who trust and are committed to the efficacy of nonscientific healthcare interventions. In addition, the social worker may experience conflict when advocating a competent patient's right to make seemingly poor decisions about treatment.

Although these situations raise legitimate professional concerns, competent ethical consultation can prevail.

The social worker's recognition of sociocultural differences can contribute to the consultation team's ability to identify conflicts inherent in diverse cultural beliefs about healthcare. The clinical goal is to minimize the effect of this potential barrier to constructive ethical consultation and maximize the patient's and family's ability to make informed choices. This goal can be accomplished by involving the patient and family in decision making in a culturally sensitive manner.

To ensure that medical social workers and other consultation team members respect patients' cultural values, Congress and Lyons suggest that they should do the following:[24]

- Increase their sensitivity to culturally diverse beliefs.
- Learn more about, and incorporate into practice, patients' beliefs.
- Avoid stereotyping and emphasize individual differences in assessments.
- Increase the ability of culturally diverse patients to make choices.

Medical social workers have always explored patients' perceptions regarding illness and treatment. Whether patients are rich, poor, recent immigrants, or highly educated, failing to respect their cultural beliefs will undoubtably raise the potential for conflict between the patient/family and the multidisciplinary healthcare team.

TRUST OF THE HEALTHCARE SYSTEM

Conflicts related to the patient and family's trust of the healthcare system are difficult to differentiate from those related to cultural diversity. For purposes of this discussion, issues of diversity are seen as grounded in belief systems and values, while issues of trust are seen as the result of actual or perceived events. Not surprisingly, the segments of society that have been historically denied access to equal opportunity are the most mistrusting of the healthcare system. A lack of trust is often the underlying cause of conflict between the healthcare team and the patient/family, making productive ethical consultation—especially regarding code status and withdrawal of futile care—most difficult.

The health of people and the quality of medical treatment they receive often reflect their status in society. Dula reports that more than twice as many African-American babies than white babies are born premature. Additionally, the mortality rate for heart disease in African-

American males is twice that of white males. Furthermore, the higher cancer mortality rate for black males is often related to delays in detection. Finally, on average, African Americans live five fewer years than their white counterparts.[25]

Although many economic, institutional, and attitudinal variables contribute to the apparent gap in healthcare for blacks and whites, African Americans are less likely than whites to be satisfied with physician treatment and hospital care and more likely to believe that their hospital stay was too short.[26] It is not unusual for dedicated healthcare professionals to become defensive when confronted with these facts. In fact, mistrust is often minimized or overlooked as a source of potential conflict between the patient/family and the healthcare team or as an obstacle in the ethics consultation process. Still, bioethics is rarely completely unrelated to the economic, political, and social order.[27]

Dula has identified the following sources of African Americans' mistrust of the American healthcare system:[28]

- slaves used in medical experiments
- the Tuskegee experiments
- sickle-cell screening
- involuntary sterilization.

As slaves, African Americans contributed to medical progress, often without informed consent. For example, through painful experimentation, slave women played an important role in perfecting the cesarian section and testing various medications.[29]

Many African Americans still point to the Tuskegee syphilis experiments as a blatant example of whites' disregard for black lives. During this project, hundreds of African-American men participated in a government study isolating the effects of untreated syphilis. The experiment, and its denial of treatment to African-American men, was regularly reported in the medical academic community with no apparent outcry.

The sickle-cell screening program in the 1970s is another event that contributed to African Americans' suspicion of the healthcare system. The preventive goals of the program were quickly overridden by confusion and discrimination. "Carriers" were fired from work, banned from participating in the armed forces, and denied insurance. The self-esteem of young African Americans was compromised as they were labeled and stigmatized.[30]

Finally, historical sterilization initiatives have greatly diminished African Americans' trust of the healthcare system. Instances have been reported where family planning services resulted in unwanted sterilization and where physicians' involvement with the delivery of minority new-borns was contingent on subsequent maternal sterilization.[31]

Other ethnic groups show a similar distrust of the U.S. healthcare system. Hispanics, one of the fastest growing populations in the United States, face many barriers to healthcare, including language gaps and subsequent misunderstandings between the patient and the healthcare team, high medical costs, and culturally insensitive institutional policies.[32] In addition, many recent immigrants have fled horrific situations that have destroyed their ability to trust those outside their immediate family.

Given these situations and perceptions, cultural minorities' lack of trust in the healthcare system should come as no surprise.[33] Although there is likely no quick, clinical fix that can mitigate years of institutional racism, it is imperative for social workers to assess the "trust issue" as a source of potential conflict and as a barrier to productive ethical consultation.

Furthermore, it is equally important that the issue of trust be raised and discussed with the family. Failure to acknowledge the obvious "elephant in the room" precludes the possibility of useful consultation or discussion. Given the historical backdrop of racism, unequal access to healthcare, and unethical experimentation, it is unrealistic to expect unilateral understanding of and comfort with discussions about code status and withdrawal of treatment.

PSYCHOLOGICAL ISSUES

Several psychological scenarios can spark conflict between the patient/family and the healthcare team. These include patient/families that are in crisis, in denial, and those with historical dysfunctional behavior and coping patterns. A general understanding of the psychological sequela often encountered in the ICU can help the social worker and multidisciplinary team to avoid or overcome conflict that can impede the ethics consultation process.

Crisis Reaction. The psychological reaction most common to the intensive care setting is the crisis reaction. The ICU environment, alone, creates a potential crisis situation for the patient and the family. The potential loss of a loved one further exacerbates an already high-stress situation. Crisis occurs when a person faces obstacles to important life goals that seem insurmountable with customary methods of problem solving. At a time of crisis, the patient and/or family loses equilibrium and then strives to regain emotional control. Medical emergencies can overwhelm patients and families, making it difficult to cope, reason, and integrate medical information. Unless this crisis stage is constructively resolved, the family's ability to trust and engage productively with the ethics consultation team is greatly diminished.

Fortunately, crises typically have a time frame during which an intervention can affect future events and interactions. It is within this window of opportunity that social workers can make a contribution. The main goal of crisis intervention is to identify and reinforce the strengths and coping skills of the patient and family. The social worker's ability to anticipate, understand, and give therapeutic direction to the crisis reaction and the concerns of family members helps to bring around a successful crisis resolution.[34] During crisis intervention, the social worker continually assesses and reassesses family dynamics, coping ability, and the degree and accuracy of the family's ability to integrate medical information. One must avoid overwhelming an already strained family. Attempting to ascertain a brief family history can be useful on three levels. First, one can better understand how the family has historically dealt with stress. Second, it engages the family in an active task, thus assisting to alleviate feelings of helplessness. Third, it helps serve as a primer to more direct discussions regarding the patient's wishes and advance directives.

The timing of intervention is critical. It is common for families of critically ill patients to keep an anxious vigil in the ICU waiting room. Over time, exhaustion and the barrage of ICU environmental stimuli make intervention difficult. A delayed assessment of crisis following an unsuccessful ethics consultation is not useful. At the initial time of crisis the family is likely to be open and receptive to outside stimuli; once saturated, the family will close, making intervention more difficult.[35]

Denial. Although not as prevalent as a crisis reaction, psychological *denial* by families of ICU patients is not uncommon. Denial, one of the major defense mechanisms, is typically defined as an unconscious, selective blindness to unpleasant facts that protects the individual from the necessity of facing intolerable thoughts or situations. To shield themselves psychologically from the devastation of losing a loved one, the family may not intellectually and emotionally accept what is apparent to the healthcare team. This "reality gap" is a source of potential conflict. Not surprising, a family in denial is likely to demand futile treatment and have unrealistic expectations of the healthcare team. Discussions concerning advance directives, code status, and other end-of-life decisions appear absurdly premature to the family that is in denial.

Denial differs from crisis in that it tends to exist beyond a first-reaction shock. Still, denial is usually a temporary defense that can be constructively broken through gentle reality testing; repeated communication of medical facts; and a trusting, short-term counseling protocol. The therapeutic goal is for the family to replace the defense mechanism of denial with participation in a process that ensures their loved one dies with dignity, without pain, and in a manner consistent with the patient's wishes. In most cases, effective denial resolution paves the way for a successful bioethics consultation.

Dysfunctional or impaired family. The least common, but most difficult to resolve, psychological barrier encountered in the ICU is the historically dysfunctional or impaired family. Dysfunctional families often exhibit patterns of distrust, suspiciousness, and detachment. There is typically a history of instability in interpersonal relationships and marked impulsivity. These family traits, coupled with the stressful nature of the intensive care environment, make clinical engagement and productive relationships with the healthcare team unlikely.

By definition a historically dysfunctional family represents an enduring pattern of thinking, feeling, and behaving. Therefore, it is unrealistic to expect a dramatic change in the family's ability to function, trust, and relate. Still, the techniques used during brief, task-focused psychotherapy can increase a family's ability to address the dilemma at hand. By exploring underlying values, communication patterns, and belief systems, the social worker may be successful in clarifying, addressing, and mitigating variables (such as guilt and anger) that often provoke conflict and undermine the relationship between the family and healthcare team.

COMMUNICATION ISSUES

The issue of communication pervades all of the previously discussed obstacles to productive bioethics consultation and sources of conflict between the healthcare team and the patient and family. Communication issues range from obvious language barriers to the more subtle components of dysfunctional communication.

Although healthcare providers are aware of the growing number of non-English-speaking patients, their solutions to communication barriers are short-sighted.[36] Often the healthcare team, finding itself in a bind, attempts to enlist the first available language resource. Such people, while proficient in the patient's language, may not be trained interpreters. Non-professional interpreters are prone to interfere with the interview or consultation process by interjecting their own opinions and biases. This interference is compounded when a member of the patient's family is asked to serve in the role of interpreter.

At times, the healthcare team overestimates the bilingual ability of a member or members of the patient's family. Often, family members falsely acknowledge a full understanding about what has been communicated. Whenever a patient's or family's fluency is unclear, it is best to include a skilled, trained interpreter in the bioethics consultation process.

Sometimes when a patient or family is in crisis, functional communication fails to achieve expected outcomes. However, most conflicts and misunderstandings in the ICU arise from poor communication. Often, what presents as an ethical issue is later found to be an issue of communication. Healthcare professionals are noted for their wide range of bedside manners. A large component of this trait is the professional's comfort and ability to communicate. If discussion of diagnosis and prognosis is avoided or overly softened, future conflict—specifically with decisions at the end of life—should be expected. Another potential conflict exists when staff communicates inconsistent or mixed messages regarding treatment plans and prognosis. Finally, staff may consistently and accurately communicate but fail to allow time for questions and processing. This "one-foot-out-of-the-door" technique often results in the family's failure to integrate medical information.

Communication can be framed and presented to families in a variety of forms and manners. Often family members are presented with double-binds from which there are no acceptable options or solutions. A common example in the ICU involves the question, "Do you want us to do everything?" This question is often asked the same way, regardless of advance directives and identified medical goals. To place the active burden of deciding upon a plan of care on the parents of a vegetative, head-injured patient is not useful and borders on maleficence. However, if one frames the question in a discussion of the patient's wishes, futility, and medical goals, the polarization often inherent in end-of-life decisions can be avoided. The question to be asked is, "Given the circumstances, do you want us to do everything we deem medically logical, while keeping the patient in total comfort?"

In the scientifically advanced environment of the ICU, common sense and skillful communication are often just as valuable as modern technology. Poor communication can exacerbate dormant issues of lack of trust inherent in relationships among patients, families, and the healthcare system.

ETHICAL ISSUES AND TRAINING
FOR THE SOCIAL WORKER-ETHICIST

The medical social worker must balance the sometimes competing needs of patient, family, and hospital. In fact, as a member of the hospital-based bioethics consultation team, the social worker may be confronted with his or her own, profession-specific ethical dilemmas. In general, social work ethics is concerned not only with conflicts between professional obligations involving two competing goods, but with the philosophical base and value framework of the profession.[37] The National Association of Social Workers' "Code of Ethics" operationalizes this philosophical base and value framework. The "Code of Ethics" underpins professional practice and outlines the social worker's ethical responsibility to clients, colleagues, the social work profession, and the employing organization.[38]

The "Code of Ethics" is an important symbolic document, but it was not designed to provide definitive practice guidelines to social workers facing difficult ethical choices.[39] Additionally, issues unique to the social worker-ethicist may be eclipsed by the generic critical care bioethics process. For example, during ethical consultation, the social worker may face complex decisions regarding limitations of patients' rights to confidentiality, self-determination, and allocation of limited resources. Medical social workers may face cases in which family members demand futile care for a loved one or a patient with acquired immunodeficiency syndrome (AIDS) requests that his diagnosis be kept from his primary caregiver.

Perhaps the most powerful ethical dilemma confronting the hospital-based social worker-ethicist is the potential conflict of interest regarding discharge planning. With decreased reimbursement from third-party payers, hospitals must maximize their profits by reducing overall hospital length of stay. This has increased the need for accountability in surviving hospital-based social work departments. At a time when external and community social welfare resources are declining, which makes the challenge of safely transferring patients out of acute care hospital beds more complex and urgent, medical social workers must be careful not to use the bioethics consultation process to conduct utilization and review studies nor to resolve complex discharge problems.

Although the above discussion is not an attempt to exclude issues of justice, scarce resources, futility, and finances from the consultation evaluation, it would be inappropriate for the social worker who is dealing with a complex discharge challenge to also consult on that case's ethical issues (particularly code status and withdrawal of treatment). If not intimately familiar with the nuances of the medical social worker's role, ethics team members will be unaware of this apparent conflict. In many instances, social workers must police themselves. Therefore, it is important to examine training issues related to social workers' involvement with bioethics consultation.

Does the training and education of a licensed, graduate-level critical care social worker adequately prepare a person to engage in bedside bioethics practice? La Puma and Priest write that success as a bioethics consultant does not correlate with a particular degree or graduate background. They consider the key predictors of competent practice to be ability to perform case management, advocacy skills, negotiation skills, and education.[40] Foster and colleagues completed an extensive survey of perceived social work bioethics training needs. More than 200 social workers from 10 urban teaching hospitals were surveyed regarding 21 practice situations. Responses were analyzed in terms of clinical participation and preparedness to handle ethical dilemmas. Not surprisingly, perceived training needs were greater in practice situations that presented problems more bioethical than psychosocial in nature. Additionally, prior ethics education or training, along with prior experience on hospital-based ethics committees, was associated with preparedness.[41]

Social workers are among the multidisciplinary healthcare professionals who must constantly reexamine the ethical-clinical relationship.[42] While, in practice, ethical and clinical problems may include each other, one must differentiate what is clinically possible from what is ethical and legal.[43] Furthermore, the social worker-ethics consultant must be clear that the bioethics consultation is driven by ethical principles.

To limit role confusion, social workers engaging in bioethics consultations should seek additional training. Before engaging in actual case consultation, each social work consultant at the Washington Hospital Center is required to complete a 10-week course in bioethics. Participants learn theoretical principles as well as a model of ethical decision making. In addition, trainees observe, firsthand, consultation completed by an experienced team. This didactic and field experience allows trainees the opportunity to become familiar with the roles and skills used by bioethics consultants.

CONCLUSION

Social work's historical concern for justice, coupled with the field's clinical and psychosocial knowledge base, allows for a natural partnership between social workers and the bioethics consultation team. Opportunities exist for medical social workers to assume an expanded, consultative role that assists in integrating the sound theoretical underpinning of bioethics consultation with productive clinical practice.

NOTES

1. L.W. Foster et al., "Bioethics: Social Work's Response and Training Needs," *Social Work in Health Care* 19, no. 1 (1993): 15-38.

2. M. Freeman, "Helping Home Bound Elderly Clients Understand and Use Advance Directives," *Social Work in Health Care* 20, no. 2 (1994): 61-73.

3. H. Bartlett, "Toward Clarification and Improvement of Social Work Practice," *Social Work* 3, no. 2 (1958): 3-9.

4. Commission of Social Work Practice, National Association of Social Workers, "Working Definition of Social Work Practice," *Social Work* 3, no. 2 (1958): 5.

5. N. Fox and E. Silverman, "Hospital-Based Bioethics: Social Worker as Consultant" (Unpublished manuscript, 1995).

6. S. Blumenfield and G. Rosenberg, "Toward a Network of Social Health Services: Redefining Discharge Planning and Expanding the Social Work Domain," *Social Work in Health Care* 13, no. 4 (1988): 31-48.

7. I. M. Cannon, *Social Work in Hospitals* (New York: Russell Sage Foundation, 1913); see note 6 above.

8. B. Phillips, "Social Workers in the Health Services," *Social Work Encyclopedia* (Silver Spring, Md.: National Assoication of Social Workers, 1977), 615-24.

9. Ibid.

10. J.P. Donnelly, "A Frame for Defining Social Work in a Hospital Setting," *Social Work in Health Care* 18, no. 1 (1992): 107-18.

11. B. Butcher. Memo to members of Society for Hospital Social Work Directors Re: Council on Social Work Education Curriculum Policy Statement, 10 July 1991.

12. S. Blazk and M. Canavan, "Managing the Discharge Crisis Following Catastrophic Illness or Injury," *Social Work in Health Care* 11, no. 4 (1986): 19-32.

13. See note 8 above.

14. R. Estes, "Social Workers in Health Care," in *Health Care and the Social Services*, ed. R. Estes (St. Louis, Mo.: Warren W. Green, 1984), 3-22.

15. C. Germain, *Social Work Practice in Health Care: An Ecological Perspective* (New York: Free Press, 1984).

16. S.H. Kuenzi and M.U. Fenton, "Crisis Intervention in Acute Care Areas," *American Journal of Nursing* 75 (1975): 830-34.

17. K. Slaiken, *Crisis Intervention* (Boston: Allyn and Bacon, 1984).

18. J. Ross, *Handbook for Hospital Ethics Committees* (Chicago: American Hospital Publishing, 1986).

19. F.G. Reamer, "Ethics Committees in Social Work," *Social Work* 32, no. 3 (1987): 188-92.

20. R. Angel and P. Thoits, "The Impact of Culture on the Cognitive Structure of Illness," *Culture, Medicine, and Psychiatry* 2 (1987): 465-94.

21. E.P. Congress and B.P. Lyons, "Cultural Differences in Health Beliefs: Implications for Social Work Practice in Health Care Settings," *Social Work in Health Care* 17, no. 3 (1992): 81-96.

22. D. DeAnda, "Bicultural Socialization Factors Affecting the Minority Experience," *Social Work* 29 (1984): 101-07.

23. See note 21 above.

24. Ibid.

25. A. Dula, "African American Suspicion of the Health Care System Is Justified: What Do We Do about It?" *Cambridge Quarterly of Healthcare Ethics* 3 (1994): 347-57; A. Dula, "Bioethics: The Need for a Dialogue with African Americans," in *It Ain't Fair: The Ethics of Health Care for African Americans*, ed. A. Dula and S. Goering (Westport, Conn.: Praeger, 1994), 11-20.

26. R.J. Blendon et al., "Access to Medical Care for White and Black Americans: A Matter of Continuing Concern," *Journal of the American Medical Association* 261, no. 2 (1989): 278-81.

27. See note 25 above.

28. Ibid.

29. Ibid.

30. R.F. Murray, "Public Health Perspectives on Screening and Problems in Counseling Sickle Cell Anemia," in *Genetic Issues in Public Health Medicine*, ed. A. Cohen, A. Lilenfield, and R. Glass (Springfield, Ill.: Charles C. Thomas, 1978), 264-79.

31. See note 25 above.

32. National Coalition of Hispanic Health and Human Service Organizations, "Overcoming Language Barriers: Working with Interpreters," *Across Cultures* 2, no. 4 (1988): 1-2.

33. See note 15 above.

34. M. Epperson, "Families in Sudden Crisis: Process and Intervention in a Critical Care Center," *Social Work in Health Care* 2 (1977): 265-73.

35. E. Silverman, "The Social Worker's Role in Shock Trauma Units," *Social Work* 31, no. 4 (1986): 311-13.

36. See note 32 above.

37. M.V. Joseph, "Social Work Ethics: Historical and Contemporary Perspectives," *Social Thought* 15, no. 3-4 (1989): 4-17.

38. National Association of Social Workers (NASW), *Code of Ethics* (Washington, D.C.: NASW, 1988).

39. See note 19 above.

40. J. La Puma and E.R. Priest, "Medical Staff Privileges for Ethics Consultants: An Institutional Model," *Quality Review Bulletin* 18, no. 1 (1992): 17-20.

41. See note 1 above.

42. Ibid.

43. R.G. Dean and M.L. Rhodes, "Ethical-Clinical Tensions in Clinical Practice," *Social Work* 37, no. 2 (1992): 128-32.

27

No Time for Ethics?
The Prehospital Environment

Sue Shevlin Edwards
and Andrew B. Edwards

INTRODUCTION

It is generally recognized that the "goal" of ethical decision making is the determination of what ought to be done (that is, what would be the most ethically appropriate course of action) in a specific set of circumstances. More often than not, these circumstances are sufficiently complicated that the decision to be made is a difficult, or at least morally uncomfortable, one. After all, if the choice to be made were simple, there would not be an ethical dilemma. Thus, the process of making such decisions is recognized as requiring a great deal of careful thought and deliberation to reason through the situation and arrive at some sort of ethically justifiable resolution. Such a reflective process would appear to require both a reasonably calm setting and a certain amount of time, elements that are noticeably lacking in any emergency situation and most especially in the prehospital setting (generally understood as the environment in which medical care, usually of an urgent or emergency nature, is provided outside of or prior to the arrival at a hospital or other appropriate healthcare facility).

Consequently, some have suggested that ethics in such a setting is an "oxymoron,"[1] and that the application of an ethical decision-making process to the unique problems of emergency medicine is simply not possible. Given the need to think and act quickly if harm (or, more likely, further harm) is to be avoided, some argue that an appeal to a thoughtful and considered decision-making process cannot occur—thus necessitating that certain decisions be made on the basis of clinical, legal, or other criteria. Proponents of such a view claim that, in a crisis, there is no time for ethics.

This need not be the case, however. Although it is true that the realities of the prehospital emergency environment can make lengthy ethical deliberations on the scene quite difficult (if not impossible), it does not necessarily follow that there is no way to address the ethical concerns that inevitably arise in the context of these situations. The process of ethical analysis can still be of great assistance, even in urgent or critical circumstances.[2] What is required, however, is an adaptation of the conventional process such that it can account for the unique aspects of emergency medical care and, consequently, provide assistance to those who are faced with ethical dilemmas in medical emergencies.

WHAT MAKES MEDICAL EMERGENCIES DIFFERENT?

Medical emergencies—situations in which "the life or future physical functioning of patients is immediately threatened, or when patients are suffering severe pain"[3]—are different. They imply a "special" situation, an exception to the rules of normal action in light of the seriousness of the situation and its urgent nature. Such emergencies generally occur very quickly and without warning. They call for immediate action of some kind in order to avoid serious or even dire consequences, even at the risk of overlooking considerations that would otherwise be very important. The fact that one finds oneself faced with a bona fide emergency—especially one in which medical treatment of the victims will be necessary—seems to call for a shift in focus to an often single-minded, action-oriented approach in behavior. Nowhere is this more true than in the prehospital environment.

Medical services provided in the out-of-hospital setting clearly possess several characteristics that differentiate them from care delivered in other healthcare settings, even the emergency department. It is the prehospital care providers—first responders (persons with various levels of medical training who are notified of an emergency and respond to the scene but who do not generally transport patients, such as police officers or firefighters), emergency medical technicians (EMTs), or paramedics—who first encounter the victim and begin to render needed care. They can arrive in the midst of the critical incident (such as during a fire or while the drowning person is still in the water) or immediately thereafter (such as following a motor vehicle accident or a shooting). Some providers, depending upon their skills and level of training, may even be required to perform certain nonmedical duties (such as extrication from a damaged vehicle or burning building) in addition to the necessary medical assistance. Because these are the people who the rest of us call when there is an emergency, it stands to reason that they are also the ones who most directly experience the unique and demanding characteristics of such crises. These characteristics include lack of time, limited access to necessary information, and absence of control. All of these contribute to the sense that the normal "rules" do not apply and, consequently, many of the elements that are often taken for granted in the provision of other forms of healthcare are simply not possible or are altered significantly in the prehospital environment.

THE ELEMENT OF CHOICE

One of the major differences that is encountered regarding medical care provided in emergency situations is the lack of choice that often exists, from the perspective of the patient as well as the healthcare provider. In contrast to most other situations in which medical care is sought and in which patients usually have the ability to select their care providers, individuals who require urgent medical attention often have no such choice. Because of the immediacy of the situation, it is often imperative that care be sought (or provided) by the first available source, regardless of personal preference. Patients may, in certain cases, even find themselves in the awkward (and uncomfortable) position of being transported by some external force to receive care that is not necessarily desired (such as court-ordered care, treatment relating to suicide attempts, or services provided to persons of questionable cognitive abilities). Understandably, the patient's initial reaction may be one of fear or anger. He or she may react irrationally as a result of disbelief or denial of the seriousness of the situation,[4] thus making it even more difficult to provide needed medical attention. Clearly, these sorts of situations represent a significant departure from the "norm," in terms of our perceptions regarding the delivery of healthcare.

Emergency situations may impose certain choice limitations on healthcare providers as well. The American Medical Association's *Principles of Medical Ethics* directs (in a statement whose sentiment is shared in other professional codes) that, "[a] physician shall, in the provision of appropriate patient care, *except in emergencies* [emphasis added] be free to choose whom to serve, with whom to associate, and the environment in which to provide medical services."[5] In other areas of healthcare, providers are generally thought to have some discretion over who they will treat and in what setting. But, in an emergency, such discretion no longer exists; treatment must be provided to those in need.

This is especially true for prehospital care providers for whom this lack of choice is an inherent part of their job. By virtue of their roles, these persons are usually the first persons to respond. They are also required physically to go to the individuals who have suffered an illness or injury, unlike those who work in an emergency department, whose patients come to them. EMTs and paramedics may be called to a wide variety of localities that are frequently dangerous, remote, or otherwise uninviting. They may also be required to deliver care to patients in less-than-optimal circumstances or to those who are potentially dangerous (for example, patients who are intoxicated, mentally unstable, or combative). Although there are limits to the extent of the risks that healthcare providers can reasonably be expected to undertake in providing emergency care, the obligations that they assume when they take on the role of emergency healthcare providers can be extensive and often require placing themselves in perilous or even potentially life-threatening positions.

ABSENCE OF PATIENT-PROVIDER RELATIONSHIP

Further, it can be difficult, if not impossible, to establish or maintain a typical "patient-provider" relationship, given the unique aspects of a medical emergency. Often absent are the trust, comfort, knowledge of medical history and patient (and provider) values, and continuity of relationship that are central to the contemporary norm of collaboration regarding the relationship between healthcare providers and patients.[6] In the prehospital setting, especially, there is rarely an opportunity for the provider to get to know the patient; on the contrary, providers must often interact with patients they do not know anything about, who did not choose them as care providers, and who do not like or even trust them.[7]

In addition, other elements such as the patient's fear, pain, and/or anxiety—an often natural result of finding oneself in a medical emergency—may contribute to the difficulties inherent in establishing a meaningful relationship between patient and provider. For instance, the transient nature of medical care provided in emergency situations may be a significant factor. Patients may present themselves for treatment of a specific urgent problem, be treated, and never be seen by that provider again. The problem is exacerbated in situations where the patient is initially treated by an EMT or paramedic, transported to a hospital where responsibility for the patient's care is transferred to the emergency department staff, and subsequently transferred to a medical floor or intensive care unit (ICU). It can be difficult for patients to feel connected to these providers (and vice versa) with whom they spend very little time and will most likely never again interact.

Furthermore, the lack of time and the need for immediate action in an emergency can produce the undesirable, but often unavoidable, consequence of the providers' ignoring the stated wishes of the patient in an effort to provide the needed medical intervention as quickly as possible. This paternalistic attitude—although sometimes justifiable—does nothing to improve patient-provider relations. Moreover, it is not uncommon for patients to be unconscious, unresponsive, confused, or uncommunicative—thus precluding completely any sort of participatory relationship. In such instances, providers can gain no insight or knowledge regarding the patient other than the information they can obtain through observation, which may be incomplete, misleading, or erroneous. Providers in such circumstances must proceed as best they can with only the commitment to the patient's best interests—however those may be determined—to guide them.

UNPREDICTABLE SITUATIONS

Unlike other forms of medical care, which are provided in a relatively organized fashion, emergency medical care is almost defined by the unexpected and the unknown. Emergency care providers, in both the prehospital and emergency department environments, have no way of knowing or controlling how many patients they will have at any given time. They must often coordinate the care of many patients at once and do their best to ensure that no patient's quality of care is compromised.[8] Moreover, injured or sick individuals in an emergency setting may not "present" the way one might expect. Depending upon what has transpired and the nature of the injury, the patient's condition may be significantly more (or less) critical than it initially appears.

One of the strange aspects of out-of-hospital medicine is that things do not always appear as they should. It is difficult to explain how someone with two bullet holes in the chest can walk up to the healthcare provider and say that he or she has been shot and doesn't really feel well. Just because the patient is not lying on the ground bleeding to death does not mean the provider can sit and visit with him or her for the next 10 minutes.[9] This potential for patients' conditions to change suddenly can result in the unexpected need for additional medical attention or a sudden and immediate change in the original plan of treatment.

Of additional concern is the difficulty created by the sometimes limited availability of resources. In any emergency medical situation, and especially in the prehospital environment, providers may not have access to many of the things they need to provide the best possible care. Depending upon the nature of the emergency as well as the location in which it has occurred (for example, a motor vehicle accident in which the car has rolled down into a ravine, a skiing accident in which the victims are trapped as the result of an avalanche, or a flood in which the victims are trapped in the middle of a swollen river), specialized medical or extrication equipment may not be readily accessible, appropriate assistance may not be available, and significant delays may be encountered in providing the needed aid. Providers may therefore be left feeling frustrated and inadequate by the absence of necessary elements of providing care.

PATIENT AND PROVIDER STRESS

It is not uncommon for a high level of stress to accompany the provision of emergency medical care. In many cases, such as that of a motor vehicle or other accident, there may be a great deal of activity taking place at the scene, including the presence of a number of people engaged in a variety of activities, some who are involved in providing medical care and others who are not. If multiple victims are involved, the necessity may arise for some sort of triage decisions to be made about who can and cannot be treated and how quickly they will receive attention. Communication (among providers, between providers and patients, and so forth) may also be limited or even impossible, depending upon the circumstances, resulting in increased anxiety on the part of the victims and the would-be rescuers. For the patient, the stress incurred in these kinds of situations can produce several understandable but often counterproductive reactions—including fear, anxiety, anger, belligerence, noncompliance, and violence—which can have the unfortunate result of complicating an already critical situation and making the provision of care that much more difficult.

EMTs and paramedics must be prepared to deal with such circumstances on a day-to-day basis. Furthermore, those in need of assistance are depending upon these providers to "get them out" and to provide the necessary treatment. This reliance can produce a certain amount of pressure on these individuals who—although well-trained and thoroughly professional in their jobs—are human too and may be subject to the influences of a variety of factors, such as personality traits, physical health, the dynamic of interactions among people, hunger, fatigue, pride, feelings of invulnerability (or vulnerability), and concern for others.[10] Providers may also be particularly affected by the realization that a great deal is depending upon their actions—namely, the lives and health of the people that they rescue. The provision of care in medical emergencies is particularly unforgiving of mistakes.

THE EMS SYSTEM

The provision of prehospital care is unique with respect to its dependence upon interrelationships between a number of healthcare providers at a variety of levels of training. Stephen Frew describes this phenomenon by noting: "The provision of emergency medical services is based on the concept of delegated practice and requires the exercise of medical direction and physician control over the EMS system and prehospital providers."[11]

The emergency medical services (EMS) system is viewed as a complex healthcare system that is composed of many different individuals, including dispatchers (a communications center), prehospital care providers (first responders, EMTs, paramedics, flight nurses, and so forth), emergency department staff (physicians, nurses, technicians, and so forth), as well a variety of support personnel. All of these individuals must work together in the context of a coordinated approach to provide a continuum of care in medical emergencies that occur outside of the hospital. Clearly, in order to avoid chaos, a certain "chain of command" must be followed. This is accomplished via the establishment of a medical director and the notion of medical control that governs the actions of the actual providers in the field. Two methods have been established by which prehospital providers can access medical control: "direct medical control" (direct communication with a physician) and "indirect medical control" (the use of protocols, training and education, and quality assurance that helps provide a standard for accountability).[12] Emergency care rendered by EMTs and paramedics is therefore provided under the direction of a physician, allowing them to be considered in some sense as "physician extenders." It is important to recognize, however, that the physician serving in the capacity of medical control has no direct contact with the patients being treated. Thus, despite the availability of medical control, it is often the prehospital providers who must confront the difficult decisions that arise in a medical emergency and who must choose how to proceed. This can result in disagreements between the providers and their medical-control physician about what is the appropriate course of action given the circumstances. Such conflicts can result in awkward relationships among individuals who must work together on an ongoing basis.

ETHICAL ISSUES IN THE PREHOSPITAL SETTING

Although a number of ethical concerns arise in the context of providing medical care in the prehospital environment, the following issues represent some of those that are most often encountered, and are most troubling, to prehospital providers.

INFORMED CONSENT/CAPACITY

The issue of informed consent is one of the most common sources of ethical conflicts for EMS providers,[13] as well as one of the most complicated. In general, our society accepts the rights of rational adults to make decisions about their medical treatment and to refuse any therapy if they so choose. Furthermore, it is asserted that persons should give "informed consent" for any treatment that is provided—that is, adult individuals who are capable of making decisions should be given appropriate and understandable information about the proposed course of action and then be allowed to choose freely whether to proceed with the intervention. To be considered capable of giving valid informed consent, patients should possess the ability to (1) understand relevant information about the treatment in question; (2) appreciate the nature of their current condition and its potential consequences; (3) engage in a rational decision-making process; and (4) make and communicate a choice (see Exhibit 27-1).[14] However, as a result of patients' injuries or medical condition, patients' decision-making capacities and, thus their ability to give informed

---

Exhibit 27-1
Valid Informed Consent

Requires patients to be able to:
1.   Understand relevant information about the treatment in question
2.   Appreciate the nature of their current condition and its potential consequences
3.   Engage in a rational decision-making process
4.   Make and communicate a choice

---

consent, may be questioned. Situations involving patients who are in pain, who are having difficulty breathing, who have experienced a period of unconsciousness, or who are in shock are examples of circumstances in which providers may be uncomfortable regarding patients' decisions about their treatment.

EMS providers often find themselves in a quandary about how to proceed with patients whose mental capacities may be diminished. Although they may acknowledge that rational adults generally have the right to make their own decisions, EMS providers may also believe that they have a duty to provide treatment to those who need it. When patients refuse what the providers feel is necessary treatment, the providers may feel obligated to discount this refusal, arguing that the patient is not capable of making a rational decision in his or her current debilitated state. The overwhelming desire to do what may be perceived as being in the patient's best interest is seen as a legitimate reason to proceed despite the patient's objections. Failure to provide necessary treatment in such a case may be viewed not only as violation of one's professional obligations but also as good grounds for a lawsuit.

Unfortunately, in their well-intentioned (but sometimes misplaced) desire to serve the best interest of the patient, prehospital providers may assume a lack of decision-making capacity where none exists. In cases involving elderly or intoxicated patients, for example, the presumption may be made that the individual cannot make an informed decision and should therefore be treated and transported regardless of his or her wishes. Because these patients' decisions do not agree with providers' perceptions that immediate intervention is required, the argument may be made that the ability of such patients to make appropriate decisions must obviously be compromised. Rather than take the chance that the patient might actually be making a reasonable and informed decision and then later be proven wrong when the patient gets worse or dies, providers often feel that the safest course of action, for both the patient and themselves, is to provide needed treatment and transportation to the hospital, regardless of the patient's objections.

Such reasoning has a long history in the tradition of emergency medicine, and it may not be entirely unfounded. There is a great deal of credibility in the assertion that in the face of uncertainty it is generally better to provide treatment that will save a patient's life despite the patient's objections. More often than not, patients are grateful to be alive after the crisis has passed; and in situations where they are not, it may be possible to provide support or necessary assistance for the patient's benefit. By the same token, this does not mean that patients' desires can simply be discounted in emergency situations where they happen to disagree with providers' perceptions of what would be best. Although time is often limited in such situations, it may still be possible to make a good-faith effort to ascertain whether the patient possesses the ability to make rational decisions. Certainly, saving the patient's life should be the primary concern; however, respect for his or her autonomy should also be considered.

PRIVACY/CONFIDENTIALITY

Maintaining the confidentiality of patients' private information is a special challenge in the prehospital environment. Often, very little information is available regarding the individuals whom the EMTs and paramedics are called to treat; consequently, providers may focus on obtaining whatever details of the patient's history they can, sometimes with little concern for the protection of what may be personal or private information. The intention of the providers is not to be insensitive to maintaining patients' confidences, but rather to do whatever is necessary to provide the best medical care for those patients.

Confidentiality issues may also occur as a result of, or in relation to, the commission of some illegal offense. For example, a patient who is being treated at the scene of a motor-vehicle accident may "confess" to the EMT treating him that the collision was his fault but then ask the EMT to promise not to tell the police. Or a woman may tearfully reveal to the paramedic treating her child who "fell" down a flight of stairs that the child's intoxicated father actually pushed the little girl, insisting that the paramedic not report the father lest he return and do the same thing (or worse) to her. In some cases, such as situations involving child abuse or gunshot wounds, prehospital providers are legally required to report whatever information they have to the proper authorities. However, in other situations there may be no such clear-cut guidelines and providers must determine the extent of their duty to maintain confidentiality. As in other healthcare settings, there is a significant obligation to protect the patient's private information; however, this obligation is not absolute and may be overridden in the interest of stronger, more compelling moral considerations, such as prevention of harm to specified others.[15]

DECISIONS AT THE END OF LIFE

Prehospital advance directives and DNR orders. Ethical conflicts involving dying patients are among the most dramatic and emotionally difficult for prehospital providers (although they do not occur as often as one might think, given the amount of attention they have received). The major focus of prehospital care has traditionally been the saving of lives that would otherwise be lost due to unexpected illness or injury. The EMT or paramedic's job was to do whatever it took to preserve the life of the patient and then to transport the patient to the appropriate healthcare facility for further care. In general, it was safe to assume that most individuals for whom an ambulance was called were interested in continued life and would therefore desire that everything possible be done to accomplish this goal.

In the early days of EMS, prior to the 1960s, the services provided in the prehospital setting were minimal. When an emergency situation that required medical care arose, victims were transported to the hospital by whoever happened to be available, often family members, members of local fire department rescue squads who had little (if any) medical training, or funeral-home-operated ambulance services. In 1966, however, "Accidental Death and Disability: The Neglected Disease of Modern Society" (commonly referred to as "The White Paper") was published, which described the inadequacies of emergency medical care and made recommendations regarding how care in both the prehospital and emergency room setting could be improved.[16] In the years that followed, training programs for EMTs and paramedics were developed, as were national standards regarding the provision of emergency medical care. As medical knowledge and technology have progressed, so too have the abilities of prehospital providers to render more advanced and effective treatment.

Prehospital medicine, like other areas of healthcare, is now faced with patients who are terminally ill and do not desire lifesaving treatment. Moreover, some of these dying patients wish to receive care that will help alleviate suffering in the dying process. In an effort to respect the patient's wishes regarding how he or she wishes to die, care that can be provided may vary from simply helping the patient to achieve a more comfortable position as he peacefully expires to administering pain medication, ventilatory support, and any aggressive measures other than actual cardiopulmonary resuscitation (CPR).

This points out the obvious complexities inherent in the prehospital provision of end-of-life care. Because of the time and information limits imposed in the emergency environment, some type of uniform, simple, and definitive written statement must be immediately available to EMS providers that indicates the patient's wishes regarding what treatment, if any, is desired. In an effort to meet this need and to simplify the medical and legal issues surrounding the use of advance directive in the prehospital setting, a number of states have implemented *prehospital* advance directives (initiated by the patient) or *prehospital* do-not-resuscitate (DNR) orders (physicians' orders). These instruments are specifically designed to communicate the required information in a form that can be quickly and easily interpreted by EMS providers. The standardized forms, which were developed specifically for use in the prehospital environment, are designed to avoid the confusion that often results from using advance directives and DNR orders intended for use in other healthcare settings. Because such general forms are not designed to facilitate immediate recognition of the patient's wishes in a crisis situation, they usually do not contain the sort of simple and specific direction necessary to the prehospital provider. Instead, they frequently include a significant amount of information regarding the patient's overall value system, which—although important to other healthcare providers in ascertaining the patient's wishes for care and goals for treatment at the end of life—simply requires too much time for the EMS provider to read through in the face of an emergency situation. Further, an advance directive or a DNR order can be written in many ways, using a variety of different forms (such as those available from healthcare institutions, the local hospital association, the state bar association, or commercial publishers for general use) or no form at all (that is, simply written on a piece of paper and signed). The use of a standard form eliminates the necessity of providers having to determine which forms are appropriate for use in their jurisdiction (since there is only one state-approved prehospital form) and having to read through a lengthy and cumbersome document in order to ascertain what the patient does or does not want done.

Futility. It has traditionally been accepted that treatment of patients in medical emergencies should be initiated except in cases of "obvious death" (that is, rigor mortis, dependent lividity, decapitation or transection of the body, and/or incineration).[17] (See Exhibit 27-2.)

Exhibit 27-2
EMS Cases of Obvious Death Not Requiring Resuscitation Attempts

---

1.   Rigor mortis
2.   Dependent lividity
3.   Decapitation
4.   Transection of body
5.   Incineration

In some cases, however, the initiation or continuation of life-sustaining treatment may be futile. Recent studies[18] have indicated that certain patients (for example, patients with specific heart rhythms, patients with previous existing medical conditions, patients who do not receive CPR within the appropriate time frame, and so on) do not respond to prehospital advanced life support efforts and rarely benefit from ongoing resuscitation in the hospital. This finding has lead to significant discussion, particularly in the EMS community, regarding the appropriate use of basic and advanced cardiac life support. In some cases, it is argued, it is medically and ethically inappropriate to initiate or continue to provide resuscitative efforts to those patients who have little or no likelihood of benefitting from them. In fact, the preface of the 1994 edition of the American Heart Association's (AHA's) Advanced Cardiac Life Support (ACLS) textbook notes that "most . . . ACLS efforts for people with cardiac arrest will fail. The majority of resuscitation attempts end with death."[19] Given this fact, healthcare providers, including those in the prehospital environment, need to recognize those situations in which continued CPR is not warranted. "For many people the last beat of the heart should be the last beat of the heart . . . CPR and ECC are meant to reverse premature death. They should restore the process of living, not prolong the process of dying. When people reach the end of life, continued resuscitative efforts are inappropriate, futile, undignified, and demeaning to both the patient and rescuers."[20]

In light of the limited expected benefits associated with resuscitation in certain circumstances, as well as the substantial commitment of human and other resources such efforts require, it has been suggested that serious discussion is needed regarding the creation of standards to deal with the issues surrounding futile care of patients in the prehospital setting. Recommendation for dealing with these concerns may include developing protocols by EMS authorities for initiation and withdrawal of resuscitative efforts,[21] developing legislation regarding prehospital advance directives and DNR orders, and encouraging advance-care planning for persons with end-stage or terminal disease processes.

SAFETY

Prehospital providers face threats from several fronts as a result of the individuals with whom they interact as well as the environments in which they must function. The unique nature of prehospital emergency care is vividly described by the ethics committee of the National Association of Emergency Medical Services Physicians: "The pre-hospital provider must frequently interact and negotiate with reluctant patients, counsel those patients who ask for advice or refuse care, . . . assume some degree of personal risk in the care of agitated, uncooperative, or infectious patients, deal with social and psychiatric challenges, and respond to a variety of unusual requests which may not be medical in nature."[22] All of these factors can clearly affect EMTs and paramedics and affect their ability to provide effective care.

Assaults on providers in the prehospital environment are a growing cause for concern. A 1994 study concluded that occupational violence is an increasing problem for EMS providers.[23] EMTs and paramedics must be acutely aware of the potential for individuals to become angry and strike out at them as a result of the confusion, pain, or anxiety that often accompanies illness or injury. Increasing violence in U.S. urban areas further subjects providers to an increased risk of injury from attacks in which they may not even be the intended victim (as in the case of drive-by shootings or incidents of domestic violence). Moreover, hostile, combative, confused, agitated, or mentally unstable patients are by no means uncommon in this environment and may present substantial challenges to providers.

In addition, certain inherent risks are associated with the provision of healthcare in general, which are exacerbated by the characteristics of prehospital medicine. As in the case of other healthcare providers, those working in EMS may become unwittingly infected by patients with diseases such as hepatitis, tuberculosis, human immunodeficiency virus (HIV), or meningitis. However, the opportunity for those in the prehospital setting to determine the extent of this risk is extremely limited, given the lack of time, privacy, and diagnostic facilities that exist outside of a hospital or other clinical setting. It is also possible that those patients who present a cause for concern to the provider will not even be transported to the hospital, where effective evaluation of their health status could be made, because they refuse or do not require further medical treatment. In some cases, the source of the risk may not be the patient at all, but rather another individual at the scene or an object (such as an unseen needle, a knife, or a piece of broken glass). Exposure to potentially infected blood or body fluids from any of these sources could result in the development of a serious or life-threatening disease.

Prehospital workers may also experience certain difficulties that are not often encountered by other healthcare providers regarding their ability to protect themselves from the danger of disease transmission. In an effort to protect themselves adequately in the frequently unsafe surroundings in which they must work, EMS providers are supposed to wear heavy, thick protective gear that makes effective assessment and treatment quite difficult. To allow greater ease of movement (and, thus, to facilitate more effective patient care), providers sometimes choose to wear thinner, lightweight equipment that satisfies the requirements of universal precautions but provides little protection from the environment. The implications of this choice are highlighted in situations such as the scene of a motor-vehicle accident (which involves working around sharp metal and large amounts of broken glass in the confined space of a badly damaged automobile) or the provision of care in an area of high intravenous-drug use (where needles are routinely left and may be hidden from direct view).

There is an additional exposure risk faced by those in prehospital settings that is rarely experienced by other healthcare workers. This is the potential contamination of individuals from hazardous materials that may be present at the scene to which EMS providers are called. Many chemicals are quite toxic and may, in some be cases, be difficult to detect. Moreover, the potential danger may not even be recognized until after the exposure has already occurred. This is a significant cause for concern, because many of these materials have potentially serious, even lethal, long-term effects.

RESEARCH

There has been a great deal of concern expressed regarding the issue of medical research performed in the emergency setting. Patients in such situations are often unable, as a result of their medical condition, to give consent for the proposed experimental treatments. The problem is accurately described in the Consensus Statement from the Coalition Conference of Acute Resuscitation and Critical Care Researchers in the following passage: "Prospective informed consent in the emergency setting is often impractible and sometimes impossible when patients have sustained cardiac arrest, severe head injury, drug overdose, or other catastrophic medical or traumatic event. The medical condition may develop rapidly and without warning and may render the patient unable to give consent."[24]

Traditionally, in research situations where the patient is not able to give consent, a suitable proxy (such as a relative or guardian) has been sought. However, such surrogates are often not available in emergency settings due to time and other constraints; thus researchers seem to be left with the options of either not conducting the studies at all or doing so without proper informed consent.

One attempt to address this conflict is the notion of "deferred consent," which was suggested by Fost and Robertson in 1980.[25] This procedure would allow patients who meet the protocol inclusion criteria to be preliminarily enrolled in a study without informed consent in certain, specific circumstances. Continued participation of such individuals would then have to be authorized within a specified amount of time by an appropriate surrogate or by the patient him- or herself, should that become possible. Without such authorization, the patient's inclusion in the protocol would be discontinued.

The concept of deferred consent was initially well received in the research community. As Robert Levine notes, "Although there were arguments about the ethical and legal rationale for its justification, no federal official challenged the validity of its use in research funded or regulated by the federal government."[26] This changed, however, in 1993 when the Office for Protection from Research Risks (OPRR) at the National Institutes of Health (NIH) issued a notice that institutional review boards (IRBs) were no longer to approve studies that contained more than a "minimal risk" (defined as an anticipated probability of harm that does not exceed what an individual would probably encounter during a routine physical examination or in daily life) to participants if researchers could not prospectively obtain informed consent. Because the types of treatments or interventions to be studied in the provision of emergency medical care are generally considered likely to present more than this "minimal risk," this statement by the OPRR resulted in a halt to much of the research in this area. (See chapter 8, "Ethics in Critical Care Research," for further discussion of emergency research.)

This was unfortunate, especially in light of the significant potential benefits of research conducted (and the previous lack of research efforts), particularly in the prehospital emergency setting. Many of the medical advances that have occurred (such as the use of automatic defibrillators or thrombolytics in the field) are the result of emergency research, research that was, by necessity, conducted on patients in the prehospital environment. In addition, in some cases the experimental intervention may be the only available option for treatment of certain medical conditions. If researchers are not given the ability to continue to perform studies on these treatments, the likelihood of developing further lifesaving techniques for use in the emergency setting becomes extremely low.

Furthermore, medical treatment that is provided in the field may differ significantly form the same types of treatment delivered in the ICU or in the emergency department. For this reason, studies conducted in the prehospital environment are especially important, as they allow researchers to evaluate the effectiveness of the proposed interventions in exactly the sorts of situations in which they will be required to function. After all, it is one thing to have data indicating that a certain thrombolytic agent works when given in the emergency department within one hour of the onset of an acute myocardial infarction (heart attack). It is quite another to extrapolate from that data the projected effectiveness of the same agent when administered under field conditions, for example, when given by a paramedic less than 10 minutes after the cardiac event. Without appropriate research on the specific treatment modalities as they are used in prehospital situations, EMS providers must work virtually "in the dark," which prevents them from delivering the best possible care to their patients.

Moreover, it is not only new procedures that need to be studied, but also current standards of care already in use, in order to assess their effectiveness and safety. Some procedures that may have been accepted over time as clinically beneficial interventions are now being questioned (for example, pneumatic antishock trousers and fluid resuscitation). Without further research, it is not possible to assess the value of such treatments adequately. As Dr. Michael Callaham notes, "The harm of applying effective treatments to the wrong patients is not merely an academic concern. . . . Knowing nothing else about efficacy, the laws of probability guarantee that [applying treatments that have not been appropriately studied] will lead to decreasing effectiveness and increasing harm."[27]

Clearly, there are potential areas of concern with respect to research conducted in the prehospital environment. In addition to the previously stated difficulty regarding the obtaining of consent from incapacitated or unconscious patients, there is the further complication involved in trying to conduct any sort of reasonable informed consent process in the midst of a crisis. Even if the patient is capable of making decisions (a questionable proposition, at best, given the stress he or she is likely to be under as a result of the pain and anxiety associated with the illness or injury), there are other aspects of the situation that must be considered. These include the potentially coercive nature of the circumstances surrounding the request for consent, such that what the patient may essentially be presented with is a choice between agreeing to the experimental intervention that could save his or her life, or receiving a treatment that, although it is the standard, is considered less effective. It would be difficult for most, especially in the tense and rushed setting of a medical emergency, to objectively weigh the risks, benefits, and alternative options that have been presented.

In addition, there is the concern raised by the fact that, in many situations, the information about the research being conducted must be given to the patient by the EMS provider. The role of obtaining informed consent for research studies is one with which many EMTs and paramedics are not overly familiar (or comfortable), thus leading to questions about whether they are capable of adequately accomplishing this task. Concerns have been expressed regarding prehospital providers' abilities to understand and appropriately explain the protocol and to answer questions or problems articulated by patients or families. In response to this, however, James Adams has pointed out that, while these may be legitimate concerns, there are ways to address them effectively. He suggests that, with the participation and support of medical control, diligent IRB oversight, and the commitment of EMS providers, "there is no ethical or medical reason that good research cannot be carried out in the prehospital setting."[28]

After much discussion and consideration of these issues in the literature, both the Department of Health and Human Services (HHS) and the Food and Drug Administration (FDA) acknowledged the importance of conducting research in the emergency setting. In October of 1996 they announced their joint approval of a waiver of the informed consent requirements for "a strictly limited class of research."[29] The waiver, which is referred to as the "Emergency Research Consent Waiver," releases researchers from the requirement to obtain and document informed consent in research activities involving persons who are in need of emergency treatment but who cannot consent for themselves (because of their medical condition) and have no legally authorized person available to represent them.[30] The Emergency Research Consent Waiver outlines very specific criteria which must be met (see Exhibit 27-3), which include the requirement to inform the patient or the patient's family member that he or she has been enrolled in the study AND that they (the patient or family) may discontinue the subject's participation at any time.[31] Even in light of these strict criteria (and perhaps even because of them), the approval of the waiver by both the HHS and FDA, which took effect 1 November 1996, was a significant accomplishment for those conducting research in the emergency setting, especially given the acknowledgment

Exhibit 27-3
Emergency Research Consent Waiver

Pursuant to Section 46.101(i), the Secretary, HHS, has waived the general requirements for informed consent at 45 CFR 46.116(a) and (b) and 46.408, to be referred to as the "Emergency Research Consent Waiver" for a class of research consisting of activities, each of which have met the following strictly limited conditions detailed under *either* (a) or (b) below:

- **(a) Research subject to FDA regulation**
  The IRB responsible for the review, approval, and continuing review of the research activity has approved both the activity and a waiver of informed consent and found and documented:
- (1) That the research activity *is subject* to regulations codified by the Food and Drug Administration (FDA) (see **Federal Register**, vol. 61, pp. 51498-51531) at Title 21 CFR Part 50 and will be carried out under an FDA investigational new drug application (IND) or an FDA investigational device exemption (IDE), the application for which has clearly identified the protocols that would include subjects who are unable to consent, and
- (2) That the requirements for exception from informed consent for emergency research detailed in **21 CFR Section 50.24** have been met relative to those protocols, **or**
- **(b) Research not subject to FDA regulation**
  The IRB responsible for the review, approval, and continuing review of the research has approved both the research and a waiver of informed consent and has (i) found and documented that the research *is not subject* to regulations codified by the FDA at 21 CFR Part 50, and (ii) found and documented and reported to the OPRR that the following conditions have been met relative to the research:
- (1) The human subjects are in a life-threatening situation, available treatments are unproven or unsatisfactory, and the collection of valid scientific evidence, which may include evidence obtained through randomized placebo-controlled investigations, is necessary to determine the safety and effectiveness of particular interventions.
- (2) Obtaining informed consent is not feasible because:
  - (i) the subjects will not be able to give their informed consent as a result of their medical condition;
  - (ii) the intervention involved in the research must be administered before consent from the subjects' legally authorized representatives is feasible; and
  - (iii) there is no reasonable way to identify prospectively the individuals likely to become eligible for participation in the research.
- (3) Participation in the research holds out the prospect of direct benefit to the subjects because:
  - (i) subjects are facing a life-threatening situation that necessitates intervention;
  - (ii) appropriate animal and other preclinical studies have been conducted, and the information derived from those studies and related evidence support the potential for the intervention to provide a direct benefit to the individual subjects; and
  - (iii) risks associated with the research are reasonable in relation to what is known about the therapy, if any, and what is known about the risks and benefits of the prosed intervention or activity.

- (4) The research could not practicably be carried out without the waiver.
- (5) The proposed research protocol defined the length of the potential therapeutic window based on scientific evidence, and the investigator has committed to attempting to contact a legally authorized representative for each subject within that window of time and, if feasible, to asking the legally authorized representative contacted for consent within that window rather than proceeding without consent. The investigator will summarize efforts made to contact representatives and make this information available to the IRB at the time of continuing review.
- (6) The IRB has reviewed and approved informed consent procedures and an informed consent document in accord with Sections 46.116 and 46.117 of 45 CFR Part 46. These procedures and the informed consent document are to be used with subjects or their legally authorized representatives in situations where use of such procedures and documents is feasible. The IRB has reviewed and approved procedures and information to be used when providing an opportunity for a family member to object to a subject's participation in the research consistent with paragraph (b)(7)(v) of this waiver.
- (7) Additional protections of the rights and welfare of the subjects will be provided, including, at least:
    - (i) consultation (including, where appropriate, consultation carried out by the IRB) with representatives of the communities in which the research will be conducted and from which the subjects will be drawn;
    - (ii) public disclosure to the communities in which the research will be conducted and from which the subjects will be drawn, prior to initiation of the research, of plans for the research and its risks and expected benefits;
    - (iii) public disclosure of sufficient information following completion of the research to apprise the community and researchers of the study, including the demographic characteristics of the research population, and its results;
    - (iv) establishment of an independent data monitoring committee to exercise oversight of the research and;
    - (v) if obtained informed consent is not feasible and a legally authorized representative is not reasonably available, the investigator has committed, if feasible, to attempting to contact within the therapeutic window the subject's family member who is not a legally authorized representative, and asking whether he or she objects to the subject's participation in the research. The investigator will summarize efforts made to contact family members and make this information available to the IRB at the time of continuing review.

In addition, the IRB is responsible for ensuring that procedures are in place to inform, at the earliest feasible opportunity, each subject, or if the subject remains incapacitated, a legally authorized representative of the subject, or if such a representative is not reasonably available, a family member, of the subject's inclusion in the research, the details of the research and other information contained in the informed consent document. The IRB shall also ensure that there is a procedure to inform the subject, or if the subject remains incapacitated, a legally authorized representative of the subject, or if such a representative is not reasonably available, a family member, that he or she may discontinue the subject's participation at any time without penalty or loss of benefits to which the subject is otherwise entitled. If a legally authorized representative or family member is told about the research and the subject's condition improves, the subject is also to be informed as soon as feasible. If a subject is entered into research with a waived consent and the subject dies before a legally authorized representative or family member can be contacted, information about the research is to be provided to the subject's legally authorized representative or family member, if feasible.

For the purpose of this waiver "family member" means any one of the following legally competent persons: spouses; parents; children (including adopted children); brothers; sisters; and spouses of brothers and sisters; and any individual related by blood or affinity whose close association with the subject is the equivalent of a family relationship.

Source: the website < http://www.nih.gov/grants/oprr/hsdc97-01.htm >, "Emergency Research Consent Waiver," *Federal Register* 61, sec. 46.101(i), 51531-51533.

that, "The Secretary, HHS, is authorizing this waiver in response to grow-ing concerns that current regulations, absent this waiver, are making high quality research in emergency circumstances difficult or impossible to carry out at a time when the need for such research is increasingly recognized."[32]

DEALING WITH ETHICAL CONFLICTS IN THE PREHOSPITAL ENVIRONMENT

Without a doubt, decision making—especially ethical decision mak-ing in medical emergencies that occur outside of the hospital setting—is a difficult undertaking. There are a number of reasons for this, most of which are related to the unique features of these situations. It is not that the ethical issues that arise, or even that the process by which one would address them, is especially unusual or atypical; rather, it is the high-stress, crisis-oriented environment in which they occur that creates the difficul-ties encountered by EMS providers. Thus it becomes necessary to think in slightly different terms when "doing ethics" in these situations.

At the theoretical level, this implies a need to alter the paradigm. In much the same way that healthcare providers change focus in acute care medicine when the patient enters the dying process (from curing the patient's disease to providing palliative or comfort care and easing the dying process), we must alter our focus in emergency situations as well. Instead of placing the emphasis on trying to deal with ethical conflicts at the time they occur, we must direct our efforts to developing guidelines and provisions for addressing these issues before they occur, when there is a greater possibility for thoughtful consideration and deliberation.

The recognition that the special characteristics of prehospital emergency care require a different approach regarding ethical problems further implies the need for certain actions at the practical level. Primary among these is a comprehensive educational effort directed toward a wide variety of people, including physicians, nurses, prehospital providers, and emergency department staff. Currently, most of these persons receive a fairly limited amount of education in ethics and very little (if any) regarding ethical issues in emergency medical care. Except in some more progressive programs, the subject of ethics (apart from professional ethics) is omitted entirely from the curriculum for EMTs and paramedics. Those who are faced with such difficult issues must be made aware of the kinds of issues that arise and of strategies for resolving them. Such education would clearly have to focus on hypothetical cases that address real issues that occur in the prehospital setting or on real cases that occurred in the past.

Such training would be invaluable to those who find themselves confronted with the need to make complicated and sometimes agonizing decisions in the field. Although there are no simple answers regarding what one should do in any given situation, it is certainly possible to provide persons with the information and tools necessary to examine seriously the types of issues that arise, consider them in light of various options that are available, know about the decisions that have been made in the past regarding similar situations, and provide ethically appropriate and justifiable resolutions to these problems. Every situation is different and requires individual consideration; however, through continued educational efforts, prehospital providers and others can develop their abilities to think about ethically problematic situations before they arise and thus to be better prepared to address these issues when they encounter them.

In addition, other individuals, such as patients, families, politicians, allied health professionals, and members of the community at large, must become aware of the many ethical issues that arise in the provision of prehospital and emergency medical care. Significant education needs to take place regarding how the EMS system works and how those in the community can best take advantage of EMS services. Individuals must come to recognize the importance of legislative attempts to address ethical issues such as prehospital advance directives and DNR orders that help preserve their autonomy with regard to healthcare decisions made near or at the end of life. In addition, they must be made aware of potential benefits of research conducted in the area of emergency medicine and participate in discussions about how best to implement this kind of research in their communities. Most importantly, individuals need to recognize and acknowledge the value of EMS to the integrity of the community as well as to its individual members and to strongly support an EMS system that provides the best possible care to all members of society.

NOTES

1. J. Ducharme, "Ethics and Emergency Medicine: An Oxymoron?" *Calyx* 4, no. 3 (1994): 1.

2. D. Mathieu, "General Introduction," in *Ethics in Emergency Medicine*, 2nd ed., ed. K.V. Iserson, A.B. Sanders, and D. Mathieu (Tucson, Ariz.: Galen Press, 1995), 3-6.

3. M.P. Battin, "The Manipulative Patient, The Irresponsible Family, and The Nursing Home 'Dump,' " in *Ethics in Emergency Medicine*, 2nd ed., ed. K.V. Iserson, A.B. Sanders, and D. Mathieu (Tucson, Ariz.: Galen Press, 1995), 300-07, at 302.

4. J.R. Clarke, J.H. Sorenson, and J.E. Hare, "The Limits of Paternalism in Emergency Care," *Hastings Center Report* 10, no. 6 (December 1980): 20-22, at 21.

5. American Medical Association, Council on Ethical and Judicial Affairs, "Principles of Medical Ethics," in *Code of Medical Ethics* (Chicago: American Medical Association, 1994), *xiv*.

6. E.W.D. Young, "Current Ethical Issues in Emergency Care," *Journal of Emergency Nursing* 12, no. 5 (September-October 1986): 301-04.

7. A.B. Sanders, "Unique Aspects of Ethics in Emergency Medicine," in *Ethics in Emergency Medicine*, 2nd ed., ed. K.V. Iserson, A.B. Sanders, and D. Mathieu, (Tucson, Ariz.: Galen Press, 1995), 7-10, at 9.

8. American College of Emergency Physicians, "American College of Emergency Physicians Ethics Manual," *Annals of Emergency Medicine* 20, no. 10 (1991): 1153-62, at 1155.

9. M. Smith, "Up and Down the Decision Tree," *Journal of Emergency Medical Services* 20, no. 10 (October 1995): 25-26.

10. W.F. Rutherford, "When Good People Make Bad Decisions," *Air Medical Journal* 14, no. 3 (July-September 1995): 123-24, at 124.

11. S.A. Frew, "Emergency Medical Services Legal Issues for the Emergency Physician," *Emergency Medical Clinics of North America* 8, no. 1 (February 1990): 41-55, at 43.

12. B.E. Bledsoe, R.S. Porter, and B.R. Shade, eds., *Brady Paramedic Emergency Care*, 2nd ed. (Englewood Cliffs, N.J.: Prentice Hall, 1994), 21-24.

13. J.G. Adams, "Ethical Conflicts in the Prehospital Setting," *Annals of Emergency Medicine* 21, no. 10 (1992): 1259-65, at 1260.

14. P.S. Appelbaum and T. Grisso, "Assessing Patients' Capacities to Consent to Treatment," *New England Journal of Medicine* 319 (1988): 1635-38.

15. M.F. Marshall, "Respecting Privacy and Confidentiality," *Introduction to Clinical Ethics*, ed. J.C. Fletcher et al. (Frederick, Md.: University Publishing Group, 1995), 39-49, at 41.

16. Committee on Trauma and Committee on Shock, Division of Medical Services, *Accidental Death and Disability: The Neglacted Disease of Modern Society* (Washington, D.C.: National Academy of Sciences-National Research Council, 1966).

17. J.D. Heckman, ed., *Emergency Care and Transportation of the Sick and Injured*, 5th ed. Rosemont, Ill.: American Academy of Orthopaedic Surgeons, 1993), 78-79.

18. For further information on this, see W.A. Gray, "Prehospital Resuscitation: The Good, the Bad, and the Futile," *Journal of the American Medical Association* 270, no. 12 (1993): 1472; G. Lombardi, J. Gallagher and P. Glennis, "Outcomes of Out-of-Hospital Cardiac Arrest in New York City," *Journal of the American Medical Association* 271, no. 9 (1994):678-83; S. Glazer and W.A. Gray, "Futile Care: What is the Endpoint of Unsuccessful Field Resuscitation?" *Emergency Medical Services* (July 1995):65-66, 75; D.S. Siscovick, "Challenges in Cardiac Arrest Research Data," *Annals of Emergency Medicine* 22, no. 1 (1993): 92-98; M.J. Bonnin et al., "Distinct Criteria for Termination of Resuscitation in the Out-of-Hospital Setting," *Journal of the American Medical Association* 270, no. 12 (1993): 1457-62; A.L. Kellerman, B.B. Hackman, and G. Somes, "Predicting the Outcome of Unsuccessful Prehospial Advanced Cardiac Life Support," *Journal of the American Medical Association* 270, no. 12 (1993): 1433-36; W.D. Weaver, "Resuscitation Outside the Hospital: What's Lacking?" *New England Journal of Medicine* 325 (1991): 1393-98; W.A. Gray, R.J. Capone, and A.S. Most, "Unsuccessful Emergency Resuscitation: Are Continued Efforts in the Emergency Department Justified?" *New England Journal of Medicine* 325 (1991):1393-98; and J. Gallagher, G. Lombardi, and P. Glennis, "Effectiveness of Bystander Cardiopulmonary Resuscitation and Survival Following Out-of-Hospital Cardiac Arrest," *Journal of the American Medical Association* 274, no. 24 (1995): 1922-25.

19. American Heart Association, *Textbook of Advanced Cardiac Life Support* (Dallas, Tex.: AHA National Center, Emergency Cardiovascular Care Programs, 1997-99), *ix*.

20. Ibid., 1-71.

21. Ibid., 16-4.

22. Ethics Committee, National Association of Emergency Medical Services Physicians, "Ethical Challenges in Emergency Medical Services," *Prehospital and Disaster Medicine* 8, no. 2 (April-June 1993): 179-82, at 179.

23. D.W. Walsh, "Vested Interest: Why You Need Body Armor," *Journal of Emergency Medical Services* 19, no. 9 (1994): 62-65.

24. M.H. Biros et al., "Informed Consent in Emergency Research," *Journal*

of the American Medical Association 273, no. 16 (1995): 1283-87, at 1284.

25. N. Fost and J.A. Robertson, "Deferring Consent with Incompetent Patients in an Intensive Care Unit," *IRB: A Review of Human Subjects Research* 2, no. 7 (1980): 5-6.

26. R.J. Levine, "Research in Emergency Situations: The Role of Deferred Consent," *Journal of the American Medical Association* 273, no. 16 (1995): 1300-02, at 1301.

27. M. Callaham, "Quantifying the Scanty Science of Prehospital Emergency Care," *Annals of Emergency Medicine* 30, no. 6 (1997): 785-90, at 789.

28. J. Adams, "Prehospital Research and Informed Consent," in *Ethics in Emergency Medicine*, 2nd ed., ed. K.V. Iserson, A.B. Sanders, and D. Mathieu (Tucson, Ariz.: Galen Press, 1995), 142-46, at 145.

29. http://www.nih.gov/grants/oprr/hsdc97-01.htm, "Emergency Research Consent Waiver," *Federal Register* 61, sec. 46.101(i), 51531-51533.

30. Ibid., at page 1 of 4.

31. Ibid., at page 3 of 4.

32. Ibid.

28

Ethical Issues in Emergency Medicine

Kenneth V. Iserson

THE NATURE OF EMERGENCY MEDICINE

Good ethical decisions begin with good information. One of the unique aspects of emergency medical care is that clinicians often must act decisively without the benefit of good information. With the most critically ill and injured patients, they must often act in the patient's best interest without knowing what the patient or the patient's surrogate wants. Sometimes these interventions leave intensive care physicians with the uncomfortable duty of withdrawing medical treatments that emergency clinicians have started. To be effective, however, emergency clinicians, in both the prehospital and emergency department (ED) settings, must act within the short time period they have and with the sparse (and often inaccurate) information they receive. These imperatives may lead to professional conflicts between the emergency clinician and the intensive care practitioner if both do not understand the different ethical and medical imperatives each works under.

COMPONENTS OF EMERGENCY MEDICINE

Emergency medicine comprises two distinct practice environments—the prehospital arena and the ED. Prehospital care most commonly involves patients for whom ambulances have been called. These patients may be in homes, in long-term care facilities, or in public places. They may suffer from acute or chronic illnesses or injuries. Although the most acutely ill patients generally come from their homes or nursing homes, most seriously injured patients come from the street—the "knife and gun club" or motor-vehicle accidents.

Ambulance providers have varied skill levels and training. Although the following description varies from state to state, it is a reasonable classification for ambulance personnel. Some areas still have first responders who often have little more than very basic first aid training. Most communities now staff their ambulances with at least emergency medical technicians (EMTs), who have completed an approximately 100-hour course in basic stabilization, emergency childbirth, and cardiopulmonary resuscitation (CPR). Usually the only medication they can administer is oxygen.

Intermediate emergency medical technicians (IEMTs), who go by a variety of names across the country, have EMT training plus the ability to start intravenous lines, intubate, cardiovert arrhythmias, and administer a limited number of drugs (such as naloxone, thiamine, glucose, and sublingual nitroglycerin). Paramedics can do all the above plus read rhythm strips, give a wide variety of medications, and, in some areas, do cricothyrotomies and needle thoracostomies.

The prehospital environment also includes "wilderness" medicine—those areas distant from normal avenues of medical care where there may commonly be adverse interactions between people and the environment (such as undersea, space, mountains, deserts, caves, and woodlands). See Chapter 27 for a discussion of the prehospital environment.

The ED is the terminus of emergency medical systems. For critically ill or injured patients, this may not be the first ED to which they are brought. Smaller hospitals often send patients to tertiary-care EDs, which may be a long distance away. Transferring patients, even by air, may take several hours. The receiving facility often has little control over what is done for patients before they arrive. The transfer also places one additional barrier between clinicians and the information they need to make patient-oriented decisions.

NATURE OF EMERGENCY CARE

Emergency medical practitioners treat sudden, unexpected medical events. They also treat more mundane medical and surgical problems that could as well be treated in clinics. Often, this is because the patients do not have access to other sources of medical care. This is usually due to lack of funds but may also be because their normal source of care is unavailable (such as during the night, on weekends, and on holidays).

The nature of the emergency patient-clinician interaction differs significantly from the normal patient-clinician paradigm. Patients presenting in crisis to emergency medical services (EMS) or the ED often do not choose the ambulance they use or the hospital to which they go. When someone calls 911, the closest available ambulance is dispatched and, if the patient is *in extremis,* he or she is taken to the closest appropriate ED. Usually that means the closest ED, but in some communities it means specialized trauma, burn, or pediatric centers. Such patients do not know their clinicians, either in the ambulance or at the ED, and the clinicians similarly do not know their patients. Even if patients are aware, they have little way of knowing what qualifications the treatment team has, nor can they easily get other practitioners to treat them initially. Unlike in most medical situations, clinicians have little or no access to the patient's records—either because they do not know the patient's identity, no such records exist at the institution, the records cannot be located (the most common excuse is that they are checked out to a clinician), or they cannot be sent to the ED promptly. This often leaves emergency clinicians with little knowledge about a critical patient's medical history or his or her wishes about treatment. Due to the nature of the information provided and the manner in which it is passed on in emergencies (often third- or fourth-hand information), what information clinicians do get about the patient is often wrong—including even the circumstances surrounding the current problem.

Despite or because of this lack of information, emergency clinicians must act quickly and decisively. Physiological constraints impel emergency clinicians to act immediately if they are to restore breathing, stabilize cardiac activity, stop bleeding, or otherwise shore up a critically ill patient's condition. Intervening to save lives in the face of limited knowledge about patients or their medical condition is a hallmark of emergency medicine. Exhibit 28-1 describes the differences between emergency and primary care practices.

Although emergency clinicians also see nonemergency patients, where patients' lack of funding has them seeking most of their medical treatment in EDs, this constitutes a major distributive justice problem. This problem has been recognized and debated on a national scale, but emergency clinicians continue to act as the "safety net" within the U.S. healthcare "nonsystem."[1] This ethical dilemma is not one of emergency medicine, but of our entire society. Emergency clinicians just happen to be the recipients of our refusal to deal with the problem.

MEDICAL AND MORAL IMPERATIVES IN EMERGENCY MEDICINE

Emergency clinicians, in both the prehospital care and ED environments, operate with four imperatives: to save lives when possible, to

---

Exhibit 28-1

Differences between Emergency Practice and Primary Care Practice

Emergency Department	Primary Care
Patient often brought in by ambulance, police, etc.	Patient chooses to enter medical care system.
Patient does not choose a physician.	Patient chooses a physician.
ED personnel must gain the patient's trust.	Physician and nurse already enjoy patient's confidence and trust.
ED personnel do not know patient, family, values, etc.	Physician and nurse often know patient, family, values, etc.
Patient experiences an acute change in health.	Patient suffers from chronic medical problems.
Anxiety, pain, alcohol, and altered mental status are frequent.	Anxiety, pain, alcohol, and altered mental status are less frequent.
Decisions are made quickly.	There is usually time for reflection and deliberation.
Physician makes decisions on his or her own.	Physician has a greater opportunity to consult with patient, family, other physicians, ethics committees, lawyers, courts, ethicists, etc.
Physician represents institution and medical staff.	Physician represents himself, herself, or medical group.
Work environment is open and less controlled.	Work environment is private and controlled.
ED personnel frequently have a stressful work schedule.	Work schedule often set or cancelled by physician.

Reprinted from K.V. Iserson, A.B. Sanders, and D. Mathieu, *Ethics in Emergency Medicine,* 2nd ed. (Tucson, Ariz.: Galen Press, 1995). © 1995, Galen Press. Used with permission.

relieve pain and suffering, to comfort patients and families, and to protect staff and patients from injury. All but the last of these is also the imperative of most other clinicians, although saving lives may occur more often and more dramatically in emergency medical settings than in most other settings.

The imperative to save lives causes the most conflict between emergency and intensive care unit (ICU) clinicians. Emergency physicians know that some of the intubations and resuscitations they perform are unwanted by patients or their surrogates. Nearly all emergency physicians have gotten calls from irate intensivists or private practitioners berating them for resuscitating patients "who should not have been resuscitated." Many families have heard physicians berate the ED and ambulance staffs for their overly aggressive resuscitative efforts. Yet the life-saving imperative begins when the ambulance is called.

EMS personnel are required to attempt resuscitation except when there is no chance that life exists (for example, with decapitation, rigor mortis, person charred beyond recognition, or decomposition). They usually have little leeway about whom to resuscitate. The real answer is for primary physicians to educate their homebound or hospice patients' families not to call the ambulance (or police) when the person dies but rather to call the clinician to pronounce the person dead.

Recently, the emergency medicine community has developed a method to avoid medical interventions, even when the ambulance is inadvertently called. Variously termed prehospital advance directives or prehospital do-not-resuscitate (DNR) orders (the former is patient/surrogate directed while the latter is a physician's order), have proved very successful where they have been implemented.[2] They usually specify that intubation, artificial ventilation, cardioversion, and CPR should not be performed. (Only Arizona statute allows their use for children.)[3]

The last imperative, safety, is nearly unique within medicine to emergency medical clinicians. Both in the prehospital and in ED settings, clinicians often encounter dangerous situations from the environment (such as fires, wilderness, floods), patients, or families. Although most clinicians try to accommodate patients' rights, their priorities, when safety questions arise, are their own safety, the safety of their coworkers, and then the patient's safety. That does not imply that clinicians should ignore the patient's safety; however, if clinicians and their colleagues are at risk (often from the patient), they should first ensure their own safety.

SPECIFIC SITUATIONS

Although many ethical issues exist in emergency medicine, emergency clinicians and intensive care clinicians most commonly interact in the situations described below.

NONTRAUMATIC CARDIAC ARREST (ADULT OR CHILD)

CPR is one of the most dramatic events in emergency care. Begun at the home, at the place of work, or in the streets, CPR and advanced life support demonstrate that modern medicine can snatch people from the brink of death. Unfortunately, even with adequate CPR, the number of people who are successfully resuscitated is quite small. Even fewer leave the hospital with their brain function intact. However, without explicit and valid instructions to the contrary, emergency clinicians must give patients the benefit of CPR and advanced life support.

Emergency clinicians, on the scene or in EDs, must rely primarily on the response to their resuscitation attempts to determine who continues to receive therapy. While EMS personnel may avoid initiating CPR where the dying process clearly cannot be reversed (for example, with decapitation or the presence of rigor or livor mortis), in most situations this is not obvious. EMS personnel often have only a rough idea of how long patients have "been down" (which can mean unconscious, in cardiac arrest, or simply on the ground, depending on the observers) or of how much time has passed since the patient was last seen alive. They must act immediately if the person has any hope of resuscitation and cannot delay initiating resuscitation procedures to learn details of the patient's history. The simple fact that they were called for help mandates that they attempt to resuscitate the patient if a standard prehospital advance directive is not present.

This resuscitation continues into the ED, where emergency physicians act under the same constraints. Most often, unless EMS personnel revive the patient in the field or there are unusual predisposing circumstances (such as electrocution, hypothermia, or an inability to use cardioversion in the field), patients who arrive in the ED in cardiac arrest do not do well. Some do, however, and it is often impossible to know which ones will survive. That often causes strife between emergency physicians and intensive care physicians, such as when heart-lung-resuscitated patients with little chance of significant brain function occupy ICU beds. Knowledge of subsequent brain function is, however, a *post hoc* determination. Emergency clinicians have the professional and societally expected imperative to save lives. Their actions must be consistent with this inescapable requirement.

One of the most tragic events in an ED is the child in cardiac arrest. Although some arrests are the result of long-standing diseases, many result from sudden infant death syndrome (SIDS), drownings, other causes of suffocation, or overwhelming infections. Respiratory distress can often be easily remedied in children, but once cardiac arrest occurs secondary to noncardiac causes, the child has virtually no chance of a meaningful recovery (unlike adults, who often have a primary cardiac arrest). Yet emergency clinicians often spend inordinate time trying to resuscitate these children and often restore cardiac activity long enough to get them to the ICU, where they most often die or, occasionally, go into a persistent vegetative state. Emergency clinicians' attitudes in these cases stem from a mix of remorse for the child and parents, the normal uncertainty about inciting events, and a group feeling that they must try "extra hard" because the patient is a child. Pediatric intensive care physicians may have problems with this attitude. The only way they may effect a change is by educating the ED team about the outcomes of, and the research demonstrating the dismal prognoses of, such children.

TRAUMATIC CARDIAC ARREST

Patients presenting in cardiac arrest from trauma cannot normally be resuscitated. Cases where these patients are successfully resuscitated are either mistakes in diagnosis (not in cardiac arrest, but in shock with a controllable bleeding site) or patients with easily reversible lesions (such as tension pneumothorax). The ethical dilemmas stemming from traumatic "codes" result from the inappropriate use of prehospital, ED, and, sometimes, operating room and ICU resources. Only a small number of patients can be successfully resuscitated from traumatic cardiac arrests (that is, leave the hospital with cognitive abilities), and the number of ground- and air-ambulance personnel injured or killed transporting patients in traumatic cardiac arrest probably equals or exceeds this number. Because it is usually the base-station emergency physician's responsibility to direct whether these patients should be transported or pronounced dead in the field, he or she should follow the imperative for safety and normally should not transport them.

If these patients do arrive in the ED, either because they "coded" en route or there was no ability to stop the transport, how many resources should be expended for them? As with nontraumatic cardiac-arrest patients, it will depend on their response to initial therapy. In these cases, however, reason suggests that therapy should normally be limited to establishing a controlled airway, ascertaining that the patient's heart has indeed stopped, and checking for easily reversible problems. If there is no response, any further resource expenditure is futile. Recognizing this may be emotionally difficult, but it is ethically essential to prevent individual tragedies, such as what happened with Nancy Cruzan and to preserve limited medical resources, including the lives of EMS personnel.

RESPIRATORY FAILURE AND "CRASHING" CANCER PATIENTS

Adults in respiratory distress comprise many of the patients intubated in the ED. Many of these patients are in the final stage of pulmonary insufficiency and have had difficult ICU courses on ventilators in the past. Others have acute illnesses, such as repeat episodes of pneumonia due to immunodeficiency, that may render intervention difficult, if not futile.

Cancer patients who seem to be dying imminently commonly are brought to EDs by their families. Often they are sent by ambulance, without either family or any past medical history available. They too may be in respiratory distress or in shock.

If these patients have decision-making capacity, they may request appropriate medical interventions—despite any prior agreements with their families or physicians. This has often been the case with patients with acquired immunodeficiency syndrome (AIDS) who have completed advance directives specifying no intubation or artificial ventilation; many still ask to be intubated when they go into respiratory distress. Many other patients cannot communicate when they arrive in the ED, or have already been intubated, or have had resuscitation begun in the prehospital arena. With the mandate to help patients who request help (usually by calling 911 or coming to the ED), emergency clinicians must try to resuscitate these patients. If these patients or their surrogates do not want this intervention, then they must not ask for EMS intervention. Their physicians are responsible for educating them about this.

The twist in this scenario is that patients should always have access to comfort care. Pain relief is a service that emergency clinicians always can and should provide. The key here, however, is to be clear about what the patient wants and about the limits of the emergency clinician's interventions. Ideally, emergency clinicians would not be involved with these patients, because the patients' primary care physician would care for their needs. That concept, however, belongs in a more ideal world than ours.

SUICIDE ATTEMPTS

Emergency clinicians routinely treat adult patients for the results of incomplete or unsuccessful suicide attempts (overdoses, motor-vehicle injuries, gunshot and stab wounds, and so forth) against their will. With unconscious patients, physicians can use presumed consent, since a case can be made that most patients would want such intervention; however, this argument may be difficult to make in cases of chronically painful or terminal diseases. With the awake patient who resists any intervention, this argument can only be made if all patients who attempt suicide are considered to lack decision-making capacity. This position is difficult to justify. It leads to a tension between patient autonomy (which includes a right to make foolish choices) and physician paternalism.

The law is a nasty little rock to hide behind; its relationship to ethics is often hazy. Yet most emergency clinicians point to their state laws to justify these actions. Some also point to the reason for state intervention through laws: to preserve lives. Yet there is an ethical justification for intervening in these cases. Not only does the emergency clinician lack knowledge about the patient's true motives for attempting suicide, but the clinician also knows that after resuscitation and psychiatric intervention (if warranted), the patient may complete the act if he or she still wants to. This may not be a highly palatable idea, but it is the measure of autonomy that all competent adults have.

RESTRAINING PATIENTS

Emergency medicine clinicians frequently face physical threats from patients who are drunk, drugged, or deranged. Many clinicians rapidly intervene with physical or chemical restraints to lessen this danger. Such restraint, however, removes a patient's autonomy. On balance, however, safety is the key imperative for these clinicians. Often the patient's safety and the ability to provide healthcare benefit from such restraint.

Although the use of restraints is neither new nor novel in any ED, the lack of sedation and restraints—often precipitated by a concern for patient autonomy—has probably led to deaths. The most frequent scenario for this is with trauma patients (often with Glasgow Coma Scores of 10 to 13) who only seem drunk and belligerent or who seem to "make a little sense." Time wasted talking to these patients, rather than rapidly sedating (often intubating) them and assessing their injuries, can lead to a worsening of their injuries. Both in using restraints and in dealing with suicidal patients, paternalism, safety, and common sense override patient autonomy.

ETHICAL DECISION-MAKING MODEL
FOR EMERGENCY CLINICIANS

Emergency clinicians often must make ethical decisions with little time for reflection or consultation. Although bioethics committees now have an increasing ability to give limited "stat" consultations, even these often do not meet the need for a rapid response. For that reason, a rapid decision-making model for emergency clinicians was developed, based on accepted biomedical theories and techniques. On occasion, this model may also be applicable to those working in critical care.[4]

The following "rules of thumb" give the emergency medicine practitioner a process to use for emergency ethical decision making, even in cases where there is not time to go through a detailed, systematic process of ethical deliberation. Although it is somewhat oversimplified, this approach offers guidance to those who are under severe time pressures and who wish to make ethically appropriate decisions (see Exhibit 28-2).

When using this approach, the practitioner must first ask, "Is this ethical problem an instance of a type of ethical problem for which I have already worked out a rule?" Or, at least, is it similar enough to such cases that the rule could be reasonably extended to cover it? In other words, if the practitioner has had time in the past to think coolly about the issues, discuss them with colleagues, and develop some rough guidelines, can they be used in this case? If the case that the clinician is now dealing with does fit under one of those guidelines arrived at through critical reflection, and the clinician does not have time to analyze the situation any further, then the most reasonable step would be to follow that rule. In ethics, this step follows from *casuistry* or case-based learning.

Such predetermined rules, of course, *must be periodically evaluated.* Practitioners must question whether the results obtained when they follow this rule remain appropriate. Are they consonant with the intention of the rule and with the values that underlie it? This approach only emphasizes that it is unrealistic and ethically irresponsible to believe that one can work out ethical rules to be mechanically applied during an entire professional career. Similarly, it would be unrealistic and irresponsible to continue to perform a medical procedure just as one learned it in medical school, regardless of its efficacy or whether better techniques had been subsequently developed.

But suppose that the practitioner faces an emergency case that does not fit under any previously generated ethical rule. At this point, the practitioner should ask himself or herself if there exists an option that will buy time for deliberation. Is there something that can relieve the time pressure? If there is, and if it does not involve unacceptable risks to the patient, then it would be the reasonable course to take. Using that delaying tactic, there may be time for consulting with other professionals including the bioethics committee, talking with the family, and developing an ethically appropriate course of action.

If there is no delaying tactic that can be used without unreasonable risk to the patient, then a set of three tests can be applied to possible courses of action to help make a decision. These tests are often what people use instinctively when confronted with ethical issues, whether

---

Exhibit 28-2
A Rapid Approach to Ethical Problems: To Be Used for Decisions When There Is Insufficient Time for Detailed Ethical Analysis

---

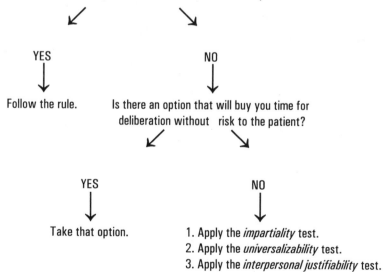

Is this a type of ethical problem for which you have already worked out a rule, or is it at least similar enough so that the rule could reasonably be extended to cover it?

YES

Follow the rule.

NO

Is there an option that will buy you time for deliberation without risk to the patient?

YES

Take that option.

NO

1. Apply the *impartiality* test.
2. Apply the *universalizability* test.
3. Apply the *interpersonal justifiability* test.

Reprinted from K.V. Iserson, A.B. Sanders, and D. Mathieu, *Ethics in Emergency Medicine,* 2nd. ed. (Tucson, Ariz.: Galen Press, 1995). © 1995, Galen Press. Used with permission.

medical or otherwise. The three tests—the impartiality test, the universalizability test, and the interpersonal-justifiability test—are drawn from three different philosophical theories.

THE IMPARTIALITY TEST

Would you be willing to have this action performed if you were in the other person's (the patient's) place? This is, in essence, a version of the Golden Rule: Do unto others as you would have done unto you. According to John Stuart Mill, this espouses "the complete spirit of the ethics of utility." It is not an infallible rule that will yield a right answer every time. It is, however, intended to correct for one obvious source of moral error—partiality, or self-interested bias. It asks practitioners to switch their point of view and to take the other person's perspective. Usually that is useful to do and can at least help avoid a grievous error.

THE UNIVERSALIZABILITY TEST

Are you willing to have this action performed in all relevantly similar circumstances? This generalizes the action and asks whether developing a universal rule for the contemplated behavior is reasonable—an application of Kant's categorical imperative. Is what you are about to do in this particular case something you would approve of if it were generalized to all cases of this sort? The usefulness of this test is that it can help eliminate not only bias and partiality but also short sightedness. In particular, it enables clinicians to evaluate a particular action by viewing it as an example of general practice in similar circumstances. In some cases we might approve of a particular action if we view it on its own account, in complete isolation, but find it unacceptable to adopt it as general practice. Because we are concerned about finding useful rules of action—focusing on types of action rather than on particular actions in isolation—this seems appropriate. Rules are always to some extent general and hence apply to types of actions. Justifying one particular instance that falls under a rule is not sufficient for justifying the practice of acting on that rule.

THE INTERPERSONAL-JUSTIFIABILITY TEST

Are you able to provide good reasons to justify your actions to others? Will peers, superiors, or the public be satisfied with the answers? Could you justify or defend your decision if it were questioned by someone else? Could you give reasons for the course of action you took? And, importantly, can you give reasons that you would be willing to state publicly? This test uses David Gauthier's basic theory of consensus values as a final screen for a proposed action.[5]

When ethical situations arise where no time exists for further deliberation, it is probably best to go ahead and act on the rule or perform the action that allows all three tests to be answered in the affirmative with some degree of confidence. Once the crisis has subsided, however, the practitioner should review the decision with the aid of colleagues and bioethicists to refine his or her emergency ethical decision-making abilities. In particular, it is crucial to ask whether the most basic ethical values have been served by the decision-making process. Were the actions taken in the emergency situation consonant with showing the kind of respect for patient autonomy that you believe appropriate? Were the ethical decisions really in the patient's best interest, or were you unduly influenced by the interests of others or considerations of your convenience or psychological comfort? Were people treated fairly, justly, and equitably?

Ethical problems, like emergency clinical problems, require *action* for resolution. Ideally, one would have extensive discussions and reflect in advance of each ethical decision. This, of course, is not possible for many emergency care decisions. Nevertheless, by making a sincere effort to anticipate recurring types of problems, subjecting them to ethical analysis in advance, and conscientiously reviewing decisions after they have been made, the emergency care professional can better fulfill his or her ethical responsibilities. Thus, an emergency decision does not have to be removed from the realm of ethical evaluation.

RESEARCH AND TEACHING IMPERATIVE

Two nonclinical ethical issues greatly affect the practice of emergency medicine, as they do critical care medicine—education and research. Both suffer from well-meaning, but uneducated, assaults by regulators and "ethicists."

One of the educational areas most under attack at present is the teaching of lifesaving procedures, such as intubation and the placement of central venous lines. Virtually all agree that teaching on unsuspecting patients, such as those undergoing surgery, is wrong. Two options remain: getting permission to teach these procedures on the living or teaching on the recently deceased. It is unclear whether many people will agree to being teaching subjects when they are already under the severe stress of being a surgical patient. Even the long-standing practices of having residents operate with attending physicians present, or of chief residents operating alone or supervising other residents, are being challenged. Going to the operating rooms for that type of training or retraining also presents logistical difficulties for emergency clinicians and intensive care clinicians. That seems to leave, at least for the present, the option of using the newly dead to teach these procedures. The arguments against this practice revolve around the concept of patient and family autonomy. Patient autonomy applies poorly to this situation, since autonomy only exists for the living. Whether families should be able to stop this practice remains unclear, since the overwhelming societal benefits gained seem to far outweigh any family discomfort. As detailed elsewhere, this practice is also the safest, most equitable, and most effective method for teaching and remaining current in lifesaving procedures.[6] Within a decade, this problem may be rendered moot with the availability of virtual-reality training techniques. For now, however, we must continue to train our emergency practitioners so they can render lifesaving medical care to those in need.

Research on many critical illnesses and injuries is also under attack. Regulators have successfully halted much of the research into new cardiac resuscitation and brain resuscitation methods, under the bizarre notion that patients would not want new therapies tried in place of the often ineffective "standard" therapies. Their theory is that, if informed consent cannot be obtained, then the research cannot proceed, even with intensive oversight by institutional review boards or others. How many future patients will be doomed to die or suffer because of this bureaucratic incompetence?[7] This, though, represents only the proverbial tip of the iceberg. Much research in emergency care is being stymied by the fallout from these decisions. Without continued research on the diseases and injuries that cause the most morbidity and mortality, emergency medical care will enter the twenty-first century with twentieth-century abilities.

CONCLUSIONS

Emergency physicians (and EMS providers), more than most others in medicine, must function with minimal knowledge about many of their sickest patients. A limited paternalism has a place in emergency medicine, due to the clinicians' lack of knowledge about their patients' wishes, patients' inadequate reflection about their sudden illnesses or injuries, a need for patients' and clinicians' safety, and families' unpreparedness for sudden catastrophic events. Emergency clinicians must often treat, assuming it will be in the patient's best interest and knowing that if they are wrong, treatment can later be withdrawn. The different set of ethical imperatives under which emergency clinicians work may place them in conflict with their colleagues who staff ICUs.

NOTES

1. K.V. Iserson and T. Kastre, "Are Emergency Departments a 'Safety Net' for the Medically Indigent?" *American Journal of Emergency Medicine* 14, no. 1 (1996): 1-5.

2. "Choice in Dying: Statutes Authorizing Do-Not-Resuscitate Orders," *Right to Die Law Digest* (June 1995); K.V. Iserson, "A Simplified Prehospital Advance Directive Law: Arizona's Approach," *Annals of Emergency Medicine* 22, no. 11 (1993): 1703-10; K.V. Iserson, A.B. Sanders, and D.R. Mathieu, eds., *Ethics in Emergency Medicine*, 2nd ed. (Tucson, Ariz.: Galen Press, 1995).

3. "Living Wills and Health Care Directives," *Arizona Revised Statutes*, Chap. 32.

4. This section is adapted with permission from K.V. Iserson, A.B. Sanders, and D. Mathieu, *Ethics in Emergency Medicine* 2nd ed. (Tucson, Ariz.: Galen Press, 1995).

5. D.P. Gauthier, *Morals by Agreement* (Oxford, England: Clarendon Press, 1986).

6. J.P. Orlowski, G.A. Kanoti, and M.J. Mehlman, "The Ethics of Using Newly Dead Patients for Teaching and Practicing Intubation Techniques," *New England Journal of Medicine* 319, no. 7 (1988): 439-41; K.V. Iserson, *Death to Dust: What Happens to Dead Bodies?* (Tucson, Ariz.: Galen Press, 1994); K.V. Iserson, "Using a Cadaver to Practice and Teach," *Hastings Center Report* 16, no. 3 (1986): 28-29; K.V. Iserson, "Postmortem Procedures in the Emergency Department: Using the Recently Dead to Practice and Teach," *Journal of Medical Ethics* 19 (1993): 92-98; K.V. Iserson, "Law versus Life: The Ethical Imperative to Practice and Teach Using the Newly Dead Emergency Department Patient," *Annals of Emergency Medicine* 25, no. 1 (1995): 91-94; K.V. Iserson, "Requiring Consent to Practice and Teach Using the Recently Dead," *Journal of Emergency Medicine* 9, no. 6 (1991): 509-10.

7. M.H. Biros et al., "Informed Consent in Emergency Research: Consensus Statement from the Coalition Conference of Acute Resuscitation and Critical Care Researchers," *Journal of the American Medical Association* 273, no. 16 (1995): 1283-87; K.V. Iserson and M. Mahowald, "Acute Care Research: Is It Ethical?" *Critical Care Medicine* 20 (1992): 1032-37; W.H. Spivey et al., "Informed

Consent for Biomedical Research in Acute Care Medicine," *Annals of Emergency Medicine* 20 (1991): 1251-65; K.V. Iserson and D.L. Lindsey, "Research on Critically Ill and Injured Patients: Rules, Reality and Ethics," *Journal of Emergency Medicine* 13, no. 4 (1995): 563-67.

29

Ethics in Critical Care: A World View

Deborah J. Nyman
and Charles L. Sprung

INTRODUCTION

The vast majority of the literature concerning ethical problems in intensive care is from North America. In order to apply ethical principles around the world, one must take into consideration differences in culture, resources, demand, religion, and level of development. Cook and colleagues reported that Canadian healthcare workers varied widely in their decisions regarding whether to withdraw life support from critically ill patients.[1] Differences were related to the values of the individual provider and also the city and province where the healthcare was provided. Even doctors working in the same institution may have different approaches to ethical issues; so it is clear that, from country to country, there may be major differences among physicians' approaches to ethical issues. All countries, however, face difficult questions regarding access to, delivery of, and payment for healthcare services, as well as the proportion of healthcare expenditures that should be appropriated for intensive care and care at the end of life.[2] The advancing age of the population will inevitably cause increased demand for medical interventions worldwide. The development of new products and devices will increase the cost of the care provided; at the same time, the capacity to meet the demand will be constrained by inadequate reimbursement, restricted growth of healthcare facilities, and personnel shortages.[3]

The principles of medical ethics are *beneficence* (acting to benefit patients by sustaining life, treating illness, and relieving pain), *nonmaleficence* (refraining from harm), *autonomy* (respecting the right of patients to determine much of their medical care), *disclosure* (providing adequate and truthful information for competent patients to make medical decisions), and *social justice* (allocating medical resources fairly and according to medical need).[4] Beneficence and nonmaleficence often collide when critical care technologies that support life also cause pain and prolong the dying process. It is hard to preserve autonomy in unconscious patients, when the situation is an emergency and the patient has no living will or other indicator of his or her prior wishes. A surrogate decision maker, even if present, may not accurately predict the patient's desires.[5] In addition, the interests of patient and society may clash over questions such as the continuation of life support in the face of a poor prognosis and lack of beds in the intensive care unit (ICU).[6]

ADMISSION TO THE ICU

One of the most frequent ethical problems that physicians face when working in the critical care unit is whom to admit and whom to exclude. These decisions often depend on the number of ICU beds available. This number varies in different countries. For instance, in the United States, approximately 8 percent of hospital beds are intensive care beds[7] whereas in Europe the numbers are much lower.[8] In the United Kingdom ICU beds are 2.6 percent of all hospital beds; in Austria, 2.8 percent; in Spain, 3 percent; in Belgium, 3.7 percent; in Switzerland, 3.8 percent; and in Denmark, 4.1 percent. In Japan and Hong Kong, ICU beds make up approximately 1 percent of hospital beds.[9]

The number of days patients spend in an ICU also varies through Europe—2.9 days in Denmark, 3 days in Switzerland and Sweden, 5.3 days in Austria, 5.6 days in France, and 5.9 days in Spain. These differences may be explained, in part, by the recovery room function of many ICUs in Europe.[10]

Although different institutions in different countries may use different strategies to solve their triage problems, most probably use some form of the guidelines for admission suggested by Teres which follow the "congestive heart failure treatment analogy" in times of limited capacity. These include:

1. *Pre-load reduction.* Keep patients in the post-anesthetic care unit or emergency room longer, postpone planned surgery, and do not transfer patients from other ICUs.

2. *Improve cardiac performance.* Perform fewer invasive procedures and transport fewer patients for investigations.
3. *Decrease afterload.* Keep unstable patients in the post-anesthesia care unit. Use intermediate units for sicker-than-usual patients, send stable, ventilator-dependent patients to general wards, and transfer "hopeless" patients.[11]

Teres maintains that "it is the responsibility of the critical care profession to articulate a just and equitable triage system during intermittent periods of high census or limited capacity."[12]

In the United States, a consensus statement on the triage of the critically ill was developed by the Society of Critical Care Medicine (SCCM) Ethics Committee. The statement puts forward several principles that should guide decision making when deciding who should receive intensive care. The statement suggests that triage should be based on a sound understanding of the probable outcome of the patient's illness, the availability of therapeutic modalities, the impact of therapy on outcome, and a judgment of the benefits and burdens of the therapy for the patient, the patient's family, and society.[13] It suggests that an explicit policy for who gains admittance and who does not should be developed and publicized, so that in acute bed shortages there would be fewer disagreements and individual patients would not suffer adverse consequences. The benefits of such a policy are for individual patients, the institution, and society. The statement declares that ethnic origin, race, sex, creed, social worth, sexual preference, or ability to pay should never be factors in triage decisions.[14] Despite these theoretical statements, ICU admission and discharge policies are either nonexistent or somewhat vague so as to allow for flexibility.[15] ICU triage policies within a hospital are typically not explicitly stated nor publicized for patients, their families, or the public.

It is surprising how few studies have been performed on the important issue of triage. In the United States, Singer and colleagues found that, during a temporary drop in coronary and ICU bed availability, the rate of ICU admissions and length of stay decreased, ICU admission was restricted to more acutely ill patients (fewer admissions for patients requiring monitoring), and patients were transferred out of the ICU sooner, without harmful consequences.[16] Strauss and colleagues also found that, during ICU bed shortages, more severely ill patients were admitted and sicker patients were discharged after a shorter stay than when more beds were available; bed availability, however, had no effect on ICU mortality rates, death after discharge, or readmission to the ICU.[17] Identifying patients who have a low risk of requiring active therapy in an ICU may be helpful. Wagner and colleagues studied 5,790 patients in 13 U.S. tertiary hospitals, of whom 1,941 patients required only monitoring. Of these patients, 70 percent were predicted to have a less than 10 percent risk of needing active treatment by routine severity-of-illness measures, and only 4.3 percent received active therapeutic interventions, with an ICU mortality of 0.5 percent.[18]

Marshall and colleagues found, however, that admitting patterns did not change and that no attempts were made to limit admissions to more severely ill patients during times of the greatest shortage of surgical ICU beds. The severity of illness of patients admitted to the surgical ICU decreased as bed availability and bed census decreased.[19] The highest percentage of all patient admissions and lowest percentage of denied admissions were for cardiothoracic surgery patients; on the other hand, the lowest percentage of admissions and the highest percentage of denied admissions were for general surgery patients, although these patients were the sickest by APACHE II scores. Surgical attending physicians rarely used other open ICU beds when surgical ICU beds were unavailable. Marshall and colleagues concluded that political power, medical provincialism, and income maximization overrode medical suitability in the provision of critical care services.[20]

In 1994, the SCCM Ethics Committee reported on a survey of physicians' attitudes concerning the distribution of ICU resources. Factors that physicians considered of little importance in making triage decisions were the patient's social worth, a previous psychiatric history, cost-benefit analysis, and the cost to society. The single most important factor considered by physicians was the quality of life as viewed by the patient. Other important factors were the probability of surviving hospitalization, the reversibility of an acute disorder, and the nature of a chronic disorder. More than 40 percent of the respondents stated that they would admit patients in a chronic vegetative state or a patient with metastatic carcinoma and a superimposed, life-threatening event. Many of the physicians surveyed felt uncomfortable discharging one patient from the ICU in order to provide care to another patient, even if the incoming patient was more likely to benefit.[21]

In 1990, Vincent conducted a survey of European physicians. Of the respondents, 57 percent said that admissions to the ICU are generally and commonly limited by the number of available beds, and 41 percent maintained that this happened only sometimes or almost never.[22] However, attitudes vary from place to place in Europe. For example, in England, exclusion criteria are much stricter and patients may be excluded merely on the basis of advanced age; in Israel, the attitude is much more toward trying to do everything for everyone, and age is not used to exclude patients from the ICU. Vincent reported that bed availability in ICUs was especially limited in Spain, Portugal, Italy, and the United Kingdom; more beds were available in Scandinavia and the Netherlands. In Europe, if ICU bed availability was limited, two categories of patients, perceived to benefit least from ICU care, were less frequently admitted: (1) patients who were less ill but might benefit from monitored care, and (2) patients with a poor quality of life or with a very poor prognosis.[23] This is also true in the United States and Israel.

Most European physicians, like their American counterparts, admitted patients to the ICUs with poor quality of life or very limited chances of survival. Spain and Portugal are the countries where the largest number of ICU physicians believe that intensive care admission should be denied to patients who have very limited chances of survival. Catholic doctors were more likely to fully treat the patient, even if this was contrary to the patient's wishes.[24]

Because severity scoring systems have not been standardized or studied for ICU triage decisions, too many patients all over the world are admitted when the ICU will not benefit them. They are admitted for monitoring or when they are so ill that even the ICU cannot save them. In addition, physicians worldwide have a problem discharging patients in whom they have forgone life-sustaining treatments.[25]

FORGOING LIFE-SUSTAINING TREATMENT

The issue of forgoing life-sustaining treatment first became prominent with the case of Karen Quinlan in 1976.[26] A U.S. court permitted the removal of a ventilator from a patient in a chronic vegetative state who was not brain dead and who physicians believed would die if the ventilator was removed. Medical standards prior to this decision did not allow the withdrawal of a ventilator for such a patient.[27] Since the Quinlan decision, it has become more and more acceptable around the world to forgo treatments in patients whose condition is terminal or vegetative.[28] Natural death acts have been enacted in the United States allowing the withholding or withdrawal of life-sustaining treatments in patients with a terminal illness.[29]

Twenty-five years ago, the majority of patients died in critical care units only after having had cardiopulmonary resuscitation (CPR) performed. Over the last decade, there has been an increase in the frequency of terminal care decisions in the ICU,[30] and more than half of the patients who die in critical care units do so after the forgoing of life-sustaining treatments.[31] In 1994, Koch and colleagues found that 79 percent of deaths in the ICU occurred after forgoing life-prolonging therapies.[32] There are, however, great differences between countries. What is adopted morally and legally in one country may not be accepted in another.[33]

The forgoing of treatments includes withholding and withdrawing CPR, intubation, mechanical ventilation, positive end-expiratory pressure, supplemental oxygen, vasopressors, blood transfusions, dialysis, surgery, antibiotics, antiarrhythmic drugs, and nutrition and fluid therapy.[34]

Although the withdrawal of ventilators and vasoactive drugs is considered passive euthanasia,[35] it is legal and accepted practice for terminally ill ICU patients in North America, Europe, and Australia.[36] Active euthanasia may be permitted in these patients in the Netherlands.[37] In Israel, however, many people consider the withdrawal of respirators and vasopressors leading to death in these patients to be unethical and illegal.[38] Thus, diverse cultural, religious, philosophical, legal, and professional attitudes may lead to great differences in attitudes and practices in various countries and even in different units within a country.[39]

Vincent found that, in Europe, do-not-resuscitate (DNR) orders are frequently used, but they are usually verbal[40] (unlike in the United States, where they are typically written).[41] Of European respondents, 31 percent discussed the order with the patient and 57 percent discussed it with the family.[42] In the United States, 95 percent of respondents discussed the order with the patient or family and only 1 percent did not,[43] but it has recently been found that only 47 percent of ICU physicians actually knew when their patients preferred not to have CPR.[44] DNR orders were reported to be least frequently used in Italy. In the United States, 87 to 96 percent of physicians reported that they have withheld or withdrawn life-sustaining treatment.[45] In Europe, 83 percent have withheld life-sustaining treatment, 63 percent have withdrawn life-sustaining treatment, and 36 percent have practiced active euthanasia.[46] Many European physicians believe that there is no real difference between withdrawal of life-supporting measures and administration of agents that result in the cessation of all organ function.[47] The majority support the principle of "limited care." Withdrawal of all support (including intravenous fluids and feeding) was usually preferred to euthanasia, and this was especially true for Catholic doctors.[48] Spain, Portugal, and Italy are the countries where DNR orders, withdrawal of life support, and euthanasia are less commonly used. In these countries, the decisions about terminal care are more often restricted to the medical staff, but the doctors usually consider that an ethics committee can help in these decisions.[49] The Netherlands, however, considered to have a permissive law on terminal care because it permits active euthanasia, does not seem to have different practices from other European countries when it comes to forgoing life-sustaining treatments.[50] According to Jewish law or *halacha,* withholding life-prolonging therapies is generally permitted, whereas withdrawing therapies that lead to death is prohibited and considered murder.[51] A recent study from Israel reported that withholding life-prolonging therapies in the ICU is very common, whereas withdrawing treatments is unusual.[52] These findings demonstrate that religious influences are important in these decisions.

Who decides to forgo life-sustaining treatments in the ICU? According to Vincent, 52 percent of European respondents indicated that the entire staff of the ICU is involved in the decision-making process, 45 percent said that participation is limited to medical staff, and 38 percent believed that an ethics consultant (or committee) could help this process. A large majority of European doctors recognized that some kind of limit to intensive care should be applied to avoid "futile therapy." When the family insisted on withholding or withdrawing life support, this had little influence on the decision; the family's preference had a stronger effect when the family insisted on full support.[53] This did not occur in the U.S. case involving Mrs. Helga Wanglie, an elderly woman in a persistent vegetative state. Her physicians wanted to remove her ventilator, but her husband wished ventilation to continue.[54] The physicians went to court, and the court decided for Mr. Wanglie.[55] Asch and colleagues reported that 34 percent of U.S. doctors continue life-sustaining treatments despite patient or surrogate wishes for discontinuation, whereas 82 percent of doctors unilaterally forgo therapies that they believe are futile. Some of these decisions are made without the knowledge or consent of the patient or surrogate, and some are made over their objections.[56]

Many European doctors feel less comfortable withdrawing than withholding treatment,[57] as do their American counterparts.[58] Christakis and Asch identified four biases in how decisions were made about forgoing treatments: physicians prefer to withdraw forms of therapy supporting organs that failed for natural rather than iatrogenic reasons, to withdraw recently instituted rather than long-standing interventions, to withdraw forms of therapy resulting in immediate death rather than delayed death; and to withdraw forms of therapy resulting in delayed death when they are confronted with diagnostic uncertainty. They found that the most likely to the least likely treatments to be withdrawn were blood products, hemodialysis, intravenous vasopressors, total parenteral nutrition, antibiotics, mechanical ventilation, tube feedings, and intravenous fluids.[59]

Asai and colleagues found that Japanese-American physicians were more likely than Japanese doctors to forgo life-sustaining treatments. Physicians answered questions with regard to a fictitious patient with metastatic gastric carcinoma. Of the Japanese physicians surveyed, 74 percent would give blood for gastrointestinal bleeding, 67 percent would give total parenteral nutrition for malnutrition, and 61 percent would give vasopressors for life-threatening hypotension (if the patient did not know the diagnosis and outlook). However, these physicians wanted a somewhat different approach for themselves. Only 29 percent would want to receive blood, 36 percent would want total parenteral nutrition, and 25 percent would want vasopressors. Of these Japanese physicians, 36 percent would override the explicit request of a competent, moribund cancer patient to withdraw all life support. Of the respondents, 42 percent would give blood, 33 percent would administer total parenteral nutrition, and 34 percent would administer vasopressors.[60]

FUTILITY

In deciding whether to continue or stop life-prolonging interventions, doctors sometimes decide to forgo therapy because it is futile or nonbeneficial.[61] There are problems using the concept of futility, including medical uncertainty[62] and the fact that any assessment of the futility of an intervention involves value judgments.[63] Lantos and colleagues argue that the claim that a treatment is futile is often used to justify a shift in the physician's ethical obligations to patients. Futile therapy is merely the end of a spectrum of therapies with very low efficacy. In medicine, it is difficult to predict with complete certainty that a treatment will provide no benefit to a particular patient.[64]

Futility determinations, like all decisions about treatment, must include clinical judgments about the chance of success of a therapy and an explicit consideration of the patient's goals for therapy. According to Prendergast, the problem is to separate utility from probability. An intervention that is not likely to help looks different if it is inexpensive, easy, and without morbidity, than if it is expensive, technologically intensive, and likely to involve great pain and suffering. Futility is how physicians describe the sense of being compelled to proceed with intensive care for marginal benefits.[65] In 1991 the American Medical Association published guidelines for the appropriate use of DNR orders. According to these guidelines: "Resuscitative efforts should be considered futile if they cannot be expected to restore cardiac or respiratory function to the patient, or to achieve the express goal of the informed patient."[66] Further, "physicians should not permit their value judgments about the quality of life to obstruct the implementation of a patient or surrogate's preferences regarding the use of CPR."[67] Despite these guidelines, decisions to continue or stop therapies are often based on soft scientific information, and medical uncertainty abounds.[68] Abuses occur when futility is inconsistently applied and expanded.[69]

The issue of futility has become more important because of the emphasis upon cost containment, the proliferation of managed-care plans, and a greater interest in societal needs. If the medical profession becomes more interested in societal necessities than the needs of their own patients, there will be a reduced drive for finding reversible illnesses, a correct diagnosis, or new potentially expensive drugs.[70] Physicians should not develop societal policies at the expense of an individual patient while they are acting as that patient's primary care physician. A further concern is that solutions to problems of medical practice are being dictated by courts, hospital administrators, risk managers, hospital attorneys, and insurance companies.[71]

Decisions about treatment should be made by physicians, nurses, and patients or families at the bedside. In fact, recently, physicians have been told not to do everything that is in the best interest of their patient, but rather to do as much as is reasonable.[72] Society should recognize that physicians can act prospectively to define what is best for patients and society—especially within the legal system, which reacts retrospectively to specific cases. Also, what is legal may not be ethical. As Koop stated in 1987, "The purely scientific issues pale by comparison to highly sensitive issues of law, ethics, economics, morality and social cohesion that are beginning to surface."[73]

CONCLUSION

Situations in various parts of the world are very different. In North America, there is a great emphasis on patient autonomy and medical consumerism.[74] These factors are much less important in Europe, and even less so in the Middle East, where a "paternalistic" attitude still prevails amongst physicians. In these areas of the world, there seems to be greater respect for doctors, and patients and their families more willingly accept and even expect physicians to make decisions for them.

In summary, there are similar problems all over the world with regard to triage, forgoing life-sustaining treatments, and predicting outcomes in ICUs. The differences lie in the availability of resources and the cultural and religious backgrounds of the populations in question. These dictate, to a great degree, how physicians approach the difficult ethical problems facing them in the ICU.

NOTES

1. D.J. Cook et al., "Determinants in Canadian Health Care Workers of the Decisions to Withdraw Life Support from the Critically Ill," *Journal of the American Medical Association* 273 (1995): 703-08.

2. Society of Critical Care Medicine Ethics Committee, "Consensus Statement on the Triage of Critically Ill Patients," *Journal of the American Medical Association* 271 (1994): 1200-03.

3. Ibid.

4. J.M. Luce, "Ethical Principles in Critical Care," *Journal of the American Medical Association* 263 (1990): 696-700.

5. D.M. High, "All in The Family: Extended Autonomy and Expectations in Surrogate Health Care Decision Making," *Gerontologist* 28 (1988): 46.

6. See note 4 above.

7. J.S. Groeger et al., "Descriptive Analysis of Critical Care Units in the United States," *Critical Care Medicine* 20 (1992): 846-63.

8. J.L. Vincent, "International Perspectives on Critical Care Medicine," in *Principles of Critical Care,* ed. J.B. Hall, G.A. Schmidt, and L.D. Wood (New York: McGraw-Hill, 1992), 2280-304.

9. Ibid.

10. Ibid.

11. D. Teres, "Civilian Triage in the Intensive Care Unit: The Ritual of the Last Bed," *Critical Care Medicine* 21 (1993): 598-606.

12. Ibid, 605.

13. See note 2 above, p. 1201.

14. Ibid, 1201.

15. Society of Critical Care Medicine, "Task Force on Guidelines: Recommendations for Intensive Care Unit Admission and Discharge Criteria," *Critical Care Medicine* 16 (1988): 807-08.

16. D.E. Singer et al., "Rationing Intensive Care-Physician Responses to a Resource Shortage," *New England Journal of Medicine* 309 (1983): 1155-60.

17. M.J. Strauss et al., "Rationing of Intensive Care Unit Services: An Everyday Occurrence," *Journal of the American Medical Association* 255 (1986): 1143-

46.

18. D.P. Wagner, W.A. Knaus, and E.A. Draper, "Identification of Low-Risk Monitor Admissions to Medical-Surgical Intensive Care Units," *Chest* 92 (1987): 423-28.

19. M.F. Marshall et al., "Influence of Political Power, Medical Provincialism, and Economic Incentives on the Rationing of Surgical Intensive Care Unit Beds," *Critical Care Medicine* 20 (1992): 387-94.

20. Ibid.

21. Society of Critical Care Medicine Ethics Committee, "Attitudes of Critical Care Medicine Professionals Concerning Distribution of Intensive Care Resources," *Critical Care Medicine* 22 (1994): 358-62.

22. J.L. Vincent, "European Attitudes Towards Ethical Problems in Intensive Care Medicine: Results of an Ethical Questionnaire," *Intensive Care Medicine* 16 (1990): 256-64.

23. Ibid.

24. Ibid.

25. C.L. Sprung and L.A. Eidelman, "Worldwide Similarities and Differences in the Foregoing of Life-Sustaining Treatments," *Intensive Care Medicine* 22 (1996): 1003-05

26. *In the Matter of Karen Quinlan,* 70 N.J. 10, 355 A.2d 647 (1976).

27. C.L. Sprung, L.A. Eidelman, and R. Pizov, "Changes in Foregoing Life-Sustaining Treatments in the United States: Concern for the Future," *Mayo Clinic Proceedings* 71 (1996): 512-16.

28. See note 25 above.

29. President's Commission for the Study of Ethical Problems in Medicine and Biomedical and Behavioral Research, *Deciding to Forego Life-Sustaining Treatment: Ethical, Medical and Legal Issues in Treatment Decisions* (Washington, D.C.: U.S. Government Printing Office, 1983), 141-45.

30. K.A. Koch, H.D. Rodeffer, and R.L. Wears, "Changing Patterns of Terminal Care Management in an Intensive Care Unit," *Critical Care Medicine* 22 (1994): 233-43; see note 25 above.

31. See note 25 above.

32. See note 30 above.

33. See note 25 above.

34. N.G. Smedira et al., "Withholding and Withdrawal of Support from the Critically Ill," *New England Journal of Medicine* 322 (1990): 309-15.

35. R.D. Truog and C.B. Berde, "Pain, Euthanasia and Anesthesiologists," *Anesthesiology* 78 (1993): 353-60.

36. C.L. Sprung, "Changing Attitudes and Practices in Foregoing Life-Sustaining Treatments," *Journal of the American Medical Association* 263 (1990): 2211-15; E.J. Emanuel, "A Review of the Ethical and Legal Aspects of Terminating Medical Care," *American Journal of Medicine* 84 (1988): 291-301; M.M. Fisher and R.F. Raper, "Withdrawing and Withholding Treatment in Intensive Care," *Medical Journal of Australia* 153 (1990): 222-25; see note 22 above.

37. M.A.M. de Wachter, "Active Euthanasia in the Netherlands," *Journal of the American Medical Association* 262 (1989): 3316-19.

38. "Euthanasia," in F. Rosner, *Modern Medicine and Jewish Ethics* (New York: Yeshiva University Press, 1986) 189-207; *Yael Shefer v. The State of Israel,* GA 506/88. Psak Din 48(1)87.

39. See note 25 above.

40. See note 22 above.

41. R.L. Jaynes et al., "Do Not Resuscitate Orders in Intensive Care Units," *Journal of the American Medical Association* 270 (1993): 2213-17.

42. See note 22 above.

43. Society of Critical Care Medicine Ethics Committee, "Attitudes of Critical Care Professionals Concerning Foregoing Life-Sustaining Treatments," *Critical Care Medicine* 20 (1992): 320-25.

44. SUPPORT Principal Investigators, "A Controlled Trial to Improve Care for Seriously Ill Hospitalized Patients," *Journal of the American Medical Association* 274 (1995): 1591-98.

45. D.A. Asch, J. Hansen-Flaschen, and P.N. Lanken, "Decisions to Limit or Continue Life-Sustaining Treatment by Critical Care Physicians in the United States: Conflicts Between Physicians' Practices and Patients' Wishes," *American Journal of Respiratory and Critical Care Medicine* 151 (1995): 188-92; see note 43 above.

46. See note 22 above.

47. See note 8 above.

48. See note 22 above.

49. Ibid.

50. Ibid.

51. See note 38 above.

52. C.L. Sprung et al., "Foregoing Life-Sustaining Treatments in an Israeli Intensive Care Unit," *Intensive Care Medicine* 24 (1998): 162-66.

53. See note 22 above.

54. M. Angell, "The Case of Helga Wanglie: A New Kind of 'Right to Die' Case," *New England Journal of Medicine* 325 (1991): 511-12.

55. *In re Helga Wanglie,* 4th Judicial District (Dist. Ct., Probate Ct. Div.), PX-91-283, Hennepin County, Minn. (1991).

56. See note 45 above.

57. See note 22 above.

58. See note 43 above.

59. N.A. Christakis and D.A. Asch, "Biases in How Physicians Choose to Withdraw Life Support," *Lancet* 342 (1993): 642-46.

60. A. Asai, S. Fukuhara, and B. Lo, "Attitudes of Japanese and Japanese-American Physicians towards Life-Sustaining Treatment," *Lancet* 346 (1995): 356-59.

61. See note 45 above.

62. S.J. Youngner, "Orchestrating a Dignified Death in the Intensive Care

Unit," *Clinical Chemistry* 36 (1990): 1617-22.

63. S.J. Youngner, "Who Defines Futility?" *Journal of the American Medical Association* 260 (1988): 2094-95.

64. J.D. Lantos et al., "The Illusion of Futility in Clinical Practice," *American Journal of Medicine* 87 (1989): 81-84.

65. T.J. Prendergast, "Futility and the Common Cold: How Requests for Antibiotics Can Illuminate Care at the End of Life," *Chest* 107 (1995): 836-44.

66. American Medical Association Council, "Ethical and Judicial Affairs: Guidelines for the Appropriate Use of Do Not Resuscitate Orders," *Journal of the American Medical Association* 265 (1991): 1871.

67. Ibid.

68. C.L. Sprung, L.A. Eidelman, and A. Steinberg, "Is the Physician's Duty to the Individual Patient or to Society?" *Critical Care Medicine* 23 (1995): 618-20.

69. R.D. Truog, A.S. Brett, and J. Frader, "The Problem with Futility," *New England Journal of Medicine* 326 (1992): 1560-64.

70. See note 68 above.

71. C.L. Sprung, "The Future of Ethical Issues in Critical Care Medicine," in *Principles and Practice of Medical Intensive Care,* ed. R.W. Carlson and M.A. Geheb (Philadelphia: W.B. Saunders, 1993), 1740-44.

72. J.M. Luce, "The Changing Physician-Patient Relationship in Critical Care Medicine under Health Care Reform," *American Journal of Respiratory and Critical Care Medicine* 15 (1994): 266-70.

73. C.E. Koop, "Medical News and Perspectives," *Journal of the American Medical Association* 258 (1987): 2023.

74. See notes 4 and 19 above.

Contributors

DAVID H. BEYDA, MD, is Director of Pediatric Critical Care at Phoenix Children's Hospital in Phoenix, Arizona, and is a Visiting Scholar at the Center of Clinical Bioethics at Georgetown University in Washington, D.C.

PHILIP CANDILIS, MD, is an Assistant Professor of Psychiatry in the Department of Psychiatry and the Office of Ethics at the University of Massachusetts Memorial Healthcare in Worcester.

JAMES A. CHRISTENSEN is a pre-medical student at Eckerd College in St. Petersburg, Florida, majoring in Bioethics.

RUSSELL B. CONNORS, JR., STD, is an Associate Professor of Theology at the College of St. Catherine in St. Paul, Minnesota.

RONALD E. CRANFORD, MD, is Assistant Chief of the Department of Neurology, Hennepin County Medical Center; is Professor of Neurology at the University of Minnesota Medical School; and is a Faculty Associate at the University of Minnesota Center for Bioethics, Minneapolis.

ROBERT E. CUNNION, MD, is a Senior Investigator in the Critical Care Medicine Department at the National Institutes of Health in Bethesda, Maryland.

EVAN G. DERENZO, PhD, is a Bioethicist in the MedStar Health Center for Ethics at the Washington Hospital Center in Washington, D.C.

ANDREW B. EDWARDS, RN, BSN, CEN, CCRN, EMT-A, is a Clinical Nurse in the Surgical Intensive Care Units at Washington Hospital Center, Washington, D.C.; is Research Coordinator for Surgical Critical Care Research at the Medlantic Research Institute, Washington, D.C.; and is a member of the Sterling Park Volunteer Rescue Squad, Sterling, Virginia.

SUE SHEVLIN EDWARDS, PhD, is an Associate Bioethicist for the Medlantic Healthcare Group Center for Ethics and the Washington Hospital Center Department of Bioethics in Washington, D.C.

H. Tristram Engelhardt, Jr., PhD, MD, is a Member of the Center for Medical Ethics and Health Policy and a Professor at Baylor College of Medicine/Rice University in Houston, Texas.

Serena J. Fox, MD, FACP, is Medical Director of the Adult Intensive Care Unit at the Columbia Hospital for Women in Washington, D.C.

Jeffrey Frank, MD, is Director of the Neurointensive Care Program at the Cleveland Clinic Foundation in Cleveland, Ohio.

Phillip J. Goldstein, MD, is Chairman of the Department of Obstetrics and Gynecology at the Washington Hospital Center in Washington, D.C.

Paul Greve, Jr., JD, is Vice President of the Medical Protective Company in Fort Wayne, Indiana.

Sharon Imbus, RN, MSc, is Research Director at the Imbus Neurological Clinic in Pasadena, California.

Kenneth V. Iserson, MD, MBA, FACEP, is a Professor of Surgery, and is Director of the Arizona Bioethics Program at the University of Arizona College of Medicine in Tucson.

Christopher W. Johnson, MD, is Acting Director of the Department of Critical Care Medicine at Kaiser Foundation Hospital in Honolulu, Hawaii.

Dante L. Landucci, MD, is Director of the Critical Care Department at Kern Medical Center in Bakersfield, California.

John J. Lynch, MD, FACP, is Associate Medical Director of the Washington Cancer Institute at Washington Hospital Center in Washington, D.C., and is a member of the Bioethics Committee at Washington Hospital Center.

Mary Faith Marshall, PhD, is Director of the Program in Bioethics at the Medical University of South Carolina in Charleston.

William T. McGee, MD, is Director of ICU Quality Improvement in the Critical Care Division of Baystate Medical Center in Springfield,

Massachusetts, and is an Assistant Professor of Medicine and Surgery at Tufts University School of Medicine in Boston.

DEBORAH J. NYMAN, MBBS, is an Attending Physician in the Department of Anesthesiology at Sha'are Tzedek Medical Center in Jerusalem, Israel.

JAMES P. ORLOWSKI, MD, FAAP, FCCP, FCCM, is Director of Pediatric Intensive Care and Chairman of Ethics at University Community Hospital in Tampa; and is Associate Professor of Pediatrics, Critical Care Medicine, and Medical Ethics at the University of South Florida, Tampa.

EMIL P. PAGANINI, MD, is Head of the Section of Dialysis and Extracorporeal Therapy at the Cleveland Clinic Foundation in Cleveland, Ohio.

MARTIN PERLMUTTER, PhD, is a Professor in the Department of Philosophy at the College of Charleston in Charleston, South Carolina.

KATHLEEN E. POWDERLY, CNM, PhD, is Acting Director of the Division of Humanities and Medicine, and is Clinical Assistant Professor of Obstetrics and Gynecology at the State University of New York, Downstate Medical Center (Brooklyn).

MICHAEL A. RIE, MD, is an Associate Professor at the University of Kentucky College of Medicine in Lexington.

JOHN SCHUMACHER, MA, is Project Coordinator for the Cleveland Health Maintenance Study in the Department of Sociology at Case Western Reserve University in Cleveland, Ohio.

ED SILVERMAN, PhD, is Director of Social Work at the Washington Hospital Center in Washington, D.C.

HENRY SILVERMAN, MD, is a Professor of Medicine at the University of Maryland Medical Systems in Baltimore.

JACQUELYN P. SLOMKA, PhD, RN, is an Educator/Researcher at the Cleveland Clinic Foundation in Cleveland, Ohio.

MARTIN L. SMITH, STD, is a Staff Bioethicist at the Cleveland Clinic Foundation in Cleveland, Ohio.

CHARLES L. SPRUNG, MD, is Director of the General Intensive Care Unit in the Department of Anesthesiology and Critical Care Medicine at Hadassah University Medical Center, Ein Karem; and is a Professor of Medicine at the Hebrew University of Jerusalem in Israel.

CAROL TAYLOR, CSFN, PhD, MSN, RN, is an Assistant Professor at Georgetown University in Washington, D.C.

DANIEL TERES, MD, FCCM, is Director of Critical Care at Baystate Medical Center in Springfield, Massachusetts; and is an Associate Professor of Medicine and Surgery at Tufts University School of Medicine in Boston.

ROBERT M. WALKER, MD, is an Associate Professor of Medicine and is Director of Medical Ethics and Humanities at the University of South Florida College of Medicine in Tampa.

GINGER SCHAFER WLODY, RN, EdD, FCCM, is Chairman of the Quality Management Department, and is an Ethics Consultant at the Carl T. Hayden Veterans Administration Medical Center in Phoenix, Arizona.

BRUCE E. ZAWACKI, MA, MD, is Associate Director for Education at the Pacific Center for Health Policy and Ethics, and is an Emeritus Associate Professor of Surgery and of Religion at the University of Southern California-Los Angeles.

Index